THERAPEUTIC MODALITIES

for Allied Health Professionals

THERAPEUTIC MODALITIES
for
Allied Health
Professionals

WILLIAM E. PRENTICE, Ph.D., P.T., A.T.C.

Professor, Coordinator of Sports Medicine Specialization,
Department of Exercise and Sport Science
Clinical Professor, Division of Physical Therapy,
Department of Medical Allied Health Professions,
Associate Professor, Department of Orthopaedics
School of Medicine
The University of North Carolina,
Chapel Hill, North Carolina

Director, Sports Medicine Education and Fellowship Program
HEALTHSOUTH Rehabilitation Corporation
Birmingham, Alabama

With Case Studies and Lab Activities Contributed by:

WILLIAM S. QUILLEN, PH.D., P.T., S.C.S.

Associate Professor and Chair   Physical Therapist
Department of Physical Therapy   Sports Medicine Clinic
College of Mount St. Joseph   Children's Hospital Medical Center
Cincinnati, Ohio   Cincinnati, Ohio

FRANK UNDERWOOD, PH.D., M.P.T., E.C.S.

Associate Professor
Department of Physical Therapy
University of Evansville
Evansville, Indiana

McGraw-Hill
Health Professions Division

New York   St. Louis   San Francisco   Auckland   Bogotá   Caracas
Lisbon   London   Madrid   Mexico City   Milan   Montreal   New Delhi
San Juan   Singapore   Sydney   Tokyo   Toronto

McGraw-Hill

A Division of The **McGraw·Hill** *Companies*

THERAPEUTIC MODALITIES FOR ALLIED HEALTH PROFESSIONALS

Copyright © 1998 by the **McGraw-Hill** Companies, Inc. All rights reserved. Printed in the United States of America. Except as permitted under the United States Copyright Act of 1976, no part of this publication may be reproduced or distributed in any form or by any means, or stored in a data base or retrieval system, without the prior written permission of the publisher.

34567890 DOCDOC 99{

ISBN 0-07-050771-6

This book was set in Adobe Caslon by Better Graphics, Inc.
The editors were Stephen Zollo and Pamela Touboul;
the production supervisors were Catherine Saggese and Helene G. Landers;
the text and cover designer was James Sullivan/RepoCat Graphics and Editoral Services.
R. R. Donnelley & Sons was printer and binder.

This book is printed on acid-free paper.

Library of Congress Cataloging-in-Publication Data

Prentice, William E.
    Therapeutic modalities for allied health professionals / William
E. Prentice; with lab activities contributed by William S. Quillen,
Frank B. Underwood.
        p.   cm.
    Includes bibliographical references and index.
    ISBN 0-07-050771-6
    1. Physical therapy.   2. Allied health personnel.   I. Quillen,
William S.   II. Underwood, Frank B.   III. Title
    [DNLM: 1. Physical Therapy—methods.   WB 460 P9266t 1998]
RM700.P78   1998
615.8'2—dc21
DNLM/DLC
for Library of Congress   97-48335
                                                                   CIP

Contents

PART TWO
ELECTRICAL MODALITIES

PART THREE
THERMAL MODALITIES

Part Four
LIGHT THERAPY

PART FIVE
MECHANICAL MODALITIES

CONTRIBUTORS

Gerald W. Bell, Ed.D., P.T. A.T.C.
Professor
Department of Physical Education
University of Illinois
Urbana, Illinois

J. Marc Davis, P.T., A.T.C.
Athletic Trainer/Physical Therapist
Division of Sports Medicine
Student Health Service
The University of North Carolina
Chapel Hill, North Carolina

Craig Denegar, Ph.D., P.T., A.T.C.
Associate Professor of Physical Therapy
Penn State University
State College, Pennsylvania

David O. Draper, Ph.D., A.T.C.
Associate Professor
Brigham Young University
Provo, Utah

Phillip B. Donley, MS., P.T., A.T.C.
Director, Chester County Orthopaedic and Sports
   Physical Therapy
West Chester, Pennsylvania

Susan H. Foreman, M.Ed., P.T., A.T.C.
Assistant Athletic Trainer
University of Virginia
Charlottesville, Virginia

Daniel N. Hooker, Ph.D., P.T., ScS, A.T.C.
Coordinator of Athletic Training and Physical Therapy
Division of Sports Medicine
Student Health Service
The University of North Carolina
Chapel Hill, North Carolina

Clairbeth Lehn, P.T., A.T.C.
Athletic Trainer/Physical Therapist
Division of Sports Medicine
Student Health Service
The University of North Carolina
Chapel Hill, North Carolina

William E. Prentice, Ph.D., P.T., A.T.C.
Professor, Coordinator of Sports Medicine Specialization
Department of Physical Education, Exercise and Sport Science
Clinical Professor, Division of Physical Therapy
Department of Medical Allied Health Professions
Associate Professor, Department of Orthopaedics
School of Medicine
The University of North Carolina
Chapel Hill, North Carolina
Director Sports Medicine Education and Fellowship Program
Healthsouth Corporation
Birmingham, Alabama

William S. Quillen, Ph.D., P.T., SCS
Associate Professor and Chair
Department of Physical TherapyCollege of Mount St. Joseph
Cincinnati, Ohio
Physical Therapist
Sports Medicine Clinic
Children's Hospital Medical Center
Cincinnati, Ohio

Ethan N. Saliba, Ph.D., P.T., A.T.C.
Instructor, Currey School of Education
Assistant Athletic Trainer
University of Virginia
Charlottesville, Virginia

Frank Underwood, PhD., M.P.T., ECS
Associate Professor
Department of Physical Therapy
University of Evansville
Evansville, Indiana

PREFACE

Physical therapists, physical therapy assistants, physical therapy aides and occupational therapists use a wide variety of therapeutic techniques in the treatment and rehabilitation of their patients. A thorough treatment regimen often involves the use of therapeutic modalities. At one time or another, virtually all therapists make use of some type of modality. This may involve a relatively simple technique such as using an ice pack for an acute injury or more complex techniques such as the stimulation of nerve and muscle tissue by electrical currents. There is no question that therapeutic modalities are useful tools in injury rehabilitation. When used appropriately, these modalities can greatly enhance the patient's chances for complete recovery. Unfortunately, the therapists' rationale for using a particular modality is too often based on habit rather than on logic or analysis of effectiveness. For the therapist, it is essential to possess knowledge regarding the scientific basis and the physiologic effects of the various modalities on a specific injury. When this theoretical basis is applied to practical experience, it has the potential to become an extremely effective clinical method.

It must be emphasized that the use of therapeutic modalities in any treatment program is an inexact science. If you were to ask ten different therapists what combination of modalities and therapeutic exercise they use in a given treatment program, you would likely get ten different responses. There is no way to "cookbook" a treatment plan that involves the use of modalities. Thus what this book will attempt to do is to present the basis for use of each different type of modality and allow the therapist to make their own decisions as to which will be most effective in a given situation. Some recommended protocols developed through the experiences of the contributing authors will be presented.

The following are a number of reasons why this text should be adopted for use.

Comprehensive Coverage of Therapeutic Modalities Used in a Clinical Setting. The purpose of this text is to provide a theoretically based but practically oriented guide to the use of therapeutic modalities for the student therapist. It is intended for use in courses where various clinically oriented techniques and methods are presented.

This text is divided into six parts. Part I-Foundations of Therapeutic Modalities begins with a chapter that discusses the scientific basis for using therapeutic modalities and classifies the modalities in a logical order in relation to the electromagnetic and acoustic spectra. Guidelines for selecting the most appropriate modalities for use in different phases of the healing process are presented. Pain is discussed, in terms of neurophysiologic mechanisms of pain and the role of therapeutic modalities in pain management. Part II-The Electrical Modalities includes detailed discussions of the principles of electricity, electrical stimulating currents, iontophoresis, and biofeedback. Part III-discusses the Thermal Modalities including shortwave and microwave diathermies, infrared modalities, and ultrasound. Part IV-Light Therapy includes chapters on both low-power laser and ultraviolet therapy. Part V-Mechanical Modalities includes chapters on traction and intermittent compression. Part VI-Manual Modalities takes a look at various techniques of manual therapy including massage, joint mobilization and traction, and proprioceptive neuromuscular facilitation techniques. Each chapter discusses (1) the physiologic basis for use, (2) clinical applications, (3) specific techniques of application through the use of related laboratory activities, and (4) relevant individual case studies. A comprehensive list of manufacturers and distributors of various types of therapeutic modalities and related equipment has been provided in the appendix.

Based on Scientific Theory. This text discusses various concepts, principles, and theories that are supported by scientific research, factual evidence, and previous experience of the authors in dealing with various conditions. The material presented in this text has been carefully researched by the contributing authors to provide up-to-date information on the theoretical basis for employing a particular modality in a specific injury situation. Additionally, the manuscript for this text has been carefully reviewed by therapists, who are considered experts in their field to ensure that the material reflects factual and current concepts for modality use.

Timely and Practical. Certainly, therapeutic modalities used in a clinical setting are important tools for the therapist. This text provides the student with a comprehensive resource which should be used in student instruction on the theoretical basis and practical application of the various modalities. It should serve as a needed guide for the student therapist who is interested in knowing not only how to use a modality but also why that particular modality is most effective in a given situation.

The authors who have contributed to this text have a great deal of clinical experience. Each of these individuals has also at one time or another been involved with the formal classroom education of the student therapist. Thus this text has been directed at the student therapist who will be asked to apply the theoretical basis of modality use to the clinical setting.

Several other texts are available that discuss the use of selected physical modalities in various patient populations. This is the most comprehensive text on therapeutic modalities available in any specific discipline.

Pedagogical Aids. The aids this text uses to facilitate its use by students and instructors include:

Objectives   These goals are listed at the beginning of each chapter to introduce students to the points that will be emphasized.

Figures and Tables   Essential points on each chapter are illustrated with clear visual materials.

Summary   Each chapter has a summary that outlines the major points covered.

Glossary of Key Terms   Each chapter contains a glossary of terms for quick reference.

References   A list of up-to-date references is provided at the end of each chapter for the student who wishes to read further on the subject being discussed.

Appendices   A chart of trigger points and a comprehensive list of manufacturers of therapeutic modality equipment is provided.

Case Studies   A series of clinically based case studies are presented to enhance student understanding of how these modalities may be applied to a specific patient.

Lab Activities   Lab activities are included guide the student through the setup and application of the various modalities.

How to Use the Laboratory Activities. There are a wide variety of laboratory activities found throughout this book.

Theory, biophysical principles and range of potential clinical medicine applications for the various physical agent modalities will be found in this text. The activities are intended to provide the student or interested reader with a systematic and sequential method of completing a therapeutic modality application. The initial performance of a therapeutic procedure should proceed in a logical step-wise fashion. They are structured to allow both the instructor or supervisor and the student the ability to assess competency in a partial or complete fashion culminating in the independent ability to safely and effectively provide a therapeutic modality treatment.

Each therapeutic modality application has a separate sequential check list. Similarities will be noted in certain aspects of treatment application and completion. Space is provided for up to three separate instructors/supervisors to "sign off" (initial and date) the successful completion and demonstration of each element of the complete application. A Master Competency Check List is provided to document the successful completion of the individual therapeutic modality checklist and when the student is deemed competent to independently provide that treatment. This system documents the acquisition of skills necessary for effective physical agent modality application and ensures accountability by the student and instructor/supervisor to patients and other concerned parties.

Competency in the skillful application of therapeutic modalities is gained through diligent and frequent practice. Use of these activities in the manner described will guide the user in productive practice and successful acquisition of essential skills. Students are encouraged to practice each of the procedures on themselves first; thereby gaining an appreciation of the sensations associated with that particular modality. Further practice with a variety of lab partners will result in the development of the desired competence and confidence with any manufacturer's equipment.

ACKNOWLEDGMENTS

I would like to thank Steve Zollo for his confidence in this project from the very beginning. His advice and direction have certainly helped in its completion.

I would also like to thank my wife Tena and our two boys, Brian and Zachary for putting up with the old man when I get going with a project like this. Sometimes it's not easy.

MASTER COMPETENCY CHECK LIST

THERAPEUTIC MODALITY	Examiner		
	1	2	3
Electrical Stimulation			
Analgesia			
Muscle Reeducation			
Muscle Srengthening			
Iontophoresis			
Biofeedback			
Shortwave Diathermy			
Infrared Therapeutic Agents			
Thermotherapy			
Hyrocollator Pack			
Paraffin Bath			
Infrared Lamp			
Cryotherapy			
Ice Massage			
Ice Pack			
Gel Cold Pack			
Vapocoolant Spray			
Hydrotherapy			
Warm Whirlpool			
Cold Whirlpool			
Contrast Bath			
Fluidotherapy			
Ultrasound			
Direct Contact			
Bladder Coupling			
Underwater Coupling			
Phonophoresis			
Low-power Lasers			
Ultraviolet			
Spinal Traction			
Cervical			
Lumbar			
Intermittent Compression			
Massage			
Joint Mobilization			
Proprioceptive Neuromuscular Facilitation Techniques			

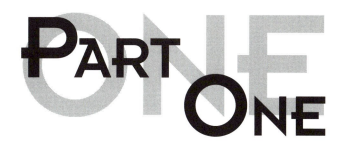

PART ONE

FOUNDATIONS OF
THERAPEUTIC MODALITIES

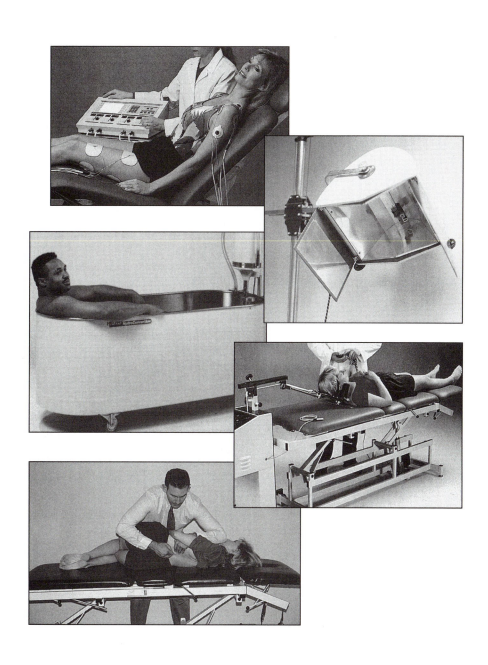

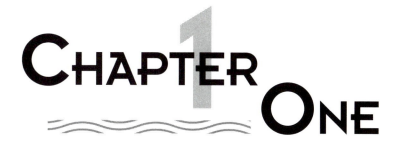

CHAPTER ONE

THE SCIENCE OF THERAPEUTIC MODALITIES

WILLIAM E. PRENTICE

OBJECTIVES

Following completion of this chapter, the student therapist will be able to:

- ✔ Discuss what radiant energy is and how it is produced.
- ✔ Describe the relationship between wavelength and frequency.
- ✔ Indicate how the therapist can make use of electromagnetic radiations to affect the biologic tissues of the body.
- ✔ Discuss the physiologic effects produced by each therapeutic modality.
- ✔ Differentiate between the electromagnetic and acoustic spectra.

There is considerable confusion among therapists regarding the relationship of the various therapeutic modalities to the **electromagnetic** and **acoustic spectra**. Electrical stimulating currents, shortwave and microwave diathermy, the infrared modalities, ultraviolet therapy, and low-power lasers are all therapeutic agents that emit a type of energy with wavelengths and frequencies that can be classified as electromagnetic radiations. **Ultrasound** is a form of radiation whose wavelength and frequency of vibration are best classified in the acoustic rather than the electromagnetic spectrum. Each of the modalities that make use of these varying types of energy will be discussed in the following chapters.

acoustic spectrum The range of frequencies and wavelengths of sound waves.

electromagnetic spectrum The range of frequencies and wavelengths associated with radiant energy.

RADIANT ENERGY

Radiation is a process by which energy in various forms travels through space. Most of us are familiar with the effects of radiation from the sun. Sunlight is a type of radiant energy, and we know that it not only makes objects visible but also produces heat. The sun emits radiant energy as a result of high-intensity chemical reactions. This radiant energy in the form of sunlight travels through space at about 300 million meters per second and eventually reaches earth where its effects may be felt or

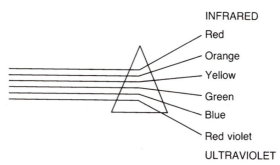

•**Figure 1-1** When a beam of light is shone through a prism, the various electromagnetic radiations in visible light are refracted and appear as a distinct band of color called a spectrum.

infrared The portion of the electromagnetic spectrum associated with thermal changes located adjacent to the red portion of the visible light spectrum.

ultraviolet The portion of the electromagnetic spectrum associated with chemical changes located adjacent to the violet portion of the visible light spectrum.

diathermy The application of high-frequency electrical energy that is used to generate heat in body tissue as a result of the resistance of the tissue to the passage of energy.

seen. However, the sun is not the only object capable of producing this radiant energy.

All matter produces energy that radiates in the form of heat. The sun produces radiation through chemical reactions. However, when a sufficiently intense chemical or electrical force is applied to any object, radiant energy in various forms can be produced by movement of electrons. Many of the therapeutic modalities to be discussed in this text produce radiant energy (i.e., the infrared modalities, the diathermies, ultraviolet, lasers, and the electrical stimulating modalities).[1,7]

If a ray of sunlight is passed through a prism, it will be broken down into various regions of colors (Fig. 1-1). Each of these colors represents a different form of radiant energy. They appear because the various forms of radiant energy are **refracted** or change direction as a result of differences in wavelength and frequency of each color, thus resulting in distinct bands of color called a spectrum. These color variations that we can detect with our eyes are referred to as visible light or luminous radiations. It becomes apparent when looking at this colorful display that there is a region of red at one end of the spectrum and a region of violet at the other end. When passed through a prism, the type of radiant energy refracted the least appears as the color red, whereas that refracted the most is violet.[7]

This beam of sunlight passing through the prism is also propagating forms of radiant energy that are not visible to our eyes. If a thermometer is placed close to the red end of the spectrum, heat will be detected. Likewise, a photographic plate placed close to the violet end of the spectrum will indicate chemical changes. The form of radiant energy that produces heat and is located in the spectrum beyond the visible red portion is referred to as the **infrared** radiation region. The form of radiant energy that produces chemical changes and is located beyond the violet end of the visible spectrum is called the **ultraviolet** radiation region (Fig. 1-2). Ultraviolet, infrared, and visible light rays are produced by heat. As the temperature increases in a particular substance, the vibration of molecules tends to increase the activity of the electrons. The movement of electrons produces electromagnetic waves. The higher the temperature, the greater the frequency of electromagnetic waves produced. These electromagnetic waves produced by heat are usually absorbed by many objects and have little penetration.[6]

It is known that other forms of radiation beyond the infrared and ultraviolet portions of the spectrum may be produced when an electrical force is applied.[7] Beyond the infrared portion of the spectrum lie several large regions of radiations known as the **diathermies**; these include radio, television, and nerve and muscle stimulating currents. Beyond the ultraviolet end of the spectrum lies the high-frequency ionizing and penetration radiation region (i.e., x-ray, alpha, beta, and gamma rays).

Region	Clinically Used Wavelength	Clinically Used Frequency*	Estimated Effective Depth of Penetration	Physiologic Effects
Electrical stimulating currents	3×10^8 Km to 75,000 Km	1–4000 Hz	Effects may occur anywhere between electrodes	Pain modulation, muscle contraction, relaxation, ion movement
Commercial radio and television				
Shortwave diathermy	22 m 11 m	13.56 MHz 27.12 MHz	3 cm	Deep tissue temperature increase, vasodilation, increased blood flow
Microwave diathermy	69 cm 33 cm 12 cm	433.9 MHz 915 MHz 2450 MHz	5 cm	Deep tissue temperature increase, vasodilation, increased blood flow
Infrared				
Cold packs (8° F)	111,000 A	2.7×10^{12} Hz		Superficial temperature decrease
Cold whirlpool (63° F)	99,514 A	3.01×10^{12} Hz		
Hot whirlpool (99° F)	93,097 A	3.22×10^{12} Hz	1 cm	Vasoconstriction— decreased blood flow
Paraffin bath (117° F)	90,187 A	3.32×10^{12} Hz		
Hydrocollar (170° F)	82,457 A	3.63×10^{12} Hz		Analgesia
Luminous IR (1341° F)	28,860 A	1.04×10^{13} Hz		Superficial temperature increase
Nonluminous IR (3140° F)	14,430 A	2.08×10^{13} Hz		Vasodilation— increased blood flow
Red Laser				
Visible light GaAs	9100 A	3.3×10^{13} Hz	5 cm	Pain modulation and wound healing
HeNe	6328 A	4.74×10^{13} Hz	10–15 mm	
Violet				
Ultraviolet				Superficial chemical changes
UV-A	3200–4000 A	9.38×10^{13}–7.5×10^{13} Hz		
UV-B	2900–3200 A	1.03×10^{14}–9.38×10^{13} Hz	2 mm	Tanning effects
UV-C	2000–2900 A	1.50×10^{14}–1.03×10^{14} Hz		Bactericidal
Ionizing radiation (x-ray, gamma rays, cosmic rays)				

*Calculated using $C = \lambda \times F$, C = velocity (3×10^8 m/sec), λ = wavelength, F = frequency.

•**Figure 1-2** Electromagnetic spectrum.

ELECTROMAGNETIC RADIATIONS

All of these various classifications of radiations collectively constitute the electromagnetic spectrum (see Fig. 1-2). All the electromagnetic radiations lying within this spectrum have several theoretical characteristics in common[2]:

1. They may be produced when sufficiently intense electrical or chemical forces are applied to any material.
2. They all travel readily through space at an equal velocity.
3. Their direction of travel is always in a straight line.
4. They may be reflected, refracted, absorbed, or transmitted, depending on the specific medium that they strike.

The luminous, infrared, and ultraviolet rays in sunlight travel in waves through a vacuum or space at a velocity of about 300 million meters per second and all reach the earth at about the same time. These rays are emitted from chemical reactions taking place on the sun, and each type of radiation processes its own individual physical characteristics. The basis of differentiation between the different regions of the electromagnetic spectrum is defined by analyzing the wavelengths and frequencies of the radiations within this spectrum.

The electromagnetic radiations produced by the different modalities all share the same physical characteristics as any other type of electromagnetic radiation. However, when these radiations come in contact with various biologic tissues, the velocity and direction of travel will be altered within the various types of tissues.

WAVELENGTH AND FREQUENCY

Wavelength is defined as the distance between the peak of one wave and the peak of either the preceding or succeeding wave. **Frequency** is defined as the number of wave oscillations or vibrations occurring in 1 second and is expressed in hertz (Hz) units.

Each of the various types of radiation in the electromagnetic spectrum has a specific wavelength and frequency of vibrations. Since it is accepted theoretically that all forms of electromagnetic radiation are produced simultaneously, travel at a constant velocity through space, and reach earth at the same time, it follows that longer wavelengths must have shorter frequencies and shorter wavelengths must have higher frequencies.

$$\text{Velocity} = \text{Wavelength} \times \text{Frequency}$$
$$C = \lambda \times F$$

Thus an inverse or reciprocal relationship exists between wavelength and frequency. Velocity is a constant 3×10^8 m/sec.[8] Therefore, if we know the wavelength, frequency can be calculated.

LAWS GOVERNING THE EFFECTS OF ELECTROMAGNETIC RADIATIONS

When electromagnetic radiations strike or come in contact with various objects, several things may happen. Some rays may be **reflected**, whereas others are **transmitted** through the tissues where they may be refracted. Still others penetrate to deeper layers where they may be **absorbed** (Fig. 1-3). Generally, those radiations that have the longest wavelengths tend to have the greatest depths of penetration regardless of their frequency. It must be added, however, that a number of other factors, which are discussed later, can also contribute to the depth of penetration.

The purpose of using therapeutic modalities is to stimulate a specific body tissue to perform its normal function. This stimulation will only occur if energy produced by the electrotherapeutic device is absorbed by the tissue. The **Arndt-Schultz principle** states that no reactions or changes can occur in the body tissues if the amount of energy absorbed is insufficient to stimulate the absorbing tissues. The goal of the therapist should be to deliver sufficient energy in one form or another to stimulate the tissues to perform their normal function while realizing that too much energy absorbed in a given period of time may seriously impair normal function and, if severe enough, may cause irreparable damage.[2]

Arndt-Schultz principle No reactions or changes can occur in the body tissues if the amount of energy absorbed is insufficient to stimulate the absorbing tissues.

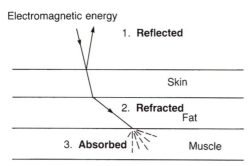

•**Figure 1-3** When electromagnetic radiations contact human tissues, they may be refracted, reflected, or absorbed. Energy that is transmitted through the tissues must be absorbed before any physiologic changes can take place.

If the therapeutic energy is not absorbed by the tissues, then according to the **Law of Grotthus-Draper**, it must be transmitted to deeper layers. The greater the amount of energy absorbed, the less transmitted and thus the less penetration.[5] The transmitted energy tends to (1) travel in a straight line; (2) come in contact with a tissue that reflects or turns away the energy; or (3) have its angle of transmission changed or refracted within the tissue.

Radiant energy is more easily transmitted to deeper tissues if the source of radiation is at a right angle to the area being radiated. Thus the smaller the angle between the propagating ray and the right angle, the less radiation reflected and the greater the absorption. This principle, known as the **cosine law**, is extremely important in the chapters dealing with the diathermies, ultraviolet light, and infrared heating, since the effectiveness of these modalities is based to a large extent on how they are positioned with regard to the patient (Fig. 1-4).

Law of Grotthus-Draper If the therapeutic energy is not absorbed by the superficial tissues it must be transmitted to deeper tissues.

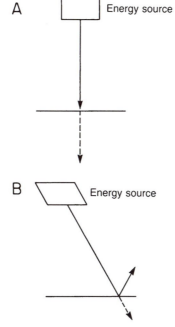

•**Figure 1-4** The cosine law states that the smaller the angle between the propagating ray and the right angle, the less radiation reflected and the greater absorbed. Thus the energy absorbed in A would be greater than in B.

The intensity of the radiation striking a particular surface is known to vary inversely with the square of the distance from the source. For example, a source of radiation that is 2 inches away from the surface will have one quarter of the intensity of a source of radiation that is 1 inch from the surface. This principle, known as the **inverse square law**, obviously is of great consequence when setting up a specific modality to achieve a desired physiologic effect (Fig. 1-5). Regardless of the path this transmitted energy takes, the physiologic effects are apparent only when the energy is absorbed by a specific tissue.

All physical modalities emitting electromagnetic radiations are subject to the relationship between **absorption** and **transmission** of energy. The modalities that emit radiations with relatively longer wavelengths have the ability to transmit energy through the superficial tissue layers, thus penetrating to the deeper tissues where it is absorbed.

Electromagnetic modalities
- Electrical stimulating currents
- Biofeedback
- Iontophoresis
- Shortwave diathermy
- Microwave diathermy
- Infrared modalities
- Ultraviolet therapy
- Low-power laser

THE APPLICATION OF THE ELECTROMAGNETIC SPECTRUM TO THERAPEUTIC MODALITIES

The therapeutic modalities discussed in detail in later chapters (with the exception of ultrasound, massage, traction, intermittent compression, mobilization, and PNF) all emit radiations with physical characteristics that may be classified as electromagnetic.

Figure 1-2 represents the electromagnetic spectrum and places all of the modalities in order based on wavelengths and corresponding frequencies. It is apparent, for example, that the electrical stimulating currents have the longest wavelength and the lowest frequency and, all other factors being equal, therefore should have the greatest depth of penetration. As we move down the chart, the wavelengths in each region become progressively shorter and the frequencies progressively higher. Shortwave and microwave diathermy, the various sources of infrared heating, and the ultraviolet regions have progressively less depth of penetration.

It should be mentioned that the regions labeled as radio and television frequencies, visible light, and high-frequency ionizing and penetrating radiations certainly fall under the classification of electromagnetic radiations. However, they do not have application as therapeutic modalities and, although extremely important to our everyday way of life, warrant no further consideration in the context of this discussion.

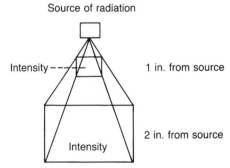

•**Figure 1-5** The inverse square law states that the intensity of the radiation striking a particular surface varies inversely with the square of the distance from the source.

ELECTRICAL STIMULATING CURRENTS

The electrical stimulating currents that affect nerve and muscle tissue have the longest wavelengths and the lowest frequencies of any of the modalities. The wavelengths of electrical stimulating units are extremely long, ranging somewhere around 15,000 km. Clinically used frequencies range from 1 to 4000 Hz. Most stimulators have the flexibility to alter the frequency output of the device to elicit a desired physiologic response. The nerve and muscle stimulating currents are capable of (1) pain modulation either through stimulation of cutaneous sensory nerves at high frequencies (TENS) or through production of β-endorphin at lower frequencies (electroaccutherapy); (2) producing muscle contraction and relaxation or tetany, depending on the type of current (alternating or direct) and frequency (Russian currents); (3) facilitating soft tissue and bone healing through the use of subsensory microcurrents (LIS); and (4) producing a net movement of ions through the use of continuous direct current and thus eliciting a chemical change in the tissues (iontophoresis; see Chapter 6).[8] The electrical stimulating currents and their various physiologic effects are discussed in detail in Chapter 5.

Electromyographic Biofeedback

Electromyographic biofeedback is a therapeutic procedure that uses electronic or electromechanical instruments to accurately measure, process, and feed back reinforcing information via auditory or visual signals. Clinically, it is used to help the patient develop greater voluntary control in terms of either neuromuscular relaxation or muscle reeducation following injury.

SHORTWAVE AND MICROWAVE DIATHERMY

The diathermies are considered to be high-frequency currents because they have more than 1 million cycles per second. When impulses of such a short duration come in contact with human tissue there is not sufficient time for ion movement to take place. Consequently, there is no stimulation of either motor or sensory nerves. The energy of this rapidly vibrating electrical current produces heat as it passes through tissue cells, resulting in a temperature increase. Shortwave diathermy may be either continuous or pulsed. Both continuous shortwave as well as microwave diathermy are used primarily for their thermal effects, whereas pulsed shortwave is used for its nonthermal effects.

The electrotherapeutic shortwave and microwave devices have preset frequencies and wavelengths that cannot be altered. Shortwave diathermy units are set at either (1) 13.56 MHz (1 MHz = 10 million Hz) with a corresponding wavelength of 22 m; or (2) 27.12 MHz with a wavelength of 11 m.[2]

Microwave units have shorter wavelengths than do shortwave diathermy units and are set at wavelengths of 33 or 12 cm with respective frequencies of 915 or 2450 MHz. The depth of penetration with microwave is a bit deeper than with shortwave because the amount of energy when using microwave is concentrated in one spot rather than spread out over a large area.[2] This is discussed in more detail in Chapter 8.

INFRARED MODALITIES

Perhaps the greatest confusion over the relationship between electromagnetic radiations and therapeutic modalities is associated with the infrared region. We tend to think of the infrared modalities as being the luminous and nonluminous infrared

Treatment Tip
When treating low back pain the therapist may choose to use infrared heating modalities, shortwave or microwave diathermy, or ultrasound, all of which have the ability to produce heat in the tissues. Ultrasound has a greater depth of penetration than any of the electromagnetic modalities since acoustic energy is more effectively transmitted through dense tissue than is electromagnetic energy.

bakers or lamps only, when in fact the largest number of modalities used by therapists actually emit radiations with wavelengths and frequencies that clearly fall within this infrared region. Cold packs, hydrocollator packs, whirlpools, paraffin baths, and contrast baths are all infrared modalities.[4]

Earlier it was stated that any object heated (or cooled) to a temperature different than the surrounding environment will dissipate heat through radiation to the other materials with which it comes in contact. The infrared modalities are used to produce a local and occasionally a generalized heating or cooling of the superficial tissues. It is generally accepted that the infrared modalities have a maximum depth of penetration of 1 cm or less. The infrared modalities can elicit either increases or decreases in circulation depending on whether heat or cold is used. They are also known to have analgesic effects as a result of stimulation of sensory cutaneous nerve endings.

The infrared region of the spectrum is located adjacent to the red end of the visible light region. The wavelengths of the infrared modalities are obviously much shorter than are those of the electrical stimulating currents and the diathermies and are expressed in Angstrom (A) units; 1 A is equal to 10^{-10} meters (m).

Both the infrared and ultraviolet wavelengths are temperature-dependent. Those modalities with the lower temperature have the longer wavelength. This means that an ice pack has a longer wavelength and thus a greater depth of penetration than does a hydrocollator pack. Temperatures used with the infrared modalities range from 0°C with ice to more than 3000°C with the infrared lamps. The wavelengths in this temperature range fall between 10,000 and 105,000 A with corresponding frequencies ranging between 2×10^{12} and 4×10^{13} Hz.

It should be pointed out that an Angstrom unit is an extremely small unit of measure and thus the differences in depth of penetration are not great between any of the infrared modalities. The critical factor is the superficial increase or decrease in tissue temperature that elicits the same physiologic response regardless of wavelength.

LASER

Of the modalities discussed in this book, the low-power **laser** is certainly the newest used by the therapist. The word laser is an acronym for light amplification by stimulated emission of radiation. Laser is a form of electromagnetic radiation that is classified within both the infrared and visible light portions of the spectrum.

Lasers are either high-power or low-power. High-power lasers are used in surgery for purposes of incision, coagulation of vessels, and thermolysis, owing to their thermal effects. The low-power or cold laser produces little or no thermal effects but seems to have some significant clinical effect on soft tissue and fracture healing as well as pain management through stimulation of acupuncture and trigger points.

Two types of low-power lasers are used by therapists: the helium-neon laser (HeNe) and the gallium-arsenide laser (GaAs). The HeNe laser has a wavelength of 632.8 nm and a direct depth of penetration to 0.8 mm, although there may be some indirect effects up to 10 to 15 mm. The GaAs laser has a wavelength of 910 nm and can penetrate indirectly as much as 5 cm. The laser as a therapeutic tool is discussed in Chapter 11.

ULTRAVIOLET THERAPY

The ultraviolet portion of the electromagnetic spectrum is adjacent to the violet end of the visible light region. As stated previously, the radiations in the ultraviolet

Treatment Tip
When setting up a patient for treatment using either microwave diathermy or ultraviolet therapy it is critical that the therapist consider the angle at which the electromagnetic energy is striking the body surface to ensure that most of the energy will be absorbed and not reflected. It is also essential to know the distance that these modalities should be placed from the surface to achieve the desired amount of energy in the target tissues.

region are undetectable by the human eye. However, if a photographic plate is placed at the ultraviolet end, chemical changes will be apparent. Although an extremely hot source (7000–9000°C) is required to produce ultraviolet wavelengths, the physiologic effects of ultraviolet are mainly chemical in nature and occur entirely in the cutaneous layers of skin. The maximum depth of penetration with ultraviolet is about 1 mm. The wavelengths with ultraviolet range between 2000 and 4000 A. The ultraviolet region is subdivided into three different areas; near ultraviolet or UV- A (3200–4000 A); middle ultraviolet or UV-B (2900–3200 A); and far ultraviolet or UV-C (2000–2900 A). Clinically used frequencies with ultraviolet range between 7×10^{13} and 7×10^{14} Hz.[2,5,8] Although rarely used by the therapist, the application of ultraviolet therapy is discussed in Chapter 12.

THE ACOUSTIC SPECTRUM AND ULTRASOUND

One additional therapeutic modality frequently used by therapists is ultrasound. Ultrasound devices produce a type of energy that must be classified as acoustic rather than electromagnetic energy. Ultrasound is frequently classified along with shortwave and microwave diathermy as a deep-heating, "conversion"-type modality, and it is certainly true that all of these are capable of producing a temperature increase in human tissue to a considerable depth. However, ultrasound is a mechanical vibration, a sound wave, produced and transformed from high-frequency electrical energy.[2] Ultrasound must be considered a type of acoustic vibration rather than a type of electromagnetic radiation.

Acoustic and electromagnetic radiations have very different physical characteristics. When acoustic vibrations are produced, they travel at a velocity that is significantly lower than electromagnetic radiations. Electromagnetic waves travel at approximately 300 million meters per second, whereas sound waves travel at speeds from hundreds to several thousand meters per second.

The relationship between velocity, wavelength, and frequency is a bit different with acoustic energy than with electromagnetic energy, even though the inverse relationship between wavelength and frequency still exists. The distinction lies in the fact that the velocity of travel is much greater for electromagnetic energy than for acoustic energy. Therefore, wavelengths are considerably shorter in acoustic vibrations than in electromagnetic radiations at any given frequency.[2] For example, ultrasound traveling in the atmosphere has a wavelength of approximately 0.3 mm, whereas electromagnetic radiations have wavelengths of 297 m at a similar frequency.

We stated that electromagnetic radiations were capable of traveling through space or a vacuum. As the density of the transmitting medium is increased, the velocity of travel significantly decreases as a result of **refraction**, **reflection**, or absorption by the molecules in the medium. Acoustic vibrations will not be transmitted at all through a vacuum since they depend on conduction through molecular collisions. The more dense the transmitting medium, the greater the velocity of travel. In human tissue ultrasound has a much greater velocity of transmission in bone tissue (3500 m/s), for example, than in fat tissue (1500 m/s).

Frequencies of ultrasound wave production are between 700,000 and 1 million cycles per second. Frequencies up to around 20,000 Hz are detectable by the human ear. Thus the ultrasound portion of the acoustic spectrum is inaudible. Ultrasound generators are generally set at a standard frequency of 1 to 3 megahertz (1000 KHz). The depth of penetration with ultrasound is much greater than with any of the electromagnetic radiations. At a frequency of 1 MHz, 50 percent of the energy produced will penetrate to a depth of about 5 cm. The reason for this great

Treatment Tip
The therapist may use ultraviolet to treat skin lesions. Since the wavelength of ultraviolet energy is short, the depth of penetration is minimal, and thus the therapeutic effects are primarily superficial. Also, the ultraviolet region of the electromagnetic spectrum is known to produce chemical effects in biologic tissue, which may be helpful in facilitating healing.

depth of penetration is that ultrasound travels very well through homogeneous tissue (e.g., fat tissue), whereas electromagnetic radiations are almost entirely absorbed. Thus when therapeutic penetration to deeper tissues is desired, ultrasound is the modality of choice.[3,6]

Therapeutic ultrasound traditionally has been used to produce a tissue temperature increase through thermal physiologic effects. However, it is also capable of enhancing healing at the cellular level as a result of its nonthermal physiologic effects. The clinical usefulness of therapeutic ultrasound is discussed in greater detail in Chapter 10.

SUMMARY

1. Radiant energy may be produced when a sufficiently intense chemical or electrical force is applied to any object.

2. Electrical stimulating currents, shortwave and microwave diathermy, the infrared modalities, and ultraviolet therapy are all classified as portions of the electromagnetic spectrum according to corresponding wavelengths and frequencies associated with each region.

3. All electromagnetic radiations travel at the same velocity; thus wavelength and frequency are inversely related.

4. Radiations may be reflected, refracted, absorbed, or transmitted in the various tissues.

5. Those radiations with the longer wavelengths tend to have the greatest depth of penetration.

6. The purpose of using any therapeutic modality is to stimulate a specific tissue to perform its normal function.

7. Ultrasound is part of the acoustic spectrum and is best propagated through dense tissue (e.g., biologic); thus it is extremely effective in reaching deep tissues.

REFERENCES

1. Goldman, L.: Introduction to modern phototherapy, Springfield, Ill., 1978, Charles C Thomas, Publisher.

2. Griffin, J., and Karselis, T.: Physical agents for physical therapists, Springfield, Ill., 1978, Charles C Thomas, Publisher.

3. Lehmann, J.F., and Guy, A.W.: Ultrasound therapy. Proc Workshop on Interaction of Ultrasound and Biological Tissues. Washington, D.C., HEW Pub. (FDA 73:8008), Sept., 1972.

4. Lehmann, J., editor: Therapeutic heat and cold, ed. 2, New Haven, 1982, Elizabeth Licht, Publisher.

5. Licht, S.: Therapeutic electricity and ultraviolet radiation, New Haven, 1959, Elizabeth Licht, Publisher.

6. Schriber, W.: A manual of electrotherapy, Philadelphia, 1975, Lea & Febiger.

7. Sears, F., Zemansky, M., and Young, H.: University physics, Reading, Massachusetts, 1976, Addison-Wesley.

8. Stillwell, K.: Therapeutic electricity and ultraviolet radiation, Baltimore, 1983, Williams & Wilkins.

SUGGESTED READINGS

Goodgold, J., and Eberstein, A.: Electrodiagnosis of neuromuscular diseases, Baltimore, 1972, Williams & Wilkins.

Jehle, H.: Charge fluctuation forces in biological systems, Ann. NY Acad. Sci. 158:240–255, 1969.

Koracs, R.: Light therapy, Springfield, Ill., 1950, Charles C Thomas, Publisher.

Licht, S., editor: Electrodiagnosis and electromyography, ed. 3, New Haven, 1971, Elizabeth Licht, Publisher.

Scott, P., and Cooksey, F.: Clayton's electrotherapy and actinotherapy, London, 1962, Bailliere, Tindall and Cox.

absorption Energy that stimulates a particular tissue to perform its normal function.

acoustic spectrum The range of frequencies and wavelengths of sound waves.

Arndt-Schultz principle No reactions or changes can occur in the body if the amount of energy absorbed is not sufficient to stimulate the absorbing tissues.

cosine law Optimal radiation occurs when the source of radiation is at right angles to the center of the area being radiated.

diathermy The application of high-frequency electrical energy used to generate heat in body tissue as a result of the resistance of the tissue to the passage of energy.

electromagnetic spectrum The range of frequencies and wavelengths associated with radiant energy.

frequency The number of cycles or pulses per second.

infrared The portion of the electromagnetic spectrum associated with thermal changes located adjacent to the red portion of the visible light spectrum.

inverse square law The intensity of radiation striking a particular surface varies inversely with the square of the distance from the radiating source.

Law of Grotthus-Draper Energy not absorbed by the tissues must be transmitted.

radiation 1. The process of emitting energy from some source in the form of waves. 2. A method of heat transfer through which heat can be either gained or lost.

reflection The bending back of light or sound waves from a surface that they strike.

refraction The change in direction of a sound wave or radiation wave when it passes from one medium or type of tissue to another.

transmission The propagation of energy through a particular biologic tissue into deeper tissues.

ultrasound A portion of the acoustic spectrum located above audible sound.

ultraviolet The portion of the electromagnetic spectrum associated with chemical changes located adjacent to the violet portion of the visible light spectrum.

wavelength The distance from one point in a propagating wave to the same point in the next wave.

CHAPTER TWO

THE HEALING PROCESS AND GUIDELINES FOR USING THERAPEUTIC MODALITIES

WILLIAM E. PRENTICE

OBJECTIVES

Following completion of this chapter the student therapist will be able to:

✓ Discuss how therapeutic modalities should be used in rehabilitation of various conditions.
✓ Understand the physiologic events associated with the four phases of the healing process.
✓ Discuss specific modalities that can be used effectively during each phase of healing and provide a rationale for their use.
✓ Identify indications and contraindications for using the various modalities discussed throughout this book.

Therapeutic modalities, when used appropriately, can be extremely useful tools in the rehabilitation of the injured patient. Like any other tool, their effectiveness is limited by the knowledge, skill, and experience of the person using them. For the therapist, decisions regarding how and when a modality may be best employed should be based on a combination of theoretical knowledge and practical experience. Modalities should not be used at random, nor should their use be based on what has always been done before. Instead, consideration must be given to what should work best in a specific clinical situation.

In any program of rehabilitation, modalities should be used primarily as adjuncts to therapeutic exercise and not at the exclusion of range-of-motion and strengthening exercises. Rehabilitation protocols and progressions must be based primarily on the physiologic responses of the tissues to injury and on an understanding of how various tissues heal. Thus the therapist must understand the healing process to be effective in incorporating therapeutic modalities into the rehabilitative process.

There are many different approaches and ideas regarding the use of modalities in injury rehabilitation. Therefore, no "cookbook" exists for modality use. Instead, therapists should make their own decisions from the available options in a given clinical situation about which modality will be most effective.

UNDERSTANDING THE HEALING PROCESS

Clinical decisions on how and when therapeutic modalities may best be used should be based on recognition of signs and symptoms as well as some awareness of the time frames associated with the various phases of the healing process.[1,10] The therapist must have a sound understanding of that process in terms of the sequence of the various phases of healing that take place.

Basically, the healing process consists of the inflammatory response phase, the fibroblastic-repair phase, and the maturation-remodeling phase. It must be stressed that although the phases of healing are presented as three separate entities, the healing process is a continuum. Phases of the healing process overlap one another and have no definitive beginning or end points.[6]

INFLAMMATORY RESPONSE PHASE

Once a tissue is injured, the process of healing begins immediately (Fig. 2-1).[2] The destruction of tissue produces direct injury to the cells of the various soft tissues. Cellular injury results in altered metabolism and the liberation of materials that initiate the inflammatory response. Cellular injury is characterized symptomatically by redness, swelling, tenderness, and increased temperature.[3,9]

Inflammation is a process by means of which **leukocytes** and other **phagocytic cells** and exudate are delivered to the injured tissue. This cellular reaction generally is protective, tending to localize or dispose of injury by-products (e.g., blood, damaged cells) through phagocytosis, thus setting the stage for repair. Locally, vascular effects, disturbances of fluid exchange, and migration of leukocytes from the blood to the tissues occur.

The vascular reaction involves vascular spasm, formation of a platelet plug, blood coagulation, and growth of fibrous tissue.[13] The immediate response to damage is a vasoconstriction of the vascular walls that lasts for approximately 5 to 10 minutes. This spasm presses the opposing endothelial linings together to produce a local anemia that is rapidly replaced by hyperemia of the area owing to dilation. This increase in blood flow is transitory and gives way to slowing of the flow in the dilated vessels, which then progresses to stagnation and stasis. The initial effusion of blood and plasma lasts for 24 to 36 hours.

Three chemical mediators, *histamine*, *leucotaxin*, and *necrosin*, are important in limiting the amount of exudate and swelling following injury. Histamine released from the injured mast cells causes vasodilation and increased cell permeability, owing to swelling of endothelial cells, and then separation between the cells. Leucotaxin is responsible for margination in which leukocytes line up along the cell walls. It also increases cell permeability locally, thus affecting passage of the fluid and white blood cells through cell walls by diapedesis to form exudate. Therefore, vasodilation and active hyperemia are important in exudate (plasma) formation and supplying leukocytes to the injured area. Necrosin is responsible for phagocytic activity. The amount of swelling that occurs is directly related to the extent of vessel damage.

Platelets do not normally adhere to the vascular wall. However, injury to a vessel disrupts the endothelium and exposes the collagen fibers. Platelets adhere to the col-

Signs of Inflammation
- Redness
- Swelling
- Tenderness to touch
- Increased temperature

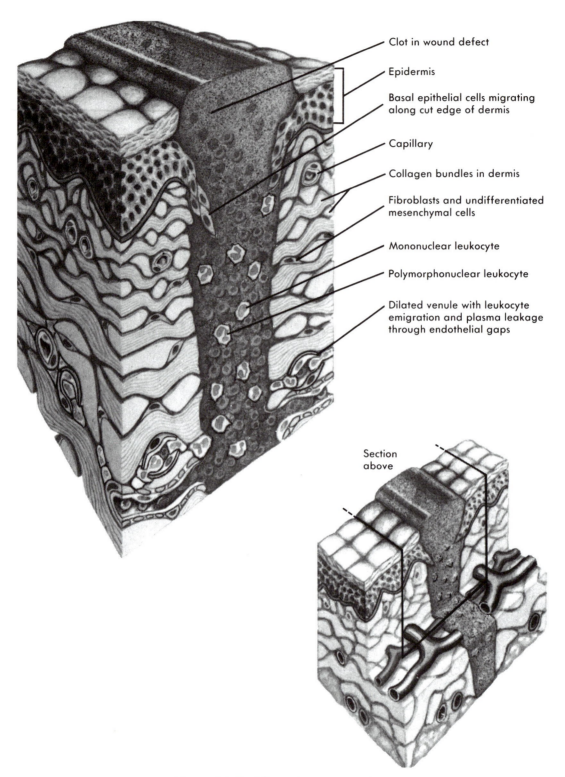

Clot in wound defect

Epidermis

Basal epithelial cells migrating along cut edge of dermis

Capillary

Collagen bundles in dermis

Fibroblasts and undifferentiated mesenchymal cells

Mononuclear leukocyte

Polymorphonuclear leukocyte

Dilated venule with leukocyte emigration and plasma leakage through endothelial gaps

Section above

•**Figure 2-1** The inflammatory response phase.

lagen fibers to create a sticky matrix on the vascular wall, to which additional platelets and leukocytes adhere and eventually form a plug. These plugs obstruct local lymphatic fluid drainage and thus localize the injury response.

The initial event that precipitates clot formation is the conversion of *fibrinogen* to *fibrin*. This transformation occurs because of a cascading effect beginning with the release of a protein molecule called *thromboplastin* from the damaged cell. Thromboplastin causes *prothrombin* to be changed into *thrombin*, which in turn causes the conversion of fibrinogen into a very sticky fibrin clot that shuts off the blood supply to the injured area. Clot formation begins around 12 hours following injury and is completed by 48 hours.

As a result of a combination of these factors, the injured area becomes walled off during the inflammatory stage of healing. The leukocytes phagocytize most of the foreign debris toward the end of the inflammatory phase, setting the stage for the fibroblastic phase. This initial inflammatory response lasts for approximately 2 to 4 days following initial injury.

Chronic Inflammation

A distinction must be made between the acute inflammatory response as described in the preceding section and chronic inflammation. Chronic inflammation occurs when the acute inflammatory response does not eliminate the injuring agent and fails to restore tissue to its normal physiologic state. Chronic inflammation involves the replacement of leukocytes with *macrophages*, *lymphocytes*, and *plasma cells*. These cells accumulate in a highly vascularized and innervated loose connective tissue matrix in the area of injury.[8]

The specific mechanisms that convert an acute to a chronic inflammatory response currently are unknown; however, they seem to be associated with situations that involve overuse or overload with cumulative microtrauma to a particular structure.[5,8] Likewise, there is no specific time frame in which the classification of acute is changed to chronic inflammation.

In Chronic Inflammation Leukocytes Are Replaced with
- Macrophages
- Lymphocytes
- Plasma cells

FIBROBLASTIC-REPAIR PHASE

During the fibroblastic phase of healing, proliferative and regenerative activity leading to scar formation and repair of the injured tissue follows the vascular and exudative phenomena of inflammation (Fig. 2-2).[7] The period of scar formation referred to as **fibroplasia** begins within the first few hours following injury and may last for as long as 4 to 6 weeks. During this period many of the signs and symptoms associated with the inflammatory response subside. The patient may still indicate some tenderness to touch and will usually complain of pain when particular movements stress the injured structure. As scar formation progresses, complaints of tenderness or pain gradually disappear.[11]

During this phase, growth of endothelial capillary buds into the wound is stimulated by a lack of oxygen. Thus, the wound is now capable of healing aerobically. Along with increased oxygen delivery comes an increase in blood flow that delivers nutrients essential for tissue regeneration in the area.[4]

The formation of a delicate connective tissue called *granulation* tissue occurs with the breakdown of the fibrin clot. Granulation tissue consists of fibroblasts, collagen, and capillaries. It appears as a reddish granular mass of connective tissue that fills in the gaps during the healing process.

Granulation Tissue Consists of
- Capillaries
- Collagen
- Fibroblasts

As the capillaries continue to grow into the area, fibroblasts accumulate at the wound site, arranging themselves parallel to the capillaries. Fibroblastic cells begin to synthesize an *extracellular matrix* that contains protein fibers of *collagen* and *elastin*, a *ground substance* that consists of nonfibrous proteins called *proteoglycans*,

The Extracellular Matrix Contains
- Collagen
- Elastin
- Ground substance

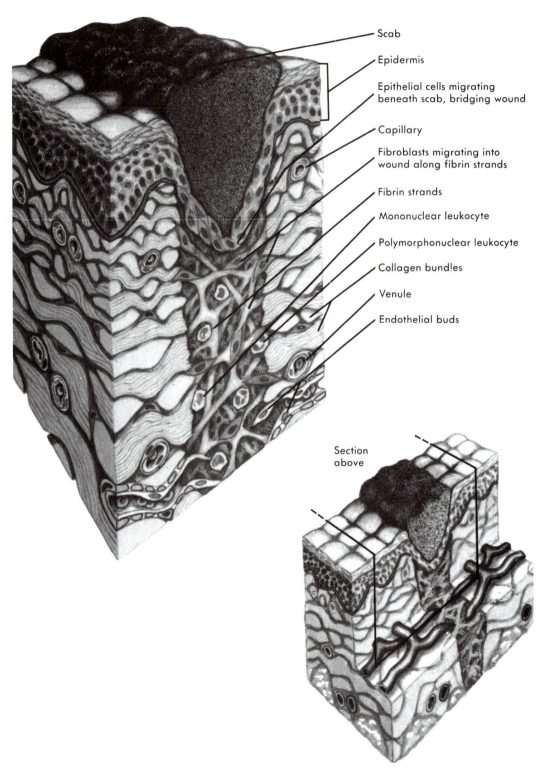

Scab

Epidermis

Epithelial cells migrating beneath scab, bridging wound

Capillary

Fibroblasts migrating into wound along fibrin strands

Fibrin strands

Mononuclear leukocyte

Polymorphonuclear leukocyte

Collagen bundles

Venule

Endothelial buds

Section above

•**Figure 2-2** The fibroblastic-repair phase.

glycosaminoglycans, and fluid. On about day 6 or 7, fibroblasts also begin producing collagen fibers that are deposited in a random fashion throughout the forming scar. As the collagen continues to proliferate, the tensile strength of the wound rapidly increases in proportion to the rate of collagen synthesis. As the tensile strength increases, the number of fibroblasts diminishes to signal the beginning of the maturation phase.

This normal sequence of events in the repair phase leads to the formation of minimal scar tissue. Occasionally, a persistent inflammatory response and continued release of inflammatory products can promote extended fibroplasia and excessive fibrogenesis that can lead to irreversible tissue damage.[14] Fibrosis can occur in synovial structures, as is the case with adhesive capsulitis in the shoulder; in extraarticular articular tissues including tendons and ligaments; in bursa; or in muscle.

fibroplasia The period of scar formation that occurs during the fibroblastic repair phase.

MATURATION-REMODELING PHASE

The maturation-remodeling phase of healing is a long-term process (Fig. 2-3). This phase features a realignment or remodeling of the collagen fibers that make up the scar tissue according to the tensile forces to which that scar is subjected. Ongoing breakdown and synthesis of collagen occur with a steady increase in the tensile strength of the scar matrix. With increased stress and strain the collagen fibers realign in a position of maximum efficiency parallel to the lines of tension. The tissue gradually assumes normal appearance and function, although a scar is rarely as strong as the normal injured tissue. Usually by the end of approximately 3 weeks, a firm, strong, contracted, nonvascular scar exists. The maturation phase of healing may require several years to be totally complete.

FACTORS THAT IMPEDE HEALING

Extent of Injury

The extent of the inflammatory response is determined by the extent of the tissue injury. **Microtears** of soft tissue involve only minor damage and most often are associated with overuse. **Macrotears** involve significantly greater destruction of soft tissue and result in clinical symptoms and functional alterations. Macrotears generally are caused by acute trauma.

Edema

The increased pressure caused by swelling retards the healing process, causes separation of tissues, inhibits neuromuscular control, produces reflexive neurologic changes, and impedes nutrition in the injured part. Edema is best controlled and managed during the initial first aid management period.[16]

Factors That Impede Healing
- Extent of injury
- Edema
- Hemorrhage
- Poor vascular supply
- Separation of tissue
- Muscle spasm
- Atrophy
- Corticosteroids
- Keloids and hypertrophic scars
- Infection
- Humidity, climate, and oxygen tension
- Health, age, and nutrition

Hemorrhage

Bleeding occurs with even the smallest amount of damage to the capillaries. Bleeding produces the same negative effects on healing as does the accumulation of edema, and its presence produces additional tissue damage and thus exacerbation of the injury.

Poor Vascular Supply

Injuries to tissues with a poor vascular supply heal poorly and slowly. This is likely related to a failure in the delivery of phagocytic cells initially and also of fibroblasts necessary for formation of scar.

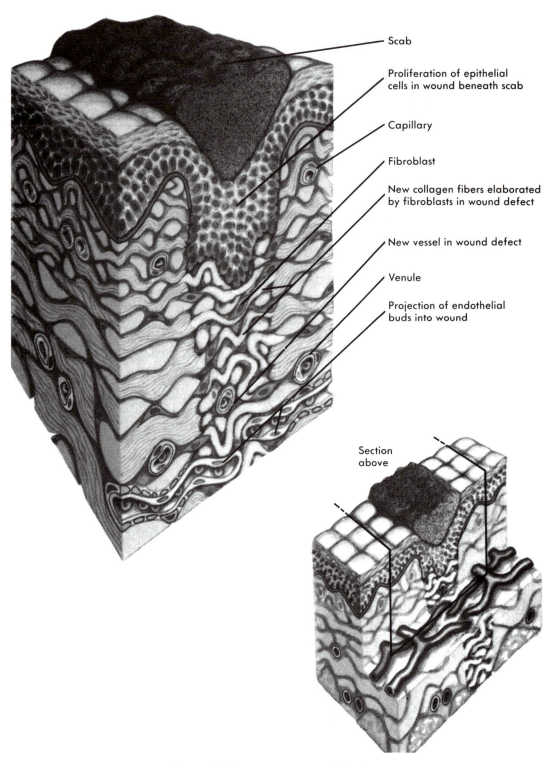

Scab

Proliferation of epithelial cells in wound beneath scab

Capillary

Fibroblast

New collagen fibers elaborated by fibroblasts in wound defect

New vessel in wound defect

Venule

Projection of endothelial buds into wound

Section above

•**Figure 2-3** The maturation-remodeling phase.

Separation of Tissue

Mechanical separation of tissue can significantly impact the course of healing. A wound that has smooth edges that are in good apposition will tend to heal by primary intention with minimal scarring. Conversely, a wound that has jagged separated edges must heal by second intention with granulation tissue filling the defect and excessive scarring.[12]

Muscle Spasm

Muscle spasm causes traction on the torn tissue, separates the two ends, and prevents approximation. Both local and generalized ischemia may result from spasm.

Atrophy

Wasting away of muscle tissue begins immediately with injury. Strengthening and early mobilization of the injured structure retards atrophy.

Corticosteroids

Use of corticosteroids in the treatment of inflammation is controversial. Steroid use in the early stages of healing has been demonstrated to inhibit fibroplasia, capillary proliferation, and collagen synthesis, and increases in tensile strength of the healing scar. Steroid use is debatable in the later stages of healing and with chronic inflammation.

Keloids and Hypertrophic Scars

Keloids occur when the rate of collagen production exceeds the rate of collagen breakdown during the maturation phase of healing. This process leads to hypertrophy of scar tissue, particularly around the periphery of the wound.

Infection

The presence of bacteria in the wound can delay healing and may cause excessive granulation tissue and large deformed scars.

Humidity, Climate, and Oxygen Tension

Humidity significantly influences the process of epithelization. Occlusive dressings stimulate the epithelium to migrate twice as fast without crust or scab formation. The formation of a scab occurs with dehydration of the wound and traps wound drainage, which promotes infection. Keeping the wound moist provides an advantage for the necrotic debris to go to the surface and be shed.

Oxygen tension relates to the neovascularization of the wound, which translates into optimal saturation and maximal tensile strength development. Circulation to the wound can be affected by ischemia, venous stasis, hematomas, and vessel trauma.

Health, Age, and Nutrition

The elastic qualities of the skin decrease with aging. Degenerative diseases such as diabetes and arteriosclerosis also become a concern of the older patient and may affect wound healing. Nutrition is important for wound healing. In particular, vitamins C (scurvy), K (clotting), and A and E (collagen synthesis); zinc for the enzyme systems; and amino acids play critical roles in the healing process.

INJURY MANAGEMENT USING MODALITIES

Traditionally in a clinical setting, injuries have been classified as being either **acute injuries** that result from trauma or **chronic injuries** that result primarily from overuse. This operational definition is not necessarily correct. If active inflammation is present that includes the classic symptoms of tenderness, swelling, redness, and so on, the injury should be considered acute and must be treated accordingly, using rest, ice, compression, and elevation. Even if active inflammation persists for months following initial injury it should still be considered acute. Classification of an injury should be made according to the existing signs and symptoms that indicate the various stages of the healing process and not according to time frames or mechanisms of injury. Once the signs of acute inflammation are no longer present the injury may be considered to be chronic. Inflammation may be considered chronic when the normal cellular response in the inflammatory process is altered, replacing leukocytes with macrophages and plasma cells, along with degeneration of the injured structure.

Based on this definition of acute and chronic injury, the rehabilitation progression following injury may be determined by the four phases of healing. These phases overlap, and the estimated time frames for each phase show extreme variability between patients. Table 2-1 summarizes the various modalities that may be used in each of the four phases.

INITIAL ACUTE INJURY PHASE

Modality use in the initial treatment phase should be directed toward limiting the amount of swelling and reducing pain that occurs acutely. The acute phase is marked by swelling, pain to touch or with pressure, and pain on both active and passive motion. In general, the less initial swelling, the less the time required for rehabilitation. Traditionally, the modality of choice has been and still is ice.

Cryotherapy is known to produce vasoconstriction, at least superficially and perhaps indirectly in the deeper tissues, and thus limits the bleeding that always occurs with injury. Ice bags, cold packs, and ice massage may all be used effectively. Cold baths should be avoided because the extremities must be placed in a gravity-dependent position. Cold whirlpools also place the extremities in the gravity-dependent position and produce a massaging action that is likely to retard clotting. The importance of applying ice immediately following injury for limiting acute swelling through vasoconstriction has probably been overemphasized. The initial use of ice is more important for producing analgesia, which occurs through stimulation of sensory cutaneous nerves that blocks or reduces pain by way of the gating mechanism.

Immediate compression has been demonstrated to be an effective technique for limiting swelling. An intermittent compression device may be used to provide even pressure around an injured extremity. The pressurized sleeve mechanically reduces the amount of space available for swelling to accumulate. Units that combine both compression and cold have been shown to be more effective in reducing swelling than using compression alone. Regardless of the specific techniques selected, cold and compression should always be combined with elevation to avoid any additional pooling of blood in the injured area owing to the effects of gravity.

Electrical stimulating currents may also be used in the initial phase for pain reduction. Parameters should be adjusted to maximally stimulate sensory cutaneous nerve fibers, again to take advantage of the gate control mechanism of pain modulation. Intensities that produce muscle contractions should be avoided because they may increase clotting time.

Ultrasound has been demonstrated to be effective in facilitating the healing process when used immediately following injury and certainly within the first

Treatment Tip
Immediately following injury the therapist should use cryotherapy, some type of compression device, along with elevation to control swelling initially. Additionally, electrical stimulating currents may be used to help provide analgesia, and ultrasound can be used to facilitate healing.

TABLE 2-1   Clinical Decision Making on the Use of Various Therapeutic Modalities in Treatment of Acute Injury

Phase	Approximate Time Frame	Clinical Picture	Possible Modalities Used	Rationale for Use
Initial acute	Injury—day 3	Swelling, pain to touch, pain on motion	CRYO ESC IC LPL ULTRA Rest	↓ Swelling, ↓ pain ↓ Pain ↓ Swelling ↓ Pain Nonthermal effects to ↑ healing
Inflammatory response	Day 2—day 6	Swelling subsides, warm to touch, discoloration, pain to touch, pain on motion	CRYO ESC IC LPL ULTRA Range of motion	↓ Swelling, ↓ pain ↓ Pain ↓ Swelling ↓ Pain Nonthermal effects to ↑ healing
Fibroblastic-repair	Day 4—day 10	Pain to touch, pain on motion, swollen	THERMO ESC LPL IC ULTRA Range of motion Strengthening	Mildly ↑ circulation ↓ Pain—muscle pumping ↓ Pain Facilitate lymphatic flow Nonthermal effects to ↑ healing
Maturation-remodeling	Day 7—recovery	Swollen, no more pain to touch, decreasing pain on motion	ULTRA ESC LPL SWD MWD Range of motion Strengthening Functional activities	Deep heating to ↑ circulation ↑ Range of motion, ↑ strength ↓ Pain ↓ Pain Deep heating to ↑ circulation Deep heating to ↑ circulation

CRYO, Cryotherapy; *ESC*, electrical stimulating currents; *IC*, intermittent compression; *LPL*, low-power laser; *MWD*, microwave diathermy; *SWD*, shortwave diathermy; *THERMO*, thermotherapy; *ULTRA*, ultrasound; ↓, decrease; ↑, increase.

48 hours. Low spatial-averaged intensities below 0.2 W/cm^2 produce nonthermal physiologic effects that alter the permeability of cell membranes to sodium and calcium ions important in healing.

The low-power laser has also been shown to be effective in pain modulation through the stimulation of trigger points and may be used acutely.

The injured part should be rested and protected for at least the first 48 to 72 hours to allow the inflammatory phase of the healing process to proceed naturally.

INFLAMMATORY RESPONSE PHASE

The inflammatory response phase begins as early as day 1 and may last as long as day 6 following injury. Clinically, swelling begins to subside and eventually stops altogether. The injured area may feel warm to the touch, and some discoloration usually is apparent. The injury is still painful to the touch, and pain is elicited on movement of the injured part.

As in the initial injury stage, modalities should be used to control pain and reduce swelling. Cryotherapy should still be used during the inflammatory stage. Ice bags, cold packs, or ice massages provide analgesic effects. The use of cold also reduces the likelihood of swelling, which may continue during this stage. Swelling subsides completely by the end of this phase.

It must be emphasized that heating an injury too soon is a bigger mistake than prolonged use of ice. Many therapists elect to stay with cryotherapy for weeks following injury; in fact, some never switch to the superficial heating techniques. This procedure is simply a matter of personal preference that should be dictated by experience. Once swelling has stopped, the therapist may elect to begin contrast baths with a longer cold to hot ratio.

An intermittent compression device may be used to decrease swelling by facilitating resorption of the by-products of the inflammatory process by the lymphatic system. Electrical stimulating currents and low-power laser can be used to help reduce pain.

After the initial stage, the patient should begin to work on active and passive range of motion. Decisions regarding how rapidly to progress with exercise should be determined by the response of the injury to that exercise. If exercise produces additional swelling and markedly exacerbates pain, then the level or intensity of the exercise is too great and should be reduced. Therapists should be aggressive in their approach to rehabilitation, but the approach will always be limited by the healing process.

Fibroblastic-Repair Phase

Once the inflammatory response has subsided, the fibroblastic-repair phase begins. During this phase of the healing process, fibroblastic cells are laying down a matrix of collagen fibers and forming scar tissue. This stage may begin as early as 4 days after the injury and may last for several weeks. At this point, swelling has stopped completely. The injury is still tender to the touch but is not as painful as during the last stage. Pain is also less on active and passive motion.

Treatments may change during this stage from cold to heat, once again using increased swelling as a precautionary indicator. Thermotherapy techniques including hydrocollator packs, paraffin, or eventually warm whirlpool may be safely employed. The purpose of thermotherapy is to increase circulation to the injured area to promote healing. These modalities can also produce some degree of analgesia.

Intermittent compression can be used once again to facilitate removal of injury by-products from the area. Electrical stimulating currents can be used to assist this process by eliciting a muscle contraction and thus inducing a muscle pumping action. This aids in facilitating lymphatic flow. Electrical currents can once again be used for modulation of pain, as can stimulation of trigger points with the low-powered laser.

The therapist must continue to stress the importance of range-of-motion and strengthening exercises and progress them appropriately during this phase.

Maturation-Remodeling Phase

The maturation-remodeling phase is the longest of the four phases and may last for several years, depending on the severity of the injury. The ultimate goal during this maturation stage of the healing process is return to activity. The injury is no longer painful to the touch, although some progressively decreasing pain may still be felt on motion. The collagen fibers must be realigned according to tensile stresses and strains placed on them. Virtually all modalities may be used safely during this stage; thus, decisions should be based on what works most effectively in a given situation.

At this point some type of heating modality is beneficial to the healing process. The deep-heating modalities of ultrasound or shortwave and microwave diathermy should be used to increase circulation to the deeper tissues. Ultrasound is particularly useful during this period since collagen absorbs a high percentage of the available acoustic energy. Increased blood flow delivers the essential nutrients to the injured area to promote healing, and increased lymphatic flow assists in breakdown and removal of waste products. The superficial heating modalities are certainly less effective at this point.

Electrical stimulating currents can be used for a number of purposes. As before, they may be used in pain modulation. They also may be used to stimulate muscle contractions for the purpose of increasing both range of motion and muscular strength.

Low-power laser can also assist in modulating pain. If pain is reduced, therapeutic exercises may be progressed more quickly.

The Role of Progressive Controlled Mobility in the Maturation Phase

Wolff's Law states that both bone and soft tissue will respond to the physical demands placed on them, causing them to remodel or realign along lines of tensile force.[15] Therefore, it is critical that injured structures be exposed to progressively increasing loads, particularly during the remodeling phase. Controlled mobilization has been shown to be superior to immobilization for scar formation, revascularization, muscle regeneration, and reorientation of muscle fibers and tensile properties in animal models.[17] However, immobilization of the injured tissue during the inflammatory response phase will likely facilitate the process of healing by controlling inflammation, thus reducing clinical symptoms. As healing progresses to the repair phase, controlled activity directed toward return to normal flexibility and strength should be combined with protective support or bracing. Generally, clinical signs and symptoms disappear at the end of this phase.

As the remodeling phase begins, aggressive active range-of-motion and strengthening exercises should be incorporated to facilitate tissue remodeling and realignment. To a great extent, pain will dictate rate of progression. With initial injury, pain is intense and tends to decrease and eventually subside altogether as healing progresses. Any exacerbation of either pain, swelling, or other clinical symptoms during or following a particular exercise or activity indicates that the load is too great for the level of tissue repair or remodeling. The therapist must be aware of the timelines required for the process of healing and realize that being overly aggressive can interfere with that process.

Treatment Tip
Therapeutic exercises should begin on day one following injury. The point is that modalities should be used to facilitate the patient's effort to actively exercise the injured part and not in place of the active exercise.

OTHER CONSIDERATIONS IN TREATING INJURY

During the rehabilitation period following injury, patients must alter their daily routines to allow the injury to heal sufficiently. Consideration must be given to maintaining levels of strength, flexibility, neuromuscular control, and cardiorespiratory endurance.

Modality use should be combined with anti-inflammatory medication, particularly during the initial acute and acute inflammatory phases of rehabilitation.

INDICATIONS AND CONTRAINDICATIONS

Table 2-2 presents a summary list of indications for use, contraindications, and precautions in using the various modalities. This list should aid the therapist in making decisions regarding the appropriate use of a therapeutic modality in a given clinical situation.

TABLE 2-2 **Indications and Contraindications for Therapeutic Modalities**

Therapeutic Modality	Physiologic Resources (Indications for Use)	Contraindications and Precautions
Electrical stimulating currents—high voltage	Pain modulation Muscle reeducation Muscle pumping contractions Retard atrophy Muscle strengthening Increase range of motion Fracture healing Acute injury	Pacemakers Thrombophlebitis Superficial skin lesions
Electrical stimulating currents—low voltage	Wound healing Fracture healing Iontophoresis	Malignancy Skin hypersensitivities Allergies to certain drugs
Electrical stimulating currents—interferential	Pain modulation Muscle reeducation Muscle pumping contractions Fracture healing Increase range of motion	Same as high-voltage
Electrical stimulating currents—Russian	Muscle strengthening	Pacemakers
Electrical stimulating currents—MENS	Fracture healing Wound healing	Malignancy Infections
Shortwave and microwave diathermy	Increase deep circulation Increase metabolic activity Reduce muscle guarding/spasm Reduce inflammation Facilitate wound healing Analgesia Increase tissue temperatures over a large area	Metal implants Pacemakers Malignancy Wet dressings Anesthetized areas Pregnancy Acute injury and inflammation Eyes Areas of reduced blood flow Anesthetized areas
Cryotherapy—cold packs, ice massage	Acute injury Vasoconstriction—decreased blood flow Analgesia Reduce inflammation Reduce muscle guarding/spasm	Allergy to cold Circulatory impairments Wound healing Hypertension
Thermotherapy—hot whirlpool, paraffin, hydrocollator, infrared lamps	Vasodilation—increased blood flow Analgesia Reduce muscle guarding/spasm Reduce inflammation Increase metabolic activity Facilitate tissue healing	Acute and postacute trauma Poor circulation Circulatory impairments Malignancy
Low-power laser	Pain modulation (trigger points) Facilitate wound healing	Pregnancy Eyes

REFERENCES

1. Arnheim, D., Prentice, W.: Principles of athletic training, ed. 9, New York, 1997, McGraw-Hill.
2. Bryant, M.: Wound healing, CIBA Clin. Symp. 29(3):2–36, 1977.
3. Carrico, T., Mehrhof, A., and Cohen, I.: Biology and wound healing, Surg. Clin. No. Am. 64(4):721–734, 1984.
4. Cheng, N.: The effects of electrocurrents on A.T.P. generation, protein synthesis and membrane transport, J. Orth. Rel. Res. 171:264–272, 1982.
5. Fantone, J.: Basic concepts in inflammation. In Leadbetter, W., Buckwalter, J., and Gordon, S., editors. Sports-induced inflammation, Park Ridge, Illinois, 1990, American Academy of Orthopaedic Surgeons.
6. Fernandez, A., Finlew, J.: Wound healing: helping a natural process, Postgrad. Med. 74(4):311–318, 1983.
7. Hettinga D.: Inflammatory response of synovial joint structures. In Gould J., Davies, G., editors: Orthopaedic and sports physical therapy, St. Louis, 1990, C.V. Mosby.
8. Leadbetter, W.: Introduction to sports-induced soft-tissue inflammation. In Leadbetter, W., Buckwalter, J., and Gordon, S., editors. Sports-induced inflammation, Park Ridge, Illinois, 1990, American Academy of Orthopaedic Surgeons.
9. Leadbetter, W., Buckwalter, J., and Gordon, S.: Sports-induced inflammation, Park Ridge, Illinois, 1990, American Academy of Orthopaedic Surgeons.
10. Marchesi, V.: Inflammation and healing. In Kissane J., editor: Anderson's pathology, ed. 8, St. Louis, 1985, C.V. Mosby.
11. Riley, W.: Wound healing, Am. Fam. Phys. 24:5, 1981.
12. Robbins, S., Cotran, R., and Kumar, V.: Pathologic basis of disease, ed. 3, Philadelphia, 1984, W.B. Saunders.
13. Rywlin, A.: Hemopoietic system. In Kissane J.M., editor: Anderson's pathology, ed. 8, St. Louis, 1985, C.V. Mosby.
14. Wahl, S., Renstrom, P.: Fibrosis in soft-tissue injuries. In Leadbetter, W., Buckwalter, J., and Gordon, S., editors. Sports-induced inflammation, Park Ridge, Illinois, 1990, American Academy of Orthopaedic Surgeons.
15. Wolff, J.: Gesetz der transformation der knochen, Berlin, 1892, Aug. Hirschwald.
16. Woo, S.L-Y., Buckwalter, J., editors. Injury and repair of musculoskeletal soft tissues, Park Ridge, Illinois, 1988, American Academy of Orthopaedic Surgeons.
17. Zachezewski, J.: Flexibility for sports. In Sanders, B., editor: Sports physical therapy, Norwalk, Connecticut, 1990, Appleton & Lange.

GLOSSARY

acute injury An injury in which active inflammation is present that includes the classic symptoms of tenderness, swelling, redness, and so on.

chronic injury An injury in which the normal cellular response in the inflammatory process is altered, replacing leukocytes with macrophages and plasma cells, along with degeneration of the injured structure.

fibroplasia The period of scar formation that occurs during the fibroblastic-repair phase.

macrotears Significant damage to soft tissues caused by acute trauma, which result in clinical symptoms and functional alterations.

microtears Minor damage to soft tissue most often associated with overuse.

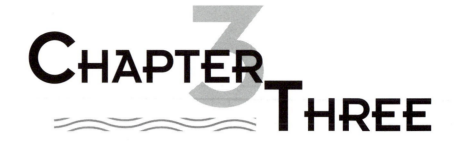

CHAPTER THREE

MANAGING PAIN WITH THERAPEUTIC MODALITIES

CRAIG R. DENEGAR and
PHILLIP B. DONLEY

OBJECTIVES

Following completion of this chapter, the student therapist will be able to:

✓ Define pain, its types, and its positive and negative effects.
✓ Describe the characteristics of sensory receptors.
✓ Describe how the nervous system relays information about painful stimuli.
✓ Describe an appropriate neurophysiologic mechanism for pain control for the therapeutic modalities used by therapists.
✓ Describe how pain perception can be modified by cognitive factors.

UNDERSTANDING PAIN

The International Association for the Study of Pain defines **pain** as "an unpleasant sensory and emotional experience associated with actual or potential tissue damage, or described in terms of such damage."[22] Pain is a subjective sensation with more than one dimension and an abundance of descriptors of its qualities and characteristics. In spite of its universality, pain is composed of a variety of human discomforts, rather than being a single entity.[21] The perception of pain can be subjectively modified by past experiences and expectations. Much of what we do to treat patients' pain is to change their perceptions of pain.[4]

Pain does have a purpose. It warns us that there is something wrong and can provoke a withdrawal response to avoid further injury. It also results in muscle spasm and guarding or protection of the injured part. However, pain can persist after it is no longer useful. It can become a means of enhancing disability and inhibiting efforts to rehabilitate the patient. Prolonged spasm, which leads to circulatory deficiency, muscle atrophy, disuse habits, and conscious or unconscious guarding, may lead to a severe loss of function.[17] Chronic pain may become a disease state in itself. Often lacking an identifiable cause, chronic pain can totally disable a patient.

Research in recent years has led to a better understanding of pain and pain relief. This research also has raised new questions, although leaving many unanswered. We now have better explanations for the analgesic properties of the physical agents we use, as well as a better understanding of the psychology of pain. However, new physical agents, such as the laser and microamperage electrical simulators, and new approaches to older agents, such as transcutaneous electrical nerve simulators, challenge our understanding of injury and pain. Not even the mechanisms for the analgesic response to heat and cold have been fully described.[31]

The control of pain is an essential aspect of caring for the injured patient. The therapist has several therapeutic agents with analgesic properties from which to choose. The selection of a therapeutic agent should be based on a sound understanding of its physical properties and physiologic effects. This chapter does not provide a complete explanation of neurophysiology, pain, and pain relief. Instead, it presents an overview of some theories of pain control, intended to provide a stimulus for therapists to develop their own rationale for using modalities in the plan of care for patients they treat. Ideally, it also will interest some in research to establish the physiologic and psychologic soundness of the use of agents for pain relief and to expand our understanding of pain. Several physiology textbooks provide extensive discussions of human neurophysiology and neurobiology to supplement this chapter.

Many of the modalities discussed in later chapters have analgesic properties. Often, they are employed to reduce pain and permit the patient to perform therapeutic exercises. Some understanding of what pain is, how it affects us, and how it is perceived is essential for the therapist who uses these modalities.

TYPES OF PAIN

Pain has been categorized as either acute or chronic. Pain lasting for more than 6 months is generally classified as chronic.[5] There is more research devoted to chronic pain and its treatment, but acute pain, or pain of sudden onset, confronts the therapist most often.

Referred pain, which also may be either acute or chronic, is pain that is perceived to be in an area that seems to have little relation to the existing pathology. For example, injury to the spleen often results in pain in the left shoulder. This pattern, known as Kehr's sign, is useful for identifying this serious injury and arranging prompt emergency care. Referred pain can outlast the causative events because of altered reflex patterns, continuing mechanical stress on muscles, learned habits of guarding, or the development of hypersensitive areas, called **trigger points**.

Irritation of nerves and nerve roots can cause radiating pain. Pressure on the lumbar nerve roots associated with a herniated disc or a contusion of the sciatic nerve can result in pain radiating down the lower extremity to the foot.

Deep somatic pain is a type that seems to be sclerotomic (associated with a **sclerotome**, a segment of bone innervated by a spinal segment). There is often a discrepancy between the site of the disorder and the site of the pain.

PAIN ASSESSMENT

Pain is a complex phenomenon that is difficult to evaluate and quantify because it is subjective and is influenced by attitudes and beliefs of the therapist and patient. Quantification is hindered by the fact that pain is a very difficult concept to put into words.[1]

Obtaining an accurate and standardized assessment of pain is problematic. Several tools have been developed. These pain profiles identify the type of pain, quantify the intensity of pain, evaluate the effect of the pain experience on the patient's level of function, and assess the psychosocial impact of pain.

The pain profiles are useful. They compel the patient to verbalize the pain and thereby provide an outlet for the patient and provide the therapist a better understanding of the pain experience. They assess the psychosocial response to pain and injury. The pain profile can assist with the evaluation process by improving communication and directing the therapist toward appropriate diagnostic tests. These assessments also assist the therapist in identifying which therapeutic agents may be effective and when they should be applied. Finally, these profiles provide a standard measure to monitor treatment progress.[12]

PAIN ASSESSMENT SCALES

The following profiles are used in the evaluation of acute and chronic pain associated with illnesses and injuries. Visual analog scales are quick and simple tests completed by the patient (Fig. 3-1). These scales consist of a line, usually 10 cm in length, the extremes of which are taken to represent the limits of the pain experience. One end is defined as "NO PAIN" and the other as "SEVERE PAIN." The patient is asked to mark the line at a point corresponding to the severity of the pain. The distance between "NO PAIN" and the mark represents pain severity. A similar scale can be used to assess treatment effectiveness by placing "NO PAIN RELIEF" at one end of the scale and "COMPLETE PAIN RELIEF" at the other. These scales can be completed daily or more often as pre- and post-treatment assessments.[15]

Pain charts can be used to establish spatial properties of pain. These two-dimensional graphic portrayals are completed by the patient to assess the location of pain and a number of subjective components. Simple line drawings of the body in several postural positions are presented to the patient (Fig. 3-2). The patient draws or colors the pictures in areas that correspond to the pain experience. Different colors are used for different sensations. For example, blue for aching pain, yellow for numbness or tingling, red for burning pain, and green for cramping pain. Descriptions can be added to the form to enhance the communication value. The form could be completed daily.[18]

Plain Assessment Techniques
- Visual analog scales
- Pain charts
- McGill Pain Questionnaire
- Activity Pattern Indicators Profile
- Numeric pain scales

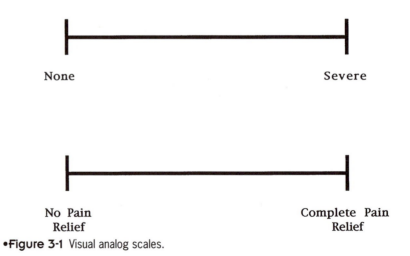

None   Severe

No Pain   Complete Pain
Relief   Relief

•**Figure 3-1** Visual analog scales.

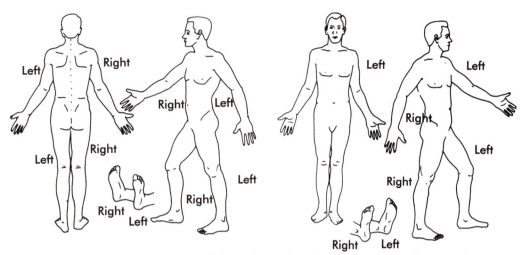

•**Figure 3-2** The pain chart. Use the following instructions: "Please use all of the figures to show me exactly where all your pains are and where they radiate to. Shade or draw with blue marker. Only the patient is to fill out this sheet. Please be as precise and detailed as possible. Use yellow marker for numbness and tingling. Use red marker for burning or hot areas and green marker for cramping. Please remember: blue = pain; yellow = numbness and tingling; red = burning or hot areas; green = cramping." (Used with permission from Melzack, R.: Pain measurement and assessment, New York, 1983, Raven Press.)

The McGill Pain Questionnaire (MPQ) is a tool with 78 words that describe pain (Fig. 3-3). These words are grouped into 20 sets that are divided into four categories, representing dimensions of the pain experience. Completion of the MPQ may take 20 minutes and is often frustrating for patients who do not speak English well. It is commonly administered to patients with low back pain. When administered every 2 to 4 weeks it has demonstrated changes in status very clearly.[21]

The Activity Pattern Indicators Pain Profile measures patient activity. It is a 64-question, self-report tool that may be used to assess functional impairment associated with pain. The instrument measures the frequency of certain behaviors such as housework, recreation, and social activities.[13]

The most common acute pain profile used in outpatient clinics today is a numeric pain scale. The patient is asked to rate his or her pain on a scale from 1 to 10, with 10 representing the worst pain experienced or could imagine. The question is asked before and after treatment. When treatments provide pain relief, patients are asked about the extent and duration of the relief. In addition, the patient may be asked to estimate the portion of the day in which he or she experiences pain and about specific activities that increase or decrease pain. When pain affects sleep, the patient may be asked to estimate the amount of sleep gotten in the previous 24 hours. In addition, the amount of medication required for pain can be noted. This information helps the therapist assess changes in pain, select appropriate treatments, and communicate more clearly with the patient about the course of recovery from injury or surgery.

All of these scales help the patient communicate the severity and duration of his or her pain and appreciate changes that occur. Often in a long recovery, patients lose sight of how much progress has been made in terms of the pain experience and return to functional activities. A review of these pain scales often can serve to reassure the patient, foster a brighter, more positive outlook, and reinforce the commitment to the plan of treatment.

Treatment Tip
There are a number of pain evaluation tools, including visual analog scales, pain charts, the McGill Pain Questionnaire, the Activity Pattern Indicators Profile, and numeric pain scales. Numeric pain scales, in which the patient is asked to rate their pain on a scale from 1 to 10, are perhaps the most widely used in the clinical setting.

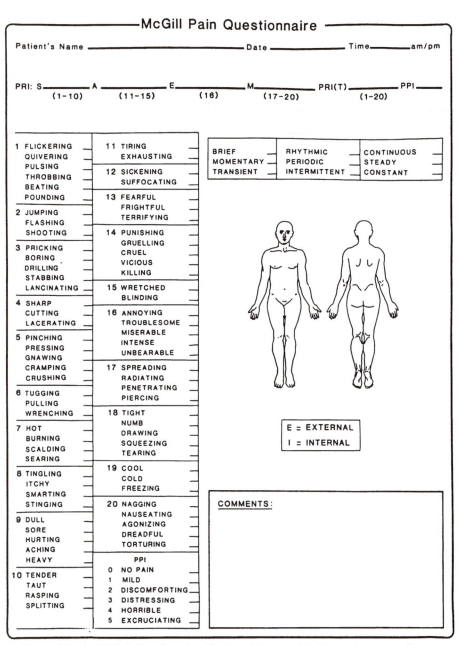

•**Figure 3-3** McGill Pain Questionnaire. The descriptors fall into four major groups: Sensory, 1 to 10; affective, 11 to 15; evaluative, 16; and miscellaneous, 17 to 20. The rank value for each descriptor is based on its position in the word set. The sum of the rank values is the pain rating index (PRI). The present pain intensity (PPI) is based on a scale of 0 to 5. (Used with permission from Melzack, R.: Pain measurement and assessment, New York, 1983, Raven Press.)

The efficacy of many of the treatments used by therapists has not been fully substantiated. These scales are one source of data that can help therapists identify the most effective approaches to managing common injuries. These assessment tools can also be useful when reviewing a patient's progress with physicians and third-party payers.

TISSUE SENSITIVITY

The four structures most sensitive to damaging (noxious) stimuli are (1) the **periosteum** and **joint capsule**; (2) subchondral bone, tendons, and ligament; (3) muscle and cortical bone; and (4) the synovium and articular cartilage. A variety of "silent" fractures produce little or no pain. Different anatomic tissues exhibit varying degrees of sensitivity to pain. **Avulsion fractures** tend to be quite painful, because they tear away the periosteum. Musculoskeletal pain usually is spread over a large area unless it is close to the surface. For example, a hamstring strain usually results in pain over the posterior thigh, whereas an acromioclavicular sprain usually localizes over the joint.

periosteum A highly vascularized and innervated membrane lining the surface of bone.

GOALS IN MANAGING PAIN

Regardless of the cause of pain, its reduction is an essential part of treatment. Pain signals the patient to seek assistance and often is useful in establishing a diagnosis. Once the injury or illness is diagnosed, pain serves little purpose. Medical or surgical treatment or immobilization is necessary to treat some conditions, but physical therapy and an early return to activity are appropriate following many injuries. The therapist's objectives are to encourage the body to heal through exercise designed to progressively increase functional capacity and to return the patient to work and recreational and other activities as swiftly and safely as possible. Pain will inhibit therapeutic exercise. The challenge for the therapist is to control acute pain and protect the patient from further injury while encouraging progressive exercise in a supervised environment.

PAIN PERCEPTION AND NEURAL TRANSMISSION

Sensory Receptors

There are several types of sensory receptors in the body, and the therapist should be aware of their existence and the types of stimuli that activate them (Table 3-1). Activation of some of these sense organs with therapeutic agents will decrease the patient's perception of pain.

Six different types of receptor nerve endings are commonly described.

1. Meissner's corpuscles are activated by light touch.
2. Pacinian corpuscles respond to deep pressure.
3. Merkel's corpuscles respond to deep pressure, but more slowly than pacinian corpuscles, and also are activated by hair follicle deflection.
4. Ruffini corpuscles in the skin are sensitive to touch, tension, and possibly heat; those in the joint capsules and ligaments are sensitive to change in position.
5. Krause's end bulbs are thermoreceptors that react to a decrease in temperature and touch.[26]
6. Pain receptors, called **nociceptors** or **free nerve endings**, are sensitive to extreme mechanical, thermal, or chemical energy.[3] They respond to noxious stimuli, namely, to impending or actual tissue damage (e.g., cuts, burns, sprains, etc.). The term **nociceptive** is from the Latin *nocere*, to damage, and is used to imply pain information. These organs respond to superficial forms of heat and cold, analgesic balms, and massage.

Proprioceptors found in muscles, joint capsules, ligaments, and tendons provide information regarding joint position and muscle tone. The muscle spindles react to

TABLE 3-1   **Some Characteristics of Selected Sensory Receptors**

Type of Sensory Receptors	Stimulus		Receptor	
	General Term	**Specific Nature**	**Term**	**Location**
Mechanoreceptors	Pressure	Movement of hair in a hair follicle	Afferent nerve fiber	Base of hair follicles
		Light pressure	Meissner's corpuscle	Skin
		Deep pressure	Pacinian corpuscle	Skin
		Touch	Merkel's touch corpuscle	Skin
Nociceptors	Pain	Distension (stretch)	Free nerve endings	Wall of gastrointestinal tract, pharynx, skin
Proprioceptors	Tension	Distension	Corpuscles of Ruffini	Skin and capsules in joints and ligaments
		Length changes	Muscle spindles	Skeletal muscle
		Tension changes	Golgi tendon organs	Between muscles and tendons
Thermoreceptors	Temperature change	Cold	Krause's end bulbs	Skin
		Heat	Corpuscles of Ruffini	Skin and capsules in joints and ligaments

From Previte JJ: *Human physiology*, New York, 1983, McGraw-Hill.

changes in length and tension when the muscle is stretched or contracted. The Golgi tendon organs also react to changes in length and tension within the muscle. See Table 3-1 for a more complete listing.

Some sensory receptors respond to phasic activity and produce an impulse when the stimulus is increasing or decreasing, but not during a sustained stimulus. They adapt to a constant stimulus. Meissner's corpuscles and pacinian corpuscles are examples of such receptors.

Tonic receptors produce impulses as long as the stimulus is present. Examples of tonic receptors are muscle spindles, free nerve endings, and Krause's end bulbs. The initial impulse is at a higher frequency than later impulses, which occur during sustained stimulation.

Adaptation is the decline in generator potential and the reduction of frequency that occurs with a prolonged stimulus or with frequently repeated stimuli. If some physical agents are used too often or for too long the receptors may adapt to or accommodate the stimulus and reduce their impulses. The **accommodation** phenomenon can be observed with the use of superficial hot and cold agents, such as ice packs and hydrocollator packs.

As a stimulus becomes stronger, the number of receptors excited increases and the frequency of the impulses increases. This provides more electrical activity at the spinal cord level, which may facilitate the effects of some physical agents.

NEURAL TRANSMISSION

afferent Conduction of a nerve impulse toward an organ.

Afferent nerve fibers transmit impulses from the sensory receptors toward the brain, whereas **efferent** fibers, such as motor neurons, transmit impulses from the brain toward the periphery. First-order or primary afferents transmit the impulses from the sensory receptor to the dorsal horn of the spinal cord (Fig. 3-4). There are four

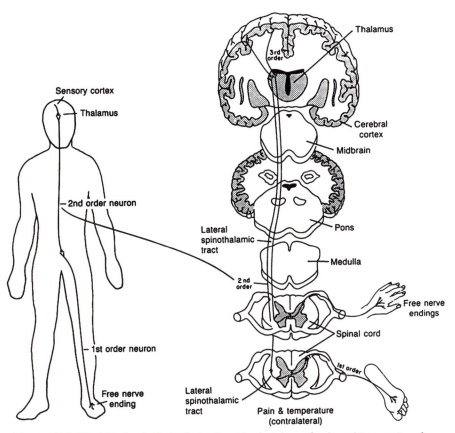

•**Figure 3-4** The lateral spinothalamic tract carries impulses of pain and temperature from the sensory receptors to the cortex.

different types of first-order neurons (Table 3-2). Note that A-alpha and A-beta fibers are characterized as being large-diameter afferents and A-delta and C fibers as small-diameter afferents.

Second-order afferent fibers carry sensory messages from the dorsal horn to the brain. Second-order afferent fibers are categorized as wide dynamic range or nociceptive-specific. The wide dynamic range second-order afferents receive input from A-beta, A-delta, and C fibers. These second-order afferents serve relatively large, overlapping receptor fields. The nociceptive-specific second-order afferents respond exclusively to noxious stimulation. They receive input only from A-delta and C fibers. These afferents serve smaller receptor fields that do not overlap. All of these neurons synapse with third-order neurons that carry information to various brain centers where the input is integrated, interpreted, and acted on.

FACILITATORS AND INHIBITORS OF SYNAPTIC TRANSMISSION

For information to pass between neurons, a transmitter substance must be released from one neuron terminal (presynaptic membrane), enter the synaptic cleft, and attach to a receptor site on the next neuron (postsynaptic membrane). In the past, all the activity within the synapse was attributed to **neurotransmitters,** such as acetylcholine. The neurotransmitters, when released in sufficient quantities, are known to

neurotransmitter Substance that passes information between neurons. It is released from one neuron terminal (presynaptic membrane) enters the synaptic cleft, and attaches (binds) to a receptor on the next neuron (postsynaptic membrane). Sustance P, enkephalins, serotonin, methionine, and leucine enkephalin are neurotransmitters.

TABLE 3-2   Classification of Afferent Neurons

Size	Type	Group	Subgroup	Diameter (Micrometers)	Conduction Velocity m/sec	Receptor	Stimulus
Large	A α	I	1a	12–20 (22)	70–120	Proprioceptive mechanoreceptor	Muscle velocity and length change, muscle shortening of rapid speed
	A α	I	1b				
	A β	II	Muscle	6–12	36–72	Proprioceptive mechanoreceptor	Muscle length information from touch and pacinian corpuscles
	A β	II	Skin			Cutaneous receptors	Touch, vibration, hair receptors
	A δ	III	Muscle	1–5 (6)	6(12)–36(80)	75% mechanoreceptors and thermoreceptors	Temperature change
Small	A δ	III	Skin			25% nociceptors, mechanoreceptors, and thermoreceptors (hot and cold)	Noxious, mechanical, and temperature (>45° C, <10° C)
	C	IV	Muscle	0.3–1.0	0.4–1.0	50% mechanoreceptors and thermoreceptors	Touch and temperature
	C	IV	Skin			50% nociceptors, 20% mechanoreceptors, and 30% thermoreceptors (hot and cold)	Noxious, mechanical, and temperature (>45° C, <10° C)

cause depolarization of the postsynaptic neuron. In the absence of the neurotransmitter, no depolarization occurs.

It is now apparent that several compounds that are not true neurotransmitters can facilitate or inhibit synaptic activity. These compounds are classified as biogenic amine transmitters or neuroactive peptides. **Serotonin** and **norepinephrine** are examples of biogenic amine transmitters. About two dozen neuroactive peptides have been identified, including **substance P**, **enkephalins**, and **β-endorphin**.[3]

Serotonin and **enkephalins** are active in descending (efferent) pathways that block the pain message.[7] Enkephalin is an **endogenous** (made by the body) **opioid** that inhibits the depolarization of second-order nociceptive nerve fibers. It is released from **interneurons**, enkephalin neurons with short axons. The enkephalins are stored in nerve-ending vesicles found in the **substantia gelatinosa** and several areas of the brain. When released, enkephalin may bind to presynaptic or postsynaptic membranes.[3]

Norepinephrine is a biogenic amine transmitter that is released by the depolarization of some neurons and that binds to the postsynaptic membranes. Norepinephrine is found in several areas of the nervous system, including a tract that descends from the pons that inhibits synaptic transmission between first-order and second-order nociceptive fibers, thus decreasing pain sensation.[16]

Other endogenous opioids may be active analgesic agents. These neuroactive peptides are released into the central nervous system and have an action similar to that of morphine, an opiate analgesic. There are specific receptors located at strategic sites, called binding sites, to receive these compounds. β-Endorphin, a 31-amino acid peptide, and **dynorphin** have potent analgesic effects. These are released within the central nervous system by mechanisms that are not fully understood at this time.

serotonin A neurotransmitter found in neurons descending in the dorsolateral tract.

enkephalin Neurotransmitter proteins that block the passage of noxious stimuli from first- to second-order afferents. They inhibit the release of substance P and are produced by enkephalinergic neurons.

endogenous opioids Opiate-like substances made by the body.

NOCICEPTION

A nociceptive neuron is a neuron that transmits pain signals. Its cell body is in the dorsal root ganglion near the spinal cord. Approximately 25 percent of the myelinated A-delta and 50 percent of the unmyelinated C fibers contact nociceptors and are considered nociceptive, afferent neurons (see Table 3-2). Once a nociceptor is stimulated, it releases a neuropeptide (substance P) that initiates the electrical impulses along the afferent fiber toward the spinal cord. Substance P also serves as a transmitter substance between the first- and second-order afferent fibers at the dorsal horn of the spinal column (Fig. 3-4).

The A-delta and C fibers that transmit sensations of pain and temperature have different diameters (A-delta are larger) and different conduction velocities (A-delta are faster). The C fibers also are connected to more of the nociceptive-specific second-order afferents. These differences result in two qualitatively different types of pain, termed fast and slow.[3] Fast pain is brief, well-localized, and well-matched to the stimulus—for example, the initial pain of an unexpected pinprick. Slow pain is an aching, throbbing, or burning sensation that is poorly localized and less specifically related to the stimulus. There is a delay in the perception of slow pain following injury, but the pain will continue long after the noxious stimulus is removed. Fast pain is transmitted over the larger, faster-conducting A-delta afferent neurons and originates from receptors located in the skin. Slow pain is transmitted by the C afferent neurons and originates from both superficial tissue (skin) and deeper tissue (ligaments and muscles).[3]

The various types of afferent fibers follow different courses as they ascend toward the brain. Some A-delta and most C afferent neurons enter the spinal cord through the dorsolateral tract of Lissauer and synapse in marginal zone (lamina 1) or

nociceptive Pain information or signals or pain stimuli.

CASE STUDY 3-1
MANAGING ACUTE PAIN

Background: Stacey is a 21-year-old college basketball player referred for physical therapy the day after athroscopic surgery to remove loose bodies and a tear in the medial meniscus of her left knee.

Impression: She is typical of patients presenting the day following acute injury and surgery. She is experiencing considerable discomfort and demonstrates inhibition of the quadriceps muscles and an unwillingness to flex and extend the knee.

Treatment: Stacey was treated with an ice bag around the knee for 20 minutes, being careful to protect the common peroneal nerve on the posterior lateral aspect of the knee. Following cold application she was encouraged to perform quadriceps setting and heel slides.

Response: Her volitional control of the quadriceps improved and she left the clinic able to perform a straight leg raise without a lag. She was also able to move the knee from extension to 50 degrees of flexion. She was sent home with instructions to use cold three to four times daily followed by the previously described exercises. Stacey demonstrated active range of motion from terminal extension to 115 degrees of flexion and good control of the quadriceps on return to the clinic 5 days later. Her rehabilitation progressed well and she returned to playing basketball within 3 weeks in preparation for the upcoming season.

Surgery results in acute pain and the associated guarding, splinting, and neuromuscular inhibition. When active muscle contractions and range of motion exercises can be performed safely, the use of therapeutic modalities can assist the patient regain function. In this case, cold was selected because of the acute presentation and the ease of use at home. TENS also would have been appropriate, either alone or in combination with cold. It is also important to appreciate the effects of pain-free movement on the recovery process. Movement lessens the sensation of stiffness postoperatively and provides large-diameter afferent input into the dorsal horn, which may relieve pain through a gating mechanism or the stimulation of enkephalin interneurons.

The rehabilitation professional employs physical agent modalities to create an optimum environment for tissue healing while minimizing the symptoms associated with the trauma or condition.

Discussion Questions

- What tissues were injured/affected?
- What symptoms were present?
- What phase of the injury-healing continuum did the patient present for care in?
- What are the physical agent modality's biophysical effects (direct/indirect/depth/tissue affinity)?
- What are the physical agent modality's indications/contraindications?
- What are the parameters of the physical agent modality's application/dosage/duration/frequency in this case study?
- What other physical agent modalities could be utilized to treat this injury or condition? Why? How?

the substantia gelatinosa (lamina 2) with a second-order neuron.[16] Most nociceptive second-order neurons ascend to higher centers along one of three tracts—(1) the lateral spinothalamic tract; (2) the spinoreticular tract; or (3) the spinoencephalic tract—with the remainder ascending along the spinocervical tract or as projections to the cuneate and gracile nuclei of the medulla.[16] Approximately 90 percent of the wide dynamic range second-order afferents terminate in the thalamus.[16] Third-order neurons project to the sensory cortex and numerous other centers in the central nervous system. These projections allow us to perceive pain. They also permit the integration of past experiences and emotions that form our response to the pain experience. These connections are also believed to be parts of complex circuits that the therapist may stimulate to manage pain. Most analgesic physical agents are believed to slow or block the impulses ascending along the A-delta and C afferent neuron pathways through direct input into the dorsal horn or through descending mechanisms. These pathways are discussed in more detail in the following section.

NEUROPHYSIOLOGIC EXPLANATIONS OF PAIN CONTROL

The neurophysiologic mechanisms of pain control through stimulation of cutaneous receptors have not been fully explained. Much of what is known and current theory are the result of work involving electroacupuncture and transcutaneous electrical nerve stimulation.[32] However, this information often provides an explanation for the analgesic response to other modalities, such as massage, analgesic balms, and moist heat.

The concepts of the analgesic response to cutaneous receptor stimulation presented here were first proposed by Melzack and Wall and Castel.[7,20] These models essentially present three analgesic mechanisms:

1. Stimulation from ascending A-beta afferents results in the blocking of impulses (pain messages) carried along A-delta and C afferent fibers.

2. Stimulation of descending pathways in the dorsolateral tract of the spinal cord by A-delta and C fiber afferent input results in a blocking of the impulses carried along the A-delta and C afferent fibers.

3. The stimulation of A-delta and C afferent fibers causes the release of endogenous opioids (β-endorphin), resulting in a prolonged activation of descending analgesic pathways.

These theories or models are not necessarily mutually exclusive. Recent evidence suggests that pain relief may result from combinations of dorsal horn and central nervous system activity.[2,9]

A decrease in input along nociceptive afferents also results in pain relief. Cooling afferent fibers decreases the rate at which they conduct impulses. Thus, a 20-minute application of cold is effective in relieving pain because of the decrease in activity, rather than an increase in activity along afferent pathways.

BLOCKING PAIN IMPULSES WITH ASCENDING A-BETA INPUT

Pain modulation caused by sensory stimulation and the resultant increase in the impulses in the large-diameter (A-beta) afferent fibers was proposed by the gate control theory of pain (Fig. 3-5).[20] Impulses ascending on these fibers stimulate the substantia gelatinosa as they enter the dorsal horn of the spinal cord. Stimulation of the substantia gelatinosa inhibits synaptic transmission in the large and small (A-delta and C) fiber afferent pathways. The "pain message" carried along the smaller-diameter fibers is not transmitted to the second-order neurons and never reaches sensory centers. The balance between the input from the small- and large-diameter afferents determines how much of the pain message is blocked or gated.

The concept of sensory stimulation for pain relief, as proposed by the gate control theory, has empirical support. Rubbing a contusion, applying moist heat, or massaging sore muscles decreases the perception of pain. The analgesic response to these treatments is attributed to the increased stimulation of large-diameter afferent fibers.

The gate control theory also proposes that A-delta and C fiber impulses inhibit the substantia gelatinosa, facilitating the perception of pain. The sensation of pain does not diminish rapidly, because free nerve endings do not accommodate and the afferent impulses from them "open the gate" to further pain message transmission.

The discovery and isolation of endogenous opioids in the 1970s led to new theories of pain relief. Castel introduced an endogenous opioid analog to the gate control theory (Fig. 3-6).[7] This theory proposes that A-beta impulses trigger a release of enkephalin from **enkephalin interneurons** found in the dorsal horn. These neu-

---

Mechanisms of Pain Control
- Blocking ascending pathways
- Blocking descending pathways
- Release of β-endorphin

Treatment Tip
The modalities that are effective in "closing the gate" to ascending pain fibers should provide a significant amount of cutaneous input that would be transmitted to the spinal cord along Aβ fibers. The modalities of choice may include various types of heat or cold, electrical stimulating currents, counterirritants (analgesic balms), or massage.

substantia gelatinosa (SG) Melzack and Wall proposed that the SG is responsible for closing the gate to painful stimuli.

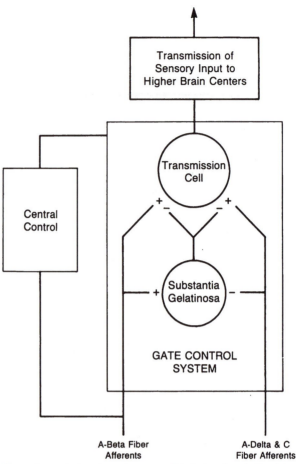

•**Figure 3-5** The gate control system. Increases A-beta input and stimulates the substantia gelatinosa that inhibits the flow of afferent input to sensory centers.

roactive amines inhibit synaptic transmission in the A-delta and C fiber afferent pathways. The end result, as in the gate control theory, is that the pain message is blocked before it reaches sensory levels.

DESCENDING PAIN CONTROL MECHANISMS

The gate control theory proposed a second analgesic mechanism that involves descending efferent fibers.[20] The central control, originating in higher centers of the central nervous system, could affect the dorsal horn gating process. Impulses from the thalamus and brain stem (**central biasing**) are carried into the dorsal horn on efferent fibers in the dorsal or dorsal lateral paths (or tracts). Impulses from the higher centers act to close the gate and block transmission of the pain message at the dorsal horn synapse. Through this system, it was theorized, previous experiences, emotional influences, sensory perceptions, and other factors could influence the transmission of the pain message and the perception of pain.

Castel offers an endogenous opioid model of descending influence over dorsal horn synapse activity (Fig. 3-7).[7] Stimulation of the **periaqueductal gray** region of the midbrain and the **raphe nucleus** in the pons and medulla by ascending neural input, especially from A-delta and C fiber afferents, and possibly central biasing, activates the descending mechanism. The periaqueductal gray stimulates the raphe nucleus, which sends impulses along serotonergic efferent fibers in the dorsal lateral

efferent Conduction of a nerve impulse away from an organ.

periaqueductal gray A midbrain structure that plays an important role in descending tracts that inhibit synaptic transmission of noxious input in the dorsal horn.

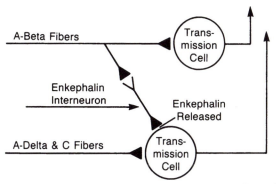

•Figure 3-6 Presynaptic inhibition of dorsal horn synapse transmission owing to A-beta fiber stimulation at enkephalin interneurons.

tract, which synapse with enkephalin interneurons. The interneurons release enkephalin into the dorsal horn, inhibiting the synaptic transmission of impulses to the second-order afferent neurons.

More recently, a second descending, norandrenergic pathway projecting from the pons to the dorsal horn has been identified.[16] The significance of these parallel pathways is not fully understood. It is also not known if these norandrenergic fibers directly inhibit dorsal horn synapses or stimulate the enkephalin interneurons.

This model provides a physiologic explanation for the analgesic response to brief, intense stimulation. The analgesia following accupressure and the use of some transcutaneous electrical nerve simulators (TENS), such as point simulators, is attributed to this descending pain control mechanism.

enkephalinergic interneurons Neurons with short axons that release enkephalin. They are widespread in the central nervous system and are found in the substantia gelatinosa, nucleus raphae magnus, and periaqueductual gray matter.

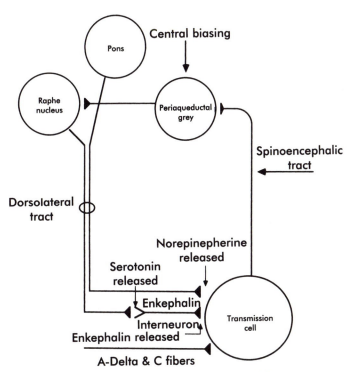

•Figure 3-7 Stimulation of the periaqueductal gray region of the midbrain and the raphe nucleus in the pons and medulla by ascending neural input, especially from A-delta and C fiber afferents, and possibly central biasing, activates the descending mechanism.

BETA-ENDORPHIN AND DYNORPHIN

There is evidence that stimulation of the small-diameter afferents (A-delta and C) can stimulate the release of other endogenous opioids.[8,10,19,23,25,27,30] Beta-endorphin (BEP) and dynorphin are neuroactive peptides with potent analgesic effects. The term **endorphin** refers to an opiatelike substance produced by the body. The mechanisms regulating the release of BEP and dynorphin have not been fully elucidated. However, it is apparent that these large endogenous substances play a role in the analgesic response to some forms of stimuli used in the treatment of patients in pain.

One of the sources of BEP is the anterior pituitary. Here it shares the prohormone propiomelanocortin (POMC) with adrenocorticotropin (**ACTH**). Prolonged (20–40 min) small-diameter afferent fiber stimulation has been thought to trigger the release of BEP from the anterior pituitary gland. Electroacupuncture, and possibly TENS with long phase durations and low pulse rates (1–5 pulses/sec), will cause small-diameter afferent fiber depolarization necessary for BEP release.[29] Recent findings do not support the anterior pituitary gland as a source of BEP in low pulse rate, long pulse width TENS-induced analgesia.[11] These results and the recognition that BEP does not readily cross the blood-brain barrier suggest that if BEP or other endogenous opioids are active analgesic agents within the central nervous system, they are released from areas within the brain.[3]

The neurons in the hypothalamus that send projections to the PAG and noradrenergic nuclei in the brain stem contain BEP. It is possible that BEP released from these neurons by stimulation of the hypothalamus is responsible for the analgesic response to the treatments (Fig. 3-8).[6]

β-endorphin A neurohormone derived from proopiomelanocortin (POMC).

ACTH Adrenocorticotrophic hormone. This hormone stimulates the release of glucocorticoids (cortisol) from the adrenal glands.

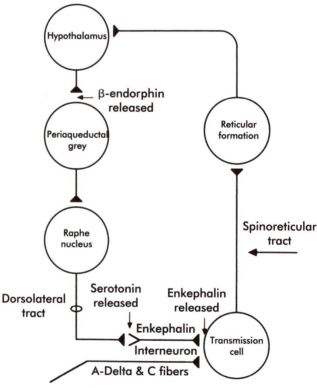

•**Figure 3-8** The neurons in the hypothalamus that send projections to the periaqueductal gray and noradrenergic nuclei in the brain stem contain β-endorphin. It is possible that β-endorphin released from these neurons by stimulation of the hypothalamus is responsible for the analgesic response to the treatments.

Dynorphin, a more recently isolated endogenous opioid, is found in the PAG, rostroventral medulla, and the dorsal horn.[16] It has been demonstrated that dynorphin is released during electroacupuncture.[14] Dynorphin may be responsible for suppressing the response to noxious mechanical stimulation.[16]

SUMMARY OF PAIN CONTROL MECHANISMS

The body's pain control mechanisms are probably not mutually exclusive. Rather, analgesia is the result of overlapping processes. It is also important to realize that the theories presented are only models. They are useful in conceptualizing the perception of pain and pain relief. These models will help the therapist understand the effects of therapeutic modalities and form a sound rationale for modality application. As more research is conducted and as the mysteries of pain and neurophysiology are solved, new models will emerge. The therapist should adapt these models to fit new developments.

COGNITIVE INFLUENCES

Pain perception and the response to a painful experience may be influenced by a variety of cognitive processes, including anxiety, attention, depression, past pain experiences, and cultural influences. These individual aspects of pain expression are mediated by higher centers in the cortex in ways that are not clearly understood. They may influence both the sensory discriminative and motivational affective dimensions of pain.

Many mental processes modulate the perception of pain through descending systems. Behavior modification, the excitement of the moment, happiness, positive feelings, **focusing** (directed attention toward specific stimuli), hypnosis, and suggestion may modulate pain perception. Past experiences, cultural background, personality, motivation to play, aggression, anger, and fear are all factors that could facilitate or inhibit pain perception. Strong central inhibition may mask severe injury for a period of time. At such times, evaluation of the injury is quite difficult.

Patients with chronic pain may become very depressed and experience a loss of fitness. They tend to be less active and may have altered appetites and sleep habits. They have a decreased will to work and exercise and often develop a reduced sex drive. They may turn to self-abusive patterns of behavior. Tricyclic drugs are often used to inhibit serotonin depletion for the patient with chronic pain.

Just as pain may be inhibited by central modulation, it may also arise from central origins. Phobias, fear, depression, anger, grief, and hostility are all capable of producing pain in the absence of local pathologic processes. In addition, pain memory, which is associated with old injuries, may result in pain perception and pain response that are out of proportion to a new, often minor, injury. Substance abuse can also alter and confound the perception of pain. Substance abuse may cause the chronic pain patient to become more depressed or may lead to depression and psychosomatic pain.

PAIN MANAGEMENT

How should the therapist approach pain? First, the source of the pain must be identified. Unidentified pain may hide a serious disorder, and treatment of such pain may delay the appropriate treatment of the disorder. Once a diagnosis has been made, many physical agents can provide pain relief. The therapist should match the thera-

CASE STUDY 3-2
MANAGING CHRONIC PAIN

Background: Linda is a 31-year-old resident in oral surgery. She was referred for physical therapy for complaints of upper back and neck pain with frequent head aches. She states that she has been experiencing the symptoms off and on for about 2 years. Her symptoms are worse at the end of the work day, especially on days she is in the operating room. There is no history of trauma to the affected region.

Physical exam reveals a forward head, rounded shoulder posture, spasm of the cervical paraspinal and trapezius muscles, and very sensitive trigger points throughout the region.

Impression: Her symptoms were consistent with pain of myofascial origin secondary to posture, job-related stress, and fatigue of the postural muscles.

Treatment: She was treated with TENS over the trigger points using a Neuroprobe, soft tissue mobilization, and instructed in a routine of postural exercises. She was encouraged to perform postural exercises and relaxation activities during breaks in her schedule. Linda returned to the clinic indicating she had experienced near complete relief following her first visit for about 6 hours. The stimulation of trigger points was repeated and Linda was instructed in the use of a TENS unit with conventional parameters over her most sensitive trigger point. She had access to the TENS unit through the surgical clinic where she worked.

Response: Linda was seen for two additional visits. She indicated her compliance with the exercise program, which was subsequently expanded into a general conditioning program with an emphasis on upper body endurance. She also indicated that her symptoms were becoming much less severe and less frequent and that the home TENS unit gave her a means of controlling her pain before it became severe enough to affect her activities. Over the subsequent several months Linda completed her residency without additional care for her neck and upper back.

Myofascial pain or pain of soft tissue origin has several causes, many of which may contribute to a single individual's symptoms. Poor posture, stress, repetitive microtrauma, and acute injuries can combine to cause a pain pattern that is often difficult to understand. The keys to management are to identify the causative factors and help the patient address them. In this case Linda had to recondition postural muscles to restore balance between antagonistic groups. Her long hours of standing over operating tables had contributed to her postural deficits. She also became more aware of how she responded to stressors and began using relaxation techniques with which she was familiar.

Her four visits to physical therapy enabled us to identify the causes of Linda's pain, break the pain spasm cycle, desensitize her trigger points, and initiate a program of progressive, pain-free exercises. Pain control is essential in the management of myofascial pain. Exercise that is painful further sensitizes trigger points and promotes the use of inefficient, antalgic movement patterns.

The rehabilitation professional employs physical agent modalities to create an optimum environment for tissue healing while minimizing the symptoms associated with the trauma or condition.

Discussion Questions

- What tissues were injured/affected?
- What symptoms were present?
- What phase of the injury-healing continuum did the patient present for care in?
- What are the physical agent modality's biophysical effects (direct/indirect/depth/tissue affinity)?
- What are the physical agent modality's indications/contraindications?
- What are the parameters of the physical agent modality's application/dosage/duration/frequency in this case study?
- What other physical agent modalities could be utilized to treat this injury or condition? Why? How?

peutic agent to each patient's situation. Casts and braces may prevent the application of ice or moist heat. However, TENS electrodes often can be positioned under a cast or brace for pain relief. Following acute injuries, ice may be the therapeutic agent of choice because of the effect of cold on the inflammatory process. There is not one "best" therapeutic agent for pain control. The therapist must select the therapeutic agent that is most appropriate for each patient, based on the knowledge of the modalities and professional judgment. In no situation should the therapist apply a therapeutic agent without first developing a clear rationale for the treatment.

In general, physical agents can be used to accomplish the following.

1. Stimulate large-diameter afferent fibers. This can be done with TENS, massage, and analgesic balms.
2. Decrease pain fiber transmission velocity with cold or ultrasound.
3. Stimulate small-diameter afferent fibers and descending pain control mechanisms with acupressure, deep massage, or TENS over acupuncture points or trigger points.[28]
4. Stimulate a release of BEP or other endogenous opioids through prolonged small-diameter fiber stimulation with TENS.[28]

Other useful pain control strategies include the following.

1. Encourage central biasing through cognitive processes, such as motivation, tension diversion, focusing, relaxation techniques, positive thinking, thought stopping, and self-control.
2. Minimize the tissue damage through the application of proper first aid and immobilization.
3. Maintain a line of communication with the patient. Let the patient know what to expect following an injury. Pain, swelling, dysfunction, and atrophy will occur following injury. The patient's anxiety over these events will increase his or her perception of pain. Often, a patient who has been told what to expect by someone he or she trusts will be less anxious and suffer less pain.
4. Recognize that all pain, even psychosomatic pain, is very real to the patient.
5. Encourage supervised exercise to encourage blood flow, promote nutrition, increase metabolic activity, and reduce stiffness and guarding, if the activity will not cause further harm to the patient.

The physician may choose to prescribe oral or injectable medications in the treatment of the patient. The most commonly used medications are classified as analgesics, anti-inflammatory agents, or both. The therapist should become familiar with these drugs and note if the patient is taking any medications. It is also important to work with the referring physician to assure that the patient takes the medications appropriately.

The therapist's approach to the patient has a great impact on the success of the treatment. The patient will not be convinced of the efficacy and importance of the treatment unless the therapist appears confident about it. The therapist must make the patient a participant rather than a passive spectator in the treatment and rehabilitation process.

The goal of most treatment programs is to encourage early pain-free exercise. The physical agents used to control pain do little to promote tissue healing. They should be used to relieve acute pain following injury or surgery or to control pain and other symptoms, such as swelling, to promote progressive exercise. The therapist should not lose sight of the effects of the physical agents or the importance of progressive exercise in restoring the patient's functional ability.

Reducing the perception of pain is as much an art as a science. Selection of the proper physical agent, proper application, and marketing are all important and will continue to be so even as we increase our understanding of the neurophysiology of pain. There is still the need for a good empirical rationale for the use of a physical agent. The therapist is encouraged to keep abreast of the neurophysiology of pain and the physiology of tissue healing to maintain a current scientific basis for selecting modalities and managing the pain experienced by his or her patients.

SUMMARY

1. Pain is a response to a noxious stimulus that is subjectively modified by past experiences and expectations.

2. Pain is classified as either acute or chronic and can exhibit many different patterns.

3. Early reduction of pain in a treatment program will facilitate therapeutic exercise.

4. Stimulation of sensory receptors via the therapeutic modalities can modify the patient's perception of pain.

5. Four mechanisms of pain control may explain the analgesic effects of physical agents:
   a. Decreased transmission of input along nociceptive pathways.
   b. Dorsal horn modulation owing to the input from large-diameter afferents through a gate control system, the release of enkephalins, or both.
   c. Descending efferent fiber activation owing to the effects of small fiber afferent input on higher centers, including the thalamus, raphe nucleus, and periaqueductal gray region.
   d. The central release of endogenous opioids including β-endorphin through prolonged small-diameter afferent stimulation.

6. Pain perception may be influenced by a variety of cognitive processes mediated by the higher brain centers.

7. The selection of a therapeutic modality for controlling pain should be based on current knowledge of neurophysiology and the psychology of pain.

8. The application of physical agents for the control of pain should not occur until the diagnosis of the injury has been established.

9. The selection of a therapeutic modality for managing pain should be based on establishing the primary cause of pain.

REFERENCES

1. Addison, R: Chronic pain syndrome, Am. J. Med. 77:54, 1985.
2. Anderson, S., Ericson, T., Holmgren, E.: Electroacupuncture affects pain threshold measured with electrical stimulation of teeth, Brain 63:393–396, 1973.
3. Berne, R., Levy, M.: Physiology, St. Louis, 1988, The C.V. Mosby Co.
4. Bishop, B.: Pain: its physiology and rationale for management, Phys. Ther. 60:13–37, 1980.
5. Bonica, J.: The management of pain, Philadelphia, 1990, Lea & Febiger.
6. Bowsher, D.: Central pain mechanisms. In Wells, P., Frampton, V., Bowsher, D., editors. Pain management in physical therapy. Norwalk, Connecticut, 1988, Appleton & Lange.
7. Castel, J.: Pain management: acupuncture and transcutaneous electrical nerve stimulation techniques, Lake Bluff, Illinois, 1979, Pain Control Services.
8. Chapman, C., Benedetti, C.: Analgesia following electrical stimulation: partial reversal by a narcotic antagonist, Life Sci. 26:44–48, 1979.
9. Cheng, R., Pomeranz, B.: Electroacupuncture analgesia could be mediated by at least two pain relieving mechanisms: endorphin and non-endorphin systems, Life Sci. 25:1957–1962, 1979.
10. Clement-Jones, V., McLaughlin, L., and Tomlin, S.: Increased beta-endorphin but not met-enkephalin levels in human cerebrospinal fluid after electroacupuncture for recurrent pain, Lancet 2:946–948, 1980.
11. Denegar, G., Perrin, D., and Rogol, A.: Influence of transcutaneous electrical nerve stimulation on pain, range of motion and serum cortisol concentration in females with induced delayed onset muscle soreness, JOSPT 11:101–103, 1989.
12. Dickerman, J.: The use of pain profiles in clinical practice, Fam. Pract. Recert. 14(3):35–44, 1992.
13. Gatchel, R.: Million behavioral health inventory: its utility in predicting physical functioning patients with low back pain. Arch. Phys. Med. Rehab. 67:878, 1986.
14. Ho, W., Wen, H.: Opioid-like activity in the cerebrospinal fluid of pain patients treated by electroacupuncture. Neuropharmacology 28:961–966, 1989.
15. Huskisson, E.: Visual analogue scales. Pain measurement and assessment. In Melzack, R., ed: Pain measurement and assessment, New York, 1983, Raven Press.

16. Jessell, T., Kelly, D.: Pain and analgesia. In Kandel, E., Schwartz, J., and Jessell T., editors. Principles of neural science, Norwalk, Connecticut, 1991, Appleton & Lange.

17. Kuland, D.N.: The injured athletes' pain. Curr. Concepts Pain 1:3–10, 1983.

18. Margoles, M.: The pain chart: spatial properties of pain. Pain measurement and assessment. In Melzack, R., editor. Pain measurement and assessment, New York, 1983, Raven Press.

19. Mayer, D., Price, D., and Rafii, A.: Antagonism of acupuncture analgesia in man by the narcotic antagonist naloxone, Brain Res. 121:368–372, 1977.

20. Melzack, R., Wall, P.: Pain mechanisms: a new theory, Science 150:971–979, 1965.

21. Melzack, R.: Concepts of pain measurement. In Melzack, R., editor. Pain measurement and assessment, New York, 1983, Raven Press.

22. Merskey, H., Albe Fessard, D., and Bonica, J.: Pain terms: a list with definitions and notes on usage, Pain 6:249–252, 1979.

23. Pomeranz, B., Paley, D.: Brain opiates at work in acupuncture, New Scientist 73:12–13, 1975.

24. Pomeranz, B., Chiu, D.: Naloxone blockade of acupuncture analgesia: enkephalin implicated, Life Sci. 19:1757–1762, 1976.

25. Pomeranz, B., Paley, D.: Electro-acupuncture hypoalgesia is mediated by afferent impulses: an electrophysiological study in mice, Exp. Neurol. 66:398–402, 1979.

26. Previte, J.: Human physiology, New York, 1983, McGraw-Hill, Inc.

27. Salar, G., Job, I., and Mingringo, S.: Effects of transcutaneous electrotherapy on CSF beta-endorphin content in patients without pain problems, Pain 10:169–172, 1981.

28. Sjolund, B., Eriksson, M.: Electroacupuncture and endogenous morphines, Lancet 2:1085, 1976.

29. Sjoland, B., Eriksson, M.: Increased cerebrospinal fluid levels of endorphins after electro-acupuncture, Acta Physiol. Scand. 100:382–384, 1977.

30. Wen, H., Ho, W., and Ling, N.: The influence of electroacupuncture on naloxone induces morphine withdrawal: elevation of immunoassayable beta-endorphin activity in the brain but not in the blood, Am. J. Clin. Med. 7:237–240, 1979.

31. Willis, W., Grossman, R.: Medical Neurobiology, ed. 3, St. Louis, 1981, C.V. Mosby.

32. Wolf, S.: Neurophysiologic mechanisms in pain modulation: relevance to TENS. In Manheimer, J., Lampe, G. editors. Clinical applications of TENS, Philadelphia, 1984, F.A. Davis.

GLOSSARY

accommodation Adaptation by the sensory receptors to various stimuli over an extended period of time.

ACTH Adrenocorticotropic hormone. This hormone stimulates the release of glucocorticoids (cortisol) from the adrenal glands.

afferent Conduction of a nerve impulse away from an organ.

avulsion fracture A fracture in which a small piece of bone is torn away by an attached tendon or ligament.

beta-endorphin A neurohormone derived from proopiomelanocortin (POMC). It is similar in structure and properties to morphine. Beta-endorphin has a half-life of 4 hours.

bradykinin A chemical formed in injured tissue as part of the inflammatory process that vasodilates small arterioles.

central biasing A theory of pain modulation where higher centers such as the cerebral cortex influence the perception of and response to pain.

dynorphin An endogenous opioid derived from the prohormone prodynorphin.

efferent Conduction of a nerve impulse toward an organ.

endogenous opioids Opiatelike substances made by the body.

endorphins Endogenous opioids whose actions have analgesic properties (i.e., β-endorphin).

enkephalin Neurotransmitter proteins that block the passage of noxious stimuli from first- to second-order afferents. They inhibit the release of substance P and are produced by enkephalinergic neurons.

enkephalinergic interneurons Neurons with short axons that release enkephalin. They are widespread in the central nervous system and are found in the substantia gelatinosa, nucleus raphae magnus, and periaqueductal gray matter.

focusing Narrowing attention to the appropriate stimuli in the environment.

interneurons Neurons contained entirely in the central nervous system. They have no projections outside the spinal cord. Their function is to serve as relay stations within the central nervous system.

joint capsule Ligamentous structure that surrounds and encapsulates a joint.

neurotransmitter Substance that passes information between neurons. It is released from one neuron terminal (presynaptic membrane), enters the synaptic cleft, and attaches (binds) to a receptor on the next neuron (postsynaptic membrane). Substance P, enkephalins, serotonin, methionine, and leucine enkephalin are neurotransmitters.

nociceptive Pain information or signals of pain stimuli.

norepinephrine A neurotransmitter.

opiate receptors Neurons that have receptors that bind to opiate substances.

periaqueductal gray A midbrain structure that plays an important role in descending tracts that inhibit synaptic transmission of noxious input in the dorsal horn.

periosteum A highly vascularized and innervated membrane lining the surface of bone.

polymodal nociceptors Small unmyelinated afferent fibers that have high threshold axons and respond only to cutaneous stimulation (i.e., pain, deep pressure, and temperature). C fibers are examples of these.

prostaglandins Irritants that are synthesized locally during injury in tissue from a fatty acid precursor (arachidonic acid). They act with bradykinin to amplify pain by sensitizing afferent neurons to chemical and mechanical stimulation. Aspirin is thought to be capable of interrupting the process. Prostaglandins are powerful vasodilators. They induce erythema, increase leakage of plasma from vessels, and attract leukocytes to an injured area.

raphe nucleus Part of the brain that is known to inhibit pain impulses being transmitted through the ascending system.

referred pain (referred myofascial pain) When nociceptive impulses reach the dorsal gray matter, they converge and their summation can depolarize internuncial neurons over several spinal segments, causing the individual to feel pain in distal areas innervated by these segments.

reticular formation A network of neurons that extends through the length of the spinal column, brain stem, and into the basal regions of the diencephalon and telencephalon. The cell bodies lie in diffuse groups within the brain stem. The reticular formation receives input from and/or sends output to most central nervous system structures.

sclerotome A segment of bone innervated by a spinal segment.

sensitization Prolonged depolarization of nociceptive neurons that results in continuous stimulation. Most sensory receptors are rendered less sensitive after prolonged stimulation. This is not the case with nociceptive neurons.

serotonin A neurotransmitter found in neurons descending in the dorsolateral tract. The dorsolateral tract is thought to play a significant role in pain control. Serotonin is found in the vesicles in nerve endings that bind when released to postsynaptic membranes. Its action is terminated by reuptake into presynaptic membranes. It is probably involved in both endogenous pain control and opiate analgesia. Increased levels of serotonin in the central nervous system are generally associated with increased analgesia.

stimulus-produced analgesia (SPA) Pain relief created by stimulation of portions of the central nervous system, either directly or indirectly. Common methods are electrical stimulation, needle, pressure, or extreme cold applied to acupuncture points, trigger points, or motor points.

substance P A peptide believed to be the neurotransmitter of small-diameter primary afferent. It is released from both ends of the neuron.

substantia gelatinosa (SG) Lamina II of the dorsal horn of the gray matter. Melzack and Wall proposed that the SG is responsible for closing the gate to painful stimuli.[20]

T cell Transmission cell or second-order neuron in the dorsal horn of the spinal cord. Principal location may be lamina V.

trigger point Localized deep tenderness in a palpable firm band of muscle is stretched, a palpating finger can snap the band like a taut string that produces local pain, a local twitch of that portion of the muscle, and a jump by the patient. Sustained pressure on a trigger point reproduces the pattern of referred pain for that site.

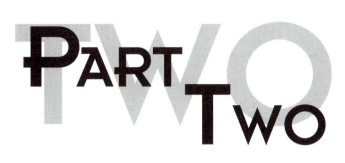

PART TWO

ELECTRICAL MODALITIES

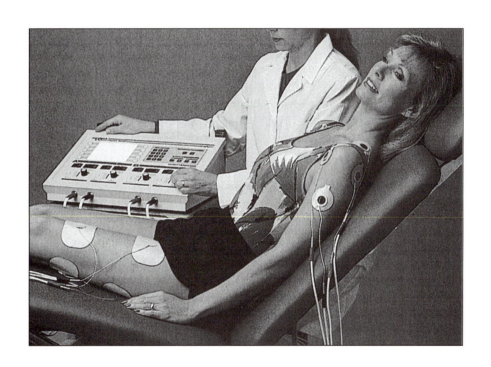

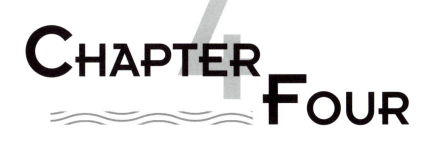

CHAPTER FOUR

BASIC PRINCIPLES OF ELECTRICITY

WILLIAM E. PRENTICE

OBJECTIVES

Following completion of this chapter, the student therapist will be able to:

- ✓ Define potential difference, ampere, volt, ohm, and watt.
- ✓ Give Ohm's law and its mathematical expression.
- ✓ Differentiate between alternating, direct, and pulsed currents.
- ✓ Discuss various waveforms and pulse characteristics.
- ✓ Discuss current modulation.
- ✓ Differentiate between series and parallel circuit arrangement.
- ✓ Discuss current flow through various types of biologic tissue.
- ✓ Discuss safety in the use of electrical equipment by the therapist.

Many of the modalities discussed in this book may be classified as electrical modalities. These pieces of equipment have the capabilities of taking the electrical current flowing from a wall outlet and modifying that current to produce a specific, desired physiologic effect in human biologic tissue.

Understanding the basic principles of electricity usually is difficult even for the therapist who is accustomed to using electrical modalities on a daily basis. To understand how current flow effects biologic tissue it is first necessary to become familiar with some of the principles that describe how electricity is produced and how it behaves in an electrical circuit.

The principles and concepts presented in this chapter can be applied to the use of all of the electrical modalities to be discussed in this book, including iontophoresis (see Chapter 6), biofeedback (see Chapter 7), the diathermies (see Chapter 8), low-power laser (see Chapter 11), ultraviolet (see Chapter 12), and even ultrasound (see Chapter 10), but are particularly applicable to Chapter 5, Electrical Stimulating Currents.

COMPONENTS OF ELECTRICAL CURRENTS

All matter is composed of atoms that contain positively and negatively charged particles called **ions**. These charged particles possess electrical energy and thus have the ability to move about. They tend to move from an area of higher concentration toward an area of lower concentration. An electrical force is capable of propelling these particles from higher to lower energy levels, thus establishing **electrical potentials**. The more ions an object has, the higher its potential electrical energy. Particles with a positive charge tend to move toward negatively charged particles, and those that are negatively charged tend to move toward positively charged particles (Fig. 4-1).[10]

electron Fundamental particles of matter possessing a negative electrical charge and very small mass.

Electrons are particles of matter possessing a negative charge and very small mass. The net movement of electrons is referred to as an **electrical current**. The movement or flow of these electrons will always go from a higher potential to a lower potential.[17] An electrical force is oriented only in the direction of the applied force. This flow of electrons may be likened to a domino reaction.

ampere Unit of measure that indicates the rate at which electrical current is flowing.

The unit of measurement that indicates the rate at which electrical current flows is the **ampere (amp)**; 1 amp is defined as the movement of 1 **coulomb** or 6.25×10^{18} electrons per second. Amperes indicate the rate of electron flow, whereas coulombs indicate the number of electrons. In the case of therapeutic modalities, **current** flow is generally described in milliamperes (1/1000 of an amp, denoted as mA) or in microamperes (1/1,000,000 of an amp, denoted as μA).

The electrons will not move unless an electrical potential difference in the concentration of these charged particles exists between two points. The electromotive force, which must be applied to produce a flow of electrons, is called a **volt (V)** and is defined as the difference in electron population (potential difference) between two points.[3]

voltage The force resulting from an accumulation of electrons at one point in an electrical circuit, usually corresponding to a deficit of electrons at another point in the circuit.

Voltage is the force resulting from an accumulation of electrons at one point in an electrical circuit, usually corresponding to a deficit of electrons at another point in the **circuit**. If the two points are connected by a suitable conductor, the potential difference (in electron population) will cause electrons to move from the area of higher population to the area of lower population.

Commercial current flowing from wall outlets produces an electromotive force of either 115 or 220 V. The electrotherapeutic devices used in injury rehabilitation modify voltages. Electrical generators are sometimes referred to as being either low- or high-volt. These terms are somewhat useless in meaning, although some older texts have referred to generators that produce less than 150 V as *low-volt* and those that produce several hundred volts as *high-volt*.[3]

Electrons can move in a current only if there is a relatively easy pathway to move along. Materials that permit this free movement of electrons are referred to as **conductors**. **Conductance** is a term that defines the ease with which current flows along a conducting medium. Metals (copper, gold, silver, aluminum) are good conductors of electricity, as are electrolyte solutions, because both are composed of large numbers of free electrons that are given up readily. Thus, materials that offer little opposition to current flow are good conductors. Materials that resist current flow are

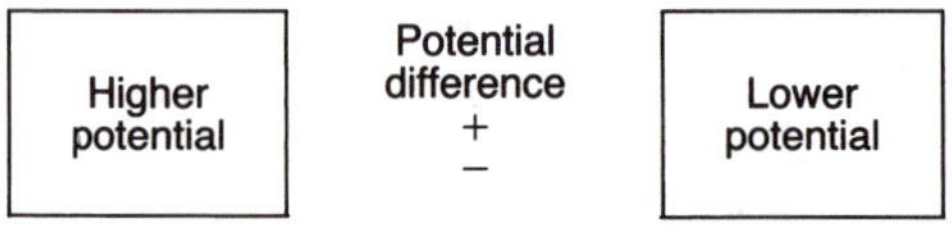

•**Figure 4-1** The difference between high potential and low potential is potential difference. Electrons tend to flow from areas of higher concentration to areas of lower concentration. A potential difference must exist if there is to be any movement of electrons.

called **insulators**. Insulators contain relatively fewer free electrons and thus offer greater resistance to electron flow. Air, wood, and glass are all considered insulators. The number of amps flowing in a given conductor is dependent both on the voltage applied and on the conduction characteristics of the material.[16]

The opposition to electron flow in a conducting material is referred to as **resistance** or **electrical impedance** and is measured in a unit known as an **ohm**. Thus, an electrical circuit that has high resistance (ohms) will have less flow (amps) than a circuit with less resistance and the same voltage.[2]

The mathematical relationship between current flow, voltage, and resistance is demonstrated in the following formula.

$$\text{Current flow} = \frac{\text{Voltage}}{\text{Resistance}}$$

This formula is the mathematical expression of **Ohm's law**, which states that the current in an electrical circuit is directly proportional to the voltage and inversely proportional to the resistance.

An analogy comparing the movement of water with the movement of electricity may help to clarify this relationship between current flow, voltage, and resistance (Table 4-1). In order for water to flow, some type of pump must create a force to produce movement. Likewise, the volt is the pump that produces the electron flow. The resistance to water flow is dependent on the length, diameter, and smoothness of the water pipe. The resistance to electrical flow depends on the characteristics of the conductor. The amount of water flowing is measured in gallons, whereas the amount of electricity flowing is measured in amperes.

The amount of energy produced by flowing water is determined by two factors: (1) the number of gallons flowing per unit of time; and (2) the pressure created in the pipe. Electrical energy or power is a product of the voltage or electromotive force and the amount of current flowing. Electrical power is measured in a unit called a **watt**.

$$\text{Watts} = \text{Volts} \times \text{Amperes}$$

Simply, the watt indicates the rate at which electrical power is being used. A watt is defined as the electrical power needed to produce a current flow of 1 amp at a pressure of 1 volt.

resistance The opposition to electron flow in a conducting material.

Ohm's law The current in an electrical circuit is directly proportional to the voltage and inversely proportional to the resistance.

ELECTROTHERAPEUTIC CURRENTS

Electrotherapeutic devices generate three different types of current that, when introduced into biologic tissue, are capable of producing specific physiologic changes. These three types of current are referred to as alternating (AC), direct (DC), or pulsed. The therapeutic effects of these various types of electrical stimulating currents are discussed in detail in Chapter 5.

Direct current, also referred to in some texts as galvanic current, has a unidirectional flow of electrons toward the positive pole (Fig. 4-2A). On most modern direct

TABLE 4-1   **Electron Flow as Analogous to Water Flow**

Electron Flow		Water Flow
Volt	=	Pump
Amperes	=	Gallons
Ohm (properties of conductor)	=	Resistance (length and distance of pipe)

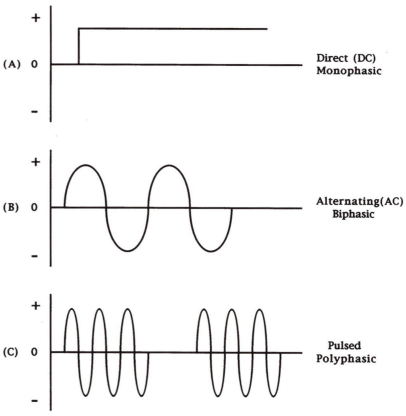

•**Figure 4-2** *A* Direct (DC) or monophasic current. *B* Alternating (AC) or biphasic current. *C* Pulsed or polyphasic current.

Types of Electrical Current
- Alternating (AC) or biphasic
- Direct (DC) or monophasic
- Pulsed or polyphasic

current devices, the polarity and thus the direction of current flow can be reversed.[2] Some generators have the capability of automatically reversing polarity, in which case the physiologic effects will be similar to AC current.[15]

In an **alternating current**, the flow of electrons constantly changes direction or, stated differently, reverses its polarity. Electrons flowing in an alternating current always move from the negative to positive pole, reversing direction when polarity is reversed (Fig. 4-2B).

Pulsed currents usually contain three or more pulses grouped together (Fig. 4-2C). These groups of pulses are interrupted for short periods of time and repeat themselves at regular intervals. Pulsed currents are used in interferential and so-called Russian currents, which are discussed in Chapter 5.[1,7]

GENERATORS OF ELECTROTHERAPEUTIC CURRENTS

A great deal of confusion has developed relative to the terminology used to describe electrotherapeutic currents. Basically, all therapeutic electrical generators, regardless of whether they deliver AC, DC, or pulsed currents through electrodes attached to the skin, are **transcutaneous electrical stimulators**. The majority of these are used to stimulate peripheral nerves and are correctly called **transcutaneous electrical nerve stimulators (TENS)**. Occasionally, the terms **neuromuscular electrical stimulators (NMES)** or electrical muscle stimulator (EMS) are used; however, these terms are only appropriate when the electrical current is being used to stimulate muscle directly, as would be the case with denervated muscle where peripheral nerves are not functioning. In recent years, a new type of transcutaneous electrical

neuromuscular electrical stimulator (NMES) Also called an electrical muscle stimulator (EMS), it is used to stimulate muscle directly, as would be the case with denervated muscle where peripheral nerves are not functioning.

stimulator has gained popularity that utilizes current intensities too small to excite peripheral nerves. The most common term used to describe these generators is **microcurrent electrical nerve stimulators (MENS)**. Most recently the term MENS has been replaced by the new term low-intensity stimulation (LIS).[1,12,14]

There is no relationship between the type of current being delivered to the patient by the generator and the type of current being used as a power source to drive the generator (i.e., a wall outlet or battery). Generators that produce electrotherapeutic currents may be driven by either alternating or direct currents. Devices that plug into the standard electrical wall outlet use alternating current. The commercially produced alternating current changes its direction of flow 120 times per second. In other words, there are 60 complete cycles per second. The number of cycles occurring in 1 second is called **frequency** and is indicated in Hertz (Hz), pulses per second (PPS), or cycles per second (CPS). The voltage of electromotive force producing this alternating directional flow of electrons is set at a standard 115 or 220 V. Thus, commercial alternating current is produced at 60 Hz with a corresponding voltage of either 115 or 220 V.

Other electrotherapeutic devices are driven by batteries that always produce direct current, ranging between 1.5 and 9 V, although the devices driven by batteries may, in turn, produce modified types of current.

To convert current coming from an AC power source to a DC current delivered to the patient is accomplished by a series of electrical components within the stimulating unit: a transformer, a rectifier, a filter, a regulator, an amplifier, and an oscillator.[5,6] A **transformer** "steps down" or reduces the amount of voltage from the power supply. The **rectifier** converts AC current to pulsating DC current. The **filter** changes the pulsating DC current to smooth DC. The **regulator** produces a specific controlled voltage output. An **output amplifier** within the stimulating unit is used to magnify or increase the amplitude of the voltage output of the generator and control it at a specific level, regardless of the electrical impedance of the remainder of the circuit (including the electrodes and patient). The **oscillator** is used to produce and output a specific waveform, which again may be different from that used to power or drive the stimulating unit.

microcurrent electrical nerve stimulator (MENS) Used primarily in tissue healing, the current intensities too small to excite peripheral nerves.

WAVEFORMS

The term **waveform** indicates a graphic representation of the shape, direction, **amplitude**, **duration**, and pulse frequency of the electrical current being produced by the electrotherapeutic device, as displayed by an instrument called an oscilloscope (Fig. 4-3).

Waveform Shapes
- Sine
- Rectangular
- Triangular

WAVEFORM SHAPE

Electrical currents may take on a sine, *rectangular*, or *triangular* waveform configurations, depending on the capabilities of the generator producing the current. (Fig. 4-4). Alternating, direct, and pulsed currents may take on any of the waveform shapes.

PULSES VERSUS PHASES AND DIRECTION OF CURRENT FLOW

On an oscilloscope, an individual waveform is referred to as a **pulse**. A pulse may contain either one or two **phases**, which is that portion of the pulse that rises above or below the baseline for some period of time. Direct current, also referred to as **monophasic current,** produces waveforms that have only a single phase in each

pulse An individual waveform is referred to as a pulse.

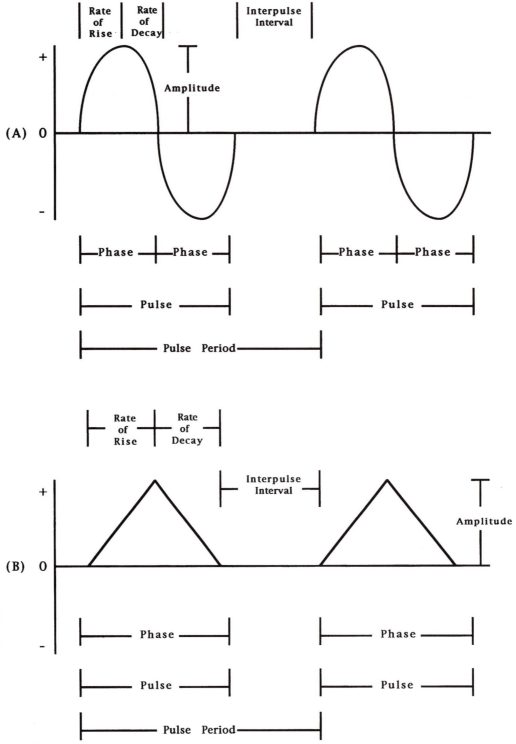

•**Figure 4-3** An individual waveform is referred to as a pulse. A pulse may contain either one or two phases, which is that portion of the pulse that rises above or below the baseline for some period of time. *A* Biphasic pulse. *B* Monophasic pulse.

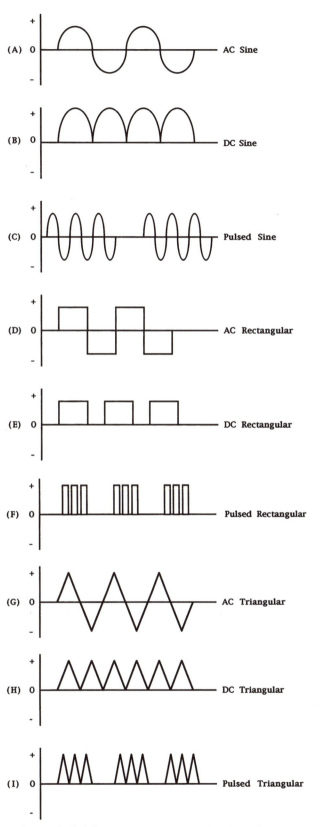

•**Figure 4-4** Waveforms of AC, DC, or pulsed current may be either sine, rectangular, or triangular in shape.

pulse. Current flow is unidirectional, always flowing in the same direction toward either the positive or negative pole (see Fig. 4-2A). Conversely, alternating current, also referred to as **biphasic current**, produces waveforms that have two separate phases during each individual pulse. Current flow is bidirectional, reversing direction or polarity once during each pulse. Biphasic waveforms may be symmetric or asymmetric. If both phases of the waveform are symmetric, the shape and size of each phase is identical (see Fig. 4-2B). Pulsed current waveforms are called **polyphasic** and are representative of electrical current that is conducted as a series of pulses of short duration (μsec) followed by a short period of time when current is not flowing called the **interpulse interval** (msec). Single pulses may be interrupted by an **intrapulse interval** (see Fig. 4-2C). Pulsed current may flow in one direction as in DC current or may reverse direction of flow as in AC current. With pulsed currents there is always some interruption of current flow.

pulse period The combined time of the pulse duration and the interpulse interval.

PULSE AMPLITUDE

The amplitude of each pulse reflects the intensity of the current, the maximum amplitude being the tip or highest point of each phase (see Fig. 4-3). The term amplitude is synonymous with the terms voltage and current intensity. The higher the amplitude, the greater the peak voltage or intensity. However, the peak amplitude should not be confused with the total amount of current being delivered to the tissues.

On electrical generators that produce short-duration pulses, the total current produced (coulombs/sec) is low compared to peak current amplitudes owing to long interpulse intervals that have current amplitudes of zero. Thus, the **average current**, or the amount of current flowing per unit of time, is relatively low, ranging from as low as 2 to as high as 100 mA on some interferential generators. Average current can be increased by either increasing pulse duration or increasing pulse frequency or by some combination of the two (Fig. 4-5).

PULSE CHARGE

pulse charge The total amount of electricity being delivered to the patient during each pulse.

The term **pulse charge** refers to the total amount of electricity being delivered to the patient during each pulse. With monophasic current, the phase charge and the pulse charge are the same and always greater than zero. With biphasic current, the pulse charge is equal to the sum of the phase charges. If the pulse is symmetric, the net pulse charge is zero. In asymmetric pulses the net pulse charge is greater than zero, which is a DC current by definition.[1]

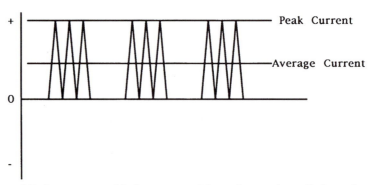

•**Figure 4-5** Average current is low compared to peak current amplitudes owing to long interpulse intervals.

PULSE RATE OF RISE AND DECAY TIMES

The **rate of rise** in amplitude, or the rise time, refers to how quickly the pulse reaches its maximum amplitude in each phase. Conversely, **decay time** refers to the time in which a pulse goes from peak amplitude to 0 V. The rate of rise is important physiologically because of the **accommodation** phenomenon, in which a fiber that has been subjected to a constant level of depolarization will become unexcitable at that same intensity or amplitude. Rate of rise and decay times are generally short, ranging from nanoseconds (billionths of a second) to milliseconds (thousandths of a second) (see Fig. 4-3).

By observing the three different waveforms it is apparent that the sine wave has a gradual increase and decrease in amplitude for alternating, direct, and pulsed currents (see Fig. 4-4, A, B, C). The rectangular wave has an almost instantaneous increase in amplitude, which plateaus for a period of time and then abruptly falls off (see Fig. 4-4, D, E, F). The triangular wave has a rapid increase and decrease in amplitude (see Fig. 4-4, G, H, I). The shape of these waveforms as they reach their maximum amplitude or intensity is directly related to the excitability of nervous tissue. The more rapid the increase in amplitude or the rate of rise, the greater the current's ability to excite nervous tissue.

Most modern DC generators make use of a twin peak triangular pulse of very short duration (170 μ) and peak amplitudes as high as 500 V (Fig. 4-6). Combining a high peak intensity with a short phase duration produces a very comfortable type of current as well as an effective means of stimulating sensory, motor, and pain fibers.[18]

The effects of the various waveforms on biologic tissue are discussed in Chapter 5.

ASYMMETRIC WAVEFORMS

Asymmetric biphasic waveforms have been used in the past but are seldom available on generators used by therapists. Occasionally, manufacturers will indicate that their equipment is producing **faradic current**. However, the true faradic waveform is no longer used. The so-called faradic current is most likely a high-frequency (> 400 Hz) pulsed wave. The original faradic waveform could only have used alternating current because there was always a reversal of direction of current flow (see Fig. 4-7A). The amplitude of the portion of the wave in the negative direction was

> Amplitude = voltage = current intensity

> **rate of rise** How quickly a waveform reaches its maximum amplitude.

> **faradic current** An asymmetric biphasic waveform seldom used on modern electrical generators.

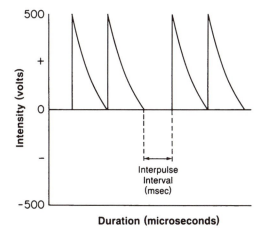

•**Figure 4-6** Most DC generators produce a twin peak triangular pulse of short duration and high amplitude.

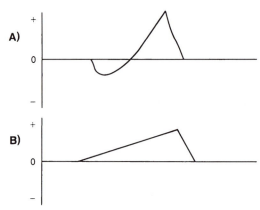

•**Figure 4-7** *A* Original faradic or asymmetric biphasic waveform. *B* Monophasic sawtooth or exponential waveform.

not great enough to produce any physiologic response. Thus, the effects of this faradic wave would be similar to those of a direct current pulsed wave (Fig. 4-7A).[8]

In the monophasic sawtooth or exponential waveform the amplitude rises very gradually and then falls abruptly (see Fig. 4-7B). Current that uses this waveform is used to stimulate denervated muscle without affecting normally innervated muscle, since the gradual rise in amplitude allows for accommodation of the normal muscle.[8]

PULSE DURATION

The **duration** of each pulse indicates the length of time current is flowing in one cycle. With monophasic current the phase duration is the same as the pulse duration and is the time from initiation of the phase to its end. With biphasic current the pulse duration is determined by the combined phase durations. In some electrotherapeutic devices the duration is preset by the manufacturer. Other devices have the capability of changing duration. The phase duration may be as short as a few microseconds or may be a long-duration direct current that flows for several minutes.

With pulsed currents, and in some instances with alternating and direct currents, the current flow is off for a period of time. The combined time of the pulse duration and the interpulse interval is referred to as the **pulse period** (see Fig. 4-3).

PULSE FREQUENCY

Pulse **frequency** indicates the number of pulses per second. Each individual pulse represents a rise and fall in amplitude. As the frequency of any waveform is increased, the amplitude tends to increase and decrease more rapidly. The muscular and nervous system responses depend on the length of time between pulses and on how the pulses or waveforms are modulated.[16] Muscle responds with individual twitch contractions to pulse rates of less than 50 pulses per second. At 50 pulses per second or greater a tetanic contraction will result, regardless of whether the current is biphasic, monophasic, or polyphasic.

Stimulators have been clinically labeled as either low-, medium-, or high-frequency generators, and a great deal of misunderstanding exists over how these frequency ranges are classified.[1] Generally, all stimulating units are low-frequency electrical generators that deliver between one and several hundred pulses per second. Recently, a number of so-called medium-frequency generators have been developed

biphasic current Another name for alternating current, in which the direction of current flow reverses direction.

frequency The number of cycles or pulses per second.

that are claimed to have frequencies of 2500 to as high as 10,000 pulses per second. However, these high-frequency pulses are in reality groups of pulses combined as **bursts** that range in frequency from 1 to 200 pulses per second. These modulated bursts are capable of producing a physiologically effective frequency of stimulation only in this 1 to 200 pulse per second range owing to the limitations of the absolute refractory period of nerve cell membranes. Therefore, many of the claims of equipment manufacturers relative to medium-frequency generators are inaccurate.[1]

CURRENT MODULATION

The physiologic responses to the various waveforms depend to a large extent on current modulation. **Modulation** refers to any alteration in the magnitude or any variation in duration of these pulses. Modulation may be continuous, interrupted, burst, or ramped.[1,9] The parameters of this modulation must be established according to various treatment goals.

Current Modulation
- Continuous
- Interrupted
- Burst
- Ramped

Continuous Modulation

Continuous modulation means that the amplitude of current flow remains the same for several seconds or perhaps minutes. Continuous modulation is usually associated with long pulse duration direct current (Fig. 4-8A). With direct current, flow is always in a uniform direction. In the discussion of physiologic responses to electrical currents, it was indicated that positive and negative ions are attracted toward poles or, in this case, electrodes of opposite polarity. This accumulation of charged ions over a period of time creates either an acidic or alkaline environment that may be of therapeutic value. This therapeutic technique has been referred to as **medical galvanism**. The technique of **iontophoresis** also uses continuous direct current to drive ions into the tissues (see Chapter 6). If the amplitude is great enough to produce a muscle contraction, the contraction will occur only when the current flow is turned on or off. Thus, with direct current continuous modulation, there will be a muscle contraction both when the current is turned on and when it is turned off.

Continuous modulation is also used with alternating current primarily for the purpose of eliciting muscle contractions.

Interrupted Modulation

With interrupted modulation, current flows for some period of time called the on time and is then periodically turned off during the off time. On most units, *on time* may be set between 1 and 60 seconds, whereas *off time* may be set between 1 and 120 seconds. Interrupted modulation is used with monophasic or biphasic currents. Current with sine, rectangular, or triangular shaped waveforms may be interrupted. Interrupted modulation is used clinically for muscle reeducation and strengthening and for improving range of motion (see Fig. 4-8B).

Burst Modulation

Burst modulation occurs when pulsed current flows for a short duration (milliseconds) and then is turned off for a short time (milliseconds) in a repetitive cycle. With polyphasic currents, sets of pulses are combined. These combined pulses are most commonly referred to in the literature as **bursts**, but they have also been called *packets*, *envelopes*, *pulse trains*, or *beats* (as is the case with interferential currents). The interruptions between individual bursts are called interburst intervals (Fig. 4-8C). The interburst interval is much too short to have any effect on a muscle contraction. Thus, the physiologic effects of a burst of pulses will be the same as with a single pulse.[1] Bursts may be used with monophasic and biphasic currents as well.

bursts A combined set of three or more pulses; also referred to as packets or envelopes.

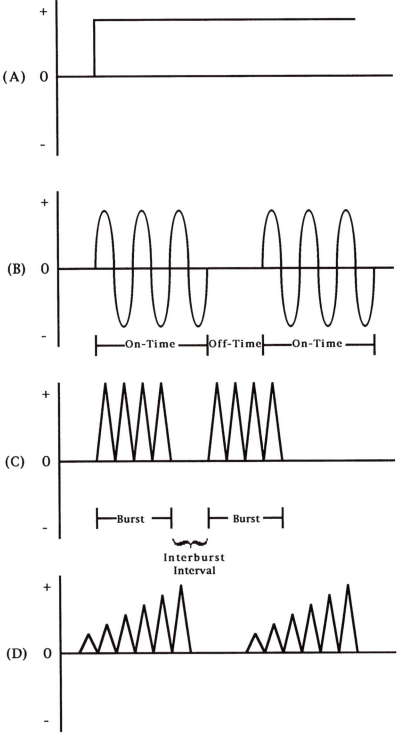

•**Figure 4-8** Current may be modulated using *A* continuous, *B* interrupted, *C* burst, or *D* ramped modes.

Ramping Modulation

ramping Another name for surging modulation, in which the current builds gradually to some maximum amplitude.

In **ramping** modulation, also called surging modulation, current amplitude will increase or ramp up gradually to some preset maximum and may also decrease or ramp down in intensity (see Fig. 4-8D). Ramp up time is usually preset at about one-third of the on time. The ramp down option is not available on all machines.

Most modern stimulators allow the therapist to set the on and off times between 1 and 10 seconds. Ramping modulation is used clinically to elicit muscle contraction and is generally considered to be a very comfortable type of current since it allows for a gradual increase in the intensity of a muscle contraction.

ELECTRICAL CIRCUITS

The path of current from a generating power source through various components back to the generating source is called an electrical **circuit**. A closed circuit is one in which electrons are flowing, and in an open circuit the current flow ceases. Electronic circuits are not ordinarily composed of single elements; they often encompass several branches or components with different resistances. The current in each branch may be easily calculated if the individual resistances are known and if the amount of voltage applied to the circuit is also known.[4]

With the development of the microelectronics industry, we all know that electrical circuits can be extremely complex. However, all electrical circuits have several basic components. There is a power source, which is capable of producing voltage. There is some type of conducting medium or pathway that current travels along and that carries the flowing electrons. Finally, there is some component or group of components that are driven by this flowing current. These driven elements provide resistance to electrical flow.[4]

SERIES AND PARALLEL CIRCUITS

The components that provide resistance to current flow may be connected to one another in one of two different patterns, a **series circuit** or a **parallel circuit**. The main difference between these two is that in a series circuit there is only one path for current to get from one terminal to another. In a parallel circuit two or more routes exist for current to pass between the two terminals.

In a series circuit the components are placed end-to-end (Fig. 4-9). The number of amperes of an electrical current flowing through a series circuit is exactly the same at any point in that circuit. The resistance to current flow in this total circuit is equal to the resistance of all the components in the circuit added together.

$$R_T = R_1 + R_2 + R_3$$

Electrical energy is required to force the current through the resistor, and this energy is dissipated in the form of heat. Consequently, there is a decrease in voltage

series circuit A circuit in which there is only one path for current to get from one terminal to another.

parallel circuit A circuit in which two or more routes exist for current to pass between the two terminals.

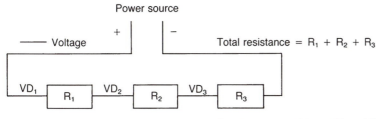

Total resistance = $R_1 + R_2 + R_3$

Total voltage = $VD_1 + VD_2 + VD_3$

•**Figure 4-9** In a series circuit, the component resistors are placed end-to-end. The total resistance to current flow is equal to the resistance of all the components added together. There is a voltage decrease at each component such that the sum of the voltage decreases is equal to the total voltage.

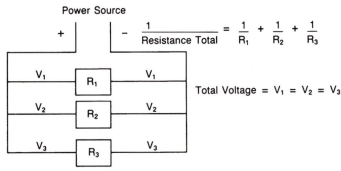

•**Figure 4-10** In a parallel circuit the component resistors are placed side by side and the ends are connected. The current flow in each of the pathways is inversely proportional to the resistance of the pathway. The total voltage is the sum of the voltages at each component.

at each component such that the total voltage at the beginning of the circuit is equal to the sum of the voltage decreases at each component.

$$V_T = VD_1 + VD_2 + VD_3$$

In a parallel circuit, the component resistors are placed side by side and the ends are connected (Fig. 4-10). Each of the resistors in a parallel circuit receives the same voltage. The current passing through each component depends on its resistance. Therefore, the total voltage will be exactly the same as the voltage at each component.

$$V_T = V_1 = V_2 = V_3$$

Each additional resistance added to a parallel circuit in effect decreases the total resistance. Adding an alternative pathway regardless of its resistance to current flow improves the ability of the current to get from one point to another. The current will, in general, choose the pathway that offers the least resistance. The formula for determining total resistance in a parallel circuit according to Ohm's law is:

$$\frac{1}{R_T} = \frac{1}{R_1} + \frac{1}{R_2} + \frac{1}{R_3}$$

Thus, component resistors connected in a series circuit have a higher resistance and lower current flow, and resistors in a parallel circuit have a lower resistance and a higher current flow.

The electrical modalities in general make use of some combination of both series and parallel circuits.[8] For example, to elicit a muscle contraction, the electrodes from an electrical stimulating unit are placed on the skin (Fig. 4-11). The current from those electrodes must pass directly through the skin and fat. The total resistance to current flow seen by the electrical stimulating unit is equal to the combined resistances at each electrode. This passage of current through the skin is basically a series circuit.

After the current passes through the skin and fat, it comes in contact with a number of different types of biologic tissues (i.e., bone, connective tissue, blood, muscle). The current has several different pathways through which it may reach the muscle to be stimulated. The total current traveling through these tissues is the sum of the currents in each different type of tissue, and since there are additional tissues through which current may travel, the total resistance is effectively reduced. Thus, in this typical application of a therapeutic modality, both parallel and series circuits are used to produce the desired physiologic effect.

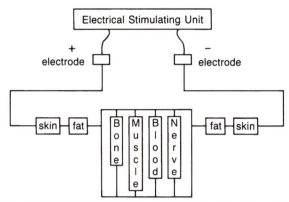

•**Figure 4-11** The electrical circuit that exists when electrons flow through human tissue is in reality a combination of a series and parallel circuit.

CURRENT FLOW THROUGH BIOLOGIC TISSUES

As stated previously, electrical current tends to choose the path that offers the least resistance to flow or, stated differently, the material that is the best conductor.[18] The conductivity of the different types of tissue in the body is variable. Typically, tissue that is highest in water content and consequently highest in ion content is the best conductor of electricity.

The skin has different layers that vary in water content, but generally the skin offers the primary resistance to current flow and is considered an insulator. Skin preparation for the purpose of reducing electrical impedance is of primary concern with electrodiagnostic apparatus, but it is also important with electrotherapeutic devices (see Chapter 7). The greater the impedance of the skin, the higher the voltage of the electrical current must be to stimulate underlying nerve and muscle. Chemical changes in the skin can make it more resistant to certain types of current. Thus, skin impedance is generally higher with direct current than with alternating current.

Blood is a biologic tissue that is composed largely of water and ions and is consequently the best electrical conductor of all tissues. Muscle is composed of about 75 percent water and depends on the movement of ions for contraction. Muscle tends to propagate an electrical impulse much more effectively in a longitudinal direction than transversely. Muscle tendons are considerably more dense than muscle, contain relatively little water, and are considered poor conductors. Fat contains only about 14 percent water and is thought to be a poor conductor. Peripheral nerve conductivity is approximately six times that of muscle. However, the nerve generally is surrounded by fat and a fibrous sheath, both of which are considered to be poor conductors. Bone is extremely dense, contains only about 5 percent water, and is considered to be the poorest biologic conductor of electrical current. It is essential for the therapist to understand that many biologic tissues will be stimulated by an electrical current. Selecting the appropriate treatment parameters is critical if the desired tissue response is to be attained.

PHYSIOLOGIC RESPONSES TO ELECTRICAL CURRENT

The effects of electrical current passing through the various tissues of the body may be thermal, chemical, or physiologic.[15]

tetany Muscle condition that is caused by hyperexcitation and results in cramps and spasms.

Treatment Tip
To produce a tetanic muscle contraction current intensity should be increased sufficiently to produce a muscle contraction and then the frequency adjusted to aproximately 50 pulses per second. This will produce a tetanic contraction regardless of whether AC, DC, or pulsed current is being used.

All electrical currents cause a rise in temperature in a conducting tissue. The tissues of the body possess varying degrees of resistance, and those of higher resistance should heat up more when electrical current passes through. As indicated in previous chapters, the diathermies generate a continuous high-frequency electrical current that is designed to produce a tissue temperature increase. The electrical currents used for stimulation of nerve and muscle have a relatively low average current flow that produces minimal thermal effects.

Basically, electrical currents are used to produce either muscle contractions or modification of pain impulses through effects on the motor and sensory nerves. This function is dependent to a great extent on selecting the appropriate treatment parameters based on the principles identified in this chapter.

Electrical currents are also used to produce chemical effects. Most biologic tissue contains negatively and positively charged ions. A direct current flow will cause migration of these charged particles toward the pole of opposite polarity. At the positive pole the negatively charged particles cause an acid reaction in which there is coagulation of protein and hardening of the tissues. At the negative pole the positively charged particles produce an alkaline reaction, liquefying protein and causing softening of the tissues.

Treatment Tip
Only a long duration continuous DC current is capable of producing ion movement. Continuous DC current can also elicit a muscle contraction when the current is turned on and off.

SAFETY IN THE USE OF ELECTRICAL EQUIPMENT

Electrical safety in the clinical setting should be of maximal concern to the professional therapist. Too often there are reports of patients being electrocuted as a result of faulty electrical circuits in whirlpools. This type of accident can be avoided by taking some basic precautions and acquiring an understanding of the power distribution system and electrical grounds.

The typical electrical circuit consists of a source producing electrical power, a conductor that carries the power to a resistor or series of driven elements, and a conductor that carries the power back to the power source.

Electrical power is carried from generating plants through high-tension powerlines carrying 2200 V. The power is decreased by a transformer and is supplied in the wall outlet at 220 or 120 V with a frequency of 60 Hz. The voltage at the outlet is alternating current, which means that one of the poles, the "hot" or "live" wire, is either positive or negative with respect to other neutral lines. Theoretically, the voltage of the neutral pole should be zero. Actually the voltage of the neutral line is about 10 V. Thus, both hot and neutral lines carry some voltage with respect to the earth, which has zero voltage. The voltage from either of these two leads may be sufficient to cause physiologic damage.

The two-pronged plug has only two leads, both of which carry some voltage. Consequently, the electrical device has no true **ground**. The term true ground literally means the electrical circuit is connected to the earth or the ground, which has the ability to accept large electrical charges without becoming charged itself. The ground will continually accept these charges until the electrical potential has been neutralized. Therefore, any electrical charge that may be potentially hazardous (i.e., any electricity escaping from the circuit) is almost immediately neutralized by the ground. If an individual were to come in contact with a short-circuited instrument that was not grounded, the electrical current would flow through that individual to reach the ground.

Electrical devices that have two-pronged plugs generally rely on the chassis or casing of the power source to act as a ground. The danger with the two-pronged plug devices is that there is no true ground. Therefore, if an individual were to touch the casing of the instrument while in contact with some object or instrument that

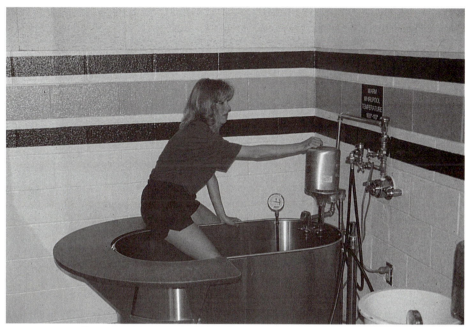

•**Figure 4-12** There is danger of electrical shock when a therapeutic device is not properly grounded. This is a major problem in a whirlpool.

has a true ground, an electrical shock may result. With three-pronged plugs, the third prong is grounded directly to the earth and all excess electrical energy theoretically should be neutralized through this.

By far the most common mechanism of injury from therapeutic devices results when there is some damage, breakdown, or short-circuit to the power cord. When this happens, the casing of the machine becomes electrically charged. In other words, there is a voltage leak, and in a device that is not properly grounded electrical shock may occur (Fig. 4-12).

The magnitude of the electrical shock is a critical factor in terms of potential health danger (Table 4-2). Shock from electrical currents flowing at 1 or less mA will not be felt and is referred to as **microshock**. Shock from a current flow greater than 1 mA is called **macroshock**. Currents that range between 1 and 15 mA produce a tingling sensation or perhaps some muscle contraction. Currents flowing at 15 to 100 mA cause a painful electrical shock. Currents between 100 and 200 mA may result in fibrillation of cardiac muscle or respiratory arrest. When current flow is above 200 mA, there is rapid burning and destruction of tissue.[11]

Most electrotherapeutic devices (e.g., muscle stimulators, ultrasound, and the diathermies) are generally used in dry environments. All new electrotherapeutic

TABLE 4-2	Physiologic Effects of Electrical Shock at Varying Magnitudes	
Intensity	**Physiologic Effects**
0–1 mA	Imperceptible
1–15 mA	Tingling sensation and muscle contraction
15–100 mA	Painful electrical shock
100–200 mA	Cardiac or respiratory arrest
>200 mA	Instant tissue burning and destruction

equipment being produced has three-pronged plugs and is thus grounded to the earth. However, in a wet or damp area the three-pronged plug may not provide sufficient protection from electrical shock.

We know that the body will readily conduct electricity because of its high water content. If the body is wet or if an individual is standing in water, the resistance to electrical flow is reduced even more. Thus if a short should occur, the shock could be as much as five times greater in this damp or wet environment. The potential danger that exists with whirlpools or tubs is obvious. The ground on the whirlpool will supposedly conduct all current leakage from a faulty motor or power cord to the earth. However, an individual in a whirlpool is actually a part of that circuit and is subject to the same current levels as any other component of the circuit. Small amounts of current therefore can be potentially harmful, no matter how well the apparatus is grounded. For this reason in 1981 the National Electrical Code required that all health care facilities using whirlpools and tubs install **ground-fault interruptors (GFI)** (Fig. 4-13). These devices constantly compare the amount of electricity flowing from the wall outlet to the whirlpool turbine with the amount returning to the outlet. If there is any leakage in current flow detected, the ground-fault circuit breaker will automatically interrupt current flow in as little as one-fortieth of a second, thus shutting off current flow and reducing the chances of electrical shock.[13] These devices may be installed either in the electrical outlet or in the circuit-breaker box.

Regardless of the type of electrotherapeutic device being used and the type of environment, the following safety practices should be considered.

1. The entire electrical system of the building or training room should be designed or evaluated by a qualified electrician. Problems with the electrical system may exist in

Treatment Tip

The National Electrical Code requires that all whirlpools have ground-fault interruptors installed to automatically shut off current flow. In addition the therapist should not allow the patient to turn the whirlpool on or off. This is especially important when the patient is already in contact with the water. Extension cords or multiple adaptors should never be used in the hydrotherapy area.

ground-fault interruptors (GFI) A safety device that automatically shuts off current flow and reducing the chances of electrical shock.

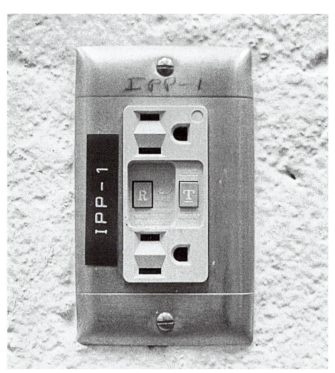

•**Figure 4-13** A typical ground-fault interruptor.

older buildings or in situations where rooms have been modified to accommodate therapeutic devices (e.g., putting a whirlpool in a locker room where the concrete floor is always wet or damp).

2. It should not be assumed that all three-pronged wall outlets are automatically grounded to the earth. The ground must be checked.

3. The therapist should become very familiar with the equipment being used and any potential problems that may exist or develop. Any defective equipment should be removed from the clinic immediately.

4. The plug should not be jerked out of the wall by pulling on the cable.

5. Extension cords or multiple adaptors should never be used.

6. Equipment should be reevaluated on a yearly basis and should conform to National Electrical Code guidelines. If a clinic or training room is not in compliance with this code, then there is no legal protection in a lawsuit.

7. Common sense should always be exercised when using electrotherapeutic devices. A situation that appears to be potentially dangerous may in fact result in injury or death.

SUMMARY

1. Electrons move along a conducting medium as an electrical current.

2. A volt is the electromotive force that produces a movement of electrons; an ampere is a unit of measurement that indicates the rate at which electrical current is flowing.

3. Ohm's law expresses the relationship between current flow voltage and resistance. The current flow is directly proportional to the voltage and inversely proportional to the resistance.

4. Electrotherapeutic devices generate three different types of current, alternating (AC) or biphasic, direct (DC) or monophasic, or pulsed or polyphasic, which are capable of producing specific physiologic changes when introduced into biologic tissue.

5. Confusion exists relative to the terminology used to describe electrotherapeutic currents, but all therapeutic electrical generators are transcutaneous electrical stimulators, regardless of whether they deliver AC, DC, or pulsed currents through electrodes attached to the skin.

6. The term pulse is synonymous with waveform, which indicates a graphic representation of the shape, direction, amplitude, duration, and pulse frequency of the electrical current being produced by the electrotherapeutic device, as displayed by an instrument called an oscilloscope.

7. Modulation refers to any alteration in the magnitude or any variation in duration of a pulse (or pulses) and may be continuous, interrupted, burst, or ramped.

8. The main difference between a series and a parallel circuit is that in a series circuit there is a single pathway for current to get from one terminal to another, and in a parallel circuit two or more routes exist for current to pass.

9. The electrical circuit that exists when electron flow is through human tissue is in reality a combination of both a series and a parallel circuit.

10. The effects of electrical current moving through biologic tissue may be chemical, thermal, or physiologic.

11. Electrical safety is critical when using electrotherapeutic devices. It is the responsibility of the therapist to make sure that all electrical modalities conform to the National Electrical Code.

REFERENCES

1. Alon, G.: Principles of electrical stimulation. In Nelson, R., Currier, D., editors. Clinical electrotherapy, Norwalk, Connecticut, 1991, Appleton & Lange.
2. Bergueld, P.: Electromedical instrumentation: a guide for medical personnel, Cambridge, 1980, Cambridge University Press.
3. Chamishion, R.: Basic medical electronics, Boston, 1964, Little, Brown.
4. Cohen, H., Brunilik, J.: Manual of electroneuromyography, ed. 2, New York, Harper & Row.
5. Cook, T., Barr, J.: Instrumentation. In Nelson, R., Currier, D., editors. Clinical electrotherapy, Norwalk, Connecticut, 1991, Appleton & Lange.
6. Cromwell, L., Arditti, M., and Weibell, F.: Medical instrumentation for health care, Englewood Cliffs, New Jersey, 1976, Prentice-Hall.
7. DeDomenico, G.: Basic guidelines for interferential therapy, Sydney, Australia, 1981, Theramed.
8. Griffin, J., Karselis, T.: Physical agents for physical therapists, Springfield, Illinois, 1988, Charles C Thomas.
9. Kloth, L., Cummings, J.: Electrotherapeutic terminology in physical therapy. Alexandria, Virginia, 1990, Section on Clinical Electrophysiology and the American Physical Therapy Association.
10. Licht, S.: Therapeutic electricity and ultraviolet radiation, vol. IV, ed. 2, Baltimore, 1969, Waverly.
11. Myklebust, B., Kloth, L.: Electrodiagnostic and electrotherapeutic instrumentation: characteristics of recording and stimulation systems and principles of safety. In Gersh, M.R.: Electrotherapy in rehabilitation, Philadelphia, 1992, F.A. Davis.
12. Myklebust, B., Robinson, A.: Instrumentation. In Snyder-Mackler, L., Robinson, A.: Clinical electrophysiology, electrotherapy and electrotherapy and electrophysiologic testing, Baltimore, 1989, Williams & Wilkins.
13. Porter, M., Porter, J.: Electrical safety in the training room, Athletic Train. 16(4):263–264, 1981.
14. Robinson, A.: Basic concepts and terminology in electricity. In Snyder-Mackler, L., Robinson, A.: Clinical electrophysiology, electrotherapy and electrotherapy and electrophysiologic testing, Baltimore 1989, Williams & Wilkins.
15. Shriber, W.: A manual of electrotherapy, ed. 4, Philadelphia, 1975, Lea & Febiger.
16. Stillwell, G.: Therapeutic electricity and ultraviolet radiation, ed. 3, Baltimore, 1983, Williams & Wilkins.
17. Watkins, A.: A manual of electrotherapy, ed. 3, Philadelphia, 1968, Lea & Febiger.
18. Wolf, S.: Electrotherapy: clinics in physical therapy, vol. 2, New York, 1981, Churchill Livingstone, Inc.

SUGGESTED READINGS

Alon, G.: High voltage stimulation: a monograph, Chattanooga, Tennessee, 1984, Chattanooga Corporation.
Alon, G.: Electrical stimulators, Chattanooga, Tennessee, 1985, Chattanooga Corporation. (Video presentation).
Alon, G., Allin, J., and Inbar, G.: Optimization of pulse duration and pulse charge during TENS, Aust. J. Physiother. 29:195, 1983.
Baker, L., McNeal, D., and Benton, L.: Neuromuscular electrical stimulation: a practical guide, Downey, California, 1993, Rancho Los Amigos Hospital.
Benton, L., Baker, L., and Bowman, B.: Functional electrical stimulation: a practical clinical guide, Downey, California, 1980, Rancho Los Amigos Hospital.
Binder, S.: In Wolf, S., editor: Electrotherapy, New York, 1981, Churchill Livingstone.
Bowman, B., Baker, L.: Effects of waveform parameters on comfort during transcutaneous neuromuscular electrical stimulation, Ann. Biomed. Eng. 13:59–74, 1985.
Brown, I.: Fundamentals of electrotherapy, course guide, Madison, Wisconsin, 1963, University of Wisconsin Press.
Campbell, J.: A critical appraisal of the electrical output characteristics of ten TENS units, Clin. Phys. Physiol. Meas. 3:141, 1982.
Geddes, L., Baler, L.: Applied biomedical instrumentation, New York, 1975, Wiley.
Geddes, L.: A short history of electrical stimulation of excitable tissue, Physiologist 27:1, 1984.
Kahn, J.: Principles and practice of electrotherapy, New York, 1994, Churchill Livingstone.
Kottke, F.: Handbook of physical medicine and rehabilitation, ed. 3, Philadelphia, 1982, W.B. Saunders.
Lane, J.: Electrical impedances of superficial limb tissues, epidermis, dermis, and muscle sheath, Ann. N.Y. Acad. Sci. 238:812, 1974.
Licht, S.: Electrodiagnosis and electromyography, vol. 1, ed. 3, Baltimore, 1971, Waverly.
Mannheimer, J., Lampe, G.: Clinical transcutaneous electrical nerve stimulation, Philadelphia, 1984, F.A. Davis.
Nelson, R., Currier, D.: Clinical electrotherapy, Norwalk, Connecticut, 1987, Appleton & Lange.
Newton, R.: Electrotherapeutic treatment: selecting appropriate wave form characteristics. Clinton, New Jersey, 1984, Preston.
Newton, R.: Electrotherapy: selecting wave form parameters, paper presented at the American Physical Therapy Association Conference, Washington, D.C., 1981.

Reismann, M.: A comparison of electrical stimulators eliciting muscle contraction, Phys. Ther. 64:751, 1984.

Scott, P: Clayton's electrotherapy and actinotherapy, eds. 5 and 7, Baltimore, 1965 and 1975, Williams & Wilkins.

Sunderland, S.: Nerves and nerve injuries, Baltimore, 1968, Williams & Wilkins.

Wadsworth, H., Chanmugan, A.: Electrophysical agents in physical therapy, Marickville, Australia, 1983, Science Press.

Ward, A.: Electricity waves and fields in therapy, Marickville, Australia, 1980, Science Press.

GLOSSARY

accommodation Adaptation by the sensory receptors to various stimuli over an extended period of time.

alternating current Current that periodically changes its polarity or direction of flow.

ampere Unit of measure that indicates the rate at which electrical current is flowing.

amplitude The intensity of current flow as indicated by the height of the waveform from baseline.

average current The amount of current flowing per unit of time.

biphasic current Another name for alternating current, in which the direction of current flow reverses direction.

bursts A combined set of three or more pulses; also referred to as packets or envelopes.

circuit The path of current from a generating source through the various components back to the generating source.

conductance The ease with which a current flows along a conducting medium.

conductors Materials that permit the free movement of electrons.

coulomb Indicates the number of electrons flowing in a current.

current The flow of electrons.

decay time The time required for a waveform to go from peak amplitude to 0 V.

direct current Galvanic current that always flows in the same direction and may flow in either a positive or negative direction.

duration Sometimes also referred to as pulse width. Indicates the length of time the current is flowing.

electrical current The net movement of electrons along a conducting medium.

electrical impedance The opposition to electron flow in a conducting material.

electrical potential The difference between charged particles at a higher and lower potential.

electron Fundamental particles of matter possessing a negative electrical charge and very small mass.

faradic current An asymmetric biphasic waveform seldom used on modern electrical generators.

filter Changes pulsating DC current to smooth DC.

frequency The number of cycles or pulses per second.

ground A wire that makes an electrical connection with the earth.

ground-fault interruptors (GFI) A safety device that automatically shuts off current flow and reduces the chances of electrical shock.

high-voltage current Current in which the waveform has an amplitude of greater than 150 V with a relatively short pulse duration.

insulators Materials that resist current flow.

interpulse interval The interruptions between individual pulses or groups of pulses.

intrapulse interval The period of time between individual pulses.

ion A positively or negatively charged particle.

iontophoresis Uses continuous direct current to drive ions into the tissues.

low-voltage current Current in which the waveform has an amplitude of less than 150 V.

macroshock An electrical shock that can be felt and has a leakage of electrical current of greater than 1 mA.

medical galvanism Creates either an acidic or alkaline environment that may be of therapeutic value.

microcurrent electrical nerve stimulator (MENS) Used primarily in tissue healing. The current intensities are too small to excite peripheral nerves.

microshock An electrical shock that is imperceptible because of a leakage of current of less than 1 mA.

modulation Refers to any alteration in the magnitude or any variation in the duration of an electrical current.

monophasic current Another name for direct current, in which the direction of current flow remains the same.

neuromuscular electrical stimulator (NMES) Also called an electrical muscle stimulator (EMS), it is used to stimulate muscle directly, as would be the case with denervated muscle where peripheral nerves are not functioning.

ohm A unit of measure that indicates resistance to current flow.

Ohm's law The current in an electrical circuit is directly proportional to the voltage and inversely proportional to the resistance.

oscillator Used to produce and output a specific waveform, which may be different from that used to power or drive the stimulating unit.

output amplifier Used to magnify or increase the amplitude of the voltage output of the generator and control it at a specific level.

parallel circuit A circuit in which two or more routes exist for current to pass between the two terminals.

phases That portion of the pulse that rises above or below the baseline for some period of time.

polyphasic current Current that contains three or more grouped phases in a single pulse and that is used in interferential and "Russian" currents.

pulse An individual waveform.

pulse charge The total amount of electricity being delivered to the patient during each pulse.

pulse period The combined time of the pulse duration and the interpulse interval.

ramping Another name for surging modulation, in which the current builds gradually to some maximum amplitude.

rate of rise How quickly a waveform reaches its maximum amplitude.

rectifier Converts AC current to pulsating DC current.

regulator Produces a specific controlled voltage output.

resistance The opposition to electron flow in a conducting material.

series circuit A circuit in which there is only one path for current to get from one terminal to another.

tetany Muscle condition that is caused by hyperexcitation and results in cramps and spasms.

transcutaneous electrical nerve stimulator (TENS) A transcutaneous electrical stimulator used to stimulate peripheral nerves.

transcutaneous electrical stimulator All therapeutic electrical generators regardless of whether they deliver AC, DC, or pulsed currents through electrodes attached to the skin.

transformer Reduces the amount of voltage from the power supply.

volt The electromotive force that must be applied to produce a movement of electrons. A measure of electrical power.

voltage The force resulting from an accumulation of electrons at one point in an electrical circuit, usually corresponding to a deficit of electrons at another point in the circuit.

watt A measure of electrical power (Watts = Volts $\times$ Amperes).

waveform The shape of an electrical current as displayed on an oscilloscope.

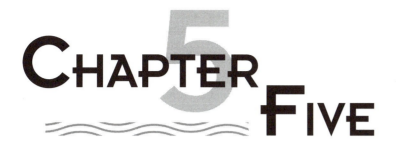

CHAPTER FIVE

ELECTRICAL STIMULATING CURRENTS

DANIEL N. HOOKER

OBJECTIVES

Following completion of this chapter, the student therapist will be able to:

- ✓ Describe muscle and nerve responses to electrical stimulation.
- ✓ Describe nonexcitatory cell and tissue responses to electrical stimulation.
- ✓ Describe the uses of electrically stimulated muscle contractions.
- ✓ Describe the various treatment parameters that must be considered with electrical stimulating currents.
- ✓ Describe the effect of noncontractable stimulation on edema.
- ✓ Describe the modulation of pain through the use of electrical stimulating currents.
- ✓ Discuss specialized electrical current generators in relation to physiologic changes and benefits.
- ✓ Identify problems that might respond to electrical stimulation.

Often the therapist uses electrical currents for treatment in an effort to create a quick cure for the physical problems suffered by his or her patients. Although electrical treatments can provide dramatic results at times, this is the exception rather than the rule. The use of electricity in treating an injury can be beneficial, but the therapist must base this use on facts about the effects of electricity on biologic tissues. The treatment program must be tailored toward influencing the problems identified in the evaluation. Electrical therapy should not be used in a "shotgun" approach if we are to maximize the effectiveness of this modality.

There has been considerable activity in the last 10 years in the commercial development of new therapeutic electrical generators. The clinical use of electrotherapy has changed as the changing technology has enabled equipment manufacturers to design and promote their latest product lines. Modern electronics have opened the doors to electronic equipment that could conceivably generate any electrical output desired. Wave shapes, amplitudes, and frequencies can be manipulated so that any combination is possible.

Research is lagging behind commercial development, as usual. Experts will continue to disagree with or challenge the interpretations of the results of the research that has been and will be conducted. Researchers in the biologic responses find it difficult to isolate one variable for experimentation and maintain control of all the other variables that could affect their results. Deciding whether the results of a study are significant for cause and effect, are merely a chance happening, or are significant but not directly caused by the manipulation of the experimental variable become very difficult decisions for the clinician. There are more questions than answers in this field of research.

Electrotherapy of the future is moving toward attempts at controlling cellular and tissue function with externally generated electrical currents. The therapist will need the concepts of **bioelectromagnetics**, the study of biologic tissues' electrical and magnetic properties, to apply and understand the therapeutic outcomes of the next generation of electrical modalities. Knowledge of the electric properties of cells, intercellular and intracellular communication, bioelectric potentials, tissue currents, strain-generated electric potentials, and the biologic effects of other nonionizing energy will be essential for the expert clinician to use present and future electrical modalities for maximum therapeutic benefit.[20,21]

PHYSIOLOGIC RESPONSE TO ELECTRICAL CURRENTS

Electricity has an effect on each cell and tissue that it passes through.[20,21,110] The type and extent of the response are dependent on the type of tissue and its response characteristics (e.g., how it normally functions and how it grows or changes under normal stress) and the nature of the current applied (i.e., direct or alternating, intensity, duration, voltage, and density). The tissue should respond to electrical energy in a manner similar to that in which it normally functions or grows. These statements are true within a certain range of current parameters, but current density above critical levels can cause coagulation and tissue destruction.[2] Clinically, therapists use electrical currents for the following reasons.

Physiologic Responses
- Excitatory
- Nonexcitatory

1. To create muscle contraction through nerve or muscle stimulations.
2. To stimulate sensory nerves to help in treating pain.
3. To create an electrical field in biologic tissues to stimulate or alter the healing process.
4. To create an electrical field on the skin surface to drive ions beneficial to the healing process into or through the skin.

As electricity moves through the body's conductive medium, changes in physiologic functioning can occur at various levels of the total system. Four levels can be readily identified from the functional standpoint.

Therapeutic Uses of Electricity
- Muscle contraction
- Sensory stimulation
- Ion movement

1. Cellular
2. Tissue
3. Segmental
4. Systematic

As in all classification systems, there is some overlap and assignment to one level may be arbitrary. The effects can be defined as follows.

1. Cellular level: This can be broken down into five major effects.
   a. Excitation of nerve cells
   b. Changes in cell membrane permeability
   c. Protein synthesis

    d. Stimulation of fibroblast, osteoblast

    e. Modification of microcirculation

2. Tissue level: This requires multiple cellular events.

    a. Skeletal muscle contraction

    b. Smooth muscle contraction

    c. Tissue regeneration

3. Segmental level: This involves a regional effect of the previous two level activities.

    a. Modification of joint mobility

    b. Muscle pumping action to change circulation and lymphatic activity

    c. An alteration of the microvascular system not associated with muscle pumping

    d. An increased movement of charged proteins into the lymphatic channels with subsequent oncotic force bringing increases in fluid to the lymph system. Lymphatic contraction increases as a result and more fluid is moved centrally.

    e. Transcutaneous electrical stimulation cannot directly stimulate lymph smooth muscle or the autonomic nervous system without also stimulating a motor nerve. It is possible that sensory stimulation may have indirectly activated the autonomic system. And the autonomic system may have released an adrenergic substance that would enhance the lymph smooth muscle contraction.

4. Systematic effects.

    a. Analgesic effects as endogenous pain suppressors are released and act at different levels to control pain.

    b. Analgesic effects from the stimulation of certain neurotransmitters to control neural activity in the presence of pain stimuli.[3]

These responses can be broken into direct and indirect effects. There is always a direct effect along the lines of current flow and under the electrodes. Indirect effects occur remote to the area of current flow and are usually the result of stimulating a natural physiologic event to occur.[3,24]

If a certain effect is desired from stimulation, goals must be established to achieve a specific physiologic response as a goal of your treatment. These responses can be grouped into two basic physiologic responses: nonexcitatory and excitatory.

The excitatory is the most obvious and the one that has been used the most often in the past in treating our patients. In the clinical setting we spend most of our time trying to get the excitatory response from the nerve cells and muscle tissue. Patients perceive excitatory responses as electric sensation, muscle contraction, and electric pain. Physiologically, the nerves that affect these perceptions fire in that order as the stimulus intensity is increased gradually. Nerves have very little discriminatory ability. They can tell only if there is electricity in sufficient magnitude to cause a depolarization of the nerve membrane. They have very little regard for the different shape and polarities of waveforms. To the nerve cell, electricity is electricity. As in all things dealing with higher level organisms, there is a big range of responses to the same stimulus depending on the environmental and systemic factors.

All perception is a product of the brain's activity of receiving the signal that a nerve has been stimulated electrically. This further enlarges the broad range of systemic effects that occur in response to the electric stimulation.

Stimulation events will change the body's perception. As the strength of the current increases and/or the duration of the current increases, more nerve cells will fire. As the strength of the stimulus increases and these events occur, certain quality judgments about the electric stimuli are made. Is the current pleasant or unpleasant? Is the intensity of the stimulus weak or strong? The broad range of individual responses to these quality judgments has a significant impact on the beneficial effects of this therapy.

MUSCLE AND NERVE RESPONSES TO ELECTRICAL CURRENTS

Presently, the major therapeutic uses of electricity center on muscle contraction or sensory stimulation or both. Let us look in a general way at the physiologic effects of electricity on nerve and muscle tissue. Specific currents or frequencies will be discussed later in the chapter.

Nerves and muscles are both excitable tissues. This excitability is dependent on the cell membrane's **voltage sensitive permeability**. The nerve or muscle cell membrane regulates the interchange of substances between the inside of the cell and the environment outside the cell. This voltage sensitive permeability produces an unequal distribution of charged ions on each side of the membrane, which in turn creates a potential difference between the charge of the interior of the cell and the exterior of the cell. The membrane then is considered to be polarized. The potential difference between the inside and outside is known as the **resting potential**, because the cell tries to maintain this electrochemical gradient as its normal homeostatic environment.[20]

Both electrical and chemical gradients are established along the cell membrane, with a greater concentration of diffusable positive ions on the outside of the membrane than on the inside. Using its active transport mechanism, the cell continually moves Na^+ from inside the cell to outside and balances this positive charge movement by moving K^+ to the inside. K^+ will have a larger concentration on the inside of the cell, but the overall charge difference produces an electrical gradient with plus charges outside and minus charges inside (Fig. 5-1). As explained by Guyton, "The potential is proportional to the difference in tendency of the ions to diffuse in one direction versus the other direction."[51] Two conditions are necessary for the membrane potential to develop: (1) The membrane must be semipermeable, allowing ions of one charge to diffuse through the pores more readily than ions of the opposite charge; and (2) the concentration of the diffusable ions must be greater on one side of the membrane than on the other side.[20,51]

The resting membrane potential is generated because the cell is an ionic battery whose concentration of ions inside and outside the cell are maintained by regulatory NA^+K^+ pumps within the cell wall. In addition to the ability of the nerve and muscle cell membranes to develop and maintain the resting potential, the membranes are excitable.[20,51]

To create transmission of an impulse in the nerve tissue, resting membrane potential must be reduced below a threshold level. Changes in the membrane's permeability then may occur. These changes create an **action potential** that will propagate the impulse along the nerve in both directions from the location of the stimulus. An action potential created by a stimulus from chemical, electrical, thermal, or mechanical means always creates the same result, membrane **depolarization**.

Not all stimuli are effective in causing an action potential and depolarization. To be an effective agent, the stimulus must have an adequate intensity and last long enough to equal or exceed the membrane's basic threshold for excitation. The stimu-

voltage sensitive permeability The quality of some cell membranes that makes them permeable to different ions based on the electric charge of the ions. Nerve and muscle cell membranes allow negatively charged ions into the cell while actively transporting some positively charged ions outside the cell membrane.

resting potential The potential difference between the inside and outside of a membrane.

action potential A recorded change in electrical potential between the inside and outside of a nerve cell, resulting in muscular contraction.

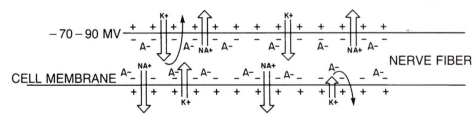

•**Figure 5-1** Nerve cell membrane with active transport mechanisms maintaining the resting membrane potential.

lus must alter the membrane so that a number of ions are pushed across the membrane, exceeding the ability of the active transport pumps to maintain the resting potentials. A stimulus of this magnitude forces the membrane to depolarize and results in an action potential.[51,119]

Depolarization

As the charged ions move across the nerve fiber membranes beneath the anode and cathode, membrane depolarization occurs. The **cathode** usually is the site of depolarization (Fig. 5-2A). As the concentration of negatively charged ions increases, the membrane's voltage potential becomes low and is brought toward its threshold for depolarization (Fig. 5-2B). The **anode** makes the nerve cell membrane potential more positive, increasing the threshold necessary for depolarization (Fig. 5-2C). The cathode in this example becomes the **active electrode**; the anode becomes the **indifferent electrode (dispersive)**. The anode and cathode may switch active and indifferent roles under other circumstances.[3,10,119] The number of ions needed to exceed the membrane pump's ability to maintain the normal membrane resting potential is tissue-dependent.

depolarization Process or act of neutralizing the cell membrane's resting potential.

Depolarization Propagation

Following excitement and propagation of the impulse along the nerve fiber, there is a brief period during which the nerve fiber is incapable of reacting to a second stimulus. This is the **absolute refractory period**, which lasts about 0.5 μsec. Excitability is restored gradually as the nerve cell membrane repolarizes itself. The nerve then is capable of being stimulated again. The maximum number of possible discharges of a nerve may reach 1000 per second, depending on fiber type.[7,10,51,119]

The difference in electrical potential between the depolarized region and the neighboring inactive regions causes the current to flow from the depolarized region through the intercellular material to the inactive membrane. The current also flows through the extracellular materials, back to the depolarized area, and finally into the

absolute refractory period Brief time period (0.5 μsec) following membrane depolarization during which the membrane is incapable of depolarizing again.

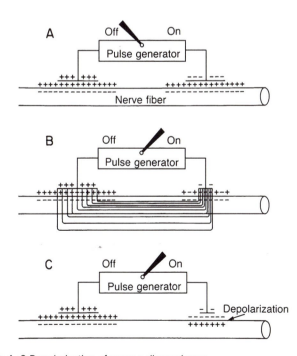

•**Figure 5-2** A–C Depolarization of nerve cell membrane.

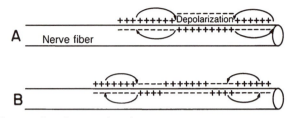

•**Figure 5-3** Propagation of a nerve impulse.

cell again. This forms a complete local circuit and makes the depolarization self-propagating as the process is repeated all along the fiber in each direction from the depolarization site. Energy released by the cell keeps the intensity of the impulse uniform as it travels down the cell.[7,10,51,119] This process is illustrated in Fig. 5-3.

Depolarization Effects

As the nerve impulse reaches its effector organ or another nerve cell, the impulse is transferred between the two at a motor end plate or synapse. At this junction, a transmitter substance is released from the nerve, rather than the impulse jumping from one to another. This transmitter substance causes the other excitable tissue to discharge (Fig. 5-4).[10,119]

In terms of muscle excitation, a **twitch muscle contraction** results. This contraction, initiated by an electrical stimulus, is the same as a twitch contraction coming from voluntary activity. Voluntary muscular activity is different only in the rate and synchrony (simultaneous response) of the muscle fiber contractions.[10,91] A graphic illustration of this threshold and propagation and contraction is the **strength-duration curve (SD)** (Fig. 5-5).

As illustrated, there is a nonlinear relationship between current duration and current intensity, in which shorter duration stimuli require increasing intensities in

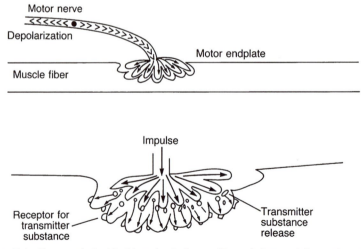

•**Figure 5-4** Change of electrical impulse to transmitter substance at the motor end plate. When activated, the muscle cell membrane will depolarize and contraction will occur.

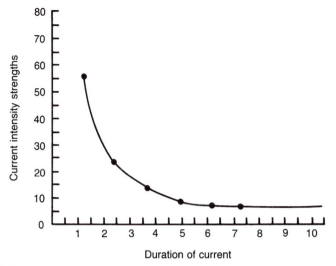

strength-duration curve A graphic illustration of the relationship between current intensity and current duration in causing depolarization of a nerve or muscle membrane.

•Figure 5-5 Strength-duration curve.

order to reach the threshold of the nerve or muscle. Nerve and muscle membrane thresholds differ significantly. Different sizes and types of nerve fibers also have different thresholds. The strength-duration curves for different classes of nerve and muscle tissue illustrate the different thresholds of excitability of these tissues. The curves are basically symmetric, but the intensity of current necessary to reach the membrane's threshold for excitation differs for each tissue (Fig. 5-6).[51,90,119,124]

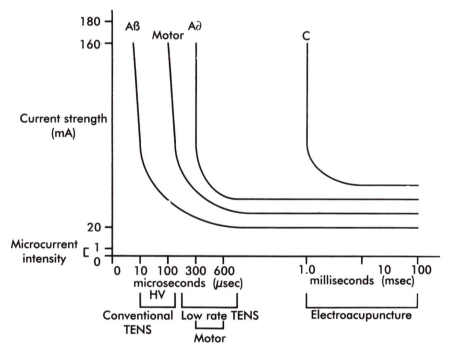

•Figure 5-6 Strength-duration curves of Aβ sensory, motor, A∂ sensory, and pain nerve fibers. Durations of several electrical stimulators are indicated along the lower axis. Corresponding intensities would be necessary to create a depolarizing stimulus for any of the nerve fibers. Microcurrent intensity is so low that the nerve fibers will not depolarize. This current travels through other body tissues to create effects.

Strength-Duration Curve

Three important concepts are represented in the strength-duration curve. These terms and ideas are used frequently in discussions on the effects of electrical currents on the nerve cellular level.[57,119]

rheobase The intensity of current necessary to cause observable tissue excitation, given a long current duration.

1. The shape of the curve relates the intensity of the electrical stimulus and the length of time (duration) necessary to cause the tissue to depolarize.
2. The **rheobase** describes the minimum intensity of current necessary to cause tissue excitation when applied for a maximum duration (Fig. 5-7).
3. **Chronaxie** describes the length of time (duration) required for a current of twice the intensity of the rheobase current to produce tissue excitation (see Fig. 5-7).

If you look at the SD curve and wish to get maximum sensory or motor response, you must use a stimulus with a high intensity and short duration. Electrical engineers have designed some units to maximize this effect. However, as the charge increases and more and more nerve fibers fire, the brain becomes more and more involved in the perceptual part of the experience.

Muscular Responses to Electrical Current

chronaxie The duration of time necessary to cause observable tissue excitation, given a current intensity of two times rheobasic current.

Stimulation of the motor nerve is the method used in most clinical applications of electrical muscular contractions. In the absence of innervation, muscle contraction can be stimulated by an electrical current that causes the muscle membrane to depolarize. This will create the same muscle contraction as a natural stimulus.

The **all-or-none response** is another important concept in applying electrical current to nerve or muscle tissue. Once a stimulus reaches a depolarizing threshold, the nerve or muscle membrane depolarizes, and propagation of the impulse or muscle contraction occurs. This reaction remains the same regardless of increases in the strength of the stimulus used. Either the stimulus causes depolarization—the all— or it does not cause depolarization—the none. There is no gradation of response; the response of the single nerve or muscle fiber is maximal or nonexistent.[10,91,119]

This all-or-none phenomenon does not mean that muscle fiber shortening and overall muscle activity cannot be influenced by changing the intensity, pulses per second, or duration of the stimulating current. Adjustments in current parameters can cause changes in the shortening of the muscle fiber and the overall muscle activity.

all or none response The depolarization of nerve or muscle membrane is the same once a depolarizing intensity threshold is reached; further increases in intensity do not increase the response.

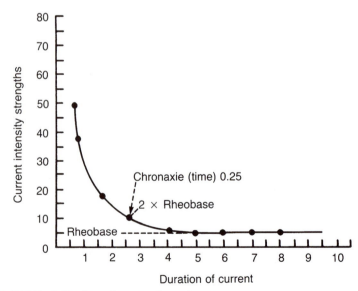

•**Figure 5-7** Excitation time of nerve cell membrane.

CASE STUDY 5-1
ELECTRICAL STIMULATING CURRENTS: STRENGTHENING OF INNERVATED MUSCLE

Background: A 22-year-old woman competitive soccer player sustained a severe grade II medial collateral ligament sprain of the left knee 3 days ago and is being treated with plaster immobilization for 3 weeks. She is not able to generate a maximal isometric quadriceps contraction voluntarily. The cast has been modified to accommodate electrodes over the femoral nerve and the motor point of the vastus medialis muscle. There are no restrictions on the amount of force she is allowed to produce during a knee extension effort.

Impression: Grade II MCL sprain of the left knee, with inability to generate maximal isometric force of the knee extensors.

Treatment Plan: A 5-day-per-week schedule of electrical stimulation was initiated. A polyphasic waveform was selected, with a 2500-Hz carrier wave, with an effective frequency of 50 Hz (10 msec on, 10 msec off). The stimulator was set to ramp the current up for 6 seconds, then maintain the current at a specific amplitude for 10 seconds, then drop to zero with no ramp; rest time was 50 seconds, giving an effective duty cycle of 1:5 (10 sec on, 50 sec off). Each treatment session began with 10 repetitions at a comfortable stimulus amplitude, followed by three sets of 10 repetitions each, with the maximal amount of current tolerable. A 2-minute rest separated the sets. During the 10 seconds on time, the current amplitude was adjusted to the maximal amount the patient was able to tolerate. The patient was encouraged to contract the quadriceps femoris muscle group as the current was delivered.

Response: The patient's tolerance for the electrical stimulation gradually increased during the first week, then reached a plateau; this plateau was maintained for the next 2 weeks. There was no measurable or visible atrophy of the left thigh on removal of the cast. A rehabilitation program of active range of motion exercises, strengthening exercises, and functional activities was initiated, and the patient returned to competition 2 weeks following cast removal.

Discussion Questions
- What tissues were injured or affected?
- What symptoms were present?
- What phase of the injury-healing continuum did the patient present for care in?
- What are the physical agent modality's biophysical effects (direct, indirect, depth, tissue affinity)?
- What are the physical agent modality's indications and contraindications?
- What are the parameters of the physical agent modality's application, dosage, duration, and frequency in this case study?
- What other physical agent modalities could be used to treat this injury or condition? Why? How?

The rehabilitation professional employs physical agent modality to create an optimum environment for tissue healing while minimizing the symptoms associated with the trauma or condition.

THE EFFECTS OF ELECTRICAL STIMULATION ON NONEXCITABLE TISSUES AND CELLS

The nonexcitatory cells respond to electric current in ways consistent with their cell type and tissue function. To understand the theory of stimulating these nonexcitatory cells, a good understanding of the cell as a part of the body's bioelectric system is needed.

Cellular Electrical Circuits
The Cell Membrane

The basic cell with cell membrane, nucleus, organelles, and so on acts like an ionic battery with the inside of the cell electrically negative and the outside electrically positive. The cell's plasma membrane is responsible for maintaining this electrochemical gradient as well as sending and receiving messages. The membrane is made up of phospholipid molecules studded with several types of proteins that project into and or through the phospholipid layers. These proteins support, transport things in and/or, receive specific molecules that alter cell functions, and promote reactions on the surface of the cell. (Fig. 5-8).

General cell electrical gradients are similar to those described for nerve cells but contain four electrical zones. The central cytoplasm area is negative and is surrounded by a narrow band of positively charged potassium ions along the inside of the cell membrane. The outer wall of the cell membrane is positively charged with sodium ions and potassium ions, and this is surrounded by a negative zone composed of sialic acid molecules (see Fig. 5-8).

The difference in potential across the membrane is maintained as described previously for nerve cell membranes with the sodium and potassium pumps in the cell membrane doing the work. Any ionic fluctuations in the cytoplasm cause the ion pumps in the membrane to activate and return the equilibrium of the cell. There are also passive ionic channels in the wall that allow passive ion movement along the electrochemical gradients (see Fig. 5-8).

The only difference between excitable and nonexcitable cell membranes is the presence of voltage-gated sodium ion channels. In the excitatory cells, these ion channels generate the action potentials once a depolarizing stimulus causes the membrane to become more permeable to the outside NA^+. The NA^+ channels are triggered to open, and NA^+ ions move into the cell causing a brief reversal of charge. The charge reversal causes these ion channels to close, and the normal membrane potential returns.

The cell membrane is not only an outside covering but also is intimately involved with internal cell structures as an intercellular membrane, surrounds organelles, and supports the internal structure of the cell. This intercellular membrane can then exercise control of the movement of substances out from the cytoplasm or into the cytoplasm from the organelles. This movement is controlled by the same type electrochemical gradients and selective ion channels as that used in maintaining the cell wall (see Fig. 5-8).[20,21]

Intercellular Structures

The internal cell structure is also made up of a dense network of hollow microtubules. These microtubules can be built and dismantled by the cell relatively rapidly and are **dipoles** with the negatively charged end directed centrally and the positive end directed peripherally. The microtubes are very active in cell function, moving materials such as neurotransmitters along the surface of the cell, making cilia move, moving organelles around within the cell, acting as sensors of the extracellular environment. The microtubes also form the mitotic spindle in the cell division process (see Fig. 5-8). Because of its ability to change rapidly and help in cell movement and intracellular movement, the microtubes are probably significant actors in the organization of the cells during wound healing and regeneration.

Normal cells are signaled and respond to changes when messages contact the outer projections of the cell wall. Likewise, messages from within the cell can be sent outside the cell. The message can be chemical, such as hormones, or possibly be an electromagnetic energy coded message. Once the message is received, the signal is conveyed across the membrane to the cell's interior. The message is then transferred to another message system or switchboard that activates the cell's response to the message. The message may speed the cell up, make it move, stimulate production of extracellular proteins, or increase the secretions of that cell (see Fig. 5-8).[20]

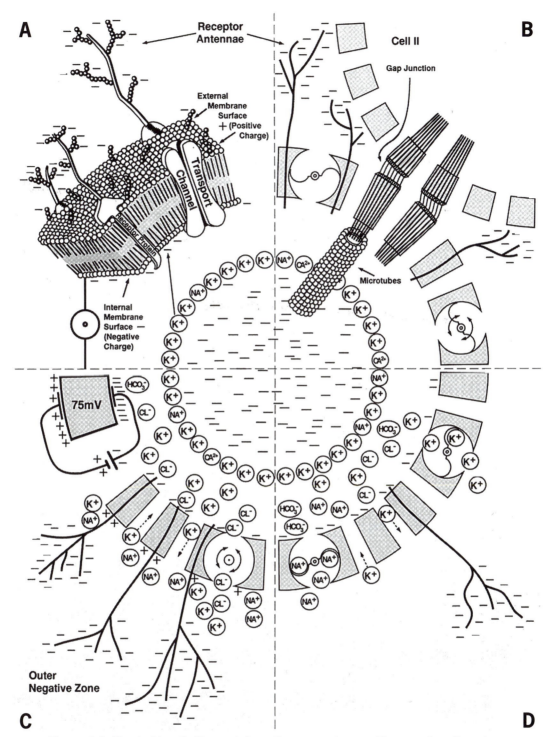

•**Figure 5-8** The electric cell with a central negative zone, an inner positive zone, the cell membrane, an outer positive zone, and an outer negative zone. Part A. Three-dimensional model of the cell membrane with transmembrane receptor proteins, receptor antennae, the outer positive surface charge, and inner negative surface charge. Part B. Gap junctions connect one cell to another and allow direct communication between cells. Receptors connect to microtubes within the cell. Part C. Cell membrane pumps and passive ion channels act as ion balancers to preserve equilibrium of the cell. Part D. Total electrochemical equilibrium acts as an ion battery creating a resting potential across the cell membrane.

Electrical Circuits in Tissue

Many cells are physically united with neighboring cells of like structure and collectively perform as one tissue. The cell membranes are bound together by junctions between the outer projections of each cell membrane. These specialized junctions allow direct communication between adjacent cells. These specialized junction areas are called **gap junctions** and contain channels for ionic, electrical, and small molecule signaling. The cells connected by gap junctions can then act together when one cell receives an extracellular message, the tissue can be coordinated in its response by the gap junction's internal message system. Embryonic and regenerating tissues are particularly rich in gap junctions, and they probably play a significant role in tissue growth and differentiation (see Fig. 5-8).

Cells are surrounded by a bonding medium of collagen, elastin, and hyaluronic acid gel. This extracellular matrix can also interact with the adjacent cell surface receptors to modify cell function, orientation and alignment, shape, movement, metabolic rate, and differentiation.[20]

Strain Related Potentials

The previous discussion on cell structure points out that every cell surface carries a charge. Every support structure within the cell, membranes, or microtubes are dipoles. In effect, cell structures have similar properties to electrets (insulators carrying a permanent charge, similar to a permanent magnet). **Electrets** are capable of **piezoelectric activity**, in which mechanical deformation of the structure causes a change in the surface electrical charge of the structure. They are also capable of **electropiezo activity**, in which changing an electric surface charge would force the electret to change shape. This becomes important when considering the piezoelectric effect of bone and connective tissue and how this change in electrical surface activity may guide or stimulate growth and healing.

Most connective tissues also generate a tissue-based electrical potential in response to strain of the tissue. Tension on surfaces or distraction on the surface creates these **strain-related potentials (SRP)**. Where there is compression, the strain-related potentials are negative. Where there is tension these SRPs are positive. Functionally, these strain related potentials have helped provide an electromechanical explanation for Wolff's law governing bone's growth in response to mechanical stress. The controlling mechanism for these events is most likely some form of the intrinsic electrochemical responses discussed earlier in this chapter, as no specific hormonal or neurologic controls have been discovered. The stress-generated potential must signal the membranes of the osteoblast, osteocytes, and osteoclasts to add or take away bone in areas of compression or tension. The cells have the necessary mechanisms to receive and decode the strain information, and intrinsically the cells can respond appropriately to maintain the integrity of the tissue (Fig. 5-9).[6,16,20]

Cells are grouped together into tissues creating segmental units, and segmental units combine into a whole system. Each cell, considered an ionic battery when added together with other cells, can collectively summate the influence and generate potential differences across the surface of the body or between different areas of the same tissue. These endogenous currents with their polarity gradients seem to play a key role in guiding the development, growth, regeneration, and repair of the cells, tissues, and segments of our bodies.[20]

Normal Bioelectric Fields

Becker demonstrated a direct current bioelectric field that could be measured in salamanders and other animals. The spatial configuration of this field coincided with

piezoelectric activity Changing electric surface charges of a structure forces the structure to change shape.

electrets Insulators carrying a permanent charge similar to a permanent magnet.

electropiezo activity Changing electric surface charges of a structure forces the structure to change shape.

strain related potentials Tissue-based electric potentials generated in response to strain for the tissue.

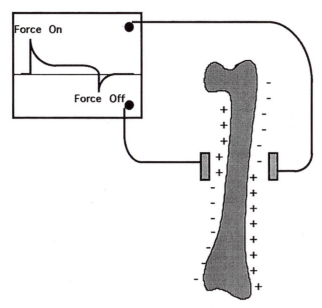

•**Figure 5-9** Electrical response of boney tissue to the momentary deforming stress of weight bearing.

the arrangement of their central nervous systems, with the positive areas being located near the major nerve cell accumulations, that is, brain, brachial, and lumbar plexus areas. The negative areas were near the major peripheral nerve outflows from these areas.[7–9,20,21]

This bioelectric field has been measured in other animals and has also been recorded for humans. The skin surface also is always negative relative to the dermis so there is a permanent electrical gradient through the skin tissue.[8,9,20] Potential difference gradients also exist on long bones with the midpoints more positive than the ends and areas of increased cellular activity, that is, epiphyseal plate area, more negative than other areas. This direct current seems to be in a continuous circuit along the length of the bone and will vary in strength according to local differences in metabolism (Fig. 5-10).[20]

Bioelectric Activity in Skin Wounds

When skin is damaged, a steady current will move from the relatively positively charged dermis into the wound area and reenter the skin just below the stratum corneum. The wound currents also generate a lateral potential difference from outside the normal area to the wound edge, forming a lateral electrical gradient. This lateral gradient appears to stimulate epithelial cells in the wound edge to regenerate and begin to grow across the wound. Once the wound edges approximate, the surface integrity is reestablished and the lateral gradient disappears. If the wound dries out, these currents will also drop because of increased resistance to electrical flow. The skin thickness is reestablished as cell layering, and the increased electric potentials return to normal (Fig. 5-11).[20,46]

Bioelectric Field Changes in Response to Injury

Becker's experiments with salamander limb injury showed that the bioelectric field gradient reversed immediately when a salamander limb was amputated. The normal current was −10 mV, and at amputation it jumped to a +20-mV current. Gradually as healing started to take place this current returned to a highly negative current of

current of injury A bioelectric current produced by any type of cellular trauma that plays a key role in stimulating healing.

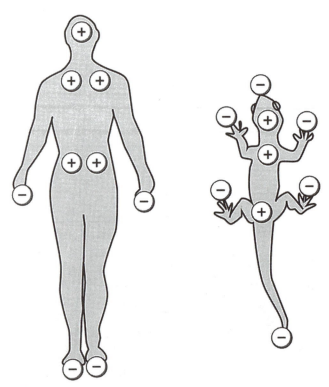

•Figure 5-10 The bioelectric field. Skin potentials in human and salamander.

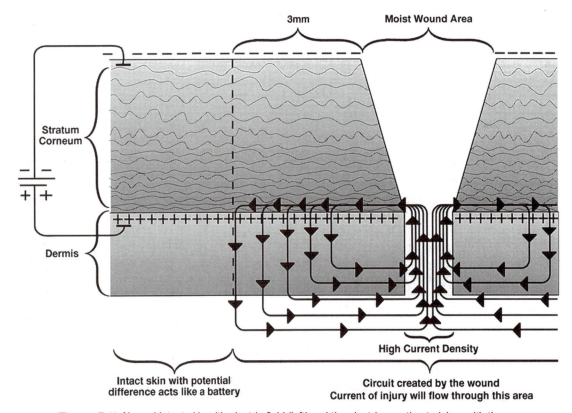

•Figure 5-11 Normal intact skin with electric field (left) and the electric reaction to injury with the current of injury path through the skin wound (right).

−30 mV and then gradually returned to baseline values as limb regeneration occurred (Fig. 5-12).[8,9]

In the frog, a nonregenerating cousin of the salamander, this bioelectric current behaved similarly upon amputation but never jumped back to a negative current. Instead it gradually moved back to the normal negative baseline values as the stump scarred over and healing became complete. Becker found this **current of injury** was produced by any type of cellular trauma and suggested that this current of injury plays a key role in stimulating healing and regeneration of tissue.[7–9]

Regeneration is more and more limited as we move up the phylogenetic ladder. Regeneration is also greatest in younger animals. Regeneration in humans is certainly limited, but certain tissues have some capacity to respond (muscle, nerve, bone, skin, connective tissue). Becker felt there were three essential ingredients for regeneration. The first is a powerful initial current of injury, initially a positive current then becoming strongly negative as the wound blastema formed and gradually returning to baseline value as the limb regenerates. The second is that a high tissue versus innervation density is a critical factor and if innervation density is below a critical level regeneration will not occur. The third ingredient needed is the presence of peripheral nerves in the wound area and the growth of these nerves to reinnervate the epithelial ingrowth at the amputation site. These neuro-epidermal junctions form at about 7 to 8 days in the wound blastema. This event seems to play a significant role in the sudden reversal of the current of injury from positive to negative (see Fig. 5-12).[9,20]

Becker and others have stimulated regeneration in nonregenerating species (frogs, rats) by applying a direct current to the amputation site that mimics the high negative current found in salamander regeneration during the blastema stage of growth, approximately 7 to 10 days postinjury. The electrode must also stay at the growing tip throughout regeneration.[7–9,20,58]

This artificial current of injury apparently causes the proliferating cells in the injured area to dedifferentiate to a more primitive cell type and then to differentiate into the appropriate cell types needed to continue the regeneration of the limb. The overall progression of the limb orientation and alignment is also probably guided by the bioelectric field, with the distal electrode being negative (see Fig. 5-12).

Becker concluded after several subsequent experiments that the bioelectric field of animals was a function of DC circuits that originated in the central nervous sys-

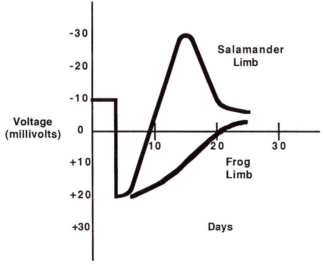

•**Figure 5-12** Voltage changes in amputated salamander and frog limbs during regeneration and healing.

tem (CNS) and returned to the CNS, indicating that there is a constant flow of DC current present in neural tissue and that the amplitude and direction of current flow are dependent on CNS activity.[9,20]

Electrical Stimulation Influence on Cellular and Tissue Activity

Cell behavior can be influenced by having extracellular molecules lock into receptor sites on the cell membrane which activate the message relay and action system within the cell (see Fig. 5-8).[88] The recognition of receptor sites and the guiding of the extracellular molecule to that destination is caused by an interaction of the electric fields from the receptor site and the extracellular molecule. Electrical stimulation of the appropriate frequency and amplitude may also be able to activate the cellular receptor site and stimulate the same cellular changes as the naturally occurring chemical molecular stimulation.

The cell functions by incorporating a multitude of chemical reactions into a living process. Enzymatic activity acclerates these reactions, and each cell contains approximately 3000 enzymes. The enzymatic activity of the cell depends on the availability of specific charged sites on the intracellular membrane surfaces. These sites may be made more or less available for enzymatic reactions by changes in shape or configuration of the surface. These changes usually occur in response to a messenger molecule but it is conceiveable that the appropriate electrical signal could also create more specific sites for enzymatic activity, thereby changing or stimulating cell function (see Fig. 5-8).[20]

The microtubules system may selectively receive and transmit electromagnetic signals through the cell. As the energy travels along the microtube the signal may stimulate organelles to activate their routine functions. The microtubule system could transmit this energy wave from cell to cell through the tight cell-to-cell contact areas at the gap junctions. This transmission could create cells working together to respond as a tissue and also allow a very small amperage current to move quickly over the length of the tissue (see Fig. 5-8).

Cells seem responsive to steady direct current gradients. The cells either move or grow toward one pole and away from the other. The electric field created by the DC current may help guide the healing process and guide the regenerative capabilities of injured or developing tissues.[20,76]

Cells also may respond to a particular frequency of current. The cell may be selectively responsive to certain frequencies and unresponsive to other frequencies. Some researchers claim that specific genes for protein manufacture can be activated by a certain shaped electrical impulse. This frequency could change in certain ways according to the cellular state. This phenomenon has been termed the **"frequency window" selectivity** of the cell.[20]

Overall we see that small-amplitude direct currents are intrinsic to the ways the body works to grow and repair. Clinically if we can duplicate some of these same signals, we may be successful in using electrotherapy in the most efficient manner. The secrets to this type of use are only beginning to be uncovered.

Hopefully, after reading this review of cell biology slanted toward the electrical components, the magnitude of the cellular electrical activity and its potential to influence cell function will become apparent. Many of the unexplained phenomena surrounding electrotherapy may become more understandable as more research promotes better understanding of the normal electrical activity at the cellular and tissue levels.

In this discussion of how electrical current influences nonexcitatory cells and tissues, we must start to rely on theory more than well-proven researched ideas. The student must understand that theories are projections of what might take place to

frequency window selectivity Cellular responses may be triggered by a certain electrical frequency range.

explain observed behavior, and the authors expect changes in these theories to occur. Therefore, beware and believe cautiously as you incorporate these theories into your clinical practice.[56]

ELECTRICAL CONCEPTS: EFFECTS OF CHANGES IN CURRENT PARAMETERS AND THEIR EFFECT ON TREATMENT PROTOCOLS

When using any of the treatment protocols aimed at the electrical stimulation of muscle or nerve tissue, several concepts must be understood for therapists to accomplish their goals:

1. Alternating versus direct current
2. Tissue impedance
3. Current density
4. Frequency of wave or pulse
5. Intensity of wave or pulse
6. Duration of wave or pulse
7. Polarity of electrodes
8. Electrode placement

Changes in these parameters affect how the electrical current changes the physiology of the body part being treated. The waveform used gives us a graphic way to measure and quantify these parameters.[125]

ALTERNATING VERSUS DIRECT CURRENT

To further understand electrically stimulated muscle contractions, we must think in terms of multiple stimuli rather than a simple direct current response. The motor nerves are not stimulated by a steady flow of direct current. The nerve repolarizes under the influence of the current and will not depolarize again until a sudden change in current intensity occurs.

If continuous direct current were the only current mode available, we would get a muscle contraction only when the current intensity rose to a stimulus threshold. Once the membrane repolarized, another change in the current intensity would be needed to force another depolarization and contraction (Fig. 5-13).

The biggest difference in the effects of alternating and direct currents is the ability of direct current to cause chemical changes. Chemical effects from using direct current usually occur only when the stimulus is continuous and applied over a period of time. These chemical changes become measurable when the duration of the stimulus reaches the 1-minute mark, but the effect is cumulative over the total treatment time. This type of current is available in most low-voltage equipment. The duration of the current in most high-voltage stimulators is nonadjustable and is too short to create any chemical effect, unless treatment time in excess of 1 hour is used.[93,119]

One theory on using direct high-voltage current in treatment of edema proposes that the direct current enhances the movement of charged proteins into the lymphatic channels. The electric field causes the charged proteins to increase their movement and migrate into the lymph channels.[30]

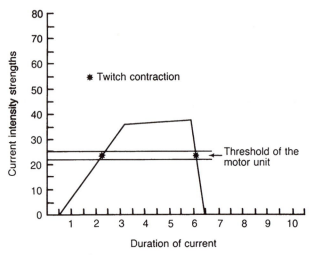

•**Figure 5-13** Direct current influence on a motor unit.

TISSUE IMPEDANCE

Impedance is the resistance of the tissue to the passage of electrical current. Bone and fat are high-impedance tissues; nerve and muscle are low-impedance tissues. If a low-impedance tissue is located under a large amount of high-impedance tissue, the current will never become high enough to cause a depolarization.[10,119]

CURRENT DENSITY

current density Amount of current flow per cubic area.

The **current density** (amount of current flow per cubic volume) at the nerve or muscle must be high enough to cause depolarization. The current density is highest where the electrodes meet the skin and diminishes as the electricity penetrates into the deeper tissues (Fig. 5-14).[10,119] If there is a large fat layer between the electrodes and the nerve, the electrical energy may not have a high enough density to cause depolarization (Fig. 5-15).

If the electrodes are spaced closely together, the area of highest current density is relatively superficial (see Fig. 5-16A). If the electrodes are spaced farther apart, the current density will be higher in the deeper tissues, including nerve and muscle (see Fig. 5-16B).

Electrode size will also change current density. As the size of one electrode relative to another is decreased, the current density beneath the smaller electrode is increased. The larger the electrode, the larger the area over which the current is spread, decreasing the current density (Fig. 5-17).[2,3,10,91,119]

Using a large (dispersive) electrode remote from the treatment area while placing a smaller (active) electrode as close as possible to the nerve or muscle motor point will give the greatest effect at the small electrode. The large electrode disperses

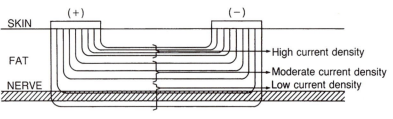

•**Figure 5-14** Current density using equal-size electrodes spaced close together.

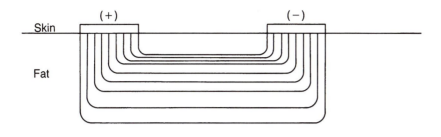

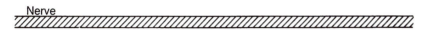

•**Figure 5-15** Equal size electrodes spaced close together on body part with thick fat layers. Thus the electrical current does not reach the nerves.

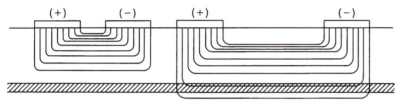

•**Figure 5-16** *A* Electrodes are very close together, producing a high-density current in the superficial tissues. *B* Increasing the distance between the electrodes increases the current density in deeper tissues.

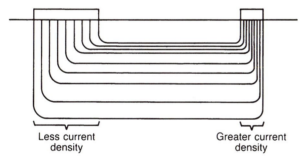

Less current density   Greater current density

•**Figure 5-17** The greatest current density is under the small or active electrode.

Treatment Tip
To increase current density in deeper tissues the size of the active electrode can be decreased, which will increase current density under that electrode. The active electrodes can be moved further apart. The current intensity can be increased. The current duration may also be increased.

the current over a large area; the small electrode concentrates the current in the area of the motor point (see Fig. 5-17).

Electrode size and placement are key elements which the therapist controls that will have great influence on your results. High current density close to the neural structure you want to stimulate makes it more certain that you will be successful with the least amount of current. Electrode placement is probably one of the biggest causes of poor results from electrical therapy.[56]

FREQUENCY

The amount of shortening of the muscle fiber and the amount of recovery allowed the muscle fiber are a function of the frequency. The mechanical shortening of the single muscle fiber response can be influenced by stimulating again as soon as the tissue membrane repolarizes. Only the membrane has the absolute refractory period; the contractile mechanism operates on a different timing sequence and is just beginning to contract. When the second stimulus is received by the muscle membrane, the myofilaments are already overlapping, and the second stimulus causes an increased mechanical shortening of the muscle fiber. This process of superimposing one twitch contraction on another is called **summation of contractions**. As the number of twitch contractions per second increases, single twitch responses cannot be distinguished, and **tetanization** of the muscle fiber is reached (Fig. 5-18). The tension developed by a muscle fiber in tetany is much greater than the tension from a twitch contraction. This muscle fiber tetany is strictly a function of the frequency of the stimulating current; it is not dependent on the intensity of the current.[10,91]

The primary difference between electrically induced muscle contraction and voluntary muscle contraction is the asynchrony of firing of motor units under voluntary control versus the synchronous firing of electrically stimulated motor units. Each time the electrical stimulus is applied, the same motor units respond. This may lead to greater fatigue in the electrically stimulated muscles. Normal firing in voluntary muscle contraction varies from one movement to the next, because some motor units are contracting while others are inactive. Voluntary contractions do not lead to muscular fatigue as early in the exercise period as do electrical contractions. This synchrony of contraction may also be important in training the muscle to use more synchronous contractions to improve muscular strength.[10,91]

INTENSITY

Increasing the intensity of the electrical stimulus in Fig. 5-19A to that in Fig. 5-19B causes the current to reach deeper into the tissue. Depolarization of more fibers then is accomplished by two methods: higher threshold fibers within the range of the first stimulus are depolarized by the higher intensity stimulus (see Fig. 5-19A); and fibers with the same threshold but deeper in the structure are depolarized by the deeper spread of the current. High-voltage stimulators are capable of deeper penetration into the tissue than low-voltage stimulators and may be desirable when stimulating deep muscle tissue. This is one of the most significant differences between high- and low-voltage generators.[3,91]

DURATION

We also can stimulate more nerve fibers with the same intensity current by increasing the length of time (duration) that an adequate stimulus is available to depolarize the membranes (see Fig. 5-19C). Greater numbers of nerve fibers then would react

summation of contractions Shortening of muscle myofilaments caused by increasing the frequency of muscle membrane depolarization.

tetanization When individual muscle twitch responses can no longer be distinguished and the responses force maximum shortening of the stimulated muscle fiber.

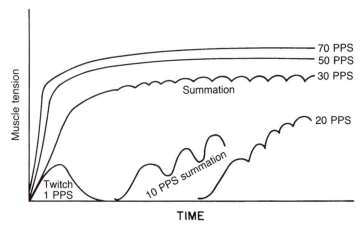

•**Figure 5-18** Summation of contractions and tetanization.

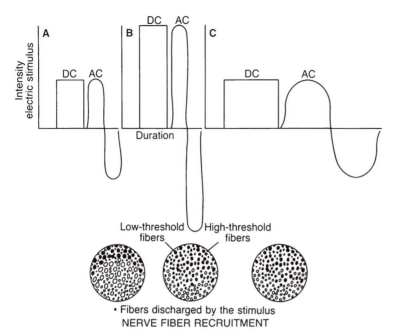

•**Figure 5-19** Recruitment of nerve fibers. *A* A stimulus pulse at a duration-intensity just above threshold will excite the closest and largest fibers. Each electrical pulse of the same intensity at the same location will cause the same fibers to fire. *B* Increasing the intensity will excite smaller fibers and fibers farther away. *C* Increasing the duration will also excite smaller fibers and fibers farther away.

to the same intensity stimulus, because the current would be available for a longer period of time.[10,57,119] This method requires the use of a stimulator with an adjustable duration. The low-voltage stimulators usually are available with this parameter, whereas the high-voltage stimulators usually have a preset pulse duration.

POLARITY

During the use of any stimulator, an electrode that has a greater level of electrons is called the negative electrode or the cathode. The other electrode in this system has a lower level of electrons and is called the positive electrode or the anode. The negative electrode attracts positive ions and the positive electrode attracts negative ions and electrons. With AC waves, these electrodes change polarity with each current cycle.

With a direct current generator, the therapist can designate one electrode as the negative and one as the positive, and for the duration of the treatment the electrodes will provide that polar effect. The polar effect can be thought of in terms of three characteristics: (1) chemical effects; (2) ease of excitation; and (3) direction of current flow.[9,10,81,91,98,119]

Chemical Effects

Changes in pH under each electrode, a reflex vasodilation, and the ability to drive oppositely charged ions through the skin into the tissue (iontophoresis) are all thought of as chemical effects. A tissue-stimulating effect is ascribed to the negative electrode. To create these effects, longer pulse durations (> 1 min) are required.[9,44,93,98] The bacteriostatic effect was achieved at either the anode or cathode with intensities in the 5 to 10 MA range, although at 1 MA or below the greatest

Chemical changes occur only with long duration continuous current.

Negative electrode = cathode
Positive electrode = anode

Muscle contraction = negative active electrode

Cathode = distal
Anode = proximal

bacteriostatic effect was found at the cathode.[51] Another study using treatment times exceeding 30 minutes found some bacteriostatic effect of high-voltage pulsed currents.[65]

Ease of Excitation of Excitable Tissue

The polarity of the active electrode usually should be negative when the desired result is a muscle contraction, because of the greater facility for membrane depolarization at the negative pole. However, current density under the positive pole can be increased rapidly enough to create a depolarizing effect. Using the positive electrode as the active electrode is not as efficient, because it will require more current intensity to create an action potential. This may cause the patient to be less comfortable with the treatment. In treatment programs requiring muscle contraction or sensory nerve stimulation, patient comfort should dictate the choice of positive or negative polarity. Negative polarity usually is the most comfortable in this instance.[35,91,119]

Direction of Current Flow

In some treatment schemes, the direction of current flow also is considered important. Generally speaking, the negative electrode is positioned distally and the positive electrode proximally. This arrangement tries to replicate the naturally occurring pattern of electrical flow in the body.[9,83]

The direction of current flow could also influence shifting of the water content of the tissues and movement of colloids (fluid suspension of the intracellular fluid). Neither of these phenomena is well documented or understood, and further study is needed before clinical treatments are designed around these concepts.[88,100,119]

True polar effects can be substantiated when they occur close to the electrodes through which the current is entering the tissue. In laboratory situations in physics and physical therapy, polar effects occur in very close proximity to the electrode. To cause these effects, the current must flow through a medium. If the tissue to be treated is centrally located between the two electrodes, results cannot be assigned to polar effects.[9,56] Clinically, polar effects are an important consideration in iontophoresis, stimulating motor points or peripheral nerves, and in the biostimulative effect on nonexcitatory cells.

ELECTRODE PLACEMENT

When using any of the treatment protocols aimed at the electrical stimulation of sensory nerves for pain suppression, there are several guidelines that will help the therapist select the appropriate sites for electrode placement. Transcutaneous electrical nerve stimulation (TENS) uses similar-sized electrodes placed according to a pattern and moved in a trial-and-error pattern until pain is decreased. The following patterns may be used.

1. Electrodes may be placed on or around the painful area.
2. Electrodes may be placed over specific dermatomes, myotomes, or sclerotomes that correspond to the painful area.
3. Electrodes may be placed close to the spinal cord segment that innervates a painful area.
4. Peripheral nerves that innervate the painful area may be stimulated by placing electrodes over sites where the nerve becomes superficial and can be stimulated easily.
5. Vascular structures contain neural tissue as well as ionic fluids that would transmit electrical stimulating currents and may be most easily stimulated by electrode placement over superficial vascular structures.
6. Electrode placement over trigger point locations.[117]

7. Both acupuncture and trigger points have been conveniently mapped out and illustrated. A reference on acupuncture and trigger areas is included in Appendix A. The therapist should systematically attempt to stimulate the points listed as successful for certain areas and types of pain. If they are effective, the patient will have decreased pain. These points also can be identified using an ohm meter point locator to determine areas of decreased skin resistance.

8. Combinations of any of the preceding systems and bilateral electrode placement also can be successful.[70,71,81,124]

9. Crossing patterns, also referred to as an interferential technique, involve electrode application such that the electrical signals from each set of electrodes add together at some point in the body and the intensity accumulates. The electrodes are usually arranged in a criss-cross pattern around the point to be stimulated (Fig. 5-20). If there is a specific superficial area (i.e., medial collateral acromioclavicular joint) that you wish to stimulate, your electrodes should be relatively close together. They should be located so the area to be treated is central to the location of the electrodes. If there is poorly localized pain (general shoulder pain) that seems to be deeper in the joint or muscle area, spread your electrodes farther apart to give more penetration to the current.

The therapist should not be limited to any one system but should evaluate electrode placement for each patient. The effectiveness of sensory stimulation is closely tied in with proper electrode placement. As in all trial-and-error treatment approaches, a

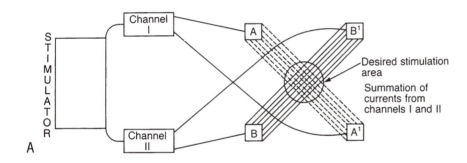

A

Treatment Tip
When using interferential current, the four electrodes should be set up in a square pattern with the target treatment area will be in the center of the square so that the maximum interference will take place where the electric field lines cross at the center of the pattern.

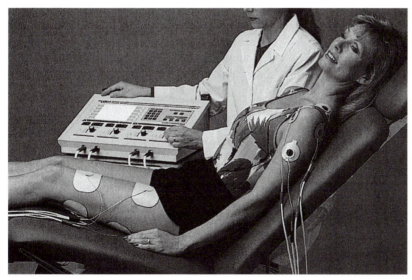

B

•**Figure 5-20** (A) Current flow would be from A to A′ and B to B′. As the currents cross the area of stimulation they summate in intensity. (B) Application of electrodes in a crossing pattern for both the thign and the shoulder.

systematic, organized search is always better than a "shotgun," hit-and-miss approach. Numerous articles have identified some of the best locations for common pain problems, and these may be used as a starting point for the first approach.[70] If the treatment is not achieving the desired results, the electrode placement should be reconsidered.

THERAPEUTIC USES OF ELECTRICALLY INDUCED MUSCLE CONTRACTION

A variety of therapeutic gains can be made by electrically stimulating a muscle contraction:

1. Muscle reeducation
2. Muscle pump contractions
3. Retardation of atrophy
4. Muscle strengthening
5. Increasing range of motion

Any electrical stimulator—high-voltage, low-voltage, alternating current, **hybrid current**, or TENS may be used to cause muscle contraction. The efficiency and effectiveness of treatment can be increased by following the protocols as closely as possible with the available equipment.

Muscle fatigue should be considered when deciding on treatment parameters. The variables that have an influence on muscle fatigue are the following.

1. Intensity: combination of the pulse stimulus' amplitude intensity and the pulse duration
2. The number of pulses or bursts per second
3. On time
4. Off time

Muscle force is varied by changing the intensity to recruit more or less motor units. Muscle force can also be varied to a certain degree by increasing the summating quality of the contraction with high burst or pulse rates. The greater the force, the greater the demands on the muscle, the greater the occlusion of muscle blood flow, the greater the fatigue. If high muscle forces are not required, the intensity and frequency can be adjusted to desired levels but fatigue can still be a factor. To minimize fatigue associated with forceful contractions, a combination of the lowest frequency and the higher intensity will keep the force constant.[12]

If high force levels are desired, then higher frequencies and intensities can be used. To keep the muscle fatigue as low as possible, the rest time between contractions should be at least 60 seconds for each 10 seconds of contraction time. A variable frequency train, in which a high-frequency, then low-frequency stimulus are used, will also help minimize fatigue in repetitive functional electric stimulation.[12]

Neuromuscular-induced contraction at the higher torques are associated with patient perceptions of pain, either from the current used or the intensity of the contraction. This is often a limiting factor in the success of any of the following protocols. Each patient needs supervision and satisfactory therapist confidence for the most effective compliance with the treatment goals.[12,34,56]

When using electrical stimulation for muscle contraction, motor point stimulation can give the best individual muscle contraction. To find the motor point of a muscle, a probe electrode should be used to stimulate the muscle. Stimulation should be started in the approximate location of the desired motor point. (See

Treatment Tip
In a conventional TENS treatment, the goals is to provide as much sensory cutaneous input as possible. Thus, both the frequency and pulse duration should be set as high as the unit will allow. The intensity should be increased until a muscle contraction is elicited, then decreased slightly until the patient feels only a tingling sensation. If using a portable unit, the treatment may continue for several hours if necessary or until the pain subsides.

Appendix A for motor point chart.) The intensity should be increased until contraction is visible, and the current intensity should be maintained at that level. The probe should be moved around until the best visible contraction for that current intensity is found; this is the motor point.[10,118] By choosing this location for stimulation, the current density can be increased in an area where numerous motor nerve fibers can be affected, maximizing the muscular response from the stimulation.

Muscle Reeducation

Muscular inhibition after surgery or injury is the primary indication for muscle reeducation. If the neuromuscular mechanisms of a muscle have not been damaged, then central nervous system inhibition of this muscle usually is a factor in loss of control. The atrophy of synaptic contacts that remain unused for long periods is theorized as a source of this sensorimotor alienation. The addition of electrical stimulation of the motor nerve provides an artificial use of the inactive synapses and helps restore a more normal balance to the system as the ascending sensory information will be reintegrated into the patient's movement control patterns. A muscle contraction usually can be forced by electrically stimulating the muscle. Forcing the muscle to contract causes an increase in the sensory input from that muscle. The patient feels the muscle contract, sees the muscle contract, and can attempt to duplicate this muscular response.[10,32,39,90]

Protocols for muscle reeducation do not list specific parameters to make this treatment more efficient, but the following criteria are essential for effective electrical stimulation.

1. Current intensity must be adequate for muscle contraction but comfortable for the patient.
2. Pulse duration must be set as close as possible to the duration needed for chronaxie of the tissue to be stimulated. This is preset on most therapeutic generators.
3. Pulses per second (pps) should be high enough to give a tetanic contraction (20–40 pulses per second).
4. Interrupted or surged current must be used.
5. On time should be 1 to 2 seconds.
6. Off time should be 4 to 10 seconds.
7. The patient should be instructed to allow just the electricity to make the muscle contract, allowing the patient to feel and see the response desired. Next, the patient should alternate voluntary muscle contractions with current-induced contractions.
8. Total treatment time should be about 15 minutes, but this can be repeated several times daily.
9. High-voltage pulsed or medium-frequency alternating current may be most effective (see Fig. 5-20).[10,32,39]

Muscle Pump Contractions

Electrically induced muscle contraction can be used to duplicate the regular muscle contractions that help stimulate circulation by pumping fluid and blood through venous and lymphatic channels back into the heart.[29] A discussion of edema formation is included in the chapter on intermittent compression. Using sensory level stimulation has also been found to decrease edema in sprain and contusion injuries in animals. That discussion is included elsewhere in this volume.

Electrical stimulation of muscle contractions in the affected extremity can help in reestablishing the proper circulatory pattern while keeping the injured part protected.

CASE STUDY 5-2
ELECTRICAL STIMULATING CURRENTS: REEDUCATION OF INNERVATED MUSCLE

Background: A 16-year-old male underwent arthroscopic partial medial meniscectomy on the right knee yesterday. He is to begin ambulation with crutches (weight bearing as tolerated) today. Clinic policy states that patients must be able to produce an active quadriceps femoris contraction prior to crutch-walking instruction. However, the patient is unable to produce an active contraction of the quadriceps femoris muscle. There is minimal pain and swelling, but after working with the patient for 15 minutes, he remains unable to contract the quadriceps femoris.

Impression: Status postarthroscopic surgery on the right knee with inhibition of quadriceps femoris control.

Treatment Plan: Using a pulsatile monophasic waveform generator, a course of electrical stimulation was initiated. The cathode (active, negative polarity) was placed over the motor point of the vastus medialis, and the anode (inactive, positive polarity) was placed on the posterior thigh. The frequency was set at 40 pps. Using an uninterrupted (1:0) duty cycle, the amplitude was set to a level that produced a visible contraction, but was below the pain threshold. After establishing the stimulus amplitude, the duty cycle was then adjusted to deliver 15 seconds of stimulus followed by 15 seconds of rest; the current was not ramped, so the effective duty cycle was 1:1. The patient was encouraged to contract the quadriceps femoris during the stimulation for the first five stimulations, then was asked to contract the quadriceps femoris before the stimulus was delivered.

Response: After 20 repetitions of the stimulus, the patient was able to initiate a contraction of the quadriceps femoris before the current was delivered. The electrical stimulation was discontinued, and the patient was able to continue to contract the quadriceps femoris voluntarily. He was then instructed in crutch walking, and routine postoperative rehabilitation was initiated.

Discussion Questions

- What tissues were injured or affected?
- What symptoms were present?
- What phase of the injury-healing continuum did the patient present for care in?
- What are the physical agent modality's biophysical effects (direct, indirect, depth, and tissue affinity)?
- What are the physical agent modality's indications and contraindications?
- What are the parameters of the physical agent modality's application, dosage, duration, and frequency in this case study?
- What other physical agent modalities could be used to treat this injury or condition? Why? How?

The rehabilitation professional employs physical agent modality to create an optimum environment for tissue healing while minimizing the symptoms associated with the trauma or condition.

The following criteria must be satisfied for the electrical treatment to be successful in helping to reduce swelling.

1. Current intensity must be high enough to provide a strong, comfortable muscle contraction.
2. Pulse duration is preset on most of the therapeutic generators. If adjustable, it should be set as close as possible to the duration needed for chronaxie of the motor nerve to be stimulated.
3. Pulses per second should be in the beginnings of tetany range (20 pps).
4. Interrupted or surged current must be used.
5. On time should be 5 to 10 seconds.
6. Off time should be 5 to 10 seconds.

7. The part to be treated should be elevated.

8. The patient should be instructed to allow the electricity to make the muscles contract. Active range of motion may be encouraged at the same time if it is not contraindicated.

9. Total treatment time should be between 20 and 30 minutes; treatment should be repeated two to five times daily.

10. High-voltage pulsed or medium-frequency alternating current may be most effective (see Fig. 5-20).[32,39,94,97,111]

11. Use this protocol in addition to the normal ice for best effect.[41,88]

Retardation of Atrophy

Prevention or retardation of atrophy has traditionally been a reason for treating patients with electrically stimulated muscle contraction. The maintenance of muscle tissue, after an injury that prevents normal muscular exercise, can be accomplished by substituting an electrically stimulated muscle contraction. The electrical stimulation reproduces the physical and chemical events associated with normal voluntary muscle contraction and helps to maintain normal muscle function.

Again, no specific protocols exist. In designing a program, the practitioner should try to duplicate muscle contractions associated with normal exercise routines. The following criteria can be used as guidelines in developing effective treatment protocols.

1. Current intensity should be as high as can be tolerated by the patient. This can be increased during the treatment as some sensory accommodation takes place. The contraction should be capable of moving the limb through the antigravity range or of achieving 25 percent or more of the normal **maximum voluntary isometric contraction (MVIC)** torque for the muscle. The higher torque readings seem to have the best results.

2. Pulse duration is preset on most of the therapeutic generators. If it is adjustable, it should be set as close as possible to the duration needed for chronaxie of the motor nerve to be stimulated.

3. Pulses per second should be in the tetany range (20–85 pps).

4. Interrupted or surge-type current should be used.

5. On time should be between 6 and 15 seconds.

6. Off time should be at least 1 minute, and preferably 2 minutes.

7. The muscle should be given some resistance, either gravity or external resistance provided by the addition of weights or by fixing the joint so that the contraction becomes isometric.

8. The patient can be instructed to work with the electrically induced contraction, but voluntary effort is not necessary for the success of this treatment.

9. Total treatment time should be 15 to 20 minutes, or enough time to allow a minimum of 10 contractions; some protocols have been successful with three sets of 10 contractions. The treatment can be repeated two times daily. Some protocols using battery-powered rather than line-powered units have advocated longer bouts with more repetitions probably because of low contraction force.

10. A medium-frequency alternating current stimulator is the machine of choice (see Fig. 5-20).[12,32–34,39,90,102,105,106]

Muscle Strengthening

Muscle strengthening from electrical muscle stimulation has been used with some good results in patients with weakness or denervation of a muscle group. The protocol is better established for this use, but more research is needed to clarify the procedures and allow us to generalize the results to other patient problems. The following summarizes the protocols used successfully.

1. Current intensity should be high enough to make the muscle develop 60 percent of the torque developed in a MVIC.

2. Pulse duration is preset on most therapeutic generators. If adjustable, it should be set as close as possible to the duration needed for chronaxie of the motor nerve to be stimulated. In general longer pulse durations should include more nerves in response.

3. Pulses per second should be in the tetany range (20–85 pps).

4. Surged or interrupted current with a gradual ramp to peak intensity is most effective.

5. On time should be in the 10- to 15-second range.

6. Off time should be in the 50-second to 2-minute range.

7. Resistance usually is applied by immobilizing the limb. The muscle is then given an isometric contraction torque equal to or greater than 25 percent of the MVIC torque. The greater the percentage of torque produced, the better the results.

8. The patient can be instructed to work with the electrically induced contraction, but voluntary effort is not necessary for the success of the treatment.

9. Total treatment time should include a minimum of 10 contractions, but mimicking normal active resistive training protocols of three sets of 10 contractions can also be productive. Fatigue is a major factor in this setup. Electrical stimulation bouts should be scheduled at least three times weekly. Generally, strength gains will continue over the treatment course, but intensities may need to increase to keep pace with the most current maximum voluntary contraction torques.

10. A medium-frequency alternating current stimulator is the machine of choice (see Fig. 5-20).[12,32–34,39,90,102,105,106]

INCREASING RANGE OF MOTION

Increasing the range of motion in contracted joints is also a possible and documented use of electrical muscle stimulation. Electrically stimulating a muscle contraction pulls the joint through the limited range. The continued contraction of this muscle group over an extended time appears to make the contracted joint and muscle tissue modify and lengthen. Reduction of contractures in patients with hemiplegia has been reported, although no studies have reported this type of use in contracted joints from athletic injuries or surgery. The protocol needed to affect joint contracture is the following.

1. Current intensity must be of sufficient intensity and duration to make a muscle contract strongly enough to move the body part through its antigravity range. Intensity should be increased gradually during treatment.

2. Pulse duration is preset on most of the therapeutic generators. If it is adjustable, it should be set as close as possible to the duration needed for chronaxie of the motor nerve to be stimulated.

3. Pulses per second should be at the beginning of the tetany range (20–30 pps).

4. Interrupted or surged current should be used.

5. On time should be between 15 and 20 seconds.

6. Off time should be equal to or greater than on time, fatigue is a big consideration.

7. The stimulated muscle group should be antagonistic to the joint contracture, and the patient should be positioned so the joint will be moved to the limits of the available range.

8. The patient is passive in this treatment and does not work with the electrical contraction.

9. Total treatment time should be 90 minutes daily. This can be broken into three 30-minute treatments.

10. High-voltage pulsed or medium-frequency alternating current stimulators are the best choices (see Fig. 5-21).

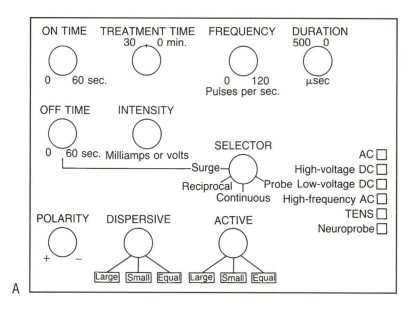

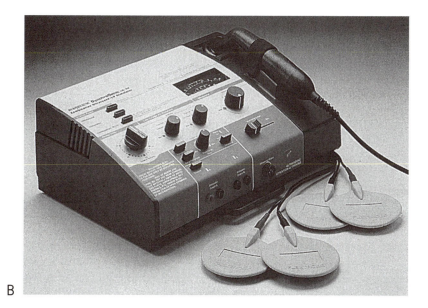

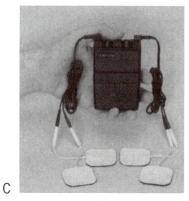

•**Figure 5-21** *A.* Electrical stimulator control panel. *B.* High-volt unit. *C.* TENS.

THE EFFECT OF NONCONTRACTILE STIMULATION ON EDEMA

Ion movement within biologic tissues is a basic theory in the electrotherapy literature. This is clearly seen in the action potential model of nerve cell depolarization. The effects of sensory level stimulation on edema has been theorized to work on this principle. Research has not documented the effectiveness of this type of treatment, and therapists should continue to use other more proven mechanisms to decrease edema. See Chapter 14 on intermittent compression for a discussion of edema formation.

Since 1987, numerous studies using rat and frog models have helped to more clearly define the effects of electrical stimulation on edema formation and reduction. The muscle pumping theory discussed elsewhere in this volume has seemed the most viable way to effect this problem. Most of the recent studies have focused on a sensory level stimulation. Early theory supported the use of sensory level direct current as a driving force to make the charged plasma protein ions in the interstitial spaces move in the direction of the oppositely charged electrode. Cook et al. demonstrated an increased lymphatic uptake of labeled albumin within rats treated with sensory level high-voltage stimulation.[29] However, there was no significant reduction in the limb volume. They hypothesized that the electric fluid introduced into the area of edema facilitated the movement of the charged proteins into the lymphatic channels. When the lymphatic channel volume increased the contraction rate of the smooth muscle in the lymphatics increase. They also hypothesize that stimulation of sensory neurons may cause an indirect activation of the autonomic nervous system. This might cause release of adrenergic substances that would also increase the rate of lymph smooth muscle contraction and lymph circulation.

1. Extended treatment times, 1 hour.
2. Direct current stimulation with polarity arranged in correct fashion.
3. Electrodes arranged to pull or push plasma proteins into the lymphatic system and be moved back into the circulatory system via the thoracic duct.

Another proposed mechanism is that a microamp stimulation of the local neurovascular components in an injured area may cause a vasoconstriction and reduce the permeability of the capillary walls to limit the migration of plasma proteins into the interstitial spaces. This would retard the accumulation of plasma proteins and the associated fluid dynamics of the edema exudate. In a study on the histamine-stimulated leakage of plasma proteins, animals treated with small doses of electrical current produced less leakage. The underlying mechanisms were a reduced pore size in the capillary walls and reduced pooling of blood in the capillaries, which could have been initiated by hormonal, neural, mechanical, or electrochemical factors.

Theory on exact mechanisms of action are cloudy but the research has given us a viable model to use in trying to stimulate and achieve the same edema control mechanisms clinically as have been proven in the laboratory. The following is an edema control sensory stimulation protocol.

1. Current intensity of 30–50 V or 10 percent less than needed to produce a visible muscle contraction is most effective.
2. Preset short-duration currents on the high-voltage equipment are effective.
3. High pulse frequencies (120 pps) are most effective.
4. Interrupted DC currents are most effective. Biphasic currents showed increases in volume.
5. The animals treated with a negative distal electrode had a significant treatment effect. The animals with a positive distal electrode showed no change.
6. Time of treatment after injury: The best results were reported when treatment began immediately after injury. Treatment started after 24 hours showed an effect on the

accumulation of new edema volume but showed no effect on the existing edema volume.

7. A 30-minute treatment showed good control of volume for 4 to 5 hours.

8. The water immersion electrode technique was effective, but using surface electrodes was not effective.

9. High-voltage pulsed generators were effective, low-voltage generators were not effective.[3,11,17,30,40,41,50,63,65,74,86–89,114,115]

STIMULATION OF DENERVATED MUSCLE

Electrical currents may be used to produce a muscle contraction in **denervated muscle**. A muscle that is denervated is one that has lost its peripheral nerve supply. The primary purpose for electrically stimulating denervated muscle is to help minimize the extent of atrophy during the period while the nerve is regenerating. Following denervation, the muscle fibers experience a number of progressive anatomic, biochemical, and physiologic changes that lead to a decrease in the size of the individual muscle fibers and in the diameter and weight of the muscle. Consequently, there will be a decrease in the amount of tension that can be generated by that muscle and an increase in the time required for the muscle to contract.[26,31] These degenerative changes progress until the muscle is reinnervated by axons regenerating across the site of the lesion. If reinnervation does not occur within 2 years, it is generally accepted that fibrous connective tissue will have replaced the contractile elements of the muscle and recovery of muscle function is not possible.[31]

A review of the literature indicates that the majority of studies support the use of electrical stimulation of denervated muscle. These studies generally indicate that muscle atrophy can be retarded, loss of both muscle mass and contractile strength can be minimized, and muscle fiber size can be maintained by the appropriate use of electrical stimulation.[27,53,55] Electrically stimulated contractions of denervated muscle may limit edema and venous stasis, thus delaying muscle fiber fibrosis and degeneration.[31] However, there also seems to be general agreement that electrical stimulation has little or no effect on the rate of nerve regeneration or muscle reinnervation.

A few studies have suggested that electrical stimulation of denervated muscle actually may interfere with reinnervation, thus delaying functional return.[76,103] These studies propose that the muscle contraction disrupts the regenerating neuromuscular junction retarding reinnervation, and that electrical stimulation may traumatize denervated muscle since it is more sensitive to trauma than normal muscle.[31,55,76]

TREATMENT PARAMETERS FOR STIMULATING DENERVATED MUSCLE

The following treatment parameters have been recommended for stimulating denervated muscle.

1. A current with an asymmetric, biphasic (faradic) waveform with a pulse duration less than 1 msec may be used during the first 2 weeks.[66]

2. After 2 weeks, either an interrupted square wave direct current, a progressive exponential wave direct current, each with a long pulse duration of greater than 10 msec, or a sine wave alternating current with a frequency lower than 10 Hz will produce a twitch contraction.[31] The length of the pulse should be as short as possible but long enough to elicit a contraction.[116]

3. The current waveform should have a pulse duration equal to or greater than the chronaxie of the denervated muscle.

4. The amplitude of the current along with the pulse duration must be sufficient to stimulate a denervated muscle with a prolonged chronaxie while producing a moderately strong contraction of the muscle fibers.

5. The pause between stimuli should be four to five times longer (about 3–6 sec) than the stimulus duration to minimize fatigue.[116]

6. Either a monopolar or bipolar electrode setup can be used with the small-diameter active electrode placed over the most electrically active point in the muscle. This may not be the motor point since the muscle is not normally innervated.

7. Stimulation should begin immediately following denervation using three stimulation treatments per day involving three sets of between 5 and 20 repetitions that can be varied according to fatigability of the muscle.[31]

THERAPEUTIC USES OF ELECTRICAL STIMULATION OF SENSORY NERVES

Clinically, efforts are made to stimulate the sensory nerves to change the patient's perception of a painful stimulus coming from an injured area. To understand how to maximally affect the perception of pain through electrical stimulation, it is necessary to understand pain perception. The gate control theory, the descending or **central biasing** theory, and the opiate pain control theory are the theoretical basis for pain reduction phenomena. These theories are covered in depth in Chapter 2.

GATE CONTROL THEORY

Electrically stimulating the large sensory fibers when there is pain in a certain area will force the central nervous system to make the brain's recognition area aware of the electrical stimuli. As long as the stimuli are applied, the perception of pain is diminished. Electrical stimulation of sensory nerves will evoke the gate control mechanism and diminish awareness of painful stimuli. As long as the stimulation is causing firing of the sensory nerves, the gate to pain should be closed. If accommodation to the electrical stimulus occurs or if the stimulus stops, the gate is then open, and pain returns to perception.[13,16,70,71,73,83,84, 101,102,106,119]

The physical dominance, enkephalin release model is used in treating pain from acute injuries, problems with the musculoskeletal system, or postoperative pain. The following criteria can be used as guidelines in developing effective treatment protocols.

1. Current intensity should be adjusted to tolerance but should not cause a muscular contraction, the higher the better.

2. Pulse duration (pulse width) should be 75 to 150 μsec or maximum possible on the machine.

3. Pulses per second should be 80 to 125, or as high as possible on the machine.

4. A transcutaneous electrical stimulator waveform should be used.

5. On time should be continuous mode.

6. Total treatment time should correspond to fluctuations in pain; the unit should be left on until pain is no longer perceived, turned off, then restarted when pain begins again.

7. If this treatment is successful, you will have some pain relief within the first 30 minutes of treatment.

8. If it is not successful, but you feel this is the best theoretical or most clinically applicable approach, change the electrode placements and try again. If this is not successful, then using a different theoretical approach may offer more help.

9. Any stimulator that can deliver this current is acceptable. Portable units are better for 24-hour pain control (see Fig. 5-20).[70,71,80]

CENTRAL BIASING THEORY

Intense electrical stimulation of the smaller fibers (C fibers or pain fibers) at peripheral sites (trigger and acupoint) for short time periods causes stimulation of descending neurons, which then affect transmission of pain information by closing the gate at the spinal cord level (see Fig. 3-5).[19]

The central biasing setup is used on sharp chronic pain or severe pathologic pain. Changing the bias of the central nervous system and increasing the descending influences on the transmission of pain are best accomplished with the following protocols.

1. Current intensity should be very high, approaching a noxious level; muscular contraction is not desirable.
2. Pulse duration should be 10 msec.
3. Pulses per second should be 80.
4. On time should be 30 seconds to 1 minute.
5. Stimulation should be applied over trigger or acupuncture points.
6. Selection and number of points used varies according to the part treated.
7. A low-frequency, high-intensity generator is the stimulator of choice for central biasing (see Fig. 5-20).[19]
8. If this treatment is successful, pain will be relieved shortly after the treatment.
9. If this treatment is not successful, try different electrode setups by expanding the treatment points used.

OPIATE PAIN CONTROL THEORY

Electrical stimulation of sensory nerves may stimulate the release of enkephalin from local sites throughout the central nervous system and the release of β-endorphin from the pituitary gland into the cerebral spinal fluid. The mechanism that causes the release and then the binding of enkephalin and β-endorphin to some nerve cells is still unclear. It is certain that a diminution or elimination of pain perception is caused by applying an electrical current to areas close to the site of pain or to acupuncture or trigger points, both local and distant to the pain area.[19,25,78,84,85,102,107,123]

To use the influence of hyperstimulation analgesia and β-endorphin release, a point stimulation setup must be used.[77] A large dispersive pad and a small pad or handheld probe point electrode are utilized in this approach. The point electrode is applied to the chosen site, and the intensity is increased until it is perceived by the patient. The probe is then moved around the area, and the patient is asked to report relative changes in perception of intensity. When a location of maximum-intensity perception is found, the current intensity is increased to maximum tolerable levels. This is much the same as finding a motor point, as described earlier.[19,95]

Beta-endorphin stimulation may offer better relief for the deep aching or chronic pain similar to overuse injury's pain. Beta-endorphin production may be stimulated using the following protocols.

1. Current intensity should be high, approaching a noxious level: muscular contraction is acceptable.
2. Pulse duration should be 200 μsec to 10 msec.
3. Pulses per second should be between 1 and 5.
4. High-voltage pulsed current should be used.
5. On time should be 30 to 45 seconds.
6. Stimulation should be applied over trigger or acupuncture points.
7. Selection and number of points used varies according to the part and condition being treated.

CASE STUDY 5-3
ELECTRICAL STIMULATING CURRENTS: PAIN MODULATION

Background: A 52-year-old woman is 9 months post-hemilaminectomy and discectomy without fusion at L5–S1 owing to a herniated disc with compromise of the S1 nerve root. The surgery resulted in relief of the peripheral pain, weakness, and sensory loss, but persistent pain in the lumbosacral spine and buttocks prevents the patient from engaging in rehabilitation exercises effectively.

Impression: Status postspinal surgery with persistent postoperative pain; no neural deficit.

Treatment Plan: The patient was already being treated with a hot pack prior to exercise; conventional TENS was added to the treatment regimen. Electrodes were placed at the L3–L4 interspace and over the greater trochanter. A pulsatile biphasic waveform was selected, with a rate of 60 pps, an amplitude between the sensory and motor thresholds, and a duty cycle of 1:0 (uninterrupted). The stimulation was delivered for the 10-minute heat application and remained in place during the therapeutic exercise, as well as for 30 minutes following the exercise.

Response: The patient experienced a 60 percent reduction in the symptoms during the exercise; this enabled the patient to perform the exercise through a greater range and with a greater effect. The effect of the TENS began to diminish after 8 weeks, but the pain had diminished to manageable levels such that the patient was able to continue the rehabilitation program without the TENS.

Discussion Questions

- What tissues were injured or affected?
- What symptoms were present?
- What phase of the injury-healing continuum did the patient present for care in?
- What are the physical agent modality's biophysical effects (direct, indirect, depth, and tissue affinity)?
- What are the physical agent modality's indications and contraindications?
- What are the parameters of the physical agent modality's application, dosage, duration, and frequency in this case study?
- What other physical agent modalities could be used to treat this injury or condition? Why? How?

The rehabilitation professional employs physical agent modality to create an optimum environment for tissue healing while minimizing the symptoms associated with the trauma or condition.

8. A high-voltage pulsed current or a low-frequency, high-intensity machine is best for this effect (see Fig. 5-20).[19,84,85]

9. If stimulation is successful, you should know at the completion of the treatment. The analgesic effect should last for several (6–7) hours.

10. If not successful, try expanding the number of stimulation sites. Add the same stimulation points on the opposite side of the body, add auricular (ear) acupuncture points, add more points on the same limb.

A combination of intense point stimulation and transcutaneous electrical nerve stimulation may be used. The transcutaneous electrical nerve stimulation applications should be used as much as needed to make the patient comfortable, and the intense point stimulation should be used on a periodic basis. Periodic use of intense point stimulation gives maximal pain relief for a period of time and allows some gains in overall pain suppression. Daily intense point stimulation may eventually bias the central nervous system and decrease the effectiveness of this type of stimulation.[57]

PLACEBO EFFECT OF ELECTRICAL STIMULATION

All three of these theories of sensory electrical stimulation produce their effects on the transmission lines of pain by interrupting or slowing the flow of pain information to the brain. The brain is the reception and interpretation center for these pain messages, and incorporating this area into your treatment can enhance the treatment's effects. This is crucial to a successful treatment because the therapist is trying to alter the patient's pain perception. This perceptual change is influenced by many factors at the cognitive and affective levels.

There is a major placebo effect in all that we do in providing any therapy to our patients. This placebo effect is a basic and extremely important tool to help us achieve the best results. Our attitude toward the patients and our presentation of the therapy to them are crucial. When the therapist demonstrates a sincere interest in the patient's problems, the patient uses that interest to add to his or her own conviction and motivation to get well.

When these factors are active, real physiologic changes occur that assist in the healing process. The therapist should not intentionally deceive the patient with a sham treatment but should use the treatment to have the best impact on the patient's perception of the problem and the treatment's effectiveness.

The treatment will work better if the patient has a profound belief in the treatment's ability to alleviate the problem. To gain the most from this effect, the patient needs to be intimately involved with the treatment. We must educate, encourage, and empower the patient to get better. Giving the patient the knowledge and ability to feel some control and to be self-determined in healing reduces the stress of injury and enhances the patient's recovery powers. In stressful situations any measure of control lessens the extent of the stress and results in the improvement of disease resistance or injury recovery factors that will improve treatment outcomes.[57]

CLINICAL USES OF LOW-VOLTAGE CONTINUOUS DIRECT CURRENT

MEDICAL GALVANISM

The application of continuous low-voltage direct current causes several physiologic changes that can be used therapeutically. The therapeutic benefits are related to the polar and vasomotor effects and to the acid reaction around the positive pole and the alkaline reaction at the negative pole. The therapist must be concerned with the damaging effects of this variety of current. Acidic or alkaline changes can cause severe skin reactions.[119] These reactions occur only with low-voltage continuous direct current and are not likely with the high-voltage pulsed generators. The pulse duration of the high-voltage pulsed generators is too short to cause these chemical changes.[93]

There is also a vasomotor effect on the skin, increasing blood flow between the electrodes. The benefits from this type of direct current are usually attributed to the increased blood flow through the treatment area.[119]

The following protocols for continuous low-voltage direct current can be used to give the greatest vasomotor effects.

1. Current intensity should be to the patient's tolerance; it should be increased as accommodation takes place. These intensities are in the mamp range.
2. Continuous direct current should be used.
3. Pulses per second should be 0.
4. A low-voltage direct current stimulator is the machine of choice.

5. Treatment time should be between a 15-minute minimum and a 50-minute maximum.

6. Equal-sized electrodes are used over gauze that has been soaked in saline solution and lightly squeezed.

7. Skin should be unbroken (see Fig. 5-20).[62,91,95]

IONTOPHORESIS

Direct current has been used for many years to drive ions from the heavy metals into and through the skin for treatment of skin infections or for a counterirritating effect. Iontophoresis is discussed in detail in Chapter 6.

TREATMENT PRECAUTIONS WITH CONTINUOUS DIRECT CURRENTS

Skin burns are the greatest hazard of any continuous direct current technique. These burns result from excessive electrical density in any area, usually from direct metal contact with skin or from setting the intensity too high for the size of the active electrode. Both these problems cause a very high density of current in the area of contact.[91,95]

FUNCTIONAL ELECTRICAL STIMULATION (FES)

Since the mid 1980s researchers have experimented with using computer-controlled electrical currents that stimulate the peripheral nervous system for the purpose of providing dynamic assistance in functional activities, such as walking or upper extremity function.[72] Used primarily in patients who have sustained spinal cord injury or suffered a stroke, **functional electrical stimulation (FES)** utilizes multiple-channel electrical stimulators controlled by a microprocessor to recruit muscles in a programmed synergistic sequence that will allow the patient to accomplish a specific functional movement pattern.[38,72] Even though this technique has been used effectively in short-term management of a variety of dysfunctions, there are many practical considerations for use that might impede or limit the long-term independent usefulness of FES by a patient.[6]

Currently, the majority of FES programs are limited to the use of surface electrodes that are difficult to adhere to the skin and to maintain positioning at the appropriate stimulation point.[54] For FES to be useful to the patient on a daily basis, the electrodes, and possibly the stimulator itself, will need to be implanted directly into the muscle or on a nerve.[1,45] Research is ongoing toward this end, but to date no acceptable system has been developed.

The existing computer control systems for FES also need to be refined if they are to be both useful and safe for the patient. The control systems must use either a preset activation sequence that will allow the patient to execute a specific task, or there must be some type of feedback from the stimulated neuromuscular systems so that the computer can make the appropriate movement corrections to ensure the safety of the patient. The development of a "closed-loop" feedback control system that would allow the computer to compensate for uneven terrain or to adjust the speed and frequency of movement presents a major challenge to researchers working in this area.[127]

Although multichannel microprocessors may be preprogrammed to execute a variety of specific movement patterns, how those programs will be activated presents another obstacle for development of FES systems. Foot switches or crutch switches

functional electrical stimulation Utilizes multiple channel electrical stimulators to recruit muscles in a programmed sequence that produces a functional movement pattern.

may potentially be used to trigger a desired response, although there are limitations to the number of switches that a spinal cord or stroke patient would actually be able to use.[38] Some of the upper extremity control devices have used movements of the contralateral shoulder to trigger a response. Verbal commands recognized by the computer also have been used to control stimulation of muscle in various functional tasks.[6]

Presently long-term independent use of FES is practical for only a few problems.[6] Certainly as new technologies continue to become available, ongoing clinical research will make FES increasingly practical for various patient populations. The future of FES holds many exciting possibilities for patients and therapists alike.

CLINICAL USES OF FES

FES has a number of clinical applications.[69] Initially, FES was used for stroke patients with a foot drop to assist dorsiflexion. Subsequently it was found to be more useful in treating patients with incomplete spinal cord injury who have good stance stability but are unable to achieve adequate flexion during the swing phase of gait.[6]

Functional electrical stimulation has been used with some success, enabling patients to stand, transfer, ambulate on level surfaces, and even ascend stairs on a limited basis using a walker or crutches in a closely supervised environment.[14,43,61,67,79,109] Spinal cord patients have used computer-controlled FES to allow them to exercise on bicycle ergometers to improve cardiorespiratory endurance and fitness.[5,15]

Control of muscles in the upper extremity using multiple-channel stimulation has allowed paraplegic patients to use the muscles of the hand and forearm of the paralyzed limb in functional grasp patterns. FES has also been used effectively in managing shoulder subluxation in the hemiplegic patient.[6]

SPECIALIZED ELECTRICAL CURRENTS

LOW-INTENSITY STIMULATORS (LIS)

Another type of low-voltage equipment are the low-intensity stimulators (LIS). The characteristic that distinguishes this type of generator is that the intensity of the stimulus is limited to 1000 μamp or less in LIS, whereas the intensity of the standard low-voltage equipment can be increased into the mamp range.

LIS < 1 mA

Generators that produce low-intensity stimulation (LIS) are among the newer electrical therapy units available to today's therapist. These units were originally called microcurrent electrical neuromuscular stimulators (MENS). However, the stimulation pathway is not the usual neural pathway, and they are not designed to stimulate a muscle contraction. Consequently, this type of generator was subsequently referred to as a microcurrent electrical stimulator (MES). Low-intensity stimulator is the most recent and currently used term in an ongoing evolution of terminology relative to this type of stimulator.

Perhaps the most important point to emphasize is that currents generated by these devices are not substantially different from the currents discussed previously. These currents still have a direction, and both AC and DC waveforms are available. The currents also have amplitude (intensity), pulse duration, and frequency.

Low-intensity stimulator currents are defined as those of less than 1 mamp or 1000 μamps. The generators can generate a variety of waveforms from modified monophasic to biphasic square waves with frequencies from 0.3 to 50 Hz. The pulse durations are also variable and may be prolonged at the lower frequencies from 1 to

500 msec. This varies as the frequency changes or is preset when pulsed currents are used. Many of these devices are made with an impedance-sensitive voltage that adapts the current to the impedance to keep the current constant as selected.[97]

If the current generator can be adjusted to allow increases of intensity above 1000 μamps the current becomes like those previously described in this text. If the current provokes an action potential in a sensory or motor nerve, the results on that tissue will be the same as previously described for other currents' sensation or muscle contraction.

Most of the literature on microcurrents and subsequently on low-intensity stimulators has been generated by researchers interested in stimulating the healing process in fractures and skin wounds. Subsequent research aimed at identifying why and how microcurrents work. The best researched areas of application of LIS-type currents is in the stimulation of bone formation in delayed union or nonunion of fractures of the long bones. Most of this research was done using implanted rather than surface electrodes, and most have used low-intensity direct current (LIDC) with the negative pole placed at the fracture site.[3,8,33] We are in danger of generalizing treatments for all problems based on success in this one area. These applications were intended to mimic the normal electrical field created during the injury and healing process.[2,40] At present these electrical changes are poorly understood, and the effects of adding additional electric current to the normal electrical activity created by the injury and healing process are still being investigated.

As can be seen in the previous sections on the bioelectric properties of cells and tissues, there are several possible theories that might explain the biostimulative effects of LIS currents and give the therapist some guidance in developing clinical protocols.

The current of injury, stress-generated potentials, cell metabolism stimulation, and bioelectric fields guiding growth are all natural events that low-intensity stimulation may augment, stimulate, or artificially replace.[20,21]

Low-intensity stimulation has been used for two major effects:

1. analgesia of the painful area; and
2. biostimulation of the healing process, either for enhancing the process or for acceleration of its stages.[36]

Analgesic Effects of Low-Intensity Stimulation

The mechanism of analgesia created by LIS current does not fit into our present theoretical framework, as sensory nerve excitation is a necessary component of all three models of electroanalgesia stimulation. At best LIS can create or change the constant direct current flow of the neural tissues, which may have some way of biasing the transmission of the painful stimulus. Low-intensity stimulation may also make the nerve cell membrane more receptive to neurotransmitters that will block transmission. The exact mechanism has not yet been established. The research is also equivocal on the effectiveness of LIS to decrease pain. This lack of consensus and disagreement in the research gives the therapist limited security in devising an effective protocol. Most of the research using delayed-onset muscle soreness (DOMS) as a pain model have found no significant difference between LIS and placebo treatments.[17,37,47,60,68,82,99,101,120,122,128]

Promotion of Wound Healing

Low-intensity direct current has been used to treat skin ulcers that have poor blood flow. The treated ulcers show accelerated healing rates when compared with untreated skin ulcers.

LIS Effects
- Analgesia
- Fracture healing
- Wound healing
- Ligament and tendon healing

The following protocol was used to promote wound healing.

1. Current intensity was 200 to 400 μamp for normal skin and 400 to 800 μamp for denervated skin.
2. Long pulse durations or continuous uninterrupted currents can be used.
3. Maximum pulse frequency.
4. Monophasic direct current is best but biphasic direct current is acceptable. Low-intensity stimulators can be used but other generators with intensities adjusted to subsensory levels also can be effective. A battery-powered portable unit is most convenient.
5. Treatment time was 2 hours followed by a 4-hour rest time.
6. Utilize two to three treatment bouts per day.
7. The negative electrode is positioned in the wound area for the first 3 days. The positive electrode should be positioned 25 cm proximal to the wound.
8. After 3 days the polarity is reversed and the positive electrode is positioned in the wound area.
9. If infection is present, the negative electrode should be left in the wound area until the signs of infection are not evident. The negative electrode remains in the wound for 3 days after the infection clears.
10. If the wound size decreases plateau, then return the negative electrode to the wound area for 3 days.

Other protocols have been successful using the anode in the wound area for the entire time. High-voltage stimulation also has been used in a manner similar to the negative-positive model presented. The intensity was adjusted to give a microamp current.

The mechanism by which LIS stimulates healing is elusive, but cells are stimulated to increase their normal proliferation, migration, motility, DNA synthesis, and collagen synthesis. Receptor levels for growth factor have also shown a significant increase when wound areas are stimulated.[18,22,23,44,46,49,58,75,90,118,121,126] The naturally occurring electrical potential gradients are enhanced following electrical stimulation.[47]

Promotion of Fracture Healing

The use of low-intensity direct current may be an adjunctive modality in the treatment of fractures, especially fractures prone to nonunion. Fracture healing may be accelerated by passing a direct current through the fracture site. Getting the current into the bony area without an invasive technique is difficult.[9,16,19,20,28,33,59,96,113]

Using a standard transcutaneous electrical nerve stimulation unit, Kahn reported favorable results in the electrical stimulation of callus formation in fractures that had nonunions after 6 months.[62] This information is based on a case study. Results of a more extensive population of nonunions have not been documented. Kahn used the following protocol.

1. Current intensity was just perceptible to the patient.
2. Pulse duration was the longest duration allowed on the unit (100–200 msec).
3. Pulses per second were set at the lowest frequency allowed on the unit (5–10 pps).
4. Standard monophasic or biphasic current in the transcutaneous electrical stimulating units were used.
5. Treatment time was from 30 minutes to 1 hour, three to four times daily.
6. A negative electrode was placed close to but distal to the fracture site. A positive electrode was placed proximal to the immobilizing device.
7. If four pads were used, the interferential placement described earlier was used.
8. Results were reassessed at monthly intervals (see Fig. 5-20).[62]

CASE STUDY 5-4
ELECTRICAL STIMULATING CURRENTS: CONTROL OF SWELLING

Background: A 43-year-old woman recreational runner sustained a grade II ankle sprain (inversion stress) approximately 4 hours prior to presentation for treatment. She is ambulatory in a touch weight-bearing mode with crutches and is not in acute distress. Positive signs are limited to the ankle, which demonstrates 3+/4 swelling, marked restriction in range of motion, and point tenderness over the anterior talofibular and calcaneal-fibular ligaments. There is no loss of ligamentous stability.

Impression: Grade II ankle sprain, with significant swelling.

Treatment Plan: In addition to therapeutic exercise, electrical stimulation was selected to assist in the reduction of the swelling. A monophasic pulsatile waveform generator was selected, and the cathode (negative polarity) was placed over the anterolateral aspect of the ankle, with the anode over the posterior leg. The pulse rate was set at 120 pps, with the amplitude between the sensory and motor thresholds. Stimulation was applied for 30 minutes daily.

Response: The swelling was reduced by approximately 30 percent after the initial treatment, but had returned the next day. Over the next 5 days, the swelling was markedly reduced following treatment, but regressed by about 50 percent by the next day. Electrical stimulation was discontinued after 7 days. A progressive rehabilitation program was initiated the first day, and the patient returned to full activity after 3 weeks.

Discussion Questions

- What tissues were injured or affected?
- What symptoms were present?
- What phase of the injury-healing continuum did the patient present for care in?
- What are the physical agent modality's biophysical effects (direct, indirect, depth, and tissue affinity)?
- What are the physical agent modality's indications and contraindications?
- What are the parameters of the physical agent modality's application, dosage, duration, and frequency in this case study?
- What other physical agent modalities could be used to treat this injury or condition? Why? How?

The rehabilitation professional employs physical agent modality to create an optimum environment for tissue healing while minimizing the symptoms associated with the trauma or condition.

Promotion of Healing in Tendon and Ligament

There are only a few research studies on the biostimulative effect of electrical stimulation on tendon or ligament healing. Both tissues have been found to generate strain-generated electric potentials naturally in response to stress. These potentials help signal the tissue to grow in response to the stress according to Wolff's law.

In an experimental study on partial division of dog patellar tendons treated with 20 μamp cathodal stimulation, the stimulated tendons showed 92 percent recovery of normal breaking strength at 8 weeks.[110]

Tendon stimulated in vitro in a culture medium showed increased fibroblastic cellular activity, tendon cellular proliferation, and collagen synthesis. The rate at which stimulated tendons demonstrated histologic repair at the injury site was also significantly accelerated over the control group.[92] Litke and Dahners studied rat medial collateral ligament (MCL) injuries treated with electrical simulation. The treated group showed statistical significance in the rupture force, stiffness, energy absorbed, and laxity.[76]

As can be seen by the previous sections, LIS current can be a valuable addition to the clinical armamentarium of the therapist, but it is untested clinically.

This is a case where more may not be better. For electricity to produce these effects (1) cells must be current-sensitive; (2) correct polarity orientation may be necessary; and (3) correct amounts of current will cause the cells to be more active in the healing process

If results are not going correctly, then reduce the current and/or change polarity. Weak stimuli may increase physiologic activity, whereas very much stronger stimuli abolish or inhibit activity.

Most generators in use today are capable of low-intensity current. Simply turn the machine on but do not increase the intensity to threshold levels. This also be a function of current density using electrode size and placement as well as intensity to keep current in the µamp range.

The therapist is certainly entitled to be very skeptical of the manufacturers' claims until more research is reported. Existing protocols for use are not well established, which leaves the therapist with an insecure feeling about this modality.

RUSSIAN CURRENTS (MEDIUM-FREQUENCY CURRENT GENERATORS)

This class of current generators was developed in Canada and the United States after the Russian scientist Yadou M. Kots presented a seminar on the use of electrical muscular stimulators to augment strength gain. The stimulators developed after this presentation were termed "Russian Current" generators. These stimulators have evolved and presently deliver a medium-frequency (2000–10,000 Hz) polyphasic AC waveform. The pulse can be varied from 50 to 250 µsec; the phase duration will be one-half of the pulse duration, or 25 to 125 µsec. As the pulse frequency increases, the pulse duration decreases.[21,40,48] There are two basic waveforms: a sine wave and a square wave cycle with a fixed intrapulse interval.

The sine wave is produced in a burst mode that has a 50 percent duty cycle. According to strength-duration curve data, to obtain the same stimulation effect as the duration of the stimulus decreases, the intensity must be increased. The intensity associated with this duration of current could be considered as painful.

To make this intensity of current tolerable, it is generated in 50-burst-per-second envelopes with an interburst interval of 10 msec. This slightly reduces the total current but allows enough of a peak current intensity to stimulate muscle very well (Fig. 5-22). If the current continued without the burst effect, the total current delivered would equal the lightly shaded area in Fig. 5-23. When generated with the burst effect, the total current is decreased. Here the total current would equal the darkly shaded area in Fig. 5-24. This allows tolerance of greater current intensity by the patient. The other factor affecting patient comfort is the effect that frequency will have on the impedance of the tissue. Higher-frequency currents reduce the resistance to the current flow, again making this type of waveform comfortable enough that the patient may tolerate higher intensities. As the intensity increases, more motor nerves are stimulated, increasing the magnitude of the contraction.

Russian Current A medium frequency (2000–10,000 Hz) polyphasic AC wave generated in 50-burst-per-second envelopes.

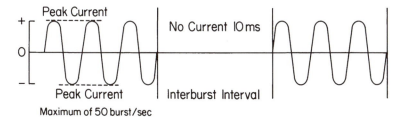

•**Figure 5-22** Russian current with polyphasic AC wave form and 10-ms interburst interval.

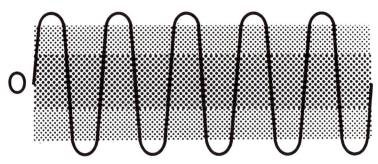

•**Figure 5-23** Russian current without an interburst interval. The light shaded area is equal to the total current.

Because it is a fast oscillating AC current, as soon as the nerve repolarizes it is stimulated again, producing a current that will maximally summate muscle contraction.

The frequency (pulses per second or, in this case, bursts per second) is also a variable that can be controlled. This would make the muscle respond with a twitch rather than a gradually increasing mechanical contraction. Gradually increasing the numbers of bursts interrupts the mechanical relaxation cycle of the muscle and causes more shortening to take place (see Fig. 5-18).[91]

INTERFERENTIAL CURRENTS

The research and use of interferential currents (IFC) has taken place primarily in Europe. An Austrian scientist, Ho Nemec, introduced the concept and suggested its therapeutic use. Nemec's concept resulted in the creation of a type of electrical generator that is difficult to understand, not because the theory is so complex, but because electrical engineers added so many options to the generator that the current can be modified substantially while still maintaining its basic waveform.

The theories and behavior of electrical waves are part of basic physics. This behavior is easiest to understand when continuous sine waves are used as an example.

With only one circuit the current behaves as described earlier; if put on an oscilloscope, it looks like generator 1 in Fig. 5-25. If a second generator is brought into the same location, the currents may interfere with each other. This interference can be summative—that is, the amplitudes of the electric wave are combined and increase (see Fig. 5-25). Both waves are exactly the same; if they are produced in phase or originate at the same time, they combine. This is called **constructive interference**.

If these waves are generated out of sync, generator 1 starts in a positive direction at the same time that generator 2 starts in a negative direction; the waves then will cancel each other out. This is called **destructive interference**; in the summation the waves end up with an amplitude of 0 (Fig. 5-26).

constructive interference The combined amplitude of two distinct circuits increases the amplitude.

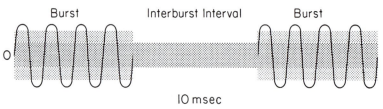

•**Figure 5-24** Russian current with an interburst interval. Dark shading represents total current, and light shading indicates total current without the interburst interval.

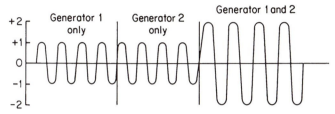

•**Figure 5-25** Sine wave from generator 1 and sine wave from generator 2 showing a constructive interference pattern.

To make this more complex, assume that one generator has a slightly slower or faster frequency and that the generators begin producing current simultaneously. Initially, the electric waves will be constructively summated; however, because the frequencies of the two waves differ, they gradually will get out of phase and become destructively summated. When dealing with sound waves, we hear distinct beats as this phenomenon occurs. We borrow the term **beat** when describing this behavior. When any waveforms are out of phase but are combined in the same location, the waves will cause a beat effect. The blending of the waves is caused by the constructive and destructive interference patterns of the waves and is called **heterodyne** (Fig. 5-27).[40,42]

The heterodyne effect is seen on an oscilloscope as a cyclic, rising and falling waveform.[112] The peaks or beat frequency in this heterodyne wave behavior occur regularly, according to the difference of each current; for example,

$$100 \text{ pps} - 90 \text{ pps} = 10 \text{ pps beat frequency}$$

In electric currents, this beat frequency is, in effect, the stimulation frequency of the waveform, because the destructive interference negates the effects of the other part of the wave. The intensity (amplitude) will be set according to sensations created by this peak.[40] When using an interference current for therapy, the therapist should select the frequencies to create a beat frequency corresponding to his or her choices of frequency when using other stimulators; 20 to 50 pps for muscle contraction, 50 to 120 pps for pain management, and 1 pps for acustim pain relief.

When the electrodes are arranged in a square alignment and interferential currents are passed through a homogeneous medium, a predictable pattern of interference will occur. In this pattern, an electric field is created that resembles a four-petaled flower, with the center of the flower located where the two currents cross and

destructive interference Combined amplitude of two distinct circuits decreases the amplitude.

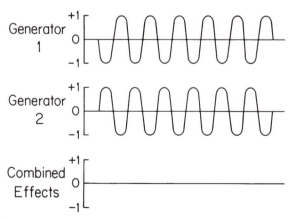

•**Figure 5-26** Sine wave from generator 1 and sine wave from generator 2 showing a destructive interference pattern.

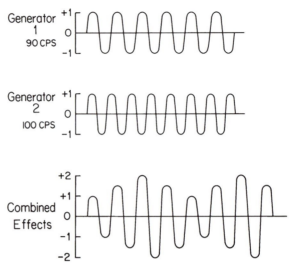

•**Figure 5-27** Sine wave from generator 1 at 90 cps and sine wave from generator 2 at 100 cps showing the heterodyne or beating pattern of interference.

the petals falling between the electric current force lines. The maximum interference effect takes place near the center, with the field gradually decreasing in strength as it moves toward the points of the petal (Fig. 5-28).[40]

Because the body is not a homogeneous medium, we cannot predict the exact location of this interference pattern; we must rely on the patient's perception. If the patient has a localized structure that is painful, locating the stimulation in the correct location is relatively easy. The therapist moves the electrode placement until the patient centers the feeling of the stimulus in the problem area.[40,42] When a patient has poorly localized pain, the task becomes more difficult. See the discussion in the electrode placement section for a general discussion on the effect of electrode movement. The engineers added features to the generators and created a scanning interferential current that moves the flower petals of force around while the treatment is taking place. This enlarges the effective treatment area. Additional technology and another set of electrodes create a three-dimensional flower effect when one looks at the electrical field. This is called a **stereodynamic interference current**.[40,42]

All these alterations and modifications are designed to spread the heterodyne effect throughout the tissue. Because it is controlled by a cyclic electrical pattern,

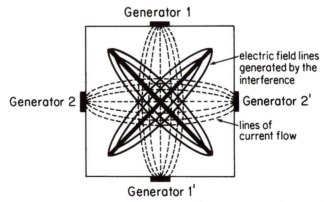

•**Figure 5-28** Square electrode alignment and interference pattern of current in a homogeneous medium.

however, we actually may be decreasing the current passed through the structures we are trying to treat. The machines seem complex but lack the versatility to do much more than the conventional TENS treatment.[91,108]

Nikolova[94] has used IFC for a variety of clinical problems and found them effective in dealing with pain problems (e.g., joint sprains with swelling; restricted mobility and pain; neuritis; retarded callus formation following fractures; pseudarthrosis).[94] These claims are supported by other researchers. Each of these researchers used slightly different protocols in treating the different clinical problems. To be successful in achieving the desired results with interferential currents, the therapist must thoroughly review existing protocols and acquire a good working knowledge of the application techniques.

The world of electrical therapy is constantly changing, owing to the advances in research, engineering, and technology and because of the competitive pressures of the marketplace. Equipment manufacturers will develop a different machine and try to market it on the basis of a single feature of their product. The old adage "let the buyer beware" is certainly good advice. The more understanding of electrical currents the therapist has, the less likely he or she is to be "snowed" or confused by the sales spiel. Even more important, the greater the understanding, the easier it becomes to manipulate the treatment protocols to optimize results for each patient.[57]

stereodynamic interference current
Three distinct circuits blending and creating a distinct electrical wave pattern.

SUMMARY

1. When an electrical system is applied to muscle or nerve tissue, the result will be tissue membrane depolarization, provided that the current has the appropriate intensity, duration, and waveform to reach the tissue's excitability threshold.

2. Nerve function and muscle contraction are the same regardless of the stimulation mechanism (i.e., natural or electrical).

3. Muscle and nerve tissue respond in an all-or-none fashion; there is no gradation of response.

4. Constant direct current has several major influences. The primary uses involve polar effects (acid or alkaline), increased blood flow, bacteriostatic effects (negative electrode), and migration and alignment of cellular building blocks in the healing processes.

5. Nonexcitatory cells and tissues respond to electric current and contain continuous direct current circuits.

6. The body responds to injury by producing changes in the local electric circuits that may guide and assist the healing process.

7. Sensory level stimulation may retard edema accumulation in traumatic injuries.

8. Muscle contraction will change according to changes in current. As the frequency of the electrical stimulus increases, the muscle will develop more tension as a result of the summation of the contraction of the muscle fiber through progressive mechanical shortening. Increases in intensity spread the current over a larger area and increase the number of motor units activated by the current. Increases in the duration of the current also will cause more motor units to be activated.

9. Electrically stimulated muscle contractions are used clinically to help with muscle reeducation, muscle contraction for muscle pumping action, reduction of swelling, prevention or retardation of atrophy, muscle strengthening, and increasing range of motion in tight joints.

10. To stimulate a given muscle, location of the muscle's motor point, size and spacing of electrodes, and impedance of the tissue between the electrodes and the motor points must be selected and adjusted to provide the most effective therapy.

11. Electrically stimulated discharges of sensory nerves help decrease pain perceptions.

12. The pain gating effect of electrical stimulation may occur at different levels in the central nervous system, depending on the type of electrical current used. Types of current similar to that used in transcutaneous electrical nerve stimulation will be gated at the spinal cord level. Hyperstimulation analgesia will stimulate central biasing with inhibitory influences descending from the brain and brain stem levels. Noxious stimuli to acupuncture or trigger areas will cause production of β-endorphin in the spinal cord and brain, with a resultant analgesic effect.

13. Specialized current waveforms (low-intensity stimulation, "Russian," interferential, etc.) all have physiologic responses that can be attributed to the characteristics of their waveforms. The differences in the waveforms and the physiologic response of each have particular effects that can be used therapeutically.

REFERENCES

1. Agnew, W., McCreery, D., and Bullara, L.: Effects of prolonged electrical stimulation of peripheral nerve. In Agnew, W., McCreery, D.: Neural prosthesis: fundamental studies, Englewood Cliffs, NJ, 1990, Prentice-Hall.

2. Alon, G.: High voltage stimulation: effects of electrode size on basic excitatory responses. Phys. Ther. 65:890, 1985.

3. Alon, G., DeDomeico, G.: High voltage stimulation: an integrated approach to clinical electrotherapy. Chattanooga, Tennessee, Chattanooga Corp., 1987.

4. American Physical Therapy Association: Electrotherapeutic terminology in physical therapy, Alexandria, Virginia, 1990, APTA Publications.

5. Arnold, P., McVey, S.: Functional electric stimulation: its efficacy and safety in improving pulmonary function and musculoskeletal fitness, Arch. Phys. Med. Rehab. 73(7):665–668, 1992.

6. Baker, L., McNeal, D., and Benton, L.: Neuromuscular electrical stimulation, Downey, California, 1993, Rancho Los Amigos Medical Center.

7. Becker, R.: The bioelectric factors in amphibian-limb regeneration, J. Bone Joint Surg. (Am): 43-A:643–656, 1961.

8. Becker, R., Bachman, C., and Friedman, H.: The direct current control system, NY J. Med. 62:1169–1176, 1962.

9. Becker, R., Selden, G.: The body electric, New York, 1985, William Morrow & Co., Inc.

10. Benton, L., Baker, L., and Bowman, B.: Functional electrical stimulation: a practical clinical guide, Downey, California, 1980, Rancho Los Amigos Hospital.

11. Bettany, J.: Influence of high voltage pulsed current on edema formation following impact injury, Phys. Ther. 70:219–224, 1990.

12. Binder-MacLeod, S., Snyder-Mackler, L.: Muscle fatigue: clinical implications for fatigue assessment and neuromuscular electrical stimulation. Phys. Ther. 73:902–910, 1993.

13. Bishop, B.: Pain: its physiology and rationale for management, Phys. Ther. 60:13–37, 1980.

14. Bogataj, U., Gros, N., and Kljajic, M.: The rehabilitation of gait in patients with hemiplegia: a comparison between conventional therapy and multichannel functional electrical stimulation therapy, Phys. Ther. 75(6):490–502, 1995.

15. Bradley, M.: The effect of participating in a functional electrical stimulation exercise program on affect in people with spinal cord injuries, Arch. Phys. Med. Rehab. 75(6):676–679, 1994.

16. Brighton, C.: Bioelectric effects on bone and cartilage, Clin. Orthop. 124:2–4, 1977.

17. Brown, S.: The effect of microcurrent on edema, range of motion, and pain in treatment of lateral ankle sprains, abstract. J. Orthop. Sports Phys. Ther. 19:55, 1994.

18. Carley, P., Wainapel, S.: Electrotherapy for the acceleration of wound healing: low-intensity direct current, Arch. Phys. Med. Rehab. 66:443–446, 1985.

19. Castel, J.: Pain management with acupuncture and transcutaneous electrical nerve stimulation techniques and photo simulation (laser). Symposium on Pain Management, Walter Reed Army Medical Center, Nov. 13, 1982.

20. Charman, R.: Bioelectricity and electrotherapy—towards a new paradigm? Part 1, the cell. Part 2, cellular reception and emission of electromagnetic signals, Physiotherapy 76:502–518; Part 3, bioelectric potentials and tissue currents, Physiotherapy 76:643–654; Part 4, strain generated potentials in bone and connective tissue, Physiotherapy 76:725–730; Part 5, exogenous currents and fields—experimental and clinical applications, Physiotherapy 76:743–750, 1990.

21. Charman, R.: Bioelectricity and electrotherapy—towards a

new paradigm. Part 6, environmental current and fields—the natural background, Physiotherapy 77:8–13; Part 7, environmental currents and fields—man made, Physiotherapy 77:129–140; Part 8, grounds for a new paradigm? Physiotherapy 77:211–221, 1991.

22. Chreng, N., Van Houf, H., and Bockx, E.: The effects of electric current on ATP generation, protein synthesis, and membrane transport in rat skin, Clin. Orthop. Relat. Res. 171:264–272, 1982.

23. Chu, C.: Weak direct current accelerates split thickness. Graft healing on tangentially excised second-degree burns, J. Burn Care Rehab. 12:285–1293, 1991.

24. Clements, F.: Effect of motor neuromuscular electrical stimulation on microvascular perfusion of stimulated rat skeletal muscle, Phys. Ther. 71:397–406, 1991.

25. Clement-Jones, V.: Increased β-endorphin but not metenkephalin levels in human cerebrospinal fluid after acupuncture for recurrent pain, Lancet, Nov. 1, 8:946–948, 1980.

26. Clemente, F., Barron, K.: Transcutaneous neuromuscular electrical stimulation effect on the degree of microvascular perfusion in autonomically denervated rat skeletal muscle. Arch. Phys. Med. Rehab. 77(2):155–160, 1996.

27. Cole, B., Gardiner, P.: Does electrical stimulation of denervated muscle continued after reinnervation, influence recovery of contractile function, Exp. Neurol. 85:52, 1984.

28. Connolly, J., Hahn, H., and Jardon, O.: The electrical enhancement of periosteal proliferation in normal and delayed fracture healing, Clin. Orthop. 124:97–105, 1977.

29. Cook, H., et al.: Effect of electrical stimulation on lymphatic flow and limb volume in the rat, Phys. Ther. 74:1040–1046, 1994.

30. Cosgrove, K., Alon, G.: The electrical effect of two commonly used clinical stimulators on traumatic edema in rats, Phys. Ther. 72:227–233, 1992.

31. Cummings, J.: Electrical stimulation of denervated muscle. In Gersch, M.: Electrotherapy in rehabilitation, Philadelphia, 1992, F.A. Davis.

32. Currier, D., Lehman, J., and Lightfoot, P.: Electrical stimulation in exercise of the quadriceps femoris muscle, Phys. Ther. 59:1508–1512, 1979.

33. Currier, D., Mann, R.: Muscular strength development by electrical stimulation in healthy individuals, Phys. Ther. 63:915–921, 1983.

34. Dallmann, S.: Preference for low versus medium frequency electrical stimulation at constant induced muscle forces, abstract R345, Phys. Ther. 725:5107, 1992.

35. Delitto, A.: A study of discomfort with electrical stimulation, Phys. Ther. 72:410–424, 1992.

36. Denegar, C.: The effects of low-volt microamperage stimulation on delayed onset muscle soreness, J. Sport Rehab. 1:95–102, 1993.

37. Denegar, C.: Influence of transcutaneous electrical nerve stimulation on pain, range of motion, and serum cortisol concentration in females experiencing delayed onset muscle soreness, J. Orthop. Sports Phys. Ther. 11:100–103, 1989.

38. DeVahl, J.: Neuromuscular electrical stimulation (NMES) in rehabilitation, In Gersh, M.: Electrotherapy in rehabilitation, Philadelphia, 1992, F.A. Davis.

39. Eriksson, E., Haggmark, T.: Comparison of isometric muscle training and electrical stimulation supplement, isometric muscle training in the recovery after major knee ligament surgery. Am. J. Sports Med. 7:169–171, 1979.

40. Fish, D.: Effect of anodal high voltage pulsed current on edema formation in frog hind limbs, Phys. Ther. 71:724–733, 1991.

41. Flicker, M.T.: An analysis of cold intermittent compression with simultaneous treatment of electrical stimulation in the reduction of postacute ankle lymphadema, unpublished master's thesis, University of North Carolina, Chapel Hill, North Carolina, May, 1993.

42. Franklin, M.E.: Effect of varying the ratio of electrically induced muscle contraction time to rest time on serum creatine kinase and perceived soreness. J. Orthop. Sports Phys. Ther. 13:310–315, 1991.

43. Gallien, P., Brisso, R., and Eyssette, M.: Restoration of gait by functional electrical stimulation for spinal cord injured patients, Paraplegia 33(11):660–664, 1995.

44. Gault, W., Gatens, P.: Use of low-intensity direct current in management of ischemic skin ulcers, Phys. Ther. 56:265–269, 1976.

45. Gellman, H., Waters, R., and Lewonski, K.: Histologic comparison of chronic implantation of nerve cuff and epineural electrodes, Adv. Ext. Control Hum. Extrem. Dubrovnick, Yugoslavia, 1990.

46. Gentzkow, G.: Electrical stimulation to heal dermal wounds, J. Derm. Surg. Oncol. 19:753–758, 1993.

47. Gersh, M.R.: Microcurrent electrical stimulation: putting it in perspective, Clin. Manage. 9(4):51–54, 1990.

48. Goodgold, J., Eberstein, A.: Electrodiagnosis of neuromuscular diseases, Baltimore, 1972, Williams & Wilkins.

49. Griffin, J.: Efficacy of high voltage pulsed current for healing of pressure ulcers in patients with spinal cord injury, Phys. Ther. 71:433–444, 1991.

50. Griffin, J.: Reduction of chronic posttraumatic hand edema: a comparison of high voltage pulsed current, intermittent pneumatic compression, and placebo treatments, Phys. Ther. 70:279–286, 1990.

51. Guyton, A.: Textbook of medical physiology, ed. 2, Philadelphia, 1961, W.B. Saunders.

52. Guffey, J., Asmussen, M.: In vitro bactericidal effects of high voltage pulsed current versus direct current against staphylococcus aureus, J. Clin. Electrophysiol. 1:5–9, 1989.

53. Gutman E., Guttman, L.: Effect of electrotherapy on denervated and reinnervated muscles in rabbit, Lancet 1:169, 1942.

54. Heller, B., Granat, M., and Andrews, B.: Swing-through gait with free-knees produced by surface functional electrical stimulation, Paraplegia 34(1):8–15, 1996.

55. Herbison, G., Jaweed, M., and Ditunno, J.: Acetylcholine sensitivity and fibrillation potentials in electrically stimulated crush-denervated rat skeletal muscle, Arch. Phys. Med. Rehab. 64:217, 1983.

56. Hooker, D.N.: personal communication, January 30, 1994.

57. Howson, D.: Report on neuromuscular reeducation, Minneapolis, 1978, Medical General.

58. Howson, D.C.: Peripheral neural excitability. Phys. Ther. 58:1467–1473, 1978.

59. Instruction manual for Electrostim. 180–182, Promatek, Canada, 1989.

60. Jeter, J., Valcenta, D.: The effects of microcurrent electrical nerve stimulation on delayed onset muscle soreness and peak torque deficits in trained weight lifters, abstract PO-R065-M. Phys. Ther. 735:5–24, 1993.

61. Kagaya, H., Shimada, Y.: Restoration and analysis of standing-up in complete paraplegia utilizing functional electrical stimulation, Arch. Phys. Med. Rehab. 76(9):876–881, 1995.

62. Kahn, J: Low-voltage technique. ed. 4, Syossett, New York, 1983, Joseph Kahn.

63. Karnes, J.: Effects of low-voltage pulsed current on edema formation in frog hind limbs following impact injury, Phys. Ther. 72:273–278, 1992.

64. Karnes, J.: Influence of high voltage pulsed current on diameters of anterioles during histamine-induced vasodilation, abstract R341, Phys. Ther. 725:5105, 1992.

65. Kincaid, C., Lavoie, K.: Inhibition of bacterial growth in vitro following stimulation with high voltage monophasic pulsed current, Phys. Ther. 69:651–655, 1989.

66. Kosman A., Osborne, S., and Ivey, A.: Comparative effectiveness of various electrical currents in preventing muscle atrophy in rat, Arch. Phys. Med. Rehab. 28:7, 1947.

67. Kralj, A., Badj, T., and Turk, R.: Enhancement of gait restoration in spinal cord injured patients by functional electrical stimulation, Clin. Orthop. 233:34, 1988.

68. Kulig, K.: Comparison of the effects of high velocity exercise and microcurrent neuromuscular stimulation on delayed onset muscle soreness, abstract R284, Phys. Ther. 715:5115, 1991.

69. Kumar, V., Lau, H., and Liu, J.: Clinical applications of functional electrical stimulation, Ann. Acad. Med. 24(3):428–435, 1995.

70. Lampe, G.: A clinical approach to transcutaneous electrical nerve stimulation in the treatment of chronic and acute pain, Minneapolis, July, 1978, Med. Gen.

71. Lampe, G.: Introduction to the use of transcutaneous electrical nerve stimulation devices, Phys. Ther. 58:1450–1454. 1978.

72. Larsson, L.: Functional electrical stimulation, Scand. J. Rehab. Ed. Supple. 30:63–72, 1994.

73. Laughman, R., Youdes, J., and Garrett, T.: Strength changes in the normal quadriceps femoris muscle as a result of electrical stimulation, Phys. Ther. 63:494–499, 1983.

74. Lea, J.: The effect of electrical stimulation on edematous rat hind paws, abstract R379, Phys. Ther. 725:5116, 1992.

75. Leffmann, D.: The effect of subliminal transcutaneous electrical stimulation on the rate of wound healing in rats, abstract R166, Phys. Ther. 725:567, 1992.

76. Litke, D., Dahners, L.: Effect of different levels of direct current on early ligament healing in a rat model, J. Orthop. Res. 12:683–688, 1994.

77. Malizia, E.: Electroacupuncture and peripheral β-endorphin and ACTH levels, Lancet, Sept 8:535–536, 1979.

78. Malezic, M., Hesse, S.: Restoration of gait by functional electrical stimulation in paraplegic patients: a modified programme of treatment, Paraplegia 33(3):126–131, 1995.

79. Mannheimer, J., Lampe, G.: Clinical transcutaneous electrical nerve stimulation, Philadelphia, 1984, F.A. Davis Co.

80. Marino, A., Becker, R.: Biologic effects of extremely low-frequency electric and magnetic fields: a review, Phys. Chem. Phys. 9:131–143, 1977.

81. Maurer, C.: The effectiveness of microelectrical neural stimulation on exercise-induced muscle trauma, abstract R200, Phys. Ther. 725:574, 1992.

82. Melzack, R.: The puzzle of pain, New York, 1973, Basic Books, Inc.

83. Melzack, R.: Prolonged relief of pain by brief, intense transcutaneous electrical stimulation, Pain 1(4):357–373, 1975.

84. Melzack, R., Stillwell, D., and Fox, E.: Trigger points and acupuncture points for pain: correlations and implications, Pain 3(1):3–23, 1977.

85. Mendel, F.: High voltage pulsed current using surface electrodes: effect on acute edema formation after hyperflexion injury in frogs, J. Orthop. Sports Phys. Ther. 16:140–144, 1992.

86. Mendel, F.: Influence of high voltage pulsed current on edema formation following impact injury in rats, Phys. Ther. 72:668–673, 1992.

87. Michlovitz, S.: Ice and high voltage pulsed stimulation in treatment of acute lateral ankle sprains, J. Orthop. Sports Phys. Ther. 9:301–304, 1988.

88. Mohr, T., Akers, T., and Landry, R.: Effect of high voltage stimulation on edema reduction in the rat hind limb, Phys. Ther. 67:1703–1707, 1987.

89. Mulder, G.: Treatment of open-skin wounds with electric stimulation, Arch. Phys. Med. Rehabil. 72:375–377, 1991.

90. Lomo, T., Slater, C.: Control of acetylcholine sensitivity and synapse formation by muscle activity, J. Physiol. 275:391, 1978.

91. Nelson, R., Currier, D.: Clinical electrotherapy. Norwalk, Connecticut, 1987, Appleton & Lange.

92. Nessler, J., Mass, P.: Direct current electrical stimulation of tendon healing in vitro, Clin. Orthop. Rel. Res. 217:303–312, 1987.

93. Newton, R., Karselis, T.: Skin pH following high voltage pulsed galvanic stimulation, Phys. Ther. 63:1593–1596, 1983.

94. Nikolova, L.: Treatment with interferential current, New York, 1987, Churchill Livingstone.

95. Notes on low volt therapy. White Plains, New York, 1966, TECA Corp.

96. Pettine, K.: External electrical stimulation and bracing for treatment of spondylolysis—a case report, Spine 188:436–439, 1993.

97. Picker, R.: Current trends: low volt pulsed microamp stimulation. Parts 1 and 2, Clin. Manage. 9:11–14; 9:(3)28–33, 1990.

98. Randall, B., Imig, C., and Hines, H.M.: Effect of electrical stimulation upon blood flow and temperature of skeletal muscles, Arch. Phys. Med. 33:73–78, 1952.

99. Rapaski, D.: Microcurrent electrical stimulation: comparison

of two protocols in reducing delayed onset muscle soreness, abstract R286, Phys. Ther. 715:5116, 1991.

100. Reed, B.: Effect of high voltage pulsed electrical stimulation on microvascular permeability to plasma proteins: a possible mechanism in minimizing edema, Phys. Ther. 68:491–495, 1988.

101. Rolle, W., Alon, G., and Nirschl, R.: Comparison of subliminal and placebo stimulation in the management of elbow epicondylitis, abstract R280, Phys. Ther. 715:5114, 1991.

102. Salar, G.: Effect of transcutaneous electrotherapy on CSF β-endorphin content in patients without pain problems, Pain 10:169–72, 1981.

103. Schimrigk, K., Mclaughlen, J., and Gruniger, W.: The effect of electrical stimulation on the experimentally denervated rat muscle, Scand. J. Rehab. Med. 9:55, 1977.

104. Selkowitz, D.: High frequency electrical stimulation in muscle strengthening. Am. J. Sport Med. 17:103–111, 1989.

105. Selkowitz, D.: Improvement in isometric strength of the quadriceps femores muscle after training with electrical stimulation, Phys. Ther. 65:186–196, 1985.

106. Siff, M.: Applications of electrostimulation in physical conditioning: a review. J. Appl. Sport Sci. Res. 4:20–26, 1990.

107. Synder-Mackler, L., Garrett, M., and Roberts, M.: A comparison of torque generating capabilities of three different electrical stimulating currents, J. Orthop. Sports Phys. Ther. 10:297–301, 1989.

108. Snyder, S.: Opiate receptors and internal opiates, Sci. Am. 236:44–56, 1977.

109. Stallard, J., Major, R.: The influence of orthosis stiffness on paraplegic ambulation and its implications for functional electrical stimulation (FES) walking, Prosth. Orthot. Int. 19(2): 108–114, 1995.

110. Stanish, W., Gunnlaugson, B.: Electrical energy and soft tissue injury healing, Sport Care and Fitness, Sept/Oct: 12–14, 1988.

111. Stillwell, G.: Therapeutic electricity and ultraviolet radiation, Baltimore, 1983, Williams & Wilkins.

112. Svacina, L.: Modified interferential technique, Pain Control, April 1978, pp. 1–2, Staodynamics, Inc.

113. Szabo, G., Illes, T.: Experimental stimulation of osteogenesis induced by bone matrix. Orthopaedics 14:63–67, 1991.

114. Taylor, K.: Effect of electrically induced muscle contraction on post traumatic edema formation in frog hind limbs. Phys. Ther. 72:127–132, 1992.

115. Taylor, K.: Effect of a single 30-minute treatment of high voltage pulsed current on edema formation in frog hind limbs, Phys. Ther. 72:63–68, 1992.

116. Thom, H.: Treatment of paralysis with exponentially progressive current, Br. J. Phys. Med. 20:49, 1957.

117. Travell, J., Simon, D.: Myofascial pain and dysfunction: the trigger point manual, Baltimore, 1983, Williams & Wilkins.

118. Unger, P.: A randomized clinical trial of the effects of HVPC on wound healing, abstract R294, Phys. Ther. 715:5118, 1991.

119. Watkins, A.: A manual of electrotherapy, ed. 3, Philadelphia, 1968, Lea & Febiger.

120. Weber, W.: The effect of MENS on pain and torque deficits associated with delayed onset muscle soreness, abstract R034, Phys. Ther. 715:535, 1991.

121. Weiss, D., Kirsner, R., and Eaglstein, W.: Electrical stimulation and wound healing, Arch. Dermatol. 126:222–225, 1990.

122. Wolcot, C.: A comparison of the effects of high voltage and microcurrent stimulation on delayed onset muscle soreness, abstract R287, Phys. Ther. 715:5116, 1991.

123. Wolf, S.: Perspectives on central nervous system responsiveness to transcutaneous electrical nerve stimulation, Phys. Ther. 58:1443–1449, 1978.

124. Wolf, S.: Electrotherapy, New York, 1981, Churchill Livingstone.

125. Wolf, S., Gersh, M., and Kutner, M.: Relationship of selected clinical variables to current delivered during transcutaneous electrical nerve stimulation, Phys. Ther. 58:1478–1483, 1978.

126. Wood, J.: A multicenter study on the use of pulsed low-intensity direct current for healing chronic stage II and stage III decubitus ulcers, Arch. Dermatol. 129:999–1009, 1993.

127. Yamamoto, T., Seireg. A.: Closing the loop: electrical muscle stimulation and feedback control for smooth limb motion, Soma 4:38, 1986.

128. Young, S.: Efficacy of interferential current stimulation alone for pain reduction in patients with osteoarthritis of the knee: a randomized placebo control clinical trial, abstract R088. Phys. Ther. 715:552, 1991.

SUGGESTED READINGS

Abdel-Moty, E., Fishbain, D., and Goldberg, M.: Functional electrical stimulation treatment of postradiculopathy associated muscle weakness, Arch. Phys. Med. Rehab. 75(6):680–686, 1994.

Akyuz, G.: Transcutaneous electrical nerve stimulation (TENS) in the treatment of postoperative pain and prevention of paralytic ileus, Clin. Rehab. 7(3):218–221, 1993.

Allen, J., Mattacola, C., and Perrin, D.: Microcurrent stimulation effect on delayed onset muscle soreness, J. Ath. Train. 31:S-47, 1996.

Alon, G., Kantor, G., and Ho, H.: Effects of electrode size on ba-sic excitatory responses and on selected stimulus parameters, J. Orthop. Sports Phys. Ther. 20(1):29–35, 1994.

Alon, G., Kantor, G., and Ho, H.: Effects of electrode size on basic excitatory responses and on selected stimulus parameters, J. Orthop. Sports Phys. Ther. 20(1):29–35, 1994.

Alon, G., Allin, T. and Inbar V.: Optimization of pulse duration and pulse charge during transcutaneous electrical stimulation, Aust. J. Physiother. 29:195, 1983.

Alon, G., Bainbridge, J., and Croson, G.: High-voltage pulsed direct current effects on peripheral blood flow, Phys. Ther. 61:678, 1981.

Alon, G.: High voltage stimulation: effects of electrode size on basic excitatory responses, Phys. Ther. 65:890, 1985.

Andersson, S., Hansson, G., and Holmgren, E.: Evaluation of the pain suppression effect of different frequencies of peripheral electrical stimulation in chronic pain conditions, Acta Orthop. Scand. 47:149, 1979.

Andersson, S.: Pain control by sensory stimulation. In Bonica, J.J., et al., editors: Advances in pain research and therapy, New York, 1979, Raven, vol. 3, pp. 569–584.

Aubin, M., Marks, R.: The efficacy of short-term treatment with transcutaneous electrical nerve stimulation for osteo-arthritic knee pain, Physiotherapy 81(11):669–675, 1995.

Baker, L.: Neuromuscular electrical stimulation in the restoration of purposeful limb movements. In Wolf, S.L., editor: Electrotherapy-clinics in physical therapy, New York, 1981, Churchill Livingstone.

Balogun, J., Onilari, O.: High voltage electrical stimulation in the augmentation of muscle strength: effects of pulse frequency, Arch. Phys. Med. Rehab. 74(9):910–916, 1993.

Bending, J.: TENS relief of discomfort, Physiotherapy 79(11): 773–774, 1993.

Benton, L., Baker, L., and Bowman, B.: Functional electrical stimulation a practical clinical guide, ed. 2, Downey, California, 1981, Professional Staff Association of Rancho Los Amigos Medical Center.

Berlandt, S.: Method of determining optimal stimulation sites for transcutaneous nerve stimulation, Phys. Ther. 64:924,1984.

Binder-Macleod, S., McDermond, L.: Changes in the force-frequency relationship of the human quadriceps femoris muscle following electrically and voluntarily induced fatigue, Phys. Ther. 72(2):95–104, 1992.

Brown, M., Cotter, M., and Hudlicka, O.: Metabolic changes in long-term stimulated fast muscles. In Howland, H., Poortmans, J.R., editors: Metabolic adaptation to prolonged physical exercise, Basel, 1975, Birkhauser.

Brown, M., Cotter, M., and Hudlicka, O.: The effects of long-term stimulation of fast muscles on their ability to withstand fatigue, J. Physiol. (Lond) 238:47, 1974.

Burr, H., Taffel, M., and Harvey, S.: An electrometric study of the healing wound in man. Yale J. Biol. Med. 12:483, 1940.

Burr, H., Harvey, S.: Bio-electric correlates of wound healing, Yale J. Biol. Med. 11:103,1938–1939, 1939.

Buxton, B., Okasaki, E., and Hetzler, R.: Self selection of transcutaneous electrical nerve stimulation parameters for pain relief in injured athletes, J. Ath. Train. 29(2):178, 1994.

Byl, N., McKenzie, A., and West, J.: Pulsed microamperage stimulation: A controlled study of healing of surgically induced wounds in Yucatan pigs, Phys. Ther. 74(3):201–211, 1994.

Caggiano, E., Emrey, T., and Shirley, S.: Effects of electrical stimulation or voluntary contraction for strengthening the quadriceps femoris muscles in an aged male population, J. Orthop. Sports Phys. Ther. 20(1): 22–28, 1994.

Campbell, J.: A critical appraisal of the electrical output characteristics of ten transcutaneous nerve stimulators, Clin. Phys. Physiol. Meas. 3:141, 1982.

Carmick, J.: Clinical use of neuromuscular electrical stimulation for children with cerebral palsy, Part 1, lower extremity, Phys. Ther. 73(8):505–513, 1993.

Carmick, J.: Clinical use of neuromuscular electrical stimulation for children with cerebral palsy, Part 2, upper extremity, Phys. Ther. 73(8):514–522, 1993.

Chan, C., Chow, S.: Electroacupuncture in the treatment of posttraumatic sympathetic dystrophy (Sudek's atrophy), Br. J. Anesth. 53:899, 1981.

Chase, J.: Elicitation of periods of inhibition in human muscle by stimulation of cutaneous nerves, J. Bone Joint Surg. (Am.) 54:173–177, 1972.

Cook, H., Morales, M., and La Rosa, E.: Effects of electrical stimulation on lymphatic flow and limb volume in the rat, Phys. Ther. 74(11):1040–1046, 1994.

Cooperman, A.: Use of transcutaneous electrical stimulation in the control of post operative pain. Results of a prospective, randomized, controlled study, Am. J. Surg. 133:185, 1977.

Curico, F., Berweger, R.: A clinical evaluation of the pain suppressor TENS, Fairleigh Dickinson University School of Dentistry, 1983. Curr. Op. Orthopaed. 4(6):105–109, 1993.

Currier, D., Mann, R.: Muscular strength development by electrical stimulation in healthy individuals, Phys. Ther. 63:915, 1983.

Currier, D., Mann, R.: Pain complaint: comparison of electrical stimulation with conventional isometric exercise, J. Orthop. Sports Phys. Ther. 5: 318, 1984.

Currier, D., Petrilli, C., and Threlkeld, A.: Effect of medium frequency electrical stimulation on local blood circulation to healthy muscle, Phys. Ther. 66:937, 1986.

Currier, D., Ray, J., and Nyland, J.: Effects of electrical and electromagnetic stimulation after anterior cruciate ligament reconstruction, J. Orthop. Sports Phys. Ther. 17(4):177–184, 1993.

DeGirardi, C., Seaborne, D., and Goulet, F.: The analgesic effect of high voltage galvanic stimulation combined with ultrasound in the treatment of low back pain: a one-group pre-test/post-test study. Physiother. Can. 36:327, 1984.

Dimitrijevic, M.: Mesh-glove. 1. A method for whole-hand electrical stimulation in upper motor neuron dysfunction. Scand. J. Rehab. Med. 26(4):183–186, 1994.

Dimitrijevic, M.: Mesh-glove. 2. Modulation of residual upper limb motor control after stroke with whole-hand electric stimulation. Scand. J. Rehab. Med. 26(4):187–190, 1994.

Eisenberg, B., Gilal, A.: Structural changes in single muscle fibers after stimulation at a low-frequency, J. Gen. Physiol. 74:1, 1979.

Eriksson, E., Haggmark, T., and Kiessling, K.H.: Effect of electrical stimulation on human skeletal muscle, Int. J. Sports Med. 2:18, 1981.

Ersek, R.: Transcutaneous electrical neurostimulation—a new modality for controlling pain. Clin. Orthop. Relat. Res. 128:314, 1977.

Faghri, P., Glaser, R., and Figoni, S.: Functional electrical stimulation leg cycle ergometer exercise: training effects on cardiorespiratory responses of spinal cord injured, Arch. Phys. Med. Rehab. 73(11):1085–1093, 1992.

Faghri, P., Rodger, M., and Glaser, R.: The effects of functional electrical stimulation on shoulder subluxation, arm function recovery, and shoulder pain in hemiplegic stroke patients, Arch. Phys. Med. Rehab. 75(1):73–79, 1994.

Ferguson, A., Granat, M.: Evaluation of functional electrical stimulation for an incomplete spinal cord injured patient, Physiotherapy 78(4):253–256, 1992.

Finlay, C: TENS: an adjunct to analgesia, Can. Nurse 88(8):24–26, 1992.

Fox, F., Melzack, R.: Transcutaneous electrical stimulation and acupuncture: comparison of treatment for low back pain, Pain 2:141, 1976.

Frank, C., Schachar, N., and Dittrich, D.: Electromagnetic stimulation of ligament healing in rabbits, Clin. Orthop. Relat. Res. 175:263, 1983.

Geddes, L.: A short history of the electrical stimulation of excitable tissue, Physiologist 27(suppl):1, 1984.

Godfrey, C., Jayawardena, H., and Quance, T.: Comparison of electro-stimulation and isometric exercise in strengthening the quadriceps muscle, Physiother. Can. 31:265, 1979.

Gotlin, R., Hershkowitz, S.: Electrical stimulation effect on extensor lag and length of hospital stay after total knee arthroplasty, Arch. Phys. Med. Rehab. 75(9):957–959, 1994.

Gould, M., Donnermeyer, D., and Gammon, G.G.: Transcutaneous muscle stimulation to retard disuse atrophy after open menisectomy. Clin. Orthop. Rel. Res. 178:190, 1983.

Granat, M.: Functional electrical stimulation and hybrid orthosis systems, Paraplegia 34(1):24–29, 1996.

Greathouse, D., Nitz, A., and Matullonis, D.: Effects of electrical stimulation on ultrastructure of rat skeletal muscles, Phys. Ther. 64:755, 1984.

Halback, J., Straus, D.: Comparison of electromyostimulation to isokinetic training in increasing power of the knee extensor mechanism, J. Orthop. Sports Phys. Ther. 2:20, 1980.

Holcomb, W., Mangus, B., and Tandy, R.: The effect of icing with the Pro-Stim Edema Management System on cutaneous cooling, J. Ath. Train. 31(2):126–129, 1996.

Ignelzi, R., Nyquist, J.: Excitability changes in peripheral nerve fibers after repetitive electrical stimulation: implications in pain modulation, J. Neurosurg. 61:824, 1979.

Indergand, H., Morgan, B.: Effect of interference current on forearm vascular resistance in asymptomatic humans, Phys. Ther. 75(5):306–312, 1995.

Indergand, H., Morgan, B.: Effects of high frequency transcutaneous electrical stimulation on limb blood flow in healthy humans, Phys. Ther. 74(4):361–367, 1994.

Jones, D., Bigland-Ritchie, B., and Edwards, R.: Excitation and frequency and muscle fatigue: mechanical responses during voluntary and stimulated contractions, Exper. Neurol. 64:401, 1979.

Kahn, J.: Low-volt technique, Syosset, New York, 1973, Joseph Kahn.

Karmel-Ross, K., Cooperman, D.: The effect of electrical stimulation on quadriceps femoris muscle torque in children with spina bifida, Phys. Ther. 72(10):723–730, 1992.

Kostov, A., Andrews, B., and Popovic, D.: Machine learning in control of functional electrical stimulation systems for locomotion, IEEE Trans. Biomed. Eng. 42(6):541–551, 1995.

Kramer, J., Mendryk, S.: Electrical stimulation as a strength improvement technique: a review, J. Orthop. Sports Phys. Ther. 4:91, 1982.

Kues, J., Mayhew, T.: Concentric and eccentric force-velocity relationships during electrically induced submaximal contractions, Phys. Ther. 76(5):S17, 1996.

Lainey, C., Walmsley, R., and Andrew, G.: Effectiveness of exercise alone versus exercise plus electrical stimulation in strengthening the quadriceps muscle, Physiother. Can. 35:5, 1983.

Lampe, G.: Introduction to the use of transcutaneous electrical nerve stimulation devices, Phys. Ther. 58:1450, 1978.

Lane, J.: Electrical impedances of superficial limb tissue, epidermis, dermis and muscle sheath. Ann. N.Y. Acad. Sci. 238:812, 1974.

Latash, M., Yee, M., and Orpett, C.: Combining electrical muscle stimulation with voluntary contraction for studying muscle fatigue, Arch. Phys. Med. Rehab. 75(1):29–35, 1994.

Laughman, R., Youdas, J., and Garrett, T.: Strength changes in the normal quadriceps femoris muscle as a result of electrical stimulation, Phys. Ther. 63:494, 1983.

LeDoux, J., Quinones, M.: An investigation of the use of percutaneous electrical stimulation m muscle reeducation, Phys. Ther. 61:678, 1981.

Leffman, D., Arnall, D., and Holmgren, P.: Effect of microamperage stimulation on the rate of wound healing in rats: A histological study, Phys. Ther. 74(3):195–200, 1994.

Levin, M., Hui-Chan, C.: Conventional and acupuncture-like transcutaneous electrical nerve stimulation excite similar afferent fibers, Arch. Phys. Med. Rehab. 74(1):54–60, 1993.

Licht, S.: History of electrotherapy. In Stillwell, G.K., editor. Therapeutic electricity and ultraviolet radiation, ed. 3, Baltimore, 1983, Williams & Wilkins.

Litke, D., Dahners, L.: Effects of different levels of direct current on early ligament healing in a rat model. J. Orthop. Res. 12:683–688, 1992.

Livesley, E.: Effects of electrical neuromuscular stimulation on functional performance in patients with multiple sclerosis. Physiotherapy 78(12):914–917, 1992.

Loeser, J.: Nonpharmacologic approaches to pain relief. In Ng, L., Bonica, J., editors: Pain, discomfort and humanitarian care, New York, 1980, Elsevier.

Loesor, J., Black, R., and Christman, A.: A relief of pain by transcutaneous stimulation, J. Neurosurg. 42:308, 1975.

Long, D.: Cutaneous afferent stimulation for relief of chronic pain, Clin. Neurosurg. 21:257, 1974.

Macdonald, A., Coates, T.: The discovery of transcutaneous spinal electroanalgesia and its relief of chronic pain, Physiotherapy 81(11):653–661, 1995.

Mannheimer, C., Lund, S., and Carlsson, C.: The effect of transcutaneous electrical nerve stimulation (TENS) on joint pain in patients with rheumatoid arthritis, Scand. J. Rheumatol. 7:13, 1978.

Mannneimer, C., Carlsson, C.: The analgesic effect of transcutaneous electrical nerve stimulation (TENS) in patients with rheumatoid arthritis. A comparative study of different pulse patterns, Pain 6:329, 1979.

Mannheimer, J.: Electrode placements for transcutaneous electrical nerve stimulation, Phys. Ther. 58:1455, 1978.

Mao, W., Ghia, J., and Scott, D.: High versus low-intensity acupuncture analgesic for treatment of chronic pain: effects on platelet serotonin, Pain 8:331, 1980.

Markov, M.: Electric current and electromagnetic field effects on soft tissue: implications for wound healing, Wounds Compen. Clin. Res. Pract. 7(3):94–110, 1995.

Marvie, K.: A major advance in the control of post-operative knee pain, Orthopedics 2:129, 1979.

Massey, B., Nelson, R., and Sharkey, B.: Effects of high frequency electrical stimulation on the size and strength of skeletal muscle, J. Sports Med. Phys. Fit. 5:136, 1965.

Mattison, J.: Transcutaneous electrical nerve stimulation in the management of painful muscle spasm in patients with multiple sclerosis, Clin. Rehab. 7(1):45–48, 1993.

McMiken, D., Todd-Smith, M., and Thompson, C.: Strengthening of human quadriceps muscles by cutaneous electrical stimulation, Scand. J. Rehab. Med. 15:25, 1983.

McQuain, M., Sinaki, M., and Shibley, L.: Effect of electrical stimulation on lumbar paraspinal muscles, Spine 18(13):1787–1792, 1993.

Meyer, G., Fields, H.: Causalgia treated by selective large fibre stimulation of peripheral nerve, Brain 95:163, 1972.

Milner-Brown, H., Stein, R.: The relation between the surface electromyogram and muscular force, J. Physiol. 246:549, 1975.

Mohr, T., Carlson, B., and Sulentic, C.: Comparison of isometric exercise and high volt galvanic stimulation on quadriceps, femoris muscle strength. Phys. Ther. 65:606, 1985.

Mostowy, D.: An application of transcutaneous electrical nerve stimulation to control pain in the elderly, J. Gerontol. Nurs 22(2):36–38, 1996.

Munsat, T., McNeal, D., and Waters, R.: Preliminary observations on prolonged stimulation of peripheral nerve in man, Arch. Neurol. 33:608, 1976.

Myklebust, J., editor: Neural stimulation, Boca Raton, Florida, 1985, CRC Press.

Naess, K., Storm-Mathison, A.: Fatigue of sustained tetanic contractions. Acta Physiol. Scand. 34:351, 1955.

Owens, J., Malone, T.: Treatment parameters of high frequency electrical stimulation as established on the electrostim 180, J. Orthop. Sports Phys. Ther. 4:162, 1983.

Packman-Braun, R.: Misconceptions regarding functional electrical stimulation, Neurol. Rept. 19(3):17–21, 1995.

Pert, V.: TENS for pain in multiple sclerosis, Physiotherapy 77(3):227–228, 1991.

Petrofsky, J.: Functional electrical stimulation, a two-year study. J. Rehab. 58(3):29–34, 1992.

Picaza, J., Cannon, B., and Hunter, S.: Pain suppression by peripheral stimulation, Part I. Observations with transcutaneous stimuli, Surg. Neurol. 4:105, 1975.

Pouran, D., Faghri, M., and Rodgers, M.: The effects of functional electrical stimulation on shoulder subluxation, arm function recovery, and shoulder pain in hemiplegic stroke patients, Arch. Phys. Med. Rehab. 75(1):73–79, 1994.

Procacci, P., Zoppi, M., and Maresca, M.: Transcutaneous electrical stimulation in low back pain: a critical evaluation, Acupunct. Electrother. Res. 7:1, 1982.

Rabischong, E., Doutrelot, P., and Ohanna, F.: Compound motor action potentials and mechanical failure during sustained contractions by electrical stimulation in paraplegic, Paraplegia 33(12):707–714, 1995.

Rack, P., Westbury, D.: The effects of length and stimulus rate on tension in the isometric cat soleus muscle, J. Physiol. 204:443, 1969.

Ray, R., Samuelson, A.: Microcurrent versus a placebo for the control of pain and edema, J. Ath. Train. 31:S-48, 1996.

Reddana, P., Moortly, C., and Govidappa, S.: Pattern of skeletal muscle chemical composition during in vivo electrical stimulations, Ind. J. Physiol. Pharmacol. 25:33, 1981.

Rieb, L., Pomeranz, B.: Alterations in electrical pain thresholds by use of acupuncture-like transcutaneous electrical nerve stimulation in pain-free subjects, Phys. Ther. 72(9):658–667, 1992.

Rochester, L.: Influence of electrical stimulation of the tibialis anterior muscle in paraplegic subjects. 1. Contractile properties, Paraplegia 33(8):437–449, 1995.

Roeser, W. et al.: The use of transcutaneous nerve stimulation for pain control in athletic medicine. A preliminary report, Am. J. Sports Med. 4(5):210, 1976.

Romero, J., Sanford, T., and Schroeder, R.: The effects of electrical stimulation of normal quadriceps on strength and girth, Med. Sci. Sports Exerc. 14:194, 1982.

Rosenberg, M., Vutyid, L., and Bourbe, D.: Transcutaneous electrical nerve stimulation for the relief of post-operative pain, Pain 5:129, 1978.

Rowley, B., McKenna, J., and Chase, G.: The influence of electrical current on an infecting microorganism in wounds, Ann. N.Y. Acad. Sci. 238:543, 1974.

Schmitz, R., Martin, D., and Perrin, D.: The effects of interferential current of perceived pain and serum cortisol in a delayed onset muscle soreness model, J. Ath. Train. 29(2):171, 1994.

Seib, T., Price, R., and Reyes, M.: The quantitative measurement of spasticity: effect of cutaneous electrical stimulation, Arch. Phys. Med. Rehab. 75(7):746–750, 1994.

Selkowitz, D.: Improvement in isometric strength of the quadricep femoris muscle after training with electrical stimulation, Phys. Ther. 65:186, 1985.

Shealey, C., Maurer, D.: Transcutaneous nerve stimulation for control of pain, Surg. Neurol. 2:45, 1974.

Simmonds, M., Wessel, J., and Scudds, R.: The effect of pain quality on the efficacy of conventional TENS, Physiotherapy (Can) 44(3):35–40, 1992.

Sjolund, B., Eriksson, M.: The influence of naloxone on analgesia produced by peripheral conditioning stimulation, Brain Res. 173:295, 1979.

Sjolund, B., Terenius, L., and Eriksson, M.: Increased cerebrospinal fluid levels of endorphin after electroacupuncture, Acta Physiol. Scand. 100:382, 1977.

Smith, B., Mulcahey, M., Betz, R.: Quantitative comparison of grasp and release abilities with and without functional neuromuscular stimulation in adolescents with tetraplegia, Paraplegia 34(1):16–23, 1996.

Smith, B., Betz, R., and Mulcahey, M.: Reliability of percutaneous intramuscular electrodes for upper extremity functional neuromuscular stimulation in adolescents with C5 injury, Arch. Phys. Med. Rehab. 75(9):939–945, 1994.

Snyder-Mackler, L., Delitto, A., Stralka, S.: Use of electrical stimulation to enhance recovery of quadriceps femoris muscle force production in patients following anterior cruciate ligament reconstruction, Phys. Ther. 74(10):901–907, 1994.

Standish, W., Valiant, G., Bonen, A.: The effects of immobilization and of electrical stimulation on muscle glycogen and myofibrillar ATPase, Can. J. Appl. Sports Sci. 7:267, 1982.

Szehi, E., David, E.: The stereodynamic interferential current—a new electrotherapeutic technique, Electromedica 48:13, 1980.

Szuminsky, N., Albers, A., and Unger, P.: Effect of narrow pulsed high voltages on bacterial viability, Phys. Ther. 74(7):660–667, 1994.

Taylor, M., Newton, R., and Personius, W.: The effects of interferential current stimulation for the treatment of subjects with recurrent jaw pain, abstract. Phys. Ther. 66:774, 1986.

Taylor, P., Hallet, M., and Flaherty, L.: Treatment of osteoarthritis of the knee with transcutaneous electrical nerve stimulation, Pain 11:233, 1981.

Terezhalmy, G., Ross, G., and Holmes-Johnson, E.: Transcutaneous electrical nerve stimulation treatment of TMJMPDS patients, Ear Nose Throat J. 61:664, 1982.

Thorsteinsson, G., Stonnington, H.: The placebo effect of transcutaneous electrical stimulation, Pain 5:31, 1978.

Walsh, D., Foster, N., and Baxter, G.: Transcutaneous electrical nerve stimulation parameters to neurophysiological and hypoalgesic effects, Phys. Ther. 76(5):552, 1996.

Weber, M., Servedio, F., and Woddall, W.: The effects of three modalities on delayed onset muscle soreness, J. Orthop. Sports Phys. Ther. 20(5): 236–242, 1994.

Wheeler, P., Wolcott, L., and Morris, J.: Neural considerations in the healing of ulcerated tissue by clinical electrotherapeutic application of weak direct current: findings and theory. In Reynolds, D., Sjoberg, A., editors: Neuroelectric research, Springfield, Illinois, 1971, Charles C Thomas, pp. 83–96.

Windsor, R., Lester, J.: Electrical stimulation in clinical practice. Phys. Sports Med. 21(2):85–86, 89–90, 91–92, 1993.

Wolf, S., Gersh, M., and Rao, V.: Examination of electrode placements and stimulating parameters in treating chronic pain with conventional transcutaneous nerve stimulation (TENS), Pain 11:37, 1981.

Wong, R., Jette, D.: Changes in sympathetic tone associated with different forms of transcutaneous electrical nerve stimulation in healthy subjects, Phys. Ther. 64:478, 1984.

Yarkony, G., Roth, E., and Cybulski, J.: Neuromuscular stimulation in spinal cord injury II: prevention of secondary complications. Part 2, Arch. Phys. Med. Rehab. 73(2):195–200, 1992.

Yarkony, G., Roth, E.: Neuromuscular stimulation in spinal cord injury: restoration of functional movement of the extremities. Part 1, Arch. Phys. Med. Rehab. 73(1):78–86, 1992.

Zecca, L., Ferrario, P., and Furia, G.: Effects of pulsed electromagnetic field on acute and chronic inflammation, Trans. Biol. Repair Growth Soc. 3:72, 1983.

GLOSSARY

absolute refractory period Brief time period (0.5 μsec) following membrane depolarization during which the membrane is incapable of depolarizing again.

action potential A recorded change in electrical potential between the inside and outside of a nerve cell, resulting in muscular contraction.

active electrode Electrode at which greatest current density occurs.

all-or-none response The depolarization of nerve or muscle membrane is the same once a depolarizing intensity threshold is reached; further increases in intensity do not increase the response. Stimuli at intensities less than threshold do not create a depolarizing effect.

anode Positively charged electrode in a direct current system.

beat Distinct wave pattern created by combining two distinct circuit electrical waves that blend into a gradual rising and falling wave.

bioelectromagnetics The study of biologic tissues' electrical and magnetic properties.

cathode Negatively charged electrode in a direct current system.

central biasing The use of hyperstimulation analgesia to bias the central nervous system against transmitting painful stimuli to the sensory recognition area. This occurs through hormonal influences created by brain stem stimulation.

chronaxie The duration of time necessary to cause observable tissue excitation, given a current intensity of two times rheobasic current.

constructive interference The combined amplitude of two distinct circuits increases the amplitude.

current density Amount of current flow per cubic area.

current of injury A bioelectric current produced by any type of cellular trauma that plays a key role in stimulating healing.

denervated muscle Muscle that has lost its peripheral nerve supply.

depolarization Process or act of neutralizing the cell membrane's resting potential.

destructive interference Combined amplitude of two distinct circuits decreases the amplitude.

dipoles Molecules whose ends carry opposite charge.

electrets Insulators carrying a permanent charge similar to a permanent magnet.

electropiezo activity Changing electric surface charges of a structure forces the structure to change shape.

frequency window selectivity Cellular responses may be triggered by a certain electrical frequency range.

functional electrical stimulation Utilizes multiple-channel electrical stimulators to recruit muscles in a programmed sequence that produces a functional movement pattern.

gap junctions Specialized junction areas connecting cells of like structure that contain channels for ionic, electrical, and small molecule signaling that pass messages from cell to cell.

heterodynes Cyclic rising and falling waveform of interferential current.

hybrid currents Currents that have waveforms containing parameters that are not classically alternating or direct.

impedance The resistance of the tissue to the passage of electrical current.

indifferent or dispersive electrode Large electrode used to spread out electrical charge and decrease current density at that electrode site.

maximum voluntary isometric contraction Peak torque produced by a muscular contraction.

piezoelectric activity Changing electric surface charges of a structure forces the structure to change shape.

resting potential The potential difference between the inside and outside of a membrane.

rheobase The intensity of current necessary to cause observable tissue excitation, given a long current duration.

Russian current A medium-frequency (2000–10,000 Hz) polyphasic AC wave generated in 50-burst-per-second envelopes.

stereodynamic interference current Three distinct circuits blending and creating a distinct electrical wave pattern.

strain-related potentials Tissue-based electric potentials generated in response to strain for the tissue.

strength-duration curve A graphic illustration of the relationship between current intensity and current duration in causing depolarization of a nerve or muscle membrane.

summation of contractions Shortening of muscle myofilaments caused by increasing the frequency of muscle membrane depolarization.

tetanization This occurs when individual muscle twitch responses can no longer be distinguished and the responses force maximum shortening of the stimulated muscle fiber.

twitch muscle contraction A single muscle contraction caused by one depolarization phenomenon.

voltage-sensitive permeability The quality of some cell membranes that makes them permeable to different ions based on the electric charge of the ions. Nerve and muscle cell membranes allow negatively charged ions into the cell while actively transporting some positively charged ions outside the cell membrane.

LAB ACTIVITY

ELECTRICAL STIMULATION: ANALGESIA

DESCRIPTION:

Electroanalgesia is arguably the most common use of therapeutic electricity. The use of therapeutic electricity for analgesia is often referred to as transcutaneous electrical nerve stimulation or TENS; however, all forms of therapeutic electricity that do not use implanted or needle electrodes are "transcutaneous," and many forms stimulate nerves. Therefore, the term TENS should be discouraged. Although there are hundreds of different types of electrical stimulators available for use, there are essentially three levels in the body that may be affected.

The first level is the spinal gate. This level is activated by increasing the input to the spinal cord from large-diameter afferent neurons. The second level is referred to as the central bias mechanism, where intense small fiber afferent input activates a negative feedback loop through connections in the midbrain. Finally, some forms of electrical stimulation appear to stimulate the production of endogenous opiates, the endorphins.

Although stimulators have many different waveforms and modulations, there is no evidence that an "optimal" waveform exists. It is impossible to predict for an individual patient what type of current, what electrode configuration, what amplitude of stimulation, and so on, will provide relief of pain. Therefore, electroanalgesia is somewhat of a trial and error phenomenon. This does not mean the approach should be haphazard; a systematic approach, based on clinical experience, is best.

Generally, there are three types of stimulation for electroanalgesia; conventional, low-frequency, and hyperstimulation. Conventional generally has a pulse rate of 10 to 100 pulses per second (pps), and is applied at an amplitude between sensory and motor thresholds. Low-frequency stimulation has a pulse rate of 1 to 5 pps, and an amplitude between motor and pain thresholds. Hyperstimulation generally uses a monophasic pulsatile current at a frequency of 1 to 128 pps, and an amplitude to pain tolerance. Hyperstimulation is often referred to as point stimulation.

PHYSIOLOGIC EFFECTS:

Depolarization of peripheral nerves

THERAPEUTIC EFFECTS:

Inhibition of pain perception

INDICATIONS:

The obvious indication for electroanalgesia is pain. However, the cause of the pain should be identified prior to the use of electrical stimulation, and it must be remembered that the modulation of pain is not treating the cause of the pain.

CONTRAINDICATIONS:

- Pregnancy
- Implanted electrical pacing devices (e.g., cardiac pacemaker, bladder stimulator, etc.)
- Cardiac arrhythmia
- Over the carotid sinus area
- Hypersensitivity (i.e., the patient who has a strong aversion to electricity, or the patient with certain types of catheters or shunts).

ELECTRICAL STIMULATION: ANALGESIA

PROCEDURE	Evaluation		
	1	2	3
1. Check supplies.			
a. Obtain towels or sheets for draping, conductant.			
b. Check stimulator, electrodes, and cables for charged battery, broken or frayed insulation, and so on.			
c. Insure the amplitude controls are at zero.			
2. Question patient.			
a. Verify identity of patient (if not already verified).			
b. Verify the absence of contraindications.			
c. Ask about previous treatments for current condition, and check treatment notes.			
3. Position patient.			
a. Place patient in a well-supported, comfortable position.			
b. Expose body part to be treated.			
c. Drape patient to preserve patient's modesty, protect clothing, but allow access to body part.			
4. Inspect body part to be treated.			
a. Check light touch perception.			
b. Assess function of body part (e.g., ROM, irritability).			
5a. Apply conventional electrical stimulation.			
a. Place conductant on electrodes as indicated, secure electrodes to patient.			
b. Remind the patient to inform you when he or she feels something. Do not tell the patient what he or she will feel; for example, do not say, "tell me when you feel a buzz or tingle."			
c. Adjust the pulse rate, pulse width, and mode of stimulation to desired settings if possible.			
d. Turn on the stimulator, and increase the amplitude slowly. Monitor the patient's response, not the stimulator.			
e. After the patient reports the onset of the stimulus, adjust the amplitude to a comfortable level, but make sure it is below motor threshold. If it is impossible to achieve suprasensory threshold stimulation without a motor response, turn the stimulator off and move the electrodes to another location.			
f. Set a timer for the appropriate treatment time and give the patient a signaling device. Make sure the patient understands how to use the signaling device.			
g. Recheck the patient after about 5 minutes. If the sensation has diminished, adjust the amplitude appropriately.			
5b. Apply low-frequency electrical stimulation.			
a. Place conductant on electrodes as indicated, secure electrodes to patient.			

PROCEDURE	Evaluation		
	1	2	3
b. Remind the patient to inform you when he or she feels something. Do not tell the patient what he or she will feel; for example, do not say, "tell me when you feel a buzz or tingle."			
c. Adjust the pulse rate, pulse width, and mode of stimulation to desired settings if possible.			
d. Turn on the stimulator, and increase the amplitude slowly. Monitor the patient's response, not the stimulator.			
e. After the patient reports the onset of the stimulus, adjust the amplitude to a comfortable level above motor threshold. The contraction should be just a twitch, not a strong contraction.			
f. Set a timer for the appropriate treatment time and give the patient a signaling device. Make sure the patient understands how to use the signaling device.			
g. Recheck the patient after about 5 minutes. If the sensation has diminished, adjust the amplitude appropriately.			
5c. Apply hyperstimulation electrical stimulation.			
a. Place conductant on "inactive" electrode, have the patient hold the electrode in his or her palm. Apply the conductant to points to be stimulated.			
b. If using electrical resistance to locate stimulation points, set sensitivity of ohm meter; set pulse rate, polarity, and length of stimulation to desired settings.			
c. Move the "active" electrode slowly in the area of the point to be stimulated until the area of minimal resistance is found; the pressure applied to the electrode must be constant.			
d. Tell the patient to report when the amplitude of stimulation is as high as he or she can tolerate. Activate the stimulation current, and increase the amplitude slowly. Monitor the patient's response, not the stimulator.			
e. After the patient reports that the stimulus is as much as he or she can tolerate, maintain constant pressure on the electrode. Stimulate the point two or three times, for 15 to 30 seconds each time.			
f. Repeat the process for each point to be stimulated.			
6. Complete treatment.			
a. When the treatment time is over, turn the intensity control to zero, and move the generator away from the patient; remove conductant with a towel.			
b. Remove material used for draping, assist the patient in dressing as needed.			
c. Have the patient perform appropriate therapeutic exercise as indicated.			
d. Clean the treatment area and equipment according to normal protocol.			
7. Assess treatment efficacy.			
a. Ask the patient how the treated area feels.			
b. Visually inspect the treated area for any adverse reactions.			
c. Perform functional tests as indicated.			

LAB ACTIVITY

ELECTRICAL STIMULATION: REEDUCATION

DESCRIPTION:

Electrical stimulation may be used to assist a patient in regaining the ability to voluntarily control a normally innervated muscle. Sometimes following surgery, a patient temporarily loses the ability to produce a muscle contraction. Probably the most common loss is of the quadriceps femoris following knee surgery. In addition, if a patient has undergone a tendon transfer, he or she may have difficulty recruiting the muscle to perform the new joint action.

The mechanism by which electrical stimulation aids in the recovery of volitional control of skeletal muscle is not clear, nor is the reason volitional control is lost following surgery. The probable method of action is via stimulation of joint, muscle, and skin proprioceptors when the muscle produces joint motion.

PHYSIOLOGIC EFFECTS:

Depolarization of peripheral nerves

THERAPEUTIC EFFECTS:

Recovery of volitional control of skeletal muscle

INDICATIONS:

The primary indication is loss of volitional control of a skeletal muscle following surgery or a tendon transfer.

CONTRAINDICATIONS:

- Pregnancy
- Implanted electrical pacing devices (e.g., cardiac pacemaker, bladder stimulator, etc.)
- Cardiac arrhythmia
- Over the carotid sinus area
- Hypersensitivity (i.e., the patient who has a strong aversion to electricity, or the patient with certain types of catheters or shunts).

ELECTRICAL STIMULATION: REEDUCATION

PROCEDURE	Evaluation		
	1	2	3
1. Check supplies.			
a. Obtain towels or sheets for draping, conductant.			
b. Check stimulator, electrodes, and cables for charged battery, broken or frayed insulation, etc.			
c. Verify that the intensity control is at zero.			
2. Question patient.			
a. Verify identity of patient (if not already verified).			
b. Verify the absence of contraindications.			
c. Ask about previous exposure to electrotherapy, check treatment notes.			

PROCEDURE	Evaluation		
	1	2	3
3. Position patient.			
a. Place patient in a well-supported, comfortable position.			
b. Expose body part to be treated.			
c. Drape patient to preserve patient's modesty, protect clothing, but allow access to body part.			
4. Inspect body part to be treated.			
a. Check light touch perception.			
b. Assess function of body part (e.g., ROM, irritability).			
5. Apply electrical stimulation for reeducation.			
a. Place conductant on electrodes as needed, secure electrodes to patient. Electrode location will vary depending on desired effect. Usually, the ideal location for the active electrode is over the motor point of the target muscle or the peripheral nerve trunk that supplies the target muscle.			
b. Remind the patient to inform you when he or she feels something. Do not tell the patient what he or she will feel; for example, do not say, "tell me when you feel a buzz or tingle."			
c. Adjust the pulse rate, pulse width, and mode of stimulation to desired settings if possible.			
d. Turn on the stimulator, and increase the amplitude slowly. Monitor the patient's response, not the stimulator.			
e. After the patient reports the onset of the stimulus, adjust the amplitude to a comfortable level above motor threshold. Encourage the patient to try to volitionally contract the muscle before the stimulator does, and increase the force during the stimulation.			
f. Continue to monitor the patient during the duration of the treatment.			
6. Complete treatment.			
a. When the treatment time is over or the patient is able to control the muscle contraction, turn the intensity to zero, and move the generator away from the patient; remove conductant with a towel.			
b. Remove material used for draping, assist the patient in dressing as needed.			
c. Have the patient perform appropriate therapeutic exercise as indicated.			
d. Clean the treatment area and equipment according to normal protocol.			
7. Assess treatment efficacy.			
a. Ask the patient how the treated area feels.			
b. Visually inspect the treated area for any adverse reactions.			
c. Perform functional tests as indicated.			

ELECTRICAL STIMULATION: STRENGTHENING

DESCRIPTION:

Electrical stimulation is often used for increasing skeletal muscle strength by itself or in conjunction with active exercise. However, there is no evidence the electrical stimulation by itself or in conjunction with active exercise is better than active exercise alone for muscle strengthening. Also, the increase in tension-developing capacity does not transfer to functional activities. Because of this, it is sometimes referred to as "electrical stimulation to increase isometric force development capacity."

PHYSIOLOGIC EFFECTS:

Depolarization of peripheral nerves

THERAPEUTIC EFFECTS:

Increase in isometric force development capacity

INDICATIONS:

The primary indication is muscle weakness. However, electrical stimulation is sometimes used in an attempt to prevent disuse atrophy during immobilization of a limb.

CONTRAINDICATIONS:

- Pregnancy
- Implanted electrical pacing devices (e.g., cardiac pacemaker, bladder stimulator, etc.)
- Cardiac arrhythmia
- Over the carotid sinus area
- Hypersensitivity (i.e., the patient who has a strong aversion to electricity, or the patient with certain types of catheters or shunts).

ELECTRICAL STIMULATION: STRENGTHENING

PROCEDURE	Evaluation		
	1	2	3
1. Check supplies.			
a. Obtain towels or sheets for draping, conductant.			
b. Check stimulator, electrodes, and cables for charged battery, broken or frayed insulation, etc.			
c. Verify that the intensity control is at zero.			
2. Question patient.			
a. Verify identity of patient (if not already verified).			
b. Verify the absence of contraindications.			
c. Ask about previous exposure to electrotherapy, check treatment notes.			
3. Position patient.			
a. Place patient in a well-supported, comfortable position.			
b. Expose body part to be treated.			
c. Drape patient to preserve patient's modesty, protect clothing, but allow access to body part.			

PROCEDURE	Evaluation		
	1	2	3
4. Inspect body part to be treated.			
a. Check light touch perception.			
b. Assess function of body part (e.g., ROM, irritability).			
5. Apply electrical stimulation for muscle strengthening.			
a. Place conductant on electrodes as indicated, secure electrodes to patient. Electrode location will vary depending on desired effect. Usually, the ideal location for the active electrode is over the motor point of the target muscle, or the peripheral nerve trunk that supplies the target muscle.			
b. Remind the patient to inform you when he or she feels something. Do not tell the patient what he or she will feel; for example, do not say, "tell me when you feel a buzz or tingle."			
c. Adjust the pulse rate, pulse width, and mode of stimulation to desired settings if possible.			
d. Turn on the stimulator, and increase the amplitude slowly. Monitor the patient's response, not the stimulator.			
e. After the patient reports the onset of the stimulus, adjust the amplitude to as high a level as the patient can tolerate.			
f. Set a timer for the appropriate treatment time and give the patient a signaling device. Make sure the patient understands how to use the signaling device.			
g. Recheck the patient after about 5 minutes. If the sensation has diminished, adjust the amplitude appropriately.			
6. Complete treatment.			
a. When the treatment time is over, turn the intensity control to zero, move the generator away from the patient; remove conductant with a towel.			
b. Remove material used for draping, assist the patient in dressing as needed.			
c. Have the patient perform appropriate therapeutic exercise as indicated.			
d. Clean the treatment area and equipment according to normal protocol.			
7. Assess treatment efficacy.			
a. Ask the patient how the treated area feels.			
b. Visually inspect the treated area for any adverse reactions.			
c. Perform functional tests as indicated.			

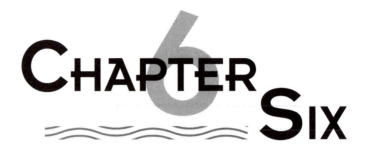

CHAPTER Six

IONTOPHORESIS

WILLIAM E. PRENTICE

OBJECTIVES

Following completion of this chapter the student therapist will be able to:

- ✓ Differentiate between iontophoresis and phonophoresis.
- ✓ Discuss the basic mechanisms of ion transfer.
- ✓ Discuss specific iontophoresis application procedures and techniques.
- ✓ Identify the different ions most commonly used in iontophoresis.
- ✓ Describe the various clinical applications for using an iontophoresis technique.
- ✓ Identify precautions and concerns about using iontophoresis treatment.

Iontophoresis is a therapeutic technique that involves the introduction of ions into the body tissues by means of a direct electrical current.[11] Originally referred to as **ion transfer**, it was first described by LeDuc in 1903 as a technique of transporting chemicals across a membrane using an electrical current as a driving force.[42] Since that time there have been increases and decreases in the popularity and use of iontophoresis as a therapeutic technique. Recently new emphasis has been placed on iontophoresis, and it has become a commonly used technique in clinical settings. Iontophoresis has several advantages as a treatment technique in that it is a painless, sterile, noninvasive technique for introducing specific ions into the tissue that has been demonstrated to have a positive effect on the healing process.

iontophoresis A therapeutic technique that involves the introduction of ions into the body tissues by means of a direct electrical current.

IONTOPHORESIS VERSUS PHONOPHORESIS

It is critical to point out the difference between iontophoresis and phonophoresis since the two techniques are often confused and occasionally the two terms are erroneously interchanged. It is true that both techniques are used to deliver chemicals to various biologic tissues. Phonophoresis, which is discussed in detail in Chapter 10, involves the use of acoustic energy in the form of ultrasound to drive whole molecules across the skin into the tissues, whereas iontophoresis uses an electrical current to transport ions into the tissues.

BASIC MECHANISMS OF ION TRANSFER

As defined in Chapter 4, **ions** are positively or negatively charged particles. Through the process of **ionization** soluble compounds such as acids, alkaloids, or salts dissociate or dissolve into ions, which are suspended in some type of solution.[12] The resulting solutions are called **electrolytes** in which ionic movement occurs. Ions will move or migrate within this solution according to the electrically charged currents acting on them. The term **electrophoresis** refers to the movement of ions in solution.

At any given instant, the electrode that has the greatest concentration of electrons is negatively charged and is referred to as the negative electrode or cathode. Conversely, the electrode with a lower concentration of electrons is called the positive electrode or anode. Negatively charged ions will be repelled from the negative electrode, and thus they move toward the positive electrode, creating an acidic reaction. Positively charged ions will tend to move toward the negative electrode and away from the positive electrode, resulting in an alkaline reaction.

The manner in which ions move in solution forms the basis for iontophoresis. Positively charged ions are driven into the tissues from the positive pole and negatively charged ions are introduced by the negative pole. Thus knowing the correct ion polarity and matching it with the appropriate electrode polarity is of critical importance in using iontophoresis.

The force that acts to move ions through the tissues is determined by both the strength of the electrical field and the electrical impedance of tissues to current flow. The strength of the electrical field is determined by the current density. The difference in current density between the active and inactive or dispersive electrodes establishes a gradient of potential difference that produces ion migration within the electrical field. (In Chapter 5 the active electrode was defined as the smaller of the two electrodes that has the greater current density. When using iontophoresis, the **active electrode** is defined as the one that is being used to drive the ion into the tissues.) Current density may be altered either by increasing or decreasing current intensity or by changing the size of the electrode. Increasing the size of the electrode will decrease current density under that electrode. It has been recommended that the current density be reduced at the cathode or negative electrode. The accumulation of positively charged ions in a small area creates an alkaline reaction that is more likely to produce tissue damage than an accumulation of negatively charged ions that produces an acidic reaction. Thus the negative electrode should be larger, perhaps twice the size of the positive electrode to reduce current density.[12,40] This size relationship should remain the same even when the negative electrode is the active electrode.

Skin and fat are poor conductors of electrical current, offering greater resistance to current flow. Higher current intensities are necessary to create ion movement in areas where the skin and fat layers are thick, further increasing the likelihood of burns particularly around the negative electrode. However, the presence of sweat glands decreases impedance, thus facilitating the flow of direct current as well as ions. The sweat ducts are the primary paths by which ions move through the skin.[31] As the skin becomes more saturated with an electrolyte and blood flow increases to the area during treatment, overall skin impedance will decrease under the electrodes.[12]

The quantity of ions transferred into the tissues through iontophoresis is determined by the intensity of the current or current density at the active electrode, the duration of the current flow, and the concentration of ions in solution.[12] The number of ions absorbed is directly proportional to the current density. In addition, the longer the current flows, the greater the number of ions transferred to the tissues. Therefore, ion transfer may be increased by increasing the intensity and duration of the treatment. Unfortunately as treatment duration increases, the skin impedance decreases, thus increasing the likelihood of burns. Even though ion concentration

ionization A process by which soluble compounds such as acids, alkaloids, or salts dissociate or dissolve into ions that are suspended in some type of solution.

acidic reaction The accumulation of negative ions under the positive pole that produces hydrochloric acid.

alkaline reaction The accumulation of positive ions under the negative electrode that produces sodium hydroxide.

effects ion transfer, concentrations greater than 1 to 2 percent are not more effective than medications at lower concentrations.[48,49]

Once the ions have passed through the skin, they recombine with existing ions and free radicals floating in the bloodstream, thus forming the necessary new compounds for favorable therapeutic interactions.[40]

IONTOPHORESIS TECHNIQUES

TYPE OF CURRENT REQUIRED

Continuous direct current has traditionally been used for iontophoresis. Direct current insures the unidirectional flow of ions that cannot be accomplished using a bidirectional or alternating current. However, a recent study has shown that drugs can be delivered by AC iontophoresis. Iontophoresis using alternating current avoids electrochemical burns, and delivery of the drug increases with duration of application.[28] Neither high-voltage direct currents nor interferential currents may be used for iontophoresis since the current is interrupted and the current duration is too short to produce significant ion movement. It should be added, however, that modulated pulsed currents have been used with some success in in vivo and in vitro studies on laboratory animals for transdermal delivery of drugs.[2,57,62]

IONTOPHORESIS GENERATORS

There are a variety of current generators available on the market that produce continuous direct current and are specifically used for iontophoresis (Fig. 6-1). It should be emphasized that any generator that has the capability of producing continuous direct current may be used for iontophoresis. Some generators are driven by batter-

Iontophoresis generators produce continuous DC current.

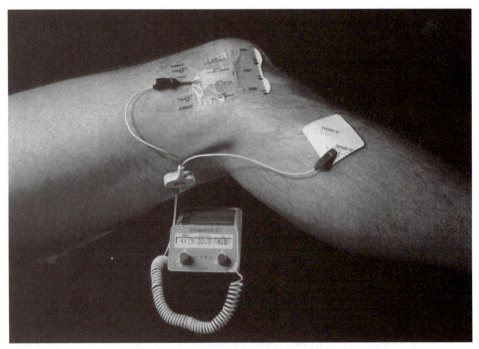

•**Figure 6-1** The Phoresor® is an example of a generator that produces continuous direct current that is specifically used for iontophoresis.

CASE STUDY 6-1
IONTOPHORESIS

Background: A 56-year-old man developed pain in the region inferior to the right patella subsequent to a fall onto the knee while playing tennis. There was immediate mild, localized swelling, which resolved with ice and rest. The acute pain subsided after about 7 days, but the patient then noted significant stiffness following rest, localized tenderness, and pain with climbing stairs, squatting, and kneeling. The physical examination was benign except for mild swelling and point tenderness of the infrapatellar tendon, as well as crepitus to palpation of the tendon during active knee extension.

Impression: Infrapatellar tendinitis.

Treatment Plan: In addition to rest and local ice application, a course of iontophoresis of dexamethasone was initiated. The area was prepared appropriately, and the cathode (negative polarity) was used as the delivery electrode. A total of 60 mA/min of current was delivered on an every-other-day schedule for a total of six treatments.

Response: There was a slight increase in the symptoms following the initial treatment, which persisted for approximately 12 hours following the second treat-

ment. The signs and symptoms then began to diminish, and the patient was symptom-free following the fifth treatment. A progressive increase in physical activity was initiated, and the patient returned to preinjury function 4 weeks later.

Discussion Questions

- What tissues were injured and affected?
- What symptoms were present?
- What phase of the injury-healing continuum did the patient present for care in?
- What are the therapeutic agent modality's biophysical effects (direct, indirect, depth, tissue affinity)?
- What are the therapeutic agent modality's indications and contraindications?
- What are the parameters of the therapeutic agent modality's application, dosage, duration, frequency in this case study?
- What other therapeutic agent modalities could be used to treat this injury or condition? Why? How?

The rehabilitation professional employs therapeutic agent modality to create an optimum environment for tissue healing while minimizing the symptoms associated with the trauma or condition.

ies, others by alternating current. Many generators produce current at a constant voltage that gradually reduces skin impedance, consequently increasing current density and thus increasing the risk of burns. The generator should deliver a constant voltage output to the patient by adjusting the output amperage to normal variations that occur in tissue impedance, thereby reducing the likelihood of burns. For safety purposes the generator should automatically shut down if the skin impedance decreases to some preset limit.

The generator should have some type of current intensity control that can be adjusted between 1 and 5 mA. There should also be an adjustable timer that can be set up to 25 minutes. Polarity of the terminals should be clearly marked, and a polarity reversal switch is desirable. The lead wires connecting the electrodes to the terminals should be well insulated and should be checked regularly for damage or breakdown.

CURRENT INTENSITY

Low-amperage currents appear to be more effective as a driving force than currents with higher intensities.[29,40,46] Higher-intensity currents tend to reduce effective penetration into the tissues. Recommended current amplitudes used for iontophoresis range between 3 and 5 mamp.[5,13,23,40] When initiating the treatment, the current intensity should always be increased very slowly until the patient reports feeling a tingling or prickly sensation. If pain or a burning sensation are elicited, the intensity is too great and should be decreased. Likewise when terminating the treatment, current intensity should be slowly decreased to zero before the electrodes are disconnected.

It has been recommended that the maximum current intensity be determined by the size of the active electrode (Fig. 6-2).[47] Current amplitude is usually set so that the current density falls between 0.1 and 0.5 mA/cm^2 of the active electrode surface.[12]

TREATMENT DURATION

Recommended treatment durations range between 10 and 20 minutes, with 15 minutes being an average. During this 15-minute treatment, the patient should be comfortable with no reported or visible signs of pain or burning. The therapist should check the patient's skin every 3 to 5 minutes during treatment, looking for signs of skin irritation. Since skin impedance usually decreases during the treatment, it may be necessary to decrease current intensity to avoid pain or burning.

ELECTRODES

The continuous direct electrical current must be delivered to the patient through some type of electrode. Many different electrodes are available to the therapist, ranging from those "borrowed" from other electrical stimulators to those that are commercially manufactured ready-to-use disposable electrodes made specifically for iontophoresis.[5,24]

The more traditional electrodes are made of tin, copper, lead, aluminum, or platinum backed by rubber and completely covered by a sponge, towel, or gauze that is in contact with the skin. The absorbent material is soaked with the ionized solu-

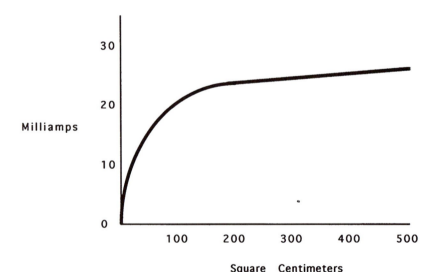

•Figure 6-2 The maximum current intensity should be determined by the size of the active electrode. Current amplitude is usually set so that the current density falls between 0.1 and 0.5 mA/cm^2 of the active electrode surface.

tion to be driven into the tissues. If the ions are contained in an ointment, it should be rubbed into the skin over the target zone and covered by some absorbent material soaked in water or saline before the electrode is applied.

The commercially produced electrodes are sold with most iontophoresis systems. These electrodes have a small chamber, into which the ionized solution may be injected, that is covered by some type of semipermeable membrane. The electrode self-adheres to the skin. (Fig. 6-3). This type of electrode has eliminated the "mess and hassles" that have been associated with electrode preparation for iontophoresis in the past.

Regardless of the type of electrode used, to ensure maximum contact of the electrodes, the skin should be shaved and cleaned prior to attachment of the electrodes. Care should be taken not to excessively abrade the skin during cleaning since damaged skin has a lower resistance to the current so that a burn may more easily occur. Also, caution should be used when treating areas that for one reason or another have reduced sensation.

Once this electrode has been prepared, it then becomes the active electrode, and the lead wire to the generator is attached such that the polarity of the wire is the same as the polarity of the ion in solution. A second electrode, the dispersive electrode, is prepared with water, gel, or some other conductive material as recommended by the manufacturer. Both electrodes must be securely attached to the skin such that uniform skin contact and pressure is maintained under both electrodes to minimize the risk of burns. Electrodes via the lead wires should not be connected to the generator unless both the generator and the amplitude or intensity control are turned off. At the end of the treatment the intensity control should be returned to zero and the generator turned off before the electrodes are detached from the patient.

The size and shape of the electrodes can cause a variation in current density and affects the size of the area treated.[20] Smaller electrodes have a higher current density and should be used to treat a specific lesion. Larger electrodes should be used when the target treatment area is not well-defined.

Recommendations for spacing between the active and dispersive electrodes seem to be variable. They should be separated by at least the diameter of the active electrode. One source has recommended spacing them at least 18 inches apart.[12] As spacing between the electrodes increases, the current density in the superficial tissues will decrease, perhaps minimizing the potential for burns.

active electrode The electrode is used to drive ions into the tissues.

The negative electrode should be larger than the positive.

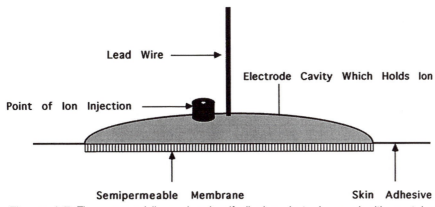

Lead Wire

Electrode Cavity Which Holds Ion

Point of Ion Injection

Semipermeable Membrane   Skin Adhesive

•**Figure 6-3** The commercially produced self-adhering electrodes used with most iontophoresis systems have a small chamber, into which the ionized solution may be injected, that is covered by some type of semipermeable membrane.

Indications and Contraindications for
Iontophoresis

Indications
  Inflammation
  Analgesia
  Muscle spasm
  Ischemia
  Edema
  Calcium deposits
  Scar tissue
  Hyperhydrosis
  Fungi
  Open skin lesions
  Herpes
  Allergic rhinitis
  Gout
  Burns
  Reflex Sympathetic Dystrophy

Contraindications
  Skin sensitivity reactions
  Sensitivity to aspirin (salicylates)
  Gastritis or active stomach ulcer (hydro-
  cortisone)
  Asthma (mecholyl)
  Sensitivity to metals (zinc, copper,
  magnesium)
  Sensitivity to seafood (iodine)

SELECTING THE APPROPRIATE ION

It is critical that the therapist be knowledgeable in the selection of the most appropriate ions for treating specific conditions. In order for a compound to penetrate a membrane such as the skin it must be soluble in both fat and water. It must be water soluble if it is to remain in an ionized state in solution. However, human skin is relatively impervious to water ions, which are soluble only in water and do not diffuse in the tissues.[7] They must be fat soluble to permeate the tissues of the body.[24] Penetration is relatively superficial and is generally less than 1 mm.[23] The majority of the ions deposited in the tissues are found primarily at the site of the active electrode, where they are stored as either a soluble or insoluble compound. They may be used locally as a concentrated source or transported by the circulating blood, producing more systemic effects.[40]

The tendency of some ions to form insoluble precipitates as they pass into the tissues inhibits their ability to penetrate. This is particularly true with heavy metal ions, including iron, copper, silver, and zinc.[14]

Negative ions accumulating at the positive pole or anode produce an acidic reaction through the formation of hydrochloric acid. Negative ions are sclerolytic, thus they produce softening of the tissues by decreasing protein density. This is useful in treating scars or adhesions. In addition, some negative ions can also produce an analgesic effect (salicylates).

The majority of the ions used for iontophoresis are positively charged. Positive ions that accumulate at the negative pole produce an alkaline reaction with the formation of sodium hydroxide. Positive ions are sclerotic and produce hardening of the tissues by increasing protein density.

Table 6-1, modified from a list compiled by Kahn, lists the ions most commonly used with iontophoresis.[37]

CLINICAL APPLICATIONS

A relatively long list of conditions for which iontophoresis is an appropriate treatment technique has been cited in the literature. Clinically, iontophoresis is most often used in the treatment of inflammatory musculoskeletal conditions. It may also be used for analgesic effects, scar modification, wound healing, and in treating edema, calcium deposits, and hyperhidrosis. Many of these published studies are case reports that attempt to establish the clinical efficacy of iontophoresis in treating various conditions.[20] Table 6-2 provides a list of studies that have treated various conditions using iontophoresis.

TREATMENT PRECAUTIONS AND CONTRAINDICATIONS

Problems that might potentially arise from treating a patient using iontophoresis techniques may be avoided for the most part if the therapist (1) has a good understanding of the existing condition to be treated; (2) uses the most appropriate ions to accomplish the treatment goal; and (3) uses appropriate treatment parameters and equipment set-up. Poor treatment technique on the part of the therapist is most often responsible for adverse reactions to iontophoresis.

TREATMENT BURNS

Perhaps the single most common problem associated with iontophoresis is a chemical burn, which usually occurs as a result of the direct current itself and not as a

---

TABLE 6-1 RECOMMENDED IONS FOR USE BY THE SPORTS THERAPIST[30]

POSITIVE

Antibiotics gentamycin sulfate (+), 8 mg/ml, for suppurative ear chondritis.

Calcium (+) from calcium chloride, 2% aqueous solution, believed to stabilize the irritability threshold in either direction, as dictated by the physiologic needs of the tissues. Effective with spasmodic conditions, tics, and "snapping fingers" (joints).

Copper (+), from a 2% aqueous solution of copper sulfate crystals; fungicide, astringent, useful with intranasal conditions, e.g., allergic rhinitis ("hay fever"), sinusitis, and also dermatophytosis ("athlete's foot").

Dexamethasone (−) from Decadron, used for treating musculoskeletal inflammatory conditions.*

Hyaluronidase (+), from Wydase crystals in aqueous solution as directed; for localized edema.

Lidocaine (+), from XYLOCAINE 5% ointment, anesthetic/analgesic, especially with acute inflammatory conditions, e.g., bursitis, tendinitis, tic doloreux, and TMJ pain.

Lithium (+), from lithium chloride or carbonate, 2% aqueous solution, effective as an exchange ion with gouty tophi and hyperuricemia.

Magnesium (+), from magnesium sulfate ("Epsom Salts"), 2% aqueous solution, an excellent muscle relaxant, good vasodilator, and mild analgesic.

Mecholyl (+), familiar derivative of acetylcholine, 0.25% ointment, is a powerful vasodilator, good muscle relaxant, and analgesic. Used with discogenic low back radiculopathies and sympathetic reflex dystrophy.

Priscoline (+), from benzazoline hydrochloride, 2% aqueous solution, reported effective with indolent ulcers.

Zinc (+), from zinc oxide ointment, 20%, a trace element necessary for healing, especially effective with open lesions and ulcerations.

NEGATIVE

Acetate (−), from acetic acid, 2% aqueous solution; dramatically effective as a sclerolytic exchange ion with calcific deposits.

Chlorine (−), from sodium chloride, 2% aqueous solution, good sclerolytic agent. Useful with scar tissue, keloids, and burns.

Citrate (−), from potassium citrate, 2% aqueous solution, reported effective in rheumatoid arthritis.

Iodine (−), from "Iodex" ointment, 4.7%, an excellent sclerolytic agent, as well as bacteriocidal, fair vasodilator. Used successfully with adhesive capsulitis ("frozen shoulder"), scars, etc.

Salicylate (−), from "Iodex with methyl salicylate," 4.8% ointment, a general decongestant, sclerolytic, and anti-inflammatory agent. If desired without the iodine, may be obtained from MYOFLEX ointment (trolamine salicylate 10%) or a 2% aqueous solution of sodium salicylate powder. Used successfully with frozen shoulder, scar tissue, warts, and other adhesive or edematous conditions.

EITHER

Ringer's solution (+/−), with alternating polarity for open decubitus lesions.

Tap water (+/−), usually administered with alternating polarity and sometimes with glycopyrronium bromide in hyperhidrosis.

*Petelenz TJ et al: Ionophoresis of dexamethasone: Laboratory Studies. *J. Control. Release* 20: 55–66, 1992.

---

result of the ion being used in treatment.[47] Passing a continuous direct electrical current through the tissues creates migration of ions, which alters the normal pH of the skin. The normal pH of the skin is between 3 and 4. In an **acidic reaction** the pH falls below 3, whereas in an **alkaline reaction** the pH is greater than 5. Although chemical burns may occur under either electrode, they most typically result from the accumulation of sodium hydroxide at the cathode. The alkaline reaction causes sclerolysis of local tissues. Initially, the burn lesion is pink and raised but within hours becomes a grayish, oozing wound.[40] Decreasing current density by increasing the size of the cathode relative to the anode can minimize the potential for chemical burn.

Treatment Tip
To minimize the likelihood of a burn the size of the cathode relative to the anode can be increased and the current density can be decreased. Also, increasing the spacing between the electrodes will decrease current intensity, thus minimizing the chances of a chemical burn.

TABLE 6-2   **Conditions Treated with Iontophoresis**

Condition	Ions Used in Treatment	Condition	Ions Used in Treatment
INFLAMMATION		**SCAR TISSUE**	
Bertolucci 1982[5]	Hydrocortisone, salicylate	Tannenbaum 1980[63]	Chlorine, iodine, salicylate
Kahn 1982[38]	Dexamethasone	Kahn 1985[41]	
Chantraine et al. 1986[9]			
Harris 1982[23]		**HYPERHIDROSIS**	
Hasson 1991[25]		Kahn 1973[40]	Tap water
Hasson et al. 1992[26]		Levit 1968[43]	
Delacerda 1982[13]		Abell et al. 1974[1]	
Glass et al. 1980[19]		Shrivastava, Sing 1977[60]	
Zawislak et al. 1996[65]		Grice et al. 1972[21]	
McEntaffer et al. 1996[44]		Hill 1976[27]	
Banta 1995[4]		Stolman 1987[61]	
Petelenz et al. 1992[51]			
Panus et al. 1996[49]	Ketoprofen	**FUNGI**	
		Kahn 1985[33]	Copper
ANALGESIA		Haggard 1939[22]	
Schaeffer et al. 1971[58]	Lidocaine, magnesium		
Russo et al. 1980[56]		**OPEN SKIN LESIONS**	
Gangarosa 1974[15]		Cornwall 1981[10]	Zinc
Gangarosa 1993[16]		Jenkinson et al. 1974[30]	
Garzione 1978[18]		Balogun et al. 1990[3]	
Pellecchia et al. 1994[50]			
Reid et al. 1993[54]		**HERPES**	
		Gangarosa et al. 1989[17]	
SPASM			
Kahn 1975[37]	Calcium, magnesium	**ALLERGIC RHINITIS**	
Kahn 1982[41]		Kahn 1985[33]	Copper
ISCHEMIA		**GOUT**	
Kahn 1985[33]	Magnesium, mecholyl, iodine	Kahn 1982[36]	Lithium
EDEMA		**BURNS**	
Kahn 1985[33]	Magnesium, mecholyl	Rapperport et al. 1965[53]	Antibiotics
Boone 1969[8]	Hyaluronidase, salicylate	Rigano et al. 1992[55]	
Magistro 1964[45]		**REFLEX SYMPATHETIC DYSTROPHY**	
Schwartz 1955[59]		Bonezzi et al. 1994[6]	Guanethidine
CALCIUM DEPOSITS			
Weider 1992[64]	Acetic acid		
Kahn 1977[35]			
Psaki 1955[52]			
Kahn 1996[32]			

Heat burns may occur as a result of high resistance to current flow created by poor contact of the electrodes with the skin. Poor contact results when the electrodes are not moist enough; when there are wrinkles in the gauze or paper towels impregnated with the ionic solution; or when there is space between the skin and electrode around the perimeter of the electrode. The patient should not be treated with body weight resting on top of the electrode since this is likely to create some ischemia (reduced circulation) under the electrode. Instead, the electrode should be held firmly in place with adhesive tape, elastic bands, or lightweight sand bags. It is recommended that both chemical burns and heat burns should be treated with sterile dressings and antibiotics.[40]

SENSITIVITY REACTIONS TO IONS

Sensitivity reactions to ions rarely occur; however, they may potentially be very serious. The therapist should routinely question the patient about known drug allergies prior to initiating iontophoresis treatment. During the treatment the therapist should closely monitor the patient, looking for either abnormal localized reactions of the skin or systemic reactions.

Patients who have sensitivity to aspirin may have a reaction when using salicylates. Hydrocortisone may adversely affect individuals with gastritis or an active stomach ulcer. In cases of asthma, mecholyl should be avoided. Patients who are sensitive to metals should not be treated with copper, zinc, or magnesium. Iodine iontophoresis should not be used with individuals who have allergies to seafood or those who have had a bad reaction to intravenous pyelograms.[40]

Treatment Tip
Dexamethasone should be placed under the positive electrode since it is a positively charged ion. Current intensity should be set between 3 and 5 mA. Treatment time should be 15 minutes. The therapist should check the skin every 3 to 5 minutes for a reaction.

SUMMARY

1. Iontophoresis is a therapeutic technique that involves the introduction of ions into the body tissues by means of a direct electrical current.

2. The manner in which ions move in solution forms the basis for iontophoresis. Positively charged ions are driven into the tissues from the positive pole and negatively charged ions are introduced by the negative pole.

3. The force that acts to move ions through the tissues is determined by both the strength of the electrical field and the electrical impedance of tissues to current flow.

4. The quantity of ions transferred into the tissues through iontophoresis is determined by the intensity of the current or current density at the active electrode, the duration of the current flow, and the concentration of ions in solution.

5. Continuous direct current must be used for iontophoresis, thus insuring the unidirectional flow of ions that cannot be accomplished using a bidirectional or alternating current.

6. Electrodes may be either reusable or commercially produced, self-adhering, prepared electrodes that must be securely attached to the skin.

7. It is critical that the therapist be knowledgeable in the selection of the most appropriate ions for treating specific conditions.

8. Clinically, iontophoresis is used in the treatment of inflammatory musculoskeletal conditions, for analgesic effects, scar modification, wound healing, and in treating edema, calcium deposits, and hyperhidrosis.

9. Perhaps the single most common problem associated with iontophoresis is a chemical burn, which usually occurs as a result of the direct current itself and not because of the ion being used in treatment.

REFERENCES

1. Abell, E., Morgan, K.: Treatment of idiopathic hyperhidrosis by glycopyrronium bromide and tap water iontophoresis, Br. J. Dermatol. 91:87, 1974.

2. Bagniefski, T., Burnette, R.: A comparison of pulsed and continuous current iontophoresis, J. Controlled Rel. 11:113–122, 1990.

3. Balogun, J., Abidoye, A., and Akala, E.: Zinc iontophoresis in the management of bacterial colonized wounds: a case report, Physiother. Can. 42(3):147–151, 1990.

4. Banta, C.: A prospective nonrandomized study of iontophoresis, wrist splinting, and antiinflammatory medication in the treatment of early mild carpal tunnel syndrome, J. Orthop. Sports Phys. Ther. 21(2):120, 1995.

5. Bertolucci, L.: Introduction of anti-inflammatory drugs by iontophoreses: a double-blind study. J. Orthop. Sports Phys. Ther. 4(2):103, 1982.

6. Bonezzi, C., Miotti, D., and Bettagilo, R.: Electromotive administration of guanethidine for treatment of reflex sympathetic dystrophy, J. Pain Sympt. Manage. 9(1):39–43, 1994.

7. Boone, D.: Applications of iontophoresis, In Wolf, S., editor. Electrotherapy, New York, 1981, Churchill Livingstone.

8. Boone, D.: Hyaluronidase iontophoresis, J. Am. Phys. Ther. Assoc. 49:139–145, 1969.

9. Chantraine, A., Lundy, J., and Berger, D.: Is cortisone iontophoresis possible? Arch. Phys. Med. Rehab. 67:380, 1986.

10. Cornwall, M.: Zinc oxide iontophoresis for ischemic skin ulcers. Phys. Ther. 61(3):359, 1981.

11. Costello, C., Jeske, A: Iontophoresis: applications in transdermal medication delivery, Phys. Ther. 75(6):554–563, 1995.

12. Cummings, J.: Iontophoresis. In Nelson, R.M., Currier, D.P., editors. Clinical electrotherapy, Norwalk, Connecticut, 1991, Appleton & Lange.

13. Delacerda, F.: A comparative study of three methods of treatment for shoulder girdle myofascial syndrome. J. Orthop. Sports Phys. Ther. 4(1):51–54, 1982.

14. Gadsby, P.: Visualization of the barrier layer through iontophoresis of ferric ions. Med. Instrum. 13:281, 1979.

15. Gangarosa, L.: Iontophoresis for surface local anesthesia. J. Am. Dent. Assoc. 88:125, 1974.

16. Gangarosa, L.: Iontophoresis in pain control, Pain Digest 3:162–174, 1993.

17. Gangarosa, L., Payne, L., and Hayakawa, K.: Iontophoretic treatment of herpetic whitlow, Arch. Phys. Med. Rehab. 70(4):336–340, 1989.

18. Garzione, J.: Salicylate iontophoresis as an alternative treatment for persistent thigh pain following hip surgery. Phys. Ther. 58 (5):570–571, 1978.

19. Glass, J., Stephen, R., and Jacobsen, S.: The quantity and distribution of radiolabeled dexamethasone delivered to tissues by iontophoresis. Int. J Dermatol. 19:519, 1980.

20. Glick, E., Synder-Mackler, L.: Iontophoresis. In Snyder-Mackler, L., Robinson, A., editors. Clinical electrophysiology and electrophysiologic testing, Baltimore, 1989, Williams & Wilkins.

21. Grice, K., Sattar, H., and Baker, H.: Treatment of idiopathic hyperhidrosis with iontophoresis of tap water and poldine methosulphate. Br. J. Dermatol. 86:72, 1972.

22. Haggard, H., Strauss, M., and Greenberg, L.: Fungus infections of hand and feet treated by copper iontophoresis. JAMA 112:1229, 1939.

23. Harris, P.: Iontophoresis: clinical research in musculoskeletal inflammatory conditions. J. Orthop. Sports Phys. Ther. 4(2): 109–112, 1982.

24. Harris, R.: Iontophoresis. In Licht, S., editor. Therapeutic electricity and ultraviolet radiation, Baltimore, 1967, Waverly.

25. Hasson, S.: Exercise training and dexamethsone intophoresis in rheumatoid arthritis: a case study, Physiotherapy (Can.) 43:11, 1991.

26. Hasson, S., Wible, C., and Reich, M.: Dexamethasone iontophoresis: effect on delayed muscle soreness and muscle function. Can. J. Sport Sci. 17:8–13, 1992.

27. Hill, B.: Poldine iontophoresis in the treatment of palmar and plantar hyperhidrosis. Aust. J. Dermatol. 17:92, 1976.

28. Howard, J., Drake, T., and Kellogg, D.: Effects of alternating current iontophoresis on drug delivery, Arch. Phys. Med. Rehab. 76(5):463–466, 1995.

29. Jacobson, S., Stephen, R., Sears, W.: Development of a new drug delivery system (iontophoresis). University of Utah, Salt Lake City, Utah, 1980.

30. Jenkinson, D., McEwan, J., and Walton, G.: The potential use of iontophoresis in the treatment of skin disorders, Vet. Rec. 94:8 Arch. Phys. Med. Rehab. 12, 1974.

31. Johnson, C., Shuster, S.: The patency of sweat ducts in normal looking skin. Br. J. Dermatol. 83:367, 1970.

32. Kahn, J.: Acetic acid iontophoresis, Phys. Ther. 76(5):S68, 1996.

33. Kahn, J.: Practices and principles of electrotherapy, New York, 1991, Churchill Livingstone.

34. Kahn, J.: Non-steroid iontophoresis, Clin. Manage. Phys. Ther. 7(1):14–15, 1987.

35. Kahn, J.: A case report: lithium iontophoresis for gouty arthritis. J. Orthop. Sports Phys. Ther. 4:113, 1982.

36. Kahn, J.: Acetic acid iontophoresis for calcium deposits. JAPTA 57(6):658, 1977.

37. Kahn, J.: Calcium iontophoresis in suspected myopathy. JAPTA 55(4):276, 1975.

38. Kahn, J.: Iontophoresis with hydrocortisone for Peyronie's disease. JAPTA 62(7):995, 1982.

39. Kahn, J.: Iontophoresis: practice tips. Clin. Manage. 2(4):37, 1982.

40. Kahn, J.: Tap-water iontophoresis for hyperhidrosis. Reprinted in Medical Group News, August, 1973.

41. Kahn, J.: Clinical electrotherapy, ed 4. Syosset, New York, 1985, J. Kahn.

42. LeDuc, S.: Electric ions and their use in medicine. Liverpool, 1903, Rebman.

43. Levit, R: Simple device for treatment of hyperhidrosis by iontophoresis. Arch Dermatol 98:505–507, 1968.

44. McEntaffer, D., Sailor, M.: The effects of stretching and iontophoretically delivered dexamethasone on plantar fasciitis, Phys. Ther. 76(5):S68, 1996.

45. Magistro, C.: Hyaluronidase by iontophoresis in the treatment of edema: A preliminary clinical report, Phys. Ther. 44:169, 1964.

46. Mandleco, C.: Research: iontophoresis.University of Utah, Salt Lake City, 1978, Institute for Biomedical Engineering.

47. Molitor, H.: Pharmacologic aspects of drug administration by ion transfer. The Merck Report: 22–29, January, 1943.

48. Murray, W., Levine L., and Seifter E.: The iontophoresis of C2 esterified glucocorticoids: Preliminary report. Phys. Ther. 43:579, 1963.

49. O'Malley, E., Oester, Y.: Influence of some physical chemical factors on iontophoresis using radioisotopes. Arch. Phys. Med. Rehabil. 36:310, 1955.

50. Pellecchia, G., Hamel, H., and Behnke, P.: Treatment of infrapatellar tendinitis: A combination of modalities and transverse friction massage versus iontophoresis, J. Sport Rehab. 3(2):135–145, 1994.

51. Petelenz, T., Buttke, J., and Bonds, C.: Iontophoresis of dexamethasone: laboratory studies, J. Controlled Rel. 20:55–66, 1992.

52. Psaki, C., Carol, J.: Acetic acid ionization: a study to determine the absorptive effects upon calcified tendinitis of the shoulder. Phys. Ther. Rev. 35:84, 1955.

53. Rapperport, A.: Iontophoresis—a method of antibiotic administration in the burn patient, Plast. Reconstr. Surg. 36(5):547–552, 1965.

54. Reid, K., Sicard-Rosenbaum, L., and Lord, D.: Iontophoresis with normal saline versus dexamethasone and lidocaine in the treatment of patients with internal disc derangement of the temporomandibular joint, Phys. Ther. 73(6):S20, 1993.

55. Rigano, W., Yanik, M., and Barone F.: Antibiotic iontophoresis in the management of burned ears, J. Burn Care Rehab.13(4):407–409, 1992.

56. Russo, J., Lipman, A., and Comstock, T.: Lidocane anesthesia: comparison of iontophoresis, injection and swabbing, Am. J. Hosp. Pharm. 37:843–847, 1980.

57. Sabbahi, M., Costello, C., and Emran, A.: A method for reducing skin irritation from iontophoresis, Phys. Ther. 74:S156, 1994.

58. Schaeffer, M., Bixler, D., and Yu, P.: The effectiveness of iontophoresis in reducing cervical hypersensitivity, J. Peridontol. 42:695, 1971.

59. Schwartz, M.: The use of hyaluronidase by iontophoresis in the treatment of lymphedema, Arch. Intern. Med. 95:662, 1955.

60. Shrivastava, S., Sing, G.: Tap water iontophoresis in palm and plantar hyperhidrosis, Br. J. Dermatol. 96:189, 1977.

61. Stolman, L.: Treatment of excess sweating of the palms by iontophoresis, Arch. Dermatol. 123:893, 1987.

62. Su, M., Srinivasan, V., and Ghanem, A.: Quantitative in vivo iontophoretic studies, J. Pharm. Sci. 83:12–17, 1994.

63. Tannenbaum, M.: Iodine iontophoresis in reduction of scar tissue. Phys. Ther. 60(6):792, 1980.

64. Weider, D.: Treatment of traumatic myositis ossificans with acetic acid iontophoresis. Phys. Ther. 72(2):133–137, 1992.

65. Zawislak, D., Rau, C., and Lee, M.: The effects of dexamethasone iontophoresis on acute inflammation using a sports model of treatment, Phys. Ther. 76(5):5–17, 1966.

SUGGESTED READINGS

Abramowitsch, D., Neoussikine, B.: Treatment by ion transfer, New York, 1946, Grune & Stratton.

Abramson, D.: Physiologic and clinical basis for histamine by ion transfer. Arch. Phys. Med. Rehab. 48:583–592, 1967.

Agostinucci, J., Powers, W.: Motoneuron excitability modulation after desensitization of the skin by iontophoresis of lidocaine hydrochloride. Arch. Phys. Med. Rehab. 73(2):190–194, 1992.

Akins, D., Meisenheimer, I., and Dobson, R.: Efficacy of the Drionic unit in the treatment of hyperhidrosis. J. Am. Acad. Dermatol. 16:828, 1987.

Brumett, A., Comeau, M.: Local anesthesia of the tympanic membrane by iontophoresis. Trans. Am. Acad. Otolaryngol. 78:453, 1974.

Cady, D., Zawislak, J., and Rau, C.: The effects of dexamethasone iontophoresis on acute inflammation using a sports model of treatment, Phys. Ther. 76(5):S17, 1996.

Comeau, M.: Anesthesia of the human tympanic membrane by iontophoresis of a local anesthetic. Laryngoscope 88:277–285, 1978.

Comeau, M.: Local anesthesia of the ear by iontophoresis. Arch. Otolaryngol. 98:114–120, 1973.

Chein, Y., Banga, A.: Iontophoretic (transdermal) delivery of drugs: overview of historical development, J. Pharm. Sci. 78:353–354, 1989.

Dellagatta, E., Thompson, E.: Changes in skin resistance produced by continuous direct current stimulation utilizing methyl nicotinate, Phys. Ther. 74(5):S12, 1994.

Falcone, A., Spadaro, J.: Inhibitory effects of electrically activated silver material on cutaneous wound bacteria, Plast. Reconstr. Surg. 77:455, 1986.

Fay, M.: Indications and applications for iontophoresis, Today's OR Nurse 11(4):10–16, 29–31, 1989.

Gangarosa, L., Park, N., and Fong, B.: Conductivity of drugs used for iontophoresis. J. Pharm. Sci. 67:1439–1443, 1978.

Gordon, A.: Sodium salicylate iontophoresis in the treatment of plantar warts. Phys. Ther. Rev. 49:869–870, 1969.

Haggard, H., Strauss, M., and Greenberg, L.: Copper, electrically injected, cures fungus diseases. Reprinted in Science Newsletter, May 6, 1939.

Hasson, S.: Exercise training and dexamethsone intophoresis in rheumatoid arthritis: a case study, Physiotherapy (Can.) 43:11, 1991.

Henley, J.: Transcutaneous drug delivery: iontophoresis, phonophoresis, Phys. Med. Rehab. 2:139, 1991.

Jarvis, C., Voita, D.: Low voltage skin burns, Pediatrics 48:831, 1971.

Kahn, J.: Phoresor adaptation, Clin. Manage. Phys. Ther. 5(4):50–51, 1985.

Kahn, J.: Iontophoresis (video tape). AREN, Pittsburgh, Pennsylvania, 1988.

Kahn, J.: Iontophoresis and ultrasound for post-surgical TMJ trismus and paresthesia. JAPTA 60(3):307, 1982.

Kahn, J.: Iontophoresis in clinical practice. Stimulus (APTA-SCE) 8(3), May, 1983.

LaForest, N., Confrancisco, C.: Antibiotic iontophoresis in the treatment of ear chondritis. JAPTA 58:32, 1978.

Langley, P.: Iontophoresis to aid in releasing tendon adhesions, Phys. Ther. 64(9):1395, 1984.

Lemming, M., Cole, R., and Howland, W.: Low voltage direct current burns, JAMA 214:1681, 1970.

McFadden, E.: Iontophoresis for pain management, J. Ped. Nurs. 10(5):331, 1995.

Nightingale, A.: Physics and electronics in physical medicine. London, 1959, F. Bell.

Nimmo, W.: Novel delivery systems: electrotransport, J. Pain Sympt. Manage. 7(3):160–162, 1992.

Panus, P., Campbell, J., and Kulkami, S.: Transdermal iontophoretic delivery of ketoprofen through human cadaver skin and in humans, Phys. Ther. 76(5):S67, 1996.

Phipps, J., Padmanabhan, R., and Lattin G.: Iontophoretic delivery of model inorganic and drug ions, J. Pharm. Sci. 78:365–369, 1989.

Puttemans, F., Massart, D., and Gilles, F.: Iontophoreses: mechanism of action studied by potentiometry and x-ray fluorescence. Arch. Phys. Med. Rehab. 63:176–180, 1982.

Sawyer, C.: Cystic fibrosis of the pancreas: a study of sweat electrolyte levels in thirty-six families using pilocarpine iontophoresis. So. Med. J. 59:197–202, 1966.

Shapiro, B.: Insulin iontophoresis in cystic fibrosis. Soc. Exp. Biol. Med. 149:592–593, 1975.

Shriber, W.: A manual of electrotherapy, 4th ed. Philadelphia, 1975, Lea & Febiger.

Sisler, H.: Iontophoresis local anesthesia for conjunctival surgery. Ann. Ophthalmol. 10:597, 1978.

Stillwell, G.: Electrotherapy. In: Kottke, F., Stillwell, G., and Lehman, J., editors. Handbook of physical medical and rehabilitation. Philadelphia, 1982, W.B. Saunders.

Tregear, R.: The permeability of mammalian skin to ions, J. Invest. Dermatol. 46:16–23, 1966.

Trubatch, J., Van Harrevel, A.: Spread of iontophoretically injected ions in a tissue, J. Theor. Biol. 36:355, 1972.

Waud, D.: Iontophoretic applications of drugs, J. Appl. Physiol. 28:128, 1967.

Zankel, H., Cress, R., and Kamin, H.: Iontophoreses studies with radioactive tracer. Arch. Phys. Med. Rehab. 40:193–196, 1959.

GLOSSARY

acidic reaction The accumulation of negative ions under the positive pole that produces hydrochloric acid.

active electrode The electrode that is used to drive ions into the tissues.

alkaline reaction The accumulation of positive ions under the negative electrode that produces sodium hydroxide.

electrolytes Solutions in which ionic movement occurs.

electrophoresis The movement of ions in solution.

ionization A process by which soluble compounds such as acids, alkaloids, or salts dissociate or dissolve into ions that are suspended in some type of solution.

ions Positively or negatively charged particles.

iontophoresis A therapeutic technique that involves the introduction of ions into the body tissues by means of a direct electrical current.

ion transfer A technique of transporting chemicals across a membrane using an electrical current as a driving force.

LAB ACTIVITY

ELECTRICAL STIMULATION: IONTOPHORESIS

DESCRIPTION:

Iontophoresis is the use of direct current electricity to introduce various drugs to subcutaneous tissues without using invasive means. Although there are many drugs that may be used, various corticosteroids and local anesthetics are the most commonly used drugs.

It is not possible to use any form of electrical current other than direct current to achieve movement of the drug; the misnamed "high-voltage galvanic stimulators" are not capable of phoresing a drug owing to the very low pulse charge. Because of the possibility of producing an electrolytic burn with direct current, it is recommended that the current amplitude remain below 0.7 mA $\times$ ð cm^2 of electrode.

There are many different electrodes available for iontophoresis. The most rudimentary is to use alligator clips to attach the cables to a tin or aluminum conductor, and use a paper towel soaked with the drug between the electrode and the patient. More commonly, electrodes developed by the manufacturer of the stimulator are used.

It is mandatory that the drug be in an ionic form; otherwise, the electrical current will not be able to move the drug. Many drugs come in both ionized forms and as a suspension. If in doubt, a PDR should be consulted.

PHYSIOLOGIC EFFECTS:

Depends on the drug

THERAPEUTIC EFFECTS:

Depends on the drug; generally, decreased inflammation and local anesthesia

INDICATIONS:

Iontophoresis is indicated when there is a need to deliver an ionized drug to localized subcutaneous tissue, and it is desirable to avoid injection of the drug with a needle. The most common types of disorders are tendinitis, bursitis, and synovitis of traumatic origin. If a local anesthetic is used, the treated area must be protected from excessive internal and external forces until normal protective mechanisms conferred by normal pain sensibility have been restored.

CONTRAINDICATIONS:

- Pregnancy
- Implanted electrical pacing devices (e.g., cardiac pacemaker, bladder stimulator, etc.)
- Cardiac arrhythmia
- Over the carotid sinus area
- Hypersensitivity (i.e., the patient who has a strong aversion to electricity, or the patient with certain types of catheters or shunts).

ELECTRICAL STIMULATION: IONTOPHORESIS			
PROCEDURE	Evaluation		
	1	2	3
1. Check supplies.			
a. Obtain towels or sheets for draping, conductant.			
b. Check stimulator, electrodes, and cables for charged battery, broken or frayed insulation, and so on.			
c. Verify that the intensity control is at zero.			
2. Question patient.			
a. Verify identity of patient (if not already verified).			
b. Verify the absence of contraindications.			

PROCEDURE	Evaluation		
	1	2	3
c. Ask about previous exposure to electrotherapy.			
3. Position patient.			
a. Place patient in a well-supported, comfortable position.			
b. Expose body part to be treated.			
c. Drape patient to preserve patient's modesty, protect clothing, but allow access to body part.			
4. Inspect body part to be treated.			
a. Check light touch perception.			
b. Assess function of body part (e.g., ROM, irritability).			
5. Apply electrical stimulation for iontophoresis.			
a. Prepare electrodes according to manufacturer's instructions, secure electrodes to patient. Electrode location will vary depending on the drug being phoresed; anionic drugs are repelled from the cathode, cations are repelled from the anode.			
b. Remind the patient to inform you when they feel something. Do not tell the patient what they will feel; for example, do not say "tell me when you feel a burning or stinging."			
c. Turn on the stimulator, and increase the amplitude slowly. Monitor the patient's response, not the stimulator.			
d. After the patient reports the onset of the stimulus, adjust the amplitude to the appropriate intensity.			
e. Continue to monitor the patient during the duration of the treatment.			
6. Complete treatment.			
a. When the treatment time is over, turn the generator off, and turn the intensity control to zero; remove conductant with a towel.			
b. Remove material used for draping, assist the patient in dressing as needed.			
c. Have the patient perform appropriate therapeutic exercise as indicated.			
d. Clean the treatment area and equipment according to normal protocol.			
7. Assess treatment efficacy.			
a. Ask the patient how the treated area feels.			
b. Visually inspect the treated area for any adverse reactions.			
c. Perform functional tests as indicated.			

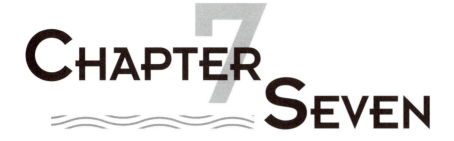

CHAPTER SEVEN

BIOFEEDBACK

WILLIAM E. PRENTICE

OBJECTIVES

After completing this chapter the student therapist will be able to:

- ✓ Define biofeedback and identify its uses in a clinical setting.
- ✓ Discuss the various types of biofeedback instruments.
- ✓ Explain physiologically how the electrical activity generated by a muscle contraction can be measured using an electromyograph (EMG).
- ✓ Explain how the electrical activity picked up by the electrodes is amplified, processed, and converted to meaningful information by the EMG unit.
- ✓ Differentiate between visual and auditory feedback.
- ✓ Discuss the equipment setup and clinical applications for EMG biofeedback.

Electromyographic biofeedback is a modality that seems to be gaining increased popularity in clinical settings. It is a therapeutic procedure that uses electronic or electromechanical instruments to accurately measure, process, and feed back reinforcing information via auditory or visual signals.[21] In clinical practice, it is used to help the patient develop greater voluntary control in terms of either neuromuscular relaxation or muscle reeducation following injury.

THE ROLE OF BIOFEEDBACK

The term biofeedback should be familiar because all therapists routinely serve as instruments of biofeedback when teaching a therapeutic exercise or in coaching a movement pattern. Using feedback can help the patient to regain function of a muscle that may have been lost or forgotten following injury.[11] Feedback includes information related to the sensations associated with movement itself as well as information related to the result of the action relative to some goal or objective. Feedback refers to the intrinsic information inherent to movement, including kinesthetic, visual, cutaneous, vestibular, and auditory signals collectively termed as response-produced feedback. However, it also refers to extrinsic information or some knowledge of results that is presented verbally, mechanically, or electronically to indicate the outcome of some movement performance. Therefore, feedback is ongoing, in a temporal sense, occurring before, during, and after any motor or movement task. Feedback from some measuring instrument that provides moment-to-moment information about a biologic function is referred to as biofeedback.[18]

biofeedback Information provided from some measuring instrument about a specific biologic function.

Perhaps the biggest advantage of biofeedback is that it provides the patient with a chance to make correct small changes in performance that are immediately noted and rewarded so that eventually larger changes or improvements in performance can be accomplished. The goal is to train the patient to perceive these changes without the use of the measuring instrument so that he or she can practice independently. Therefore, the patient learns early in the rehabilitation process to do something for him- or herself and not to totally rely on the therapist. This will help him or her to build confidence and increase feelings of self-efficacy. Treatments using biofeedback are useful, particularly in a patient who has difficulty in perceiving the initial small correct responses or who may have a faulty perception of what he or she is doing. Hopefully, the rehabilitating patient will be motivated and encouraged by seeing early signs of slight progress; thus relieving feelings of helplessness and reducing injury-related stress to some extent.[18]

To process feedback information, the patient makes use of a complicated series of interrelated feedback loops involving very complex anatomic and neurophysiologic components.[28] An in-depth discussion of these components is well beyond the scope of this text. Thus, our focus will be oriented toward how biofeedback may best be incorporated in a treatment program.

BIOFEEDBACK INSTRUMENTATION

Biofeedback Instruments Measure
- Peripheral skin temperature
- Finger phototransmission
- Skin conductance activity
- Electromyographic activity

Biofeedback instruments are designed to monitor some physiologic event, objectively quantify these monitorings, and then interpret the measurements as meaningful information.[22] There are several different types of biofeedback modalities available for use in rehabilitation. These biofeedback units cannot directly measure a physiologic event. Instead they record some aspect that is highly correlated with the physiologic event. Thus the biofeedback reading should be taken as a convenient indication of a physiologic process but should not be confused with the physiologic process itself.[22]

The most commonly used instruments include those that record _peripheral skin temperatures_, indicating the extent of vasoconstriction or vasodilation; _finger phototransmission units (photoplethysmograph)_, which also measure vasoconstriction and vasodilation; units that record _skin conductance activity_, indicating sweat gland activity; and units that measure _electromyographic activity_, indicating amount of electrical activity during muscle contraction.

There are other types of biofeedback units available also, including electroencephalographs (EEG), pressure transducers, and electrogoniometers.

PERIPHERAL SKIN TEMPERATURE

Peripheral skin temperature is an indirect measure of the diameter of peripheral blood vessels. As vessels dilate, more warm blood is delivered to a particular area, thus increasing the temperature in that area. This effect is easily seen in the fingers and toes where the surrounding tissue warms and cools rapidly. Variations in skin temperature seem to be correlated with affective states, with a decrease occurring in response to stress or fear. Temperature changes are usually measured in degrees Fahrenheit.[22]

CASE STUDY 7-1
BIOFEEDBACK

Background: A 14-year-old female subluxed her left patella while at soccer practice. There was immediate pain and a localized effusion that resolved with the use of an immobilizer, intermittent ice packs, and rest over a 7-day period. On referral for the initiation of quadriceps rehabilitation the patient reported no pain, minimal swelling, but residual stiffness and sensation of weakness in the knee joint. The physical examination was unremarkable except for limited ROM of 10 to 110 degrees and the inability of the patient to successfully initiate and sustain an isometric contraction of the quadriceps musculature.

Impression: Quadriceps inhibition secondary to injury and immobilization.

Treatment Plan: In addition to the initiation of therapeutic exercise—static (stretching) and active (assistive ROM exercise for the knee joint)—biofeedback was initiated for the quadriceps mechanism. Using the vastus medialis muscle as the target muscle, the skin was cleansed and electrodes placed in alignment with the fibers of the muscle. A microvolt threshold of detection slightly above the patient's ability to maximize auditory and visual feedback was chosen. The patient was encouraged to perform isometric quadriceps-setting exercises of 6 to 10 seconds duration, attempting to "max out" feedback for the chosen threshold level. The threshold was advanced and the process repeated.

Response: Over the course of the initial rehabilitation session, the patient advanced several threshold levels and "reacquired" the ability to initiate and sustain an isometric quadriceps muscle contraction comparable to her uninvolved extremity. She was rapidly transitioned to limited-range dynamic exercise and a functional closed-chain exercise sequence, with emphasis on terminal-range knee stability. She returned to soccer activities several weeks later.

Discussion Questions

- What tissues were injured or affected?
- What symptoms were present?
- What phase of the injury-healing continuum did the patient present for care in?
- What are the therapeutic agent modality's biophysical effects (direct, indirect, depth, and tissue affinity)?
- What are the therapeutic agent modality's indications and contraindications?
- What are the parameters of the therapeutic agent modality's application, dosage, duration, and frequency in this case study?
- What other therapeutic agent modalities could be utilized to treat this injury or condition? Why? How?

The rehabilitation professional employs therapeutic agent modalities to create an optimum environment for tissue healing while minimizing the symptoms associated with the trauma or condition.

FINGER PHOTOTRANSMISSION

The degree of peripheral vasoconstriction can also be measured indirectly using a photoplethysmograph. This instrument monitors the amount of light that can pass through a finger or toe, reflect off a bone, and pass back through the soft tissue to a light sensor. As the volume of blood in a given area increases, the amount of light detected by the sensor decreases, thus giving some indication of blood volume. Only changes in blood volume can be detected, since there are no standardized units of measure. These instruments are used most often to monitor pulse.[14]

SKIN CONDUCTANCE ACTIVITY

Sweat gland activity can be indirectly measured by determining electrodermal activity, most commonly referred to as the "galvanic skin response." Sweat contains salt that increases electrical conductivity. Thus sweaty skin is more conductive than dry skin. This instrument applies a very small electrical voltage to the skin, usually on the palmar surface of the hand or the volar surface of the fingers where there are a lot of sweat glands, and measures the impedance of the electrical current in micro-ohm units. Measuring skin conductance is a technique useful in objectively assessing psychophysiologic arousal and is most often used in "lie detector" testing.[22]

ELECTROMYOGRAPHIC BIOFEEDBACK

electromyographic biofeedback A therapeutic procedure that uses electronic or electromechanical instruments to accurately measure, process, and feed back reinforcing information via auditory or visual signals.

Electromyographic biofeedback is certainly the most typically used of all the biofeedback modalities in a clinical setting. Muscle contraction results from the more or less synchronous contraction of individual muscle fibers that compose a muscle. Individual muscle fibers are innervated by nerves that collectively comprise a motor unit. The axon of that motor unit conducts an action potential to the neuro-muscular junction where a neurotransmitter substance (acetylcholine) is released. As this neurotransmitter binds to receptor sites on the sarcolemma, depolarization of that muscle fiber occurs, moving in both directions along the muscle fiber, creating movement of ions and thus an electrochemical gradient around the muscle fiber. Changes in potential difference or voltage associated with depolarization can be detected by an electrode placed in close proximity. (Fig. 7-1).

MOTOR UNIT RECRUITMENT

The amount of tension developed in a muscle is determined by the number of active motor units. As more motor units are recruited and the frequency of discharge increases, muscle tension increases.

The pattern of motor unit recruitment varies depending on the inherent properties of specific motor neurons, the force required during the activity, and the speed of contraction. Smaller motor units are recruited first and are somewhat limited in their ability to generate tension. Larger motor units generate greater tension since more muscle fibers are recruited.

Motor units are recruited based on the force required in an activity and not on the type of contraction performed. Thus the firing rate and recruitment of the motor

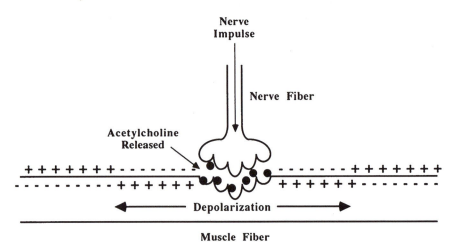

•**Figure 7-1** The nerve fiber conducts an impulse to the neuromuscular junction where acetylcholine binds to receptor sites on the sarcolemma, inducing a depolarization of the muscle fiber that creates movement of ions and thus an electrochemical gradient around the muscle fiber.

units are dependent on the external force required. The speed of contraction also influences motor unit recruitment. Fast contractions tend to excite larger and depress smaller motor units.

Measuring Electrical Activity

Despite the fact that EMG is used to determine muscle activity, it does not measure muscle contraction directly. Instead it measures electrical activity associated with muscle contraction. Movement of ions across the membrane creates a depolarization of the muscle membranes, resulting in a reversal in polarity, followed by repolarization. The various stages of membrane activity generate a triphasic electrical signal.[4] Electrical activity of the muscle is measured in volts, or more precisely, microvolts ($1 \text{ V} = 1,000,000 \text{ }\mu\text{V}$).

Measurement of electrical activity is made in standard quantitative units. Monitoring is useful in detecting changes in electrical activity, although changes cannot be quantified. The advantage of measurement over monitoring is that an objective scale is used; therefore, comparisons can be made between different individuals, occasions, and instruments. Measurement allows *procedures* to be replicated.

Unfortunately, with EMG biofeedback units there is no universally accepted standardized measurement scale. Each brand of EMG unit serves as its own reference standard. Different brands of EMG equipment may give different readings for the same degree of muscle contraction. Consequently, EMG readings can be compared only when the same equipment is used for all readings.[22]

The EMG biofeedback unit receives small amounts of electrical energy generated during muscle contraction through an electrode. It then separates or filters this electrical energy from other extraneous electrical activity on the skin and amplifies the EMG electrical energy. The amplified EMG activity is then converted to information that has meaning to the user. Figure 7-2 is a diagram of the various components of an EMG biofeedback unit.

Electrodes

Skin-surface electrodes are most often used in EMG biofeedback. Fine-wire indwelling electrodes may also be used that permit localized highly accurate mea-

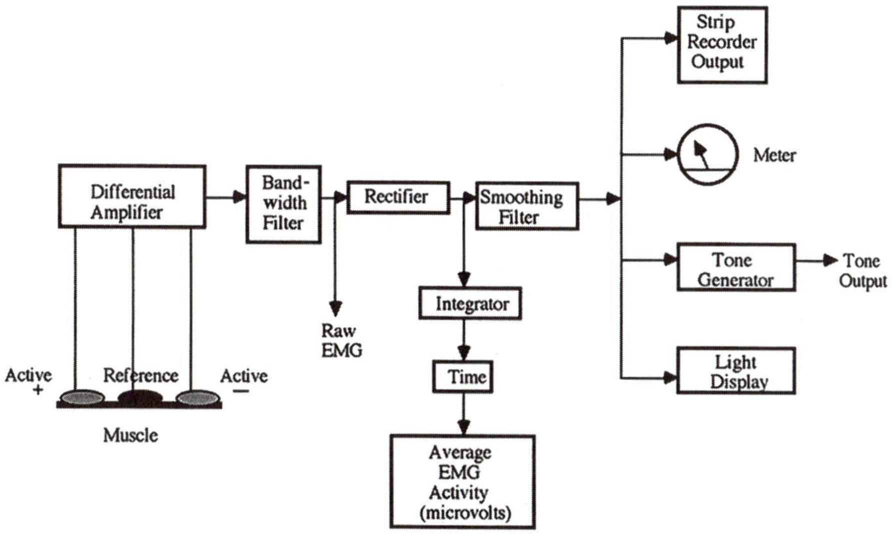

> EMG measures electrical activity of muscle and not muscle contraction.

> **Treatment Tip**
> Biofeedback units do not directly measure muscle contraction. Instead, they measure only the electrical activity associated with a muscle contraction. Thus the patient should understand that the electrical activity implies some information about the quality of a muscle contraction, but does not measure the strength of that muscle contraction specifically.

> Most biofeedback units use surface electrodes.

•**Figure 7-2** Diagram of a typical EMG biofeedback unit.

surement of electrical activity. However, these electrodes must be inserted percutaneously and thus are relatively impractical in a clinical setting.

Various types of surface electrodes are available for use with EMG biofeedback units. Electrodes are most often made of stainless steel or nickel-plated brass recessed in a plastic holder. These less expensive electrodes are effective in EMG biofeedback applications. More expensive electrodes made of gold or silver/silver chloride also have been used.[30]

The size of the electrodes may range from 4 mm in diameter for recording small muscle activity to 12.5 mm for use with larger muscle groups. Increasing the size of the electrode will not cause an increase in the amplitude of the signal.[17]

Regardless of whether or not electrodes are disposable, some type of conducting gel, paste, or cream with high salt content is necessary to establish a highly conductive connection with the skin. Disposable electrodes come with the appropriate amount of gel and an adhesive ring already applied so that the electrode can be easily connected to the skin. Nondisposable electrodes need to have a double-sided adhesive ring applied. Then enough conducting gel must be added so that it is level with the surface of the adhesive ring before the electrode is applied to the skin.

Prior to attachment of the surface electrodes, the skin must be appropriately prepared by removing oil and dead skin along with excessive hair from the surface to reduce skin impedance. Scrubbing with an alcohol-soaked prep pad is recommended.[30] However, if the skin is cleaned until it becomes irritated it may interfere with EMG recording.

Some surface electrodes are permanently attached to cable wires, whereas others may snap onto the wire. Some biofeedback units include a set of three electrodes preplaced on a Velcro™ band that may be easily attached to the skin.

Electrode Placement

The electrodes should be placed as near to the muscle being monitored as possible to minimize recording extraneous electrical activity. They should be secured with the body part in the position in which it will be monitored so that movement of the skin will not alter the positioning of the electrodes over a particular muscle (Fig. 7-3).[30]

The electrodes should be parallel to the direction of the muscle fibers to ensure that a better sample of muscle activity is monitored while reducing extraneous electrical activity.

Spacing of the electrodes is also a critical consideration. Electrodes generally detect measurable signals from a distance equal to that of the interelectrode spacing. Therefore, as the distance between the electrodes increases, the EMG signal will include electrical activity not only from muscles directly under the electrodes but also from other nearby muscles.[4]

Separation and Amplification of Electromyographic Activity

Once the electrical activity is detected by the electrodes, the extraneous electrical activity, or "**noise,**" must be eliminated before the EMG activity is amplified and subsequently objectified. This is accomplished by using two **active electrodes** and a single ground or **reference electrode** in a **bipolar arrangement** to create three separate pathways from the skin to the biofeedback unit (Fig. 7-4). The active electrodes should be placed in close proximity to one another, whereas the reference electrode may be placed anywhere on the body. Typically in biofeedback, the reference electrode is placed between the two active electrodes.

The active electrodes pick up electrical activity from motor units firing in the muscles beneath the electrodes. The magnitude of the small voltages detected by each active electrode will differ with respect to the reference electrode, creating two separate signals. These two signals are then fed to a **differential amplifier** that basi-

noise Extraneous electrical activity that may be produced by any source other than the contracting muscle.

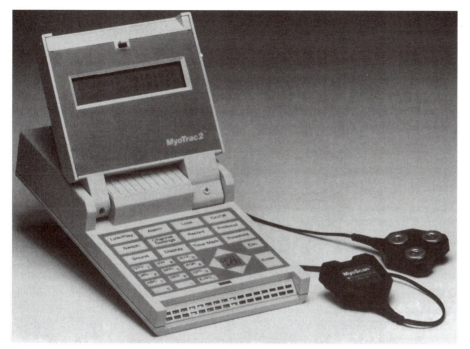

active electrode An electrode attached directly to the skin over a muscle that picks up the electrical activity produced by a muscle contraction.

•**Figure 7-3** The biofeedback unit is connected via a series of electrodes to the skin over the contracting muscle.

cally subtracts the signal of one active electrode from the other. This, in effect, cancels out or rejects any components that the two signals have in common coming from the active electrodes, thus amplifying the difference between the signals. The differential amplifier uses the reference electrode to compare the signals of the two active or recording electrodes (see Fig. 7-4).

There will always be some degree of extraneous electrical activity created by power lines, motors, lights, appliances, and so on, that is picked up by the body and eventually detected by the surface electrodes on the skin. Assuming that this extra-

reference electrode Also referred to as the ground electrode, serves as a point of reference to compare the electrical activity recorded by the active electrodes.

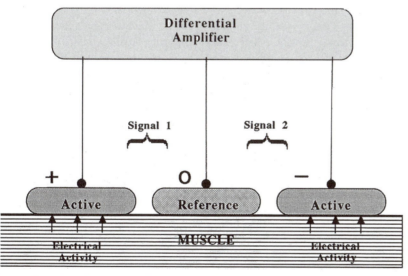

•**Figure 7-4** The differential amplifier monitors the two separate signals from the active electrodes and amplifies the difference, thus eliminating extraneous noise.

neous "noise" is detected equally by both active electrodes, the differential amplifier will subtract the noise detected by one active electrode from the noise detected by the other, leaving only the true difference between the active electrodes. The ability of the differential amplifier to eliminate the common noise between the active electrodes is called the **common mode rejection ratio (CMRR)**.

External noise can be reduced further by using **filters** that essentially make the amplifier more sensitive to some incoming frequencies and less sensitive to others. Therefore, the amplifier will pick up signals only at those frequencies produced by electrical activity in the muscle within a specific frequency range or **bandwidth**. In general, the wider the bandwidth, the higher the EMG and noise readings.

It must be noted that the therapist is interested in measuring the electrical activity within the muscle. An excessive external noise that is not eliminated by the biofeedback instrument will mask true EMG activity and will significantly decrease the reliability of the information being generated by that device.

CONVERTING ELECTROMYOGRAPHIC ACTIVITY TO MEANINGFUL INFORMATION

After amplification and filtering, the EMG signal is indicative of the true electrical activity within the muscles being monitored. This is referred to as "raw EMG" activity. **Raw EMG** is an alternating voltage that means that the direction or polarity is constantly reversing (Fig. 7-5A). The amplitude of the oscillations increases to a maximum then diminishes. Biofeedback measures the overall increase and decrease in electrical activity. To obtain this measurement the deflection toward the negative pole must be flipped upward toward the positive pole, otherwise the sum total of their deflections would cancel out one another (Fig. 7-5B) This process is referred to as **rectification** that essentially creates a pulsed direct current (DC).

Raw EMG activity may be
- Rectified
- Smoothed
- Integrated

Processing the Electromyographic Signal

The rectified EMG signal can be smoothed and integrated. **Smoothing** the EMG signal means eliminating the peaks and valleys or eliminating the high-frequency fluctuations that are produced with a changing electrical signal (Fig. 7-5C). Once the EMG has been smoothed, the signal may be integrated by measuring the area under the curve for a specified period of time. **Integration** forms the basis for quantification of EMG activity (Fig. 7-5D).

At this point it is necessary to take this rectified, smoothed, and integrated EMG signal and display the information in a form that has some meaning. Biofeedback units generally provide either visual or auditory feedback relative to the quantity of electrical activity. Some biofeedback units can provide both visual and auditory feedback, depending on the output mode selected.

Visual Feedback

Biofeedback information may be visual or auditory or both.

Raw EMG activity is usually displayed visually on an oscilloscope. On most biofeedback units, integrated EMG activity is visually presented, either as a line traveling across a monitor, as a light or series of lights that go on and off, or as a bar graph that changes dimension in response to the incoming integrated signal. Some of the newer EMG units have incorporated video games as part of their visual feedback system. If a biofeedback unit uses some type of meter, it may either be calibrated in objective units such as microvolts, or it may simply give some relative scale of measure.[30]

Meters also may be either analog or digital. Analog meters have a continuous scale and a needle that indicates the level of electrical activity within a particular range. Digital meters display only a number. They are very simple and easy to read.

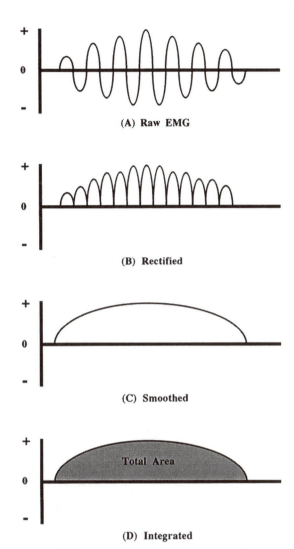

•Figure 7-5 Processing an EMG signal involves taking (A) raw EMG and then (B) rectifying, (C) smoothing, and (D) integrating it so that the information can be presented in some meaningful format.

However, the disadvantage of a digital meter is that it is more difficult to tell where the signal falls in a given range.

Audio Feedback

On some biofeedback units, raw EMG activity can be listened to and is one type of audio feedback. The majority of biofeedback units have audio feedback that produces some tone, buzzing, beeping, or clicking. An increase in the pitch of a tone, buzz, or beep, or an increase in the frequency of clicking indicates an increase in the level of EMG activity. This would be most useful for individuals who need to strengthen muscle contractions. Conversely, decreases in pitch or frequency indicating a decrease in EMG activity would be most useful in teaching patients to relax.

Setting Sensitivity

Signal sensitivity or **signal gain** may be set by the therapist on many biofeedback units. If a high gain is chosen, the biofeedback unit will have a high sensitivity for

signal gain Determines the signal sensitivity. If a high gain is chosen the biofeedback unit will have a high sensitivity for the muscle activity signal.

the muscle activity signal. Sensitivity may be set at 1, 10, or 100 μV. A 1-μV setting is sensitive enough to detect the smallest amounts of electrical activity and thus has the highest signal gain. High sensitivity levels should be used during relaxation training. Comparatively lower sensitivity levels are more useful in muscle reeducation, during which the patient may produce several hundred microvolts of EMG activity. Generally, when adjusting the sensitivity range it should be set at the lowest level that does not elicit feedback at rest.

EQUIPMENT SETUP AND APPLICATION

It is imperative that the therapist have some understanding of how biofeedback units monitor and record the electrical activity being produced in a muscle before attempting to set up and use the biofeedback unit in the treatment of a patient. Specific treatment protocols involve skin preparation, application of electrodes, selection of feedback or output modes, and selection of sensitivity settings, all of which have been previously discussed. Once these are complete, the therapist should choose to have the patient sitting, lying, or occasionally standing in a comfortable position, depending on the treatment objectives. Generally the therapist should begin with easy tasks and progressively make the activities more difficult. Teaching the patient how to appropriately use the biofeedback unit and briefly explaining what is being measured are essential. In most cases, it is recommended that the therapist attach the biofeedback unit to him- or herself and then demonstrate to the patient exactly what will be done during the treatment.[17]

CLINICAL APPLICATIONS

There are a number of clinical conditions for which biofeedback would be useful as a therapeutic modality. The primary applications for using biofeedback include: muscle reeducation, which involves regaining neuromuscular control and increasing muscle strength; relaxation of muscle spasm or muscle guarding; and pain reduction.

MUSCLE REEDUCATION

The goal in muscle reeducation is to provide feedback that will reestablish neuromuscular control or promote the ability of a muscle or group of muscles to contract. It may also be used to regain normal agonist/antagonist muscle action and for postural control retraining. EMG biofeedback is used to indicate the electrical activity associated with that muscle contraction.[13]

When biofeedback is being used to elicit a muscle contraction, the sensitivity setting should be chosen by having the patient perform a maximum isometric contraction of the target muscle. Then the gain should be adjusted such that the patient will be able to achieve the maximum on about two-thirds of the muscle contractions. If the patient cannot produce a muscle contraction, the therapist should attempt to facilitate a contraction by stroking or tapping the target muscle. It is also helpful to have the patient look at the muscle when trying to contract. It may be necessary to move the active electrodes to the contralateral limb and have the patient "practice" the muscle contraction you hope to achieve on the opposite side.

The patient should maximally contract the target muscle isometrically for 6 to 10 seconds. During this contraction, the visual or auditory feedback should be at a

---

Indications and Contraindications for Biofeedback

Indications
  Muscle reeducation
  Regaining neuromuscular control
  Increasing isometric and isotonic strength of a muscle
  Relaxation of muscle spasm
  Decreasing muscle guarding
  Pain reduction
  Psychological relaxation

Contraindications
  Any musculoskeletal condition in which a muscular contraction might exacerbate that condition.

Treatment Tip
The therapist should set the signal gain on the biofeedback unit at a high-sensitivity setting whenever the goal is relaxation, whereas a low-sensitivity setting should be used with muscle reeducation.

maximum and should be closely monitored by both the therapist and patient. Between each contraction the patient should be instructed to completely relax the muscle such that the feedback mode returns to baseline or zero prior to initiating another contraction. A period of 5 to 10 minutes working with a single muscle or muscle group is most desirable since longer periods tend to produce fatigue and boredom, neither of which is conducive to optimal learning.[16]

As increases in EMG activity occur, the patient should develop the ability to rapidly activate motor units. This can be accomplished by setting the sensitivity level to 60 to 80 percent of maximum isometric activity and instructing the patient to reach that level as many times as possible during a given time period (i.e., 10 or 30 sec). Again, total relaxation must occur between contractions.

It is essential that the treatment be functionally relevant to the patient. Attention to mobility and muscle power cannot be neglected in favor of biofeedback therapy.[16] The therapist should have the patient perform functional movements while observing body mechanics and the related EMG activity. Then recommendations can be made as to how movements can be altered to elicit normal EMG responses.[8] Biofeedback is useful in patients who perform poorly on manual muscle tests. If the patient can only elicit a fair, trace, or zero grade, then biofeedback should be incorporated. Stronger muscles generally should be given resistive exercises rather than biofeedback, although biofeedback has been recommended for increasing the strength of healthy muscle.[10,16]

Treatment Tip
Biofeedback electrodes should be placed as close to the muscle as possible to minimize "noise." They should be placed parallel to the direction of the muscle fibers. The spacing should be close enough to monitor activity from a specific muscle. If spaced too far apart then electrical activity from other anatomically close muscles may also be detected.

RELAXATION OF MUSCLE GUARDING

Often in a clinical setting, patients demonstrate a protective response in muscle that occurs owing to pain or fear of movement that is most accurately described as **muscle guarding**.

Muscle guarding must be differentiated from those neuromuscular problems arising from central nervous system deficits that result in a clinical condition known as muscle spasticity. For the therapist treating patients exhibiting muscle guarding, the goal is to induce relaxation of the muscle by reducing EMG activity through the use of biofeedback.[16]

Since muscle guarding most often involves fear of pain that may result when the muscle moves, perhaps the most important goal in treatment is to modulate pain. This is best accomplished through the use of other modalities such as ice or electrical stimulation.

Biofeedback treatments should be designed so that the patient experiences success from the first treatment. The patient is now attempting to reduce the visual or auditory feedback to zero. Initially, positioning of the patient in a comfortable relaxed position is critical to reduction of muscle guarding. A high sensitivity setting should be selected so that any electrical activity in the muscle will be easily detected.

During relaxation training the patient should be given verbal cues that will enhance relaxation of either individual muscles, muscle groups, or body segments. For example, with individual muscles or small muscle groups, the patient may be instructed to contract then relax a specific muscle or to imagine a feeling of warmth within the muscle. For larger muscle groups, using mental imagery or deep-breathing exercises may be useful.

As relaxation progresses, the spacing between the electrodes should be increased. Also, the sensitivity setting should move from low to high. Both of these changes will require the patient to relax more muscles, thus achieving greater relaxation. The patient must then apply this newly learned relaxation technique in different positions that are potentially more uncomfortable. Again, the goal is to eliminate muscle guarding during functional activities.[16]

Treatment Tip
With biofeedback units there is no universally accepted or standardized measurement scale. Different machines are likely to give different readings for the same degree of muscle contraction. Each manufacturer has its own reference standards for a particular unit. Thus, information provided from two different units cannot be compared.

PAIN REDUCTION

A number of therapeutic modalities discussed in this text are used for the purpose of reducing or modulating pain. As mentioned in the section on muscle guarding, biofeedback can be used to relax muscles that are tense secondary to fear of pain on movement. If the muscle can be relaxed, then chances are that pain will also be reduced by breaking the "pain-guarding-pain" cycle. It has been experimentally demonstrated to reduce pain in headaches and low back pain.[2,7–9,20,25] Pain modulation is often associated with techniques of imagery and progressive relaxation.

Treating Neurologic Conditions

Biofeedback has been identified as an effective technique for treating a variety of neurologic conditions, including hemiplegia following stroke, spinal cord injury, spasticity, cerebral palsy, fascial paralysis, and urinary and fecal incontinence.[1,3,5,6,12,15,19,23,24,26,27]

SUMMARY

1. Biofeedback is a therapeutic procedure that uses electronic or electromechanical instruments to accurately measure, process, and feed back reinforcing information by using auditory or visual signals.

2. Perhaps the biggest advantage of biofeedback is that it provides the patient with a chance to make correct small changes in performance that are immediately noted and rewarded so that eventually larger changes or improvements in performance can be accomplished.

3. Several different types of biofeedback modalities are available for use in rehabilitation, with EMG biofeedback being the most widely used in a clinical setting.

4. An EMG biofeedback unit measures the electrical activity produced by depolarization of a muscle fiber as an indicator of the quality of a muscle contraction.

5. The EMG biofeedback unit receives small amounts of electrical energy generated during muscle contraction through active electrodes, then separates or filters extraneous electrical energy via a differential amplifier before it is processed and subsequently converted to some type of information that has meaning to the user.

6. Biofeedback information is displayed either visually using lights or meters or auditorily using tones, beeps, buzzes, or clicks.

7. High sensitivity levels should be used during relaxation training, whereas comparatively lower sensitivity levels are more useful in muscle reeducation.

8. In a clinical setting, biofeedback is most typically used for muscle reeducation, to decrease muscle guarding, or for pain reduction.

REFERENCES

1. Amato, A., Hermomeyer, C., and Kleinman, K.: Use of electromyographic feedback to increase control of spastic muscles, Phys. Ther. 53:1063, 1973.

2. Arena, J., Bruno, G., and Hannah, S.: A comparison of frontal electromyographic biofeedback training, trapezius electromyographic biofeedback training, and progressive muscle relaxation therapy in the treatment of tension headache, Headache 35(7): 411–419, 1995.

3. Asato, H., Twiggs, D., and Ellison, S.: EMG biofeedback training for a mentally retarded individual with cerebral palsy. Phys. Ther. 61:1447–1451, 1981.

4. Basmajian, J.: Description and analysis of EMG signal. In Basmajian, J., Deluca, C., editors. Muscles alive. Their functions revealed by electromyography, Baltimore, 1985, Williams & Wilkins.

5. Brown, D., Nahai, F., and Wolf, S.: Electromyographic feed-

back in the re-education of fascial palsy, Am. J. Phys. Med. 57:183–190, 1978.

6. Brucker, B., Bulaeva, N.: Biofeedback effect on electromyography responses in patients with spinal cord injury, Arch. Phys. Med. Rehab. 77(2):133–137, 1996.

7. Budzynski, D.: Biofeedback strategies in headache treatment. In Basmajian J., editor. Biofeedback: principles and practice for clinicians, Baltimore, 1989, Williams & Wilkins.

8. Bush, C., Ditto, B., and Feuerstein, M.: Controlled evaluation of paraspinal EMG biofeedback in the treatment of chronic low back pain, Health Psychol. 4:307–321, 1985.

9. Chapman, S.: A review and clinical perspective on the use of EMG and thermal biofeedback for chronic headaches, Pain 27:1, 1986.

10. Croce, R.: The effects of EMG biofeedback on strength aquisition, Biofeedback Self Regul. 9:395, 1986.

11. Draper, V.: Electromyographic feedback and recovery in quadriceps femoris muscle function following anterior cruciate ligament reconstruction, Phys. Ther. 70:25, 1990.

12. Engardt, M.: Term effects of auditory feedback training on relearned symmetrical body weight distribution in stroke patients. A follow-up study, Scand. J. Rehab. Med. 26(2):65–69, 1994.

13. Fogel, E.: Biofeedback-assisted musculoskeletal therapy and neuromuscular re-education. In Schwartz, M.S., editor. Biofeedback: a practitioners guide. New York, 1987, The Guilford Press.

14. Jennings, J., Tahmoush, A., and Redmond, D.: Non-invasive measurement of peripheral vascular activity, In Martin I., Venables, P.H., editors. Techniques in psychophysiology, New York, 1980, Wiley.

15. Klose, K., Needham, B., and Schmidt, D.: An assessment of the contribution of electromyographic biofeedback as a therapy in the physical training of spinal cord injured persons, Arch. Phys. Med. Rehab. 74(5):453–456, 1993.

16. Krebs, D.: Neuromuscular re-education and gait training. In Schwartz, M., editor. Biofeedback: a practitioners guide, New York, 1987, The Guilford Press.

17. LeCraw, D., Wolf, S.: Electromyographic biofeedback (EMGBF) for neuromuscular relaxation and re-education, In Gersh, M., editor. Electrotherapy in rehabilitation, Philadelphia, 1992, F.A. Davis Company.

18. Miller, N.: Biomedical foundations for biofeedback as a part of behavioral medicine. In Basmajian, J., editor. Biofeedback: principles and practice for clinicians. Baltimore, 1989, Williams & Wilkins.

19. Moreland, J., Thompson, M.: Efficacy of EMG biofeedback compared with conventional physical therapy for upper extremity function in patients following stroke: a research overview and meta-analysis, Phys. Ther. 74(6):534–543, 1994.

20. Nouwen, A., Bush, C.: The relationship between paraspinal EMG and chronic low back pain, Pain 20:109–123, 1984.

21. Olson, R.: Definitions of biofeedback. In Schwartz, M., editor. Biofeedback: a practitioners guide, New York, 1987, The Guilford Press.

22. Peek, C.: A primer of biofeedback instrumentation. In Schwartz, M., editor. Biofeedback: a practitioners guide, New York, 1987, The Guilford Press.

23. Regenos, E., Wolf, S.: Involuntary single motor unit discharges in spastic muscles during EMG biofeedback training, Arch. Phys. Med. Rehab. 60:72–73, 1979.

24. Schleenbaker, R., Mainous, A.: Electromyographic biofeedback for neuromuscular reeducation in the hemiplegic stroke patient: a meta-analysis, Arch. Phys. Med. Rehab. 74(12): 1301–1304, 1993.

25. Studkey, S., Jacobs, A., and Goldfarb, J.: EMG biofeedback training, relaxation training, and placebo for the relief of chronic back pain, Percept. Mot. Skills 63:1023, 1986.

26. Sugar, E., Firlit, C.: Urodynamic feedback: a new therapeutic approach for childhood incontinence/infection, J. Urol. 128: 1253, 1982.

27. Whitehead, W.: Treatment of fecal incontinence in children with spina bifida: comparison of biofeedback and behavior modification, Arch. Phys. Med. Rehab. 67:218, 1986.

28. Wolf, S., Binder-Macleod, S.: Electromyographic feedback in the physical therapy clinic. In Basmajian, J.V., editor. Biofeedback: principles and practice for clinicians, Baltimore, 1989, Williams & Wilkins.

29. Wolf, S., Binder-Macleod, S.: Neurophysiological factors in electromyographic feedback for neuromotor disturbances. In Basmajian, J.V. editor. Biofeedback: principles and practice for clinicians, Baltimore, 1989, Williams & Wilkins.

30. Wolf, S.: Treatment of neuromuscular problems, treatment of musculoskeletal problems. In Sandweiss, J., editor. Biofeedback: review seminars, Los Angeles, 1982, University of California, 1982.

SUGGESTED READINGS

Baker, M., Regenos, E., and Wolf, S.: Developing strategies for biofeedback: applications in neurologically handicapped patients, Phys. Ther. 57:402–408, 1977.

Baker, M., Hudson, J., and Wolf, S.: "Feedback" cane to improve the hemiplegic patient's gait: suggestion from the field, Phys. Ther. 59:170, 1979.

Balliet, R., Levy, B., and Blood, K.: Upper extremity sensory feedback therapy in chronic cerebrovascular accident patients with impaired expressive aphasia and auditory comprehension, Arch. Phys. Med. Rehabil. 67:304, 1986.

Basmajian, J., Samson, J.: Special review: standardization of methods in single motor unit training, Am. J. Phys. Med. 52:250–256, 1973.

Basmajian, J., et al.: Biofeedback treatment of foot drop after stroke compared with standard rehabilitation technique: effects on voluntary control and strength, Arch. Phys. Med. Rehabil. 56:231–236, 1975.

Basmajian, J.: Learned control of single motor units. In Schwartz G.E., Beatty, J., editors, Biofeedback: theory and research, New York, 1977, Academic Press.

Basmajian, J.: Biofeedback: principles and practice for clinicians, Baltimore, 1989, Williams & Wilkins.

Basmajian, J., Blumenthal, R.: Electroplacement in electromyographic biofeedback. In Basmajian, J.V., editor. Biofeedback: principles and practice for clinicians, ed 3, Baltimore, 1989, Williams & Wilkins.

Basmajian, J., Regenos, E., and Baker, M.: Rehabilitating stroke patients with biofeedback, Geriatrics 32:85, 1977.

Basmajian, J: Biofeedback in rehabilitation: a review of principles and practice, Arch. Phys. Med. Rehabil. 62:469, 1981.

Beal, M., Diefenbach, G., and Allen, A.: Electromyographic biofeedback in the treatment of voluntary posterior instability of the shoulder, Am. J. Sports Med. 15:175, 1987.

Bernat, S., Wooldridge, P., and Marecki, M.: Biofeedback-assisted relaxation to reduce stress in labor, J. Obstet. Gynecol. Neonatal Nurs. (4):295–303, 1992.

Biedermann, H.: Comments on the reliability of muscle activity comparisons in EMG biofeedback research with back pain patients, Biofeedback Self Regul. 9:451–458, 1984.

Biedermann, H., McGhie, A., and Monga, T.: Perceived and actual control in EMG treatment of back pain, Behav. Res. Ther. 25:137–147, 1987.

Bowman, B., Baker, L., and Waters, R.: Positional feedback and electrical stimulation. An automated treatment for the hemiplegic wrist, Arch. Phys. Med. Rehabil. 60:497, 1979.

Brudny, J., Grynbaum, B., and Korein, J.: Spasmodic torticollis: treatment by feedback display of EMG, Arch. Phys. Med. Rehabil. 55:403–408, 1974.

Burke, R.: Motor unit recruitment: what are the critical factors? In Desmedt, J., editor. Progress in clinical neurophysiology, Vol 9, Basel, 1981, Karger.

Burnside, I., Tobias, H., and Bursill, D.: Electromyographic feedback in the rehabilitation of stroke patients: a controlled trial, Arch. Phys. Med. Rehab. 63:217, 1982.

Burnside, I., Tobias, H., and Bursill, D.: Electromyographic feedback in the remobilization of stroke patients: a controlled trial, Arch. Phys. Med. Rehab. 63:1393, 1983.

Carlsson, S.: Treatment of temporo-mandibular joint syndrome with biofeedback training, J. Am. Dent. Assoc. 91:602–605, 1975.

Christie, D., Dewitt, R., and Kaltenbach, P.: Using EMG biofeedback to signal hyperactive children when to relax, Except. Child. 50:547–548, 1984.

Cox, R., Matyas, T.: Myoelectric and force feedback in the facilitation of isometric strength training: a controlled comparison, Psychophysiology, 20:35–44, 1983.

Crow, J., Lincoln, N., and De Weerdt, N.: The effectiveness of EMG biofeedback in the treatment of arm function after stroke, Intern. Disabil. Stud. 11(4):155–160, 1989.

Cummings, M., Wilson, V., and Bird, E.: Flexibility development in sprinters using EMG biofeedback and relaxation training, Biofeedback Self Regul. 9:395–405, 1984.

Debacher, G.: Feedback goniometers for rehabilitation. In Basmajian, J., editor. Biofeedback: principles and practice for clinicians, Baltimore, 1983, Williams & Wilkins.

Deluca, C.: Apparatus, detection, and recording techniques. In Basmajian, J., Deluca, C., editors. Muscles alive: their functions revealed by electromyography, Baltimore, 1985, Williams & Wilkins.

Draper, V., Ballard, L.: Electrical stimulation versus electromyographic biofeedback in the recovery of quadriceps femoris muscle function following anterior cruciate ligament surgery, Phys. Ther. 71(6):455–464, 1991.

Draper, V.: Electromyographic biofeedback and recovery of quadriceps femoris muscle function following anterior cruciate ligament reconstruction, Phys. Ther. 70(1):11–17, 1990.

English, A., Wolf, S.: The motor unit: anatomy and physiology, Phys. Ther. 62:1763, 1982.

Fields, R.: Electromyographically triggered electric muscle stimulation for chronic hemiplegia, Arch. Phys. Med. Rehabil. 68:407–414, 1987.

Flom, R., Quast, J., and Boller, J.: Biofeedback training to overcome poststroke footdrop, Geriatrics 31:47–51, 1976.

Flor, H., Haag, G., and Turk, D.: Long-term efficacy of EMG biofeedback for chronic rheumatic back pain, Pain 27:195–202, 1986.

Flor, H., et al.: Efficacy of EMG biofeedback, pseudotherapy, and conventional medical treatment for chronic rheumatic back pain, Pain 17:21–31, 1983.

Gaarder, K., Montgomery, P.: Clinical biofeedback: a procedural manual, Baltimore, 1977, Williams & Wilkins.

Gallego, J., Perez de la Sota, A., and Vardon, G.: Electromyographic feedback for learning to activate thoracic inspiratory muscles, Am. J. Phys. Med. Rehabil. 70(4):186–190, 1991.

Goodgold, J., Eberstein, A.: Electrodiagnosis of neuromuscular diseases, Baltimore, 1972, Williams & Wilkins.

Green, E., Walters, E., and Green, A.: Feedback technology for deep relaxation, Psychophysiology 6:371–377, 1969.

Hijzen, T., Slangen, J., van Houweligen, H.: Subjective, clinical and EMG effects of biofeedback and splint treatment, J. Oral Rehabil. 13:529–539, 1986.

Hirasawa, Y., Uchiza, Y., and Kusswetter, W.: EMG biofeedback therapy for rupture of the extensor pollicis longus tendon, Arch. Orthop. Trauma Surg. 104:342, 1986.

Honer, L., Mohr, T., and Roth, R.: Electromyographic biofeedback to dissociate an upper extremity synergy pattern: a case report, Phys. Ther. 62:299–303, 1982.

Howard, P.: Use of EMG biofeedback to reeducate the rotator cuff in a case of shoulder impingement, JOSPT 23(1):79, 1996.

Ince, L., Leon, M.: Biofeedback treatment of upper extremity dysfunction in Guillain-Barre syndrome, Arch. Phys. Med. Rehabil. 67:30–33, 1986.

Ince, L., Leon, M., and Christidis, D.: EMG biofeedback with upper extremity musculature for relaxation training: a critical review of the literature, J. Behav. Ther. Exp. Psychiatry 16:133–137, 1985.

Ince, L., Leon, M., and Christidis, D.: Experimental foundations of EMG biofeedback with the upper extremity: a review of the literature, Biofeedback Self Regul. 9:371–383, 1984.

Inglis, J., Donald, M., and Monga, T.: Electromyographic biofeedback and physical therapy of the hemiplegic upper limb, Arch. Phys. Med. Rehabil. 65:755–759, 1984.

Johnson, H., Garton, W.: Muscle reeducation in hemiplegia by use of electromyographic device, Arch. Phys. Med. Rehabil. 54: 322–323, 1973.

Johnson, H., Hockersmith, V.: Therapeutic electromyography in chronic back pain. In Basmajian, J.V., editor. Biofeedback: principles and practice for clinicians, ed 2, Baltimore, 1983, Williams & Wilkins.

Johnson, R., Lee, K.: Myofeedback: a new method of teaching breathing exercise to emphysematous patients, J. Am. Phys. Ther. Assoc. 56:826–829, 1976.

Kelly, J., Baker, M., and Wolf, S.: Procedures for EMG biofeedback training in involved upper extremities of hemiplegic patients, Phys. Ther. 59:1500, 1979.

King, A., Ahles, T., and Martin, J.: EMG biofeedback-controlled exercise in chronic arthritic knee pain, Arch. Phys. Med. Rehabil. 65:341–343, 1984.

King, T.: Biofeedback: a survey regarding current clinical use and content in occupational therapy educational curricula, Occ. Ther. J. Res. 12(1):50–58, 1992.

Kleppe, D., Groendijk, H., and Huijing, P.: Single motor unit control in the human mm. abductor pollicis brevis and mylohyoideus in relation to the number of muscle spindles, Electromyogr. Clin. Neurophysiol. 22:21–25, 1982.

Krebs, D.: Biofeedback in neuromuscular reeducation and gait training. In Schwartz, M. editor. Biofeedback: a practitioner's guide, New York, 1987, The Guilford Press.

Large, R., Lamb, A.: Electromyographic (EMG) feedback in chronic musculoskeletal pain: a controlled trial, Pain 17:167–177, 1983.

Large, R.: Prediction of treatment response in pain patients: the illness self-concept repertory grid and EMG feedback, Pain 21: 279–287, 1985.

Lucca, J., Recchiuti, S.: Effect of electromyographic biofeedback on an isometric strengthening program, Phys. Ther. 63:200–203, 1983.

Mandel, A., Nymark, J., and Balmer, S.: Electromyographic versus rhythmic positional biofeedback in computerized gait retraining with stroke patients, Arch. Phys. Med. Rehabil. 71(9): 649–654, 1990.

Marinacci, A., Horande, M.: Electromyogram in neuromuscular reeducation, Bull. Los Angeles Neurol. Soc. 25:57–67, 1960.

Mims, H: Electromyography in clinical practice, So. Med. J. 49:804, 1956.

Morasky, R., Reynolds, C., and Clarke, G.: Using biofeedback to reduce left arm extensor EMG of string players during musical performance, Biofeedback Self Regul. 6:565–572, 1981.

Morris, M., Matyas, T., and Bach, T.: Electrogoniometric feedback: its effect on genu recurvatum in stroke, Arch. Phys. Med. Rehabil. 73(12):1147–1154, 1992.

Mulder, T., Hulstijn, W.: Delayed sensory feedback in the learning of a novel motor task, Psychol. Res. 47:203–209, 1985.

Mulder, T., Hulstijn, W., and van der Meer, J.: EMG feedback and the restoration of motor control. A controlled group study of 12 hemiparetic patients, Am. J. Phys. Med. 65:173–188, 1986.

Nafpliotis, H.: EMG feedback to improve ankle dorsiflexion, wrist extension and hand grasp, Phys. Ther. 56:821–825, 1976.

Nouwen, A.: EMG biofeedback used to reduce standing levels of paraspinal muscle tension in chronic low back pain, Pain 17:353–360, 1983.

Poppen, R., Maurer, J.: Electromyographic analysis of relaxed postures, Biofeedback Self Regul. 7:491–498, 1982.

Russell, G., Woolbridge, C.: Correction of a habitual head tilt using biofeedback techniques—a case study, Physiother. Can. 27: 181–184, 1975.

Saunders, J., Cox, D., and Teates, C.: Thermal biofeedback in the treatment of intermittent claudication in diabetes: a case study, Biofeedback Self Regul. 19(4):337–345, 1994.

Smith, D., Newman, D.: Basic elements of biofeedback therapy for pelvic muscle rehabilitation, Urol. Nurs. 14(3):130–135, 1994.

Soderback, I., Bengtsson, I., and Ginsburg, E.: Video feedback in occupational therapy: its effect in patients with neglect syndrome, Arch. Phys. Med. Rehab. 73(12):1140–1146, 1992.

Swaan, D., van Wiergen, P., and Fokkema, S.: Auditory electromyographic feedback therapy to inhibit undesired motor activity, Arch. Phys. Med. Rehabil. 55:251, 1974.

Winchester, P.: Effects of feedback stimulation training and cyclical electrical stimulation on knee extension in hemiparetic patients, Phys. Ther. 63:1097, 1983.

Wolf, S.: Fallacies of clinical EMG measures from patients with musculoskeletal and neuromuscular disorders. Paper presented at the 14th annual meeting of the Biofeedback Society of America, Denver, 1983.

Wolf, S., Binder-Macleod, S.: Electromyographic biofeedback applications to the hemiplegic patient. Changes in lower extremity neuromuscular and functional status, Phys. Ther. 63:1404–1413, 1983.

Wolf, S., Regenos, E., and Basmajian, J.: Developing strategies for biofeedback applications in neurologically handicapped patients, Phys. Ther. 57:402–408, 1977.

Wolf, S., Baker, M., and Kelly, J.: EMG biofeedback in stroke: a 1-year follow-up on the effect of patient characteristics, Arch. Phys. Med. Rehabil. 61:351–355, 1980.

Wolf, S., Baker, M., and Kelly, J.: EMG biofeedback in stroke: effect of patient characteristics, Arch. Phys. Med. Rehabil. 60:96–102, 1979.

Wolf, S.: Electromyographic biofeedback in exercise programs, Phys. Sports Med. 8:61–69, 1980.

Wolf, S., Binder-Macleod, S.: Electromyographic biofeedback applications to the hemiplegic patient: Changes in upper extremity neuromuscular and functional status, Phys. Ther. 63:1393, 1983.

Wolf, S., Hudson, J.: Feedback signal based upon force and time delay: Modification of the Krusen limb load monitor: Suggestion from the field, Phys. Ther. 60:1289, 1980.

Wolf, S., Edwards, D., and Shutter, L.: Concurrent assessment of muscle activity (CAMA): A procedural approach to assess treatment goals, Phys. Ther. 66:218, 1986.

Wolf, S., LeCraw, D., Barton, L.: A comparison of motor copy and targeted feedback training techniques for restitution of upper extremity function among neurologic patients, Phys. Ther. 69:719, 1989.

Wolf, S., Nacht, M., and Kelly, J.: EMG feedback training during dynamic movement for low back pain patients, Behav. Ther. 13:395, 1982.

Wolf, S.: Biofeedback. In Currier, D.P., Nelson, R.M., editors. Clinical electrotherapy, ed 2, Norwalk, Connecticut, 1991, Appleton & Lange.

Wolf, S.: EMG biofeedback application in physical rehabilitation: an overview, Physiother. Can. 31:65, 1979.

Wolf, S.: Essential considerations in the use of EMG biofeedback, Phys. Ther. 58:25, 1978.

Young, M.: Electromyographic biofeedback use in the treatment of voluntary posterior dislocation of the shoulder a case study, JOSPT 20(3):173–175, 1994.

GLOSSARY

active electrode An electrode attached directly to the skin over a muscle that picks up the electrical activity produced by a muscle contraction.

bandwidth A specific frequency range in which the amplifier will pick up signals produced by electrical activity in the muscle.

bipolar arrangement Two active recoding electrodes placed in close proximity to one another.

common mode rejection ratio (CMRR) The ability of the differential amplifier to eliminate the common noise between the active electrodes.

differential amplifier A device that monitors the two separate signals from the active electrodes and amplifies the difference, thus eliminating extraneous noise.

electromyographic biofeedback A therapeutic procedure that uses electronic or electromechanical instruments to accurately measure, process, and feed back reinforcing information via auditory or visual signals.

filters Devices that help to reduce external noise that essentially make the amplifier more sensitive to some incoming frequencies and less sensitive to others.

integration An EMG signal-processing technique that measures the area under the curve for a specified period of time, thus forming the basis for quantification of EMG activity.

muscle guarding A protective response in muscle that occurs owing to pain or fear of movement.

noise Extraneous electrical activity that may be produced by any source other than the contracting muscle.

raw EMG A form in which the electrical activity produced by muscle contraction may be displayed and/or recorded before the signal is processed.

rectification A signal-processing technique that changes the deflection of the waveform from the negative to the positive pole, essentially creating a pulsed direct current.

reference electrode Also referred to as the ground electrode; serves as a point of reference to compare the electrical activity recorded by the active electrodes.

signal gain Determines the signal sensitivity. If a high gain is chosen the biofeedback unit will have a high sensitivity for the muscle activity signal.

smoothing An EMG signal-processing technique that eliminates the high-frequency fluctuations that are produced with a changing electrical signal.

LAB ACTIVITY

BIOFEEDBACK

DESCRIPTION:

Biofeedback utilizes the body's self-generated motor unit action potentials (MUAP). These signals are recorded by surface electrodes, amplified, then processed and converted into audio or visual signals to allow an individual to monitor various psychophysiologic processes and recognize appropriate responses.

PHYSIOLOGIC EFFECTS:

Increase level of motor unit activation
Decrease level of motor unit activation

THERAPEUTIC EFFECTS:

Increase level of muscle activation (muscle reeducation)
Decrease level of muscle activation (reduce spasticity)
General body muscular relaxation

INDICATIONS:

Biofeedback is primarily employed by the sports therapist as an adjunct in the re-education of muscle function following injury, immobilization, or surgery or as an aid to identifying unwanted levels of muscle activity (spasticity) that may be interfering with the athlete's recovery. Sometimes biofeedback is used as a tool to assess the body's general neuromuscular status as an aid in relaxation to reduce pain and anxiety.

CONTRAINDICATIONS:

- Possible skin irritation at electrode site from coupling gel or adhesives

BIOFEEDBACK			
PROCEDURE	Evaluation		
	1	2	3
1. Check supplies.			
a. Obtain biofeedback unit, coupling gel, and tape.			
b. Insure that batteries in unit are fresh.			
2. Question patient.			
a. Verify identity of patient and review previous treatment notes.			
b. Verify the absence of contraindications.			
3. Position patient.			
a. Place patient in a well-supported, comfortable position.			
b. Select and expose appropriate muscle or /group to monitor.			
c. Drape patient to preserve patient's modesty, and protect clothing, but allow access to muscle or group.			
4. Select appropriate electrode.			

PROCEDURE	Evaluation		
	1	2	3
5. Prepare the electrode site.			
a. Clean the skin surface with alcohol or soap and water.			
6. Apply the electrodes.			
a. Secure with tape or wrap.			
7. Explain the procedure to patient.			
8. Begin the indicated procedure.			
a. Muscle reeducation			
i. Adjust unit to lowest threshold (μV) that picks up any activity (MUAPs).			
ii. Adjust audio and visual feedback.			
iii. Have patient contract target muscle to produce maximum audio and visual feedback.			
iv. Facilitate target muscle contraction as necessary by tapping, stroking, or contracting opposite like muscle.			
v. When maximum feedback is obtained for selected threshold, advance threshold and attempt again.			
vi Advance muscle or limb to other positions.			
vii. Continue muscle contractions for 10 to 15 minutes per training session or until maximal muscle activation is obtained.			
b. Spasticity inhibition			
i. Adjust unit to sensitivity threshold (μV) that picks up maximal activity (MUAPs).			
ii. Adjust audio or visual feedback.			
iii. Have patient relax target muscle to produce minimum audio or visual feedback.			
iv. Facilitate target muscle relaxation as necessary by tapping, stroking, or contracting opposite like muscle.			
v. When minimum feedback is obtained for selected threshold, reduce threshold and attempt relaxation again.			
vi. Advance muscle or limb to other functional positions.			
vii. Continue muscle relaxation for 10 to 15 minutes per training session or until muscle relaxation is obtained.			
viii. Complete the treatment.			
9. Remove the electrodes.			
a. Thoroughly clean electrode site.			
b. Record results of session.			
c. Assess treatment efficacy.			
10. Instruct the patient in any indicated exercise.			
11. Return equipment to storage after cleaning.			

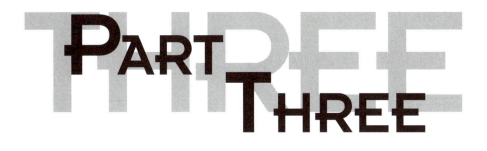

PART THREE

THERMAL MODALITIES

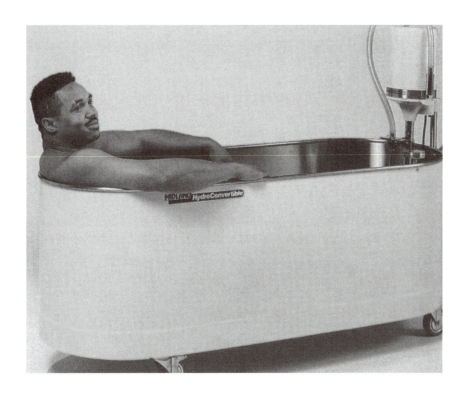

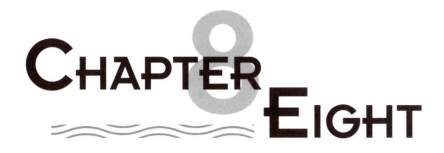

CHAPTER EIGHT

SHORTWAVE AND MICROWAVE DIATHERMY

WILLIAM E. PRENTICE and
DAVID O. DRAPER

OBJECTIVES

Following completion of this chapter the student therapist will be able to:

✓ Discuss how the diathermies may best be used in a clinical setting.
✓ Explain the physiologic effects of diathermy.
✓ Explain the difference between capacitance and induction shortwave diathermy techniques and identify the associated electrodes.
✓ Describe treatment techniques for continuous shortwave and pulsed shortwave diathermy.
✓ Explain the equipment setup and treatment technique for microwave diathermy.
✓ Discuss the various clinical applications and indications for using continuous shortwave, pulsed shortwave, and microwave diathermy.
✓ Discuss the treatment precautions for using the diathermies.
✓ List the major differences between microwave and shortwave diathermy.
✓ Discuss rate of heating and how long muscle retains the heat generated from a shortwave diathermy treatment.
✓ Compare and contrast diathermy and ultrasound as deep-heating agents.

Diathermy is the application of high-frequency electromagnetic energy that is primarily used to generate heat in body tissues. Heat is produced by resistance of the tissue to the passage of the energy. Diathermy may also be used to produce nonthermal effects.

Diathermy as a therapeutic agent may be classified as two distinct modalities, shortwave and microwave diathermy. Shortwave diathermy may be either continuous or pulsed. Continuous shortwave diathermy has been used in the treatment of a variety of conditions for some time. Recently, pulsed shortwave diathermy has received renewed interest and research documenting its clinical efficacy.[4,8,18]

To a great extent, diathermy is a modality that for one reason or another has fallen out of popularity among clinicians in the past 10 to 15 years. The current lack

diathermy The application of high-frequency electrical energy that is used to generate heat in body tissues as a result of the resistance of the tissue to the passage of energy.

of use of this modality has been based largely on the lack of available technology to reduce radio frequency interference, lack of dosimetry information, and reports of several contraindications attributed to diathermy.[18,28,29] It is important to note that most of the negative reports on this modality are attributed to microwave, not shortwave, diathermy. Equally important are the recent improvements in shielding from electromagnetic waves in the newer diathermy machines that not only protect the patient and clinician but also provide better heating of tissues.[4,8] Shortwave diathermy is a relatively safe modality that can be very effectively incorporated into clinic use.

The effectiveness of a shortwave or microwave diathermy treatment depends on the therapist's ability to tailor the treatment to the patient's needs. This requires that the therapist have an accurate evaluation or diagnosis of the patient's condition and knowledge of the heating patterns produced by various electrodes or applicators. The depth of penetration is greater than with any of the infrared modalities, yet many therapists feel that neither shortwave nor microwave diathermy produces heating at the depths desired for the treatment of musculoskeletal injuries. However, it has been determined recently that pulsed shortwave diathermy produces the same magnitude and depth of muscle heating as 1 MHz ultrasound.[8,9]

PHYSIOLOGIC RESPONSES TO DIATHERMY

THERMAL EFFECTS

The diathermies are not capable of producing depolarization and contraction of skeletal muscle since the wavelengths are much too short in duration.[6] Thus, the physiologic effects of continuous shortwave and microwave diathermy are primarily thermal, resulting from high-frequency vibration of molecules.

The primary benefits of diathermy are those of heat in general, such as tissue temperature rise, increased blood flow, dilation of the blood vessels, increased filtration and diffusion through the different membranes, increased tissue metabolic rate, changes in some enzyme reactions, alterations in the physical properties of fibrous tissues (such as those found in tendons, joints, and scars), decreased joint stiffness, a certain degree of muscle relaxation, a heightened pain threshold, and enhanced recovery from injury.[2,3,10,16,23,24,33,42,43]

Diathermy can have both thermal and non-thermal effects.

Diathermy treatment doses are not precisely controlled, and the amount of heating the patient receives cannot be accurately prescribed or directly measured. Heating occurs in proportion to the square of the current density and in direct proportion to the resistance of the tissue.

$$\text{Heating} = \text{Current density}^2 \times \text{Resistance}$$

Lehmann stated that temperature increases of 1°C can reduce mild inflammation and increase metabolism, and that moderate heating, an increase of 2 to 3°C, will decrease pain and muscle spasm. Increasing tissue temperatures more than 3 to 4°C above baseline will increase tissue extensibility, thus enabling the clinician to treat chronic connective tissue problems.[25]

There appear to be differing opinions regarding the desired temperature increases needed to enhance extensibility of collagen. Some believe that optimal heating occurs when the tissue temperature rises above 38 to 40°C, whereas others believe that a tissue temperature increase of 3 to 4°C above baseline temperature is optimal.[1,2,19,25] Presently, no research can validate one opinion over another, but it is clear that the more vigorous the heating with diathermy, the greater chance there is for collagen elongation to occur.

Why certain pathologic conditions respond better to diathermy than other forms of deep heat is not well understood or documented. It probably is more directly related either to the skill of the clinician applying the modality or to some placebo effects associated with tissue temperature increase than it is to the specific effects of diathermy itself.

NONTHERMAL EFFECTS

Pulsed shortwave diathermy has also been used for its nonthermal effects in the treatment of soft-tissue injuries and wounds.[20]

The mechanism of its effectiveness has been theorized to occur at the cellular level, relating specifically to cell membrane potential.[21] Damaged cells undergo depolarization, resulting in cell dsyfunction that might include loss of cell division and proliferation and loss of regenerative capabilities. Pulsed shortwave diathermy has been said to repolarize damaged cells, thus correcting cell dysfunction.[32]

It has also been suggested that sodium tends to accumulate in the cell because of a decrease in activity of the sodium pump during the inflammatory process, thus creating a negatively charged environment. When a magnetic field is induced, the sodium pump is reactivated, thus allowing the cell to regain normal ionic balance.[36]

SHORTWAVE DIATHERMY

A shortwave diathermy unit is basically a radio transmitter. **The Federal Communications Commission (FCC)** assigned three frequencies to shortwave diathermy units: the first is 27.12 MHz with a wavelength of 11 meters; the second is 13.56 MHz with a wavelength of 22 meters; and the third, although rarely used, is 40.68 MHz with a wavelength of 7.5 meters (see Fig. 3-2).

SHORTWAVE DIATHERMY GENERATORS

The shortwave diathermy unit consists of a power supply that provides power to a radio frequency oscillator (Fig. 8-1). This radio frequency oscillator provides stable, drift-free oscillations at the required frequency. The power amplifier generates the power required to drive the different types of electrodes. The output resonant tank

Pulsed Shortwave Diathermy
- Pulsed electromagnetic energy (PEME)
- Pulsed electromagnetic field (PEMF)
- Pulsed electromagnetic energy treatment (PEMET)

Pulsed shortwave diathermy = nonthermal effects

Treatment Tip
Pulsed shortwave diathermy is capable of heating a much larger area than ultrasound; the applicator is stationary so the heat applied to the area is more constant; the rate of temperature decay is slower following diathermy application allowing more time for stretching; using diathermy doesn't require constant monitoring.

Pulsed Shortwave diathermy uses drum electrodes.

Federal Communications Commission (FCC) Federal agency charged with assigning frequencies for all radio transmitters, including diathermies.

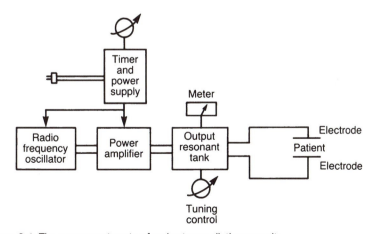

•**Figure 8-1** The component parts of a shortwave diathermy unit.

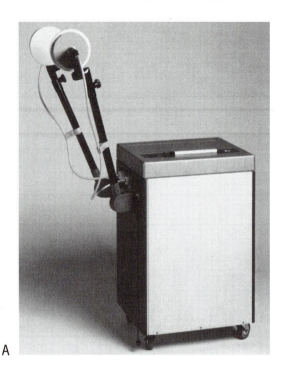

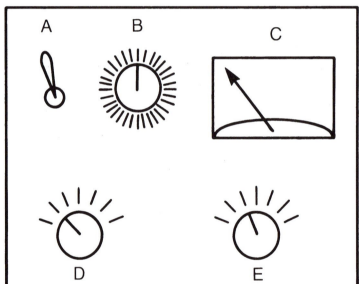

•**Figure 8-2** A. Shortwave diathermy unit. B. Control panel of a shortwave diathermy unit. A. Power switch, B. timer, C. output power meter (monitors current drawn from power supply only and not in patient circuit), D. output intensity (controls the percentage of maximum power transferred to the patient), E. tuning control (tunes the output circuit for maximum energy transfer from radio frequency oscillator).

tunes in the patient as part of the circuit and allows maximum power to be transferred to the patient.

Figure 8-2 shows the control panel of a shortwave diathermy unit. The output intensity knob controls the percentage of maximum power transferred to the patient circuit. This is similar to the volume control on a radio. The tuning control adjusts the output circuit for maximum energy transfer from the radio frequency oscillator, which is similar to tuning in a station on a radio. The power output meter monitors only the current that is drawn from the power supply and not the energy being delivered to the patient. Thus, it is only an indirect measure of the energy reaching the patient.

The power output of a shortwave diathermy unit should produce sufficient energy to raise the tissue temperature into a therapeutic range. The **specific absorption rate (SAR)** represents the rate of energy absorbed per unit area of tissue mass. Most shortwave units have a power output of between 80 and 120 watts.

Some units are not capable of this, making them safe but ineffective. It is important to remember that the tissue temperature rise with diathermy units can be offset dramatically by an increase in blood flow, which has a cooling effect in the tissue being energized. Therefore, units should be able to generate enough power to provide for an excess of the SAR.

Patient sensation provides the basis for recommendations of continuous shortwave diathermy dosage and thus varies considerably with different patients.[26,36] The following dosage guidelines have been recommended.

Dose I (lowest): No sensation of heat
Dose II (low): Mild heating sensation
Dose III (medium): Moderate (pleasant) heating sensation
Dose IV (heavy): Vigorous heating that is tolerable below the pain threshold

Some shortwave diathermy generators have manual tuning; others have automatic tuning devices. If the machine is not an automatically tuning type, it is necessary to tune the patient's circuit to resonance with the oscillating circuit of the unit. This is accomplished by placing the electrodes over the area to be treated and then setting the output intensity at 30 to 40 percent. Then, the variable capacitor in the generator's circuitry can be adjusted by using the meter on the generator to determine the peak tuning readings. These readings should not be confused as an indication of the power received by the patient. The tuning control should be adjusted until the output power meter moves to the maximum and then it should be adjusted down to patient tolerance, which is usually about 50 percent of maximum output. If more than 50 percent of the available power on the meter is used, then the patient's setup is out of tune or out of resonance. Shortwave diathermy units with automatic tuning turn off the power when the patient circuit is out of tune.

A shortwave diathermy unit that generates a high-frequency electrical current will produce both an **electrical field** and a **magnetic field** in the tissues.[12] The ratio of the electrical field to the magnetic field depends on the characteristics of the different units as well as on the characteristics of electrodes or applicators. Shortwave units with a frequency of 13.56 MHz tend to produce a stronger magnetic field than do units with the frequency of 27.12 MHz, which produces a stronger electric field. The majority of the new pulsed shortwave diathermy units use a drum electrode and produce a stronger magnetic field.

SHORTWAVE DIATHERMY ELECTRODES

Shortwave diathermy may be delivered to the patient via either capacitance or induction techniques. Each of these techniques can affect different biologic tissues, and selection of the appropriate electrodes is essential for effective treatment.

The shortwave diathermy uses several types of applicators or electrodes, including air space plates, pad electrodes, cable electrodes, or drum electrodes.

Capacitor Electrodes

The capacitance technique, using **capacitor electrodes**, creates a stronger electrical field than a magnetic field. As discussed in Chapter 6, within the body there are many free ions that are positively or negatively charged. A positively charged elec-

specific absorption rate (SAR) Represents the rate of energy absorbed per unit area of tissue mass.

electrical field The lines of force exerted on charged ions in the tissues by the electrodes that cause charged particles to move from one pole to the other.
magnetic field Created when current is passed through a coiled cable affecting surrounding tissues by inducing localized secondary currents, called eddy currents within the tissues.

Pulsed Shortwave Diathermy
• Pulsed electromagnetic energy (PEME)
• Pulsed electromagnetic field (PEMF)
• Pulsed electromagnetic energy treatment (PEMET)

Capacitor Electrodes
• Air space plates
• Pad electrodes
capacitor electrodes Air space plates or pad electrode that creates a stronger electrical field than a magnetic field.

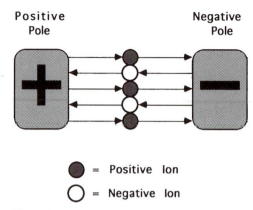

Positive Pole   Negative Pole

● = Positive Ion
○ = Negative Ion

•**Figure 8-3** A positively charged electrode or plate will repel positively charged ions and attract negatively charged ions. Conversely, the negative electrode will repel negative ions and attract positive ions.

trode or plate will repel positively charged ions and attract negatively charged ions. Conversely, the negative electrode will repel negative ions and attract positive ions (Fig. 8-3).

An electrical field is essentially the lines of force exerted on these charged ions by the electrodes that cause charged particles to move from one pole to the other (Fig. 8-4). The intensity of the electrical field is determined by the spacing of the electrodes and is greatest when they are close together. The center of this electrical field has a higher current density than regions at the periphery. When using capacitance electrodes, the patient is placed between two electrodes or plates and becomes part of the circuit. Thus, the tissue between the two electrodes is in a series circuit arrangement (see Chapter 4).

As the electrical field is created in the biologic tissues, the tissue that offers the greatest resistance to current flow tends to develop the most heat. Tissues that have a

Capacitor electrodes = strong electrical field

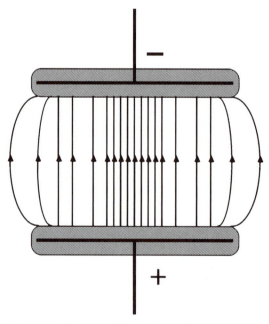

•**Figure 8-4** An electrical field is essentially the lines of force exerted on these charged ions by the electrodes that cause charged particles to move from one pole to the other. (Modified from Michlovitz, S.: Thermal agents in rehabilitation, Philadelphia, 1990, F.A. Davis.)

high fat content tend to insulate and resist the passage of an electrical field. These tissues, particularly subcutaneous fat, tend to overheat when an electrical field is used, which is characteristic of a capacitance type of electrode application.

Air Space Plates

Air space plates are an example of a capacitance (strong electrical field) technique or a capacitor electrode. This type of electrode consists of two metal plates with a diameter of 7.5 to 17.5 cm surrounded by a glass or plastic plate guard. The metal plates may be adjusted approximately 3 cm within the plate guard, thus changing the distance from the skin (Fig. 8-5).[21] Air space plates produce high-frequency oscillating current that is passed through each plate millions of times per second. When one plate is overloaded, it discharges to the other plate of the lower potential, and this is reversed millions of times per second.[14]

When air space plates are used, the area to be treated is placed between the electrodes and becomes part of the external circuit (Fig. 8-6). The sensation of heat tends to be in direct proportion to the distance of the plate from the skin. The closer the plate is to the skin, the better the energy transmission because there is less reflection of the energy. However, it should be remembered that the closer plate will also generate more surface heat in the skin and the subcutaneous fat in that area (Fig. 8-7). The greatest surface heat will be under the electrodes. Parts of the body that are low in subcutaneous fat content (e.g., hands, feet, wrists, and ankles) are best treated by this method. Patients who have a very low subcutaneous fat content can be effectively treated in other body areas.[13] This technique is also very effective for treating the spine and the ribs.

electrical field The lines of force exerted on charged ions in the tissues by the electrodes that cause charged particles to move from one pole to the other.

air space plate A capacitor type electrode in which the plates are separated from the skin by the space in a glass case. Used with shortwave diathermy.

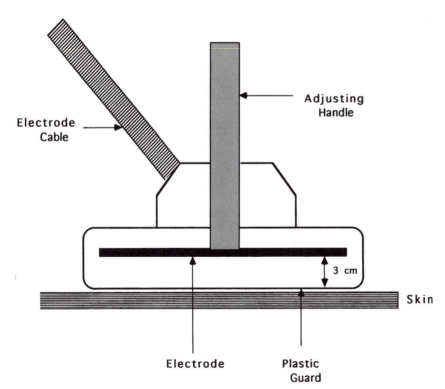

•**Figure 8-5** Air space plate electrodes consist of a metal plate enclosed in a glass or plastic plate guard. The metal plate may be adjusted approximately 3 cm within the plate guard, thus changing the distance from the skin.

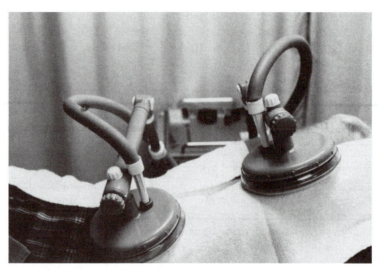

•**Figure 8-6** Treatment of the low back with air space plates. The patient is in a series setup.

pad electrodes Capacitor type electrode used with shortwave diathermy to create an electrical field.

Pad Electrodes

Pad electrodes are seldom used in the clinical setting; however, they may be available for some units. They are true capacitor electrodes, and they must have uniform contact pressure on the body part if they are to be effective in producing deep heat, as well as in avoiding skin burns (Fig. 8-8). The patient is part of the external circuit. Several layers of toweling are necessary to make sure that there is sufficient space between the skin and the pads. The pads should be separated such that they are at least as far apart as the cross-sectional diameter of the pads. In other words, if the pads are 15 cm across, then there should be at least 15 cm between the pads. The closer the spacing of the pads, the higher the current density in the superficial tissues. Increasing the space between the pads will increase the depth of penetration in the tissues (Fig. 8-9). The part of the body to be treated should be centered between the pads.[12,14,17,24]

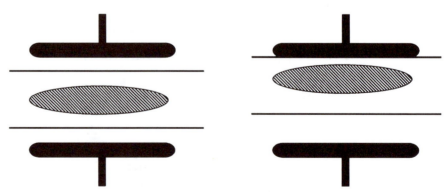

•**Figure 8-7** As the plate moves closer to the surface of the skin the electrical field shifts, generating more surface heat in the skin and the subcutaneous fat.

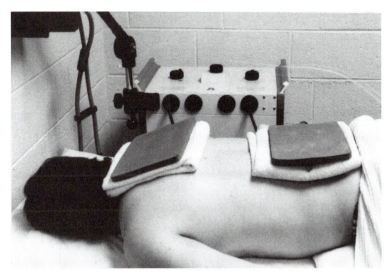

•**Figure 8-8** Pad electrodes showing correct placement and spacing.

Induction Electrodes

The inductance technique, using **induction electrodes**, creates a stronger magnetic field than an electrical field. When the induction technique is used in shortwave diathermy, a cable or coil is either wrapped circumferentially around an extremity or it is coiled within an electrode. In either case, when current is passed through a coiled cable a magnetic field is generated that can affect surrounding tissues by inducing localized secondary currents, called **eddy currents,** within the tissues (Fig. 8-10).[21] Eddy currents are small circular electrical fields, and the **intermolecular oscillation (vibration)** of tissue contents causes heat generation.

In the induction technique, the patient is in a magnetic field and is not part of the circuit. The tissues are in a parallel circuit, thus the greatest current flow is through the tissues with least resistance (see Chapter 4). When a magnetic field is used with an induction-type setup, the fat does not provide nearly as much resistance to the flow of the energy. Therefore, tissues that are high in electrolytic content (i.e., muscle and blood) respond best to the magnetic field by producing heat. It is

induction electrodes Cable electrodes or drum electrodes that create a stronger magnetic field than electrical field.

intermolecular vibration Movement between molecules that produces friction and thus heat.

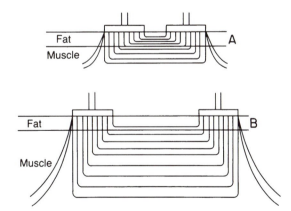

•**Figure 8-9** Pad electrodes should be separated by at least the diameter of the electrodes. A. Electrodes placed close together produce more superficial heating. B. As spacing increases, the current density increases in the deeper tissues.

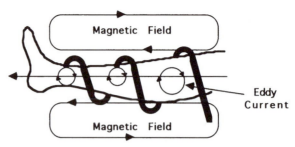

•**Figure 8-10** When current is passed through a coiled cable a magnetic field is generated that can affect surrounding tissues by inducing localized secondary currents, called eddy currents, within the tissues. (Modified from Michlovitz, S.: Thermal agents in rehabilitation, Philadelphia, 1990, F.A. Davis.)

eddy currents Small circular electrical fields induced when a magnetic field is created the result in intramolecular oscillation (vibration) of tissue contents, causing heat generation.

important to remember that if the energy is owing primarily to generation of a magnetic field, heating may not be as obvious to the patient because the magnetic field will not provide nearly as much sensation of warmth in the skin as an electrical field.

Cable Electrodes

cable electrodes An inductance type electrode in which the electrodes are coiled around a body part, creating an electromagnetic field.

The **cable electrode** is an induction electrode which produces a magnetic field (Fig. 8-11). There are two basic types of arrangements: the pancake coil and the wraparound coil. If a pancake coil is used, the size of the smaller circle should be greater than 6 inches in diameter. In either arrangement, there should be at least 1 cm of toweling between the cable and the skin. Stiff spacers should be used to keep the coils or the turns of the pancake or the wraparound coil between 5 and 10 cm between turns of the cable, thus providing spacing consistency. Both the pancake coils and the wraparound coils often provide more even heating because they both are more able to follow the contours of the skin than are the drum or the air space plates. It is important that the cables not touch each other because they will short out and cause excessive heat buildup. Diathermy units that operate on a frequency of 13.56 MHz are probably best suited to cable electrode–type applications. This is primarily because the lower frequency provides better production of a magnetic field.[13]

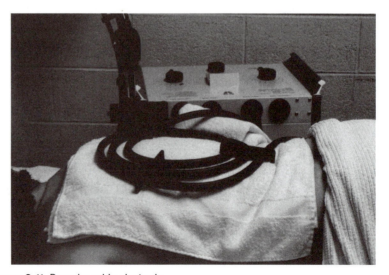

•**Figure 8-11** Pancake cable electrode.

CASE STUDY 8-1
SHORTWAVE DIATHERMY

Background: A thirty-two-year old graduate student developed the gradual onset of lumbar paravertebral muscle spasm following a self-made move of her apartment contents. The symptoms were noted the day after the move on arising and were described as a tightness and restriction of mobility in the low back. She reported no radiation of her symptoms into the buttocks or legs and no difficulty with bowel or bladder function. Physical examination revealed restriction in forward flexion and side rotation of the trunk with tenderness to palpation in the lumbar paravertebral musculature 1 week after the extensive bending and lifting.

Impression: Lumbar paravertebral muscle strain, subacute.

Treatment Plan: The patient was initiated on a course of inductive shortwave diathermy to the lumbar paravertebral musculature, followed by active and active-assisted lumbar region range of motion exercise. Treatment was provided on an every-other-day basis for 2 weeks, with increasing emphasis on mobilizing and strengthening the lumbar paravertebral musculature.

Response: The patient experienced immediate, but short duration, relief of her low back pain following the initial treatment and enthusiastically pursued her exercise sequence. With each subsequent session, the duration of relief and improved trunk mobility increased. At the 2-week point in the treatment regimen the patient was independent in the performance of her lumbar exercise regimen and scheduled to attend a back education class prior to discharge.

Discussion Questions

- What tissues were injured or affected?
- What symptoms were present?
- What phase of the injury-healing continuum did the patient present for care in?
- What are the therapeutic agent modality's biophysical effects (direct, indirect, depth, or tissue affinity)?
- What are the therapeutic agent modality's indications and contraindications?
- What are the parameters of the therapeutic agent modality's application, dosage, duration, and frequency in this case study?
- What other therapeutic agent modalities could be utilized to treat this injury or condition? Why? How?

The rehabilitation professional employs therapeutic agent modalities to create an optimum environment for tissue healing while minimizing the symptoms associated with the trauma or condition.

Drum Electrodes

The **drum electrode** also produces a magnetic field. The drum electrode is made up of one or more monoplanar coils that are rigidly fixed inside some kind of housing (Fig. 8-12). If a small area is to be treated, particularly a small flat area, then a one-drum setup is fine. However, if the area is contoured, then two or more drums, which may be on a hinged apparatus or hinged arm, may be more suitable.

Penetration into the tissues tends to be on the order of 2 to 3 cm if the skin is no more than 1 to 2 cm away from the drum.[5] The magnetic field may be significant up to 5 cm away from the drum. A light towel must be kept in contact with the skin and between the drum and the skin. The towel is used to absorb moisture because an accumulation of water droplets would tend to overheat and cause hot spots on the surface. If there is more than 2 cm of fat, there probably will be no great tissue temperature rise under the fat with a drum setup. The maximum penetration of shortwave diathermy with a drum electrode is 3 cm, provided there is no more than 2 cm of fat beneath the skin. For best absorption of energy, the housing of the drum should be in contact with the towel that is covering the skin.[13]

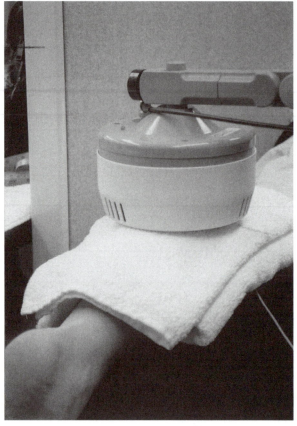

•**Figure 8-12** Drum electrode.

drum electrodes Induction electrodes that produce a strong magnetic field. Primarily used with pulsed shortwave diathermy.

PULSED SHORTWAVE DIATHERMY

Pulsed shortwave diathermy, also referred to in the literature as pulsed electromagnetic energy (PEME), pulsed electromagnetic field (PEMF), or pulsed electromagnetic energy treatment (PEMET), is a relatively new form of diathermy.[18] Pulsed diathermy is created by simply interrupting the output of continuous shortwave diathermy at consistent intervals (Fig. 8-13). Energy is delivered to the patient in a series of high-frequency bursts or pulse trains. Pulse duration is short, ranging from 20 to 400 μsec with an intensity of up to 1000 watts per pulse. The interpulse interval or off time depends on the pulse repetition rate, which ranges between 1 and 7000 Hz. The pulse repetition rate may be selected using the pulse-frequency control on the generator control panel.[21] Generally the off time is considerably longer than the on time. Therefore, even though the power output during the on time is sufficient to produce tissue heating, the long off time interval allows the heat to dissipate. This reduces the likelihood of any significant tissue temperature increase and reduces the patient's perception of heat.

pulsed shortwave diathermy Created by simply interrupting the output of continuous shortwave diathermy at consistent intervals, it is used primarily for nonthermal effects.

Pulsed diathermy is claimed to have therapeutic value and to produce nonthermal effects with minimal thermal physiologic effects, depending on the intensity of the application. When pulsed diathermy is used in intensities that create an increase in tissue temperature, its effects are no different from those of continuous shortwave diathermy. Successful treatments have largely resulted from the application of higher intensities and longer treatment times. Studies that use pulsed shortwave diathermy do not normally compare it with continuous shortwave diathermy but rather with a control group that has received no heat treatment.[24]

Treatment Tip
Pulsed shortwave diathermy is capable of heating a much larger area than ultrasound; the applicator is stationary so the heat applied to the area is more constant; the rate of temperature decay is slower following diathermy application allowing more time for stretching; using diathermy doesn't require constant monitoring.

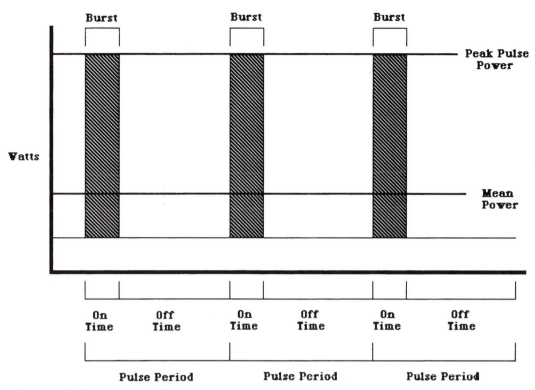

•**Figure 8-13** Pulsed diathermy is created by simply interrupting the output of continuous shortwave diathermy at consistent intervals.

With pulsed shortwave diathermy, mean power provides a measure of heat production. Mean power may be calculated by dividing peak pulse power by the pulse repetition frequency to determine the pulse period (on time plus off time).

$$\text{Pulse period} = \frac{\text{Peak pulse power (watts)}}{\text{Pulse repetition frequency (Hz)}}$$

The percentage on time is calculated by dividing the pulse duration by pulse period.

$$\text{Percentage on time} = \frac{\text{Pulse duration (msec)}}{\text{Pulse period (msec)}}$$

The mean power is then determined by dividing the peak pulse power by the percentage on time.

$$\text{Mean power} = \frac{\text{Peak pulse power (watts)}}{\text{Percentage on time}}$$

With pulsed shortwave diathermy the highest mean power output is usually lower than the power delivered with continuous shortwave diathermy.

Generators that deliver pulsed shortwave diathermy typically use a drum type of electrode (Fig. 8-14). As with continuous shortwave diathermy, the drum electrode is made of a coil wrapped in a flat circular spiral pattern and housed within a plastic case. The energy is induced in the treatment area via the production of a magnetic field.

Pulsed Shortwave diathermy uses drum electrodes.

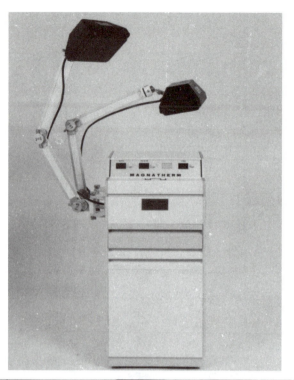

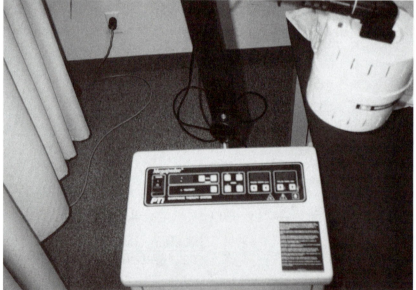

•**Figure 8-14** A. The Magnatherm (Courtesy of International Medical Electronics.) and B. The Megapulse (Courtesy of Physiotechnology, Inc.) are examples of generators capable of producing pulsed shortwave diathermy. Energy is delivered to the patient through a drum electrode.

TREATMENT TIME

Treatments lasting only 15 minutes have produced vigorous heating of the triceps surae muscle of humans.[8] A 20- to 30-minute treatment for one body area is probably all that is necessary to reach maximum physiologic effects.[13] The physiologic effects, particularly circulatory, seem to last about 30 minutes.

Treatments in excess of 30 minutes may create a circulatory rebound phenomenon in which the digital temperature may drop after the treatment because of reflex vasoconstriction. If a therapist finds that a diathermy unit has been left on in excess of 30 minutes, it would be wise to check the temperature of the toes or fingers, depending on which extremity has been treated. It was observed that pulsed shortwave diathermy administered to the triceps surae resulted in peak heating at only 15 minutes into the treatment, and the temperature actually dropped 0.3°C from the 15- to 20-minute mark.[8] Perhaps this can be explained by the increase in blood flow created by the thermal effects of diathermy. The increase in temperature and blood flow engages the body's natural cooling mechanism. Therefore, it may be more difficult to heat muscle tissue than the less vascular tendinous tissue. Perhaps tissue temperatures as high as 45°C, as postulated by other researchers, are too high for the body to tolerate.[8]

It is important to remember that as skin temperature goes up, impedance goes down. Therefore, the unit may need to be returned after 5 to 10 minutes of treatment.

MICROWAVE DIATHERMY

Microwave diathermy has two FCC-assigned frequencies in this country, 2456 and 915 MHz. Microwave has a much higher frequency and a shorter wavelength than shortwave diathermy. Microwave diathermy units generate a strong electrical field and relatively little magnetic field.

With appropriate setup of the microwave diathermy unit, less than 10 percent of the energy is lost from the machine as it is applied to the patient. The microwave applicator beams energy toward the patient, creating the potential for much of the energy to be reflected. Heating is caused by the intramolecular vibration of molecules that are high in polarity.[19] If subcutaneous fat is greater than 1 cm, the fat temperature will rise to a level that is too uncomfortable before there is a tissue temperature rise in the deeper tissues.[14] This is less of a problem if the microwave diathermy is of the frequency of 915 MHz. However, there are very few commercial units operating on that frequency. Almost all of the older units have the higher frequency of 2456 MHz. If the subcutaneous fat is 0.5 cm or less, microwave diathermy can penetrate and cause a tissue temperature rise up to 5 cm deep in the tissue. Bone tends to absorb more shortwave and microwave energy than any type of soft tissue.

MICROWAVE DIATHERMY GENERATORS

The microwave diathermy generator consists of a power supply that energizes the magnetron and timing circuitry. The magnetron control regulates output power by varying the magnetron operating voltage. The magnetron oscillator uses a magnetic field to produce high-frequency currents (Fig. 8-15).

Figure 8-16 represents the control panel of a microwave unit. The power output can be adjusted to patient tolerance. The output meter indicates the relative output in watts or the amount of transmitted and unabsorbed energy. There are two indicator lamps: The amber lamp indicates that the machine is still warming up, and the red lamp indicates that the machine is ready to output energy.

MICROWAVE DIATHERMY APPLICATORS

Electrodes for microwave diathermy are called **applicators.** The microwave energy can only be beamed to one surface at a time. The contour of that surface must be very flat, otherwise there will be considerable reflection of the energy.

Microwave Diathermy Applicators
• Circular
• Rectangular

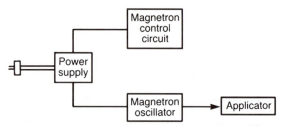

•**Figure 8-15** Component parts of a microwave diathermy unit.

Those microwave diathermy units operating on the frequency 2456 MHz will have a specified air space required between the applicator and the skin. The manufacturer-suggested distances and power output should be followed closely. A directional antenna is attached to the applicator perpendicular to the face of the applicator to assure that spacing is correct and that the energy generated from the microwave unit is striking the target treatment area at the correct angle (cosine law). Units that operate on the higher frequency may have one or more applicators of various shapes and configurations.

There are two types of applicators that may be used with microwave diathermy: circular- and rectangular-shaped. The circular-shaped applicators are either 4 or 6 inches in diameter. With circular-shaped electrodes, the maximum temperature is produced at the periphery of each radiation field (Fig. 8-17A).

Rectangular-shaped applicators are either $4\frac{1}{2} \times 5$ inches or 5×21 inches and produce the maximum temperature at the center of the radiation field (Fig. 8-17B).

In units that have a frequency of 915 MHz, the applicators are placed at a distance of 1 cm from the skin, and the air space between the antenna and the skin is built into the applicator, thus minimizing energy reflection.[24]

MICROWAVE TREATMENT TECHNIQUE

Microwave diathermy units require a period of time to warm up. This is normally built into the circuitry so that the unit power cannot be turned on until the unit is sufficiently warmed. This warm-up time is a good time for the therapist to position

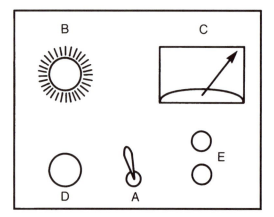

•**Figure 8-16** Control panel of a microwave diathermy unit. A. Power switch, B. timer, C. output meter (indicates relative output in watts of transmitted energy), D. power output level, E. indicator lamps (amber, standby, magnetron accelerating; red, microwaves available for output).

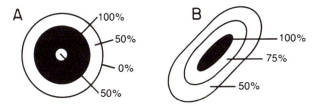

•**Figure 8-17** A. Circular-shaped microwave electrode. B. Rectangular-shaped microwave electrode.

the director and the patient (Fig. 8-18). The director should be located so that the maximum amount of energy will be penetrating at a right angle or perpendicular to the skin. Any angle greater or less than perpendicular will create reflection of the energy and significant loss of absorption (cosine law). Microwave diathermy is best used to treat conditions that exist in those areas of the body that are covered with low subcutaneous fat content. The tendons of the foot, hand, and wrist are well treated, as are the acromioclavicular and sternoclavicular joints, the patellar tendon, the distal tendons of the hamstrings, the Achilles tendon, and the costochondral joints and sacroiliac joints in lean individuals.

In review, there are some distinct differences between shortwave and microwave diathermy. Some of the major differences are as follows.

1. Microwave diathermy produces an electrical field that generates heat owing to dipole response within the cell membrane. Shortwave diathermy produces magnetic fields.
2. Microwave diathermy does not penetrate as deep as shortwave diathermy.
3. Microwave diathermy cannot penetrate the fat layer as well as shortwave diathermy. (Energy is collected by adipose tissue, rendering the effects at about one-third the depth of shortwave diathermy.)
4. No metal should be within 4 feet of microwave diathermy, since it will interfere with the signal.
5. Spacing is required between the skin and applicator with microwave diathermy, whereas the applicator on a shortwave unit can be placed in contact with the treatment area.
6. It appears that shortwave diathermy is much safer than microwave diathermy.

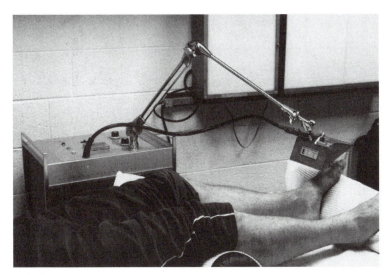

•**Figure 8-18** Typical microwave diathermy unit with rectangular applicator.

CLINICAL APPLICATIONS FOR DIATHERMY

For the most part, the clinical applications for the diathermies are similar to those of other physical agents that are capable of producing thermal effects resulting in a tissue temperature increase.[37] In addition to the diathermies, the infrared modalities discussed in Chapter 9 and ultrasound discussed in Chapter 10 are commonly used as heating modalities.

As with pulsed shortwave diathermy, there have been nonthermal effects documented with microwave diathermy; however, there does not appear to be any evidence that these nonthermal effects have any significant role in the medical application of microwave diathermy.[15,26]

The diathermies have been used in the treatment of a variety of musculoskeletal conditions, including muscle strains, contusions, ligament sprains, tendinitis, tenosynovitis, bursitis, joint contractures, and myofascial trigger points.

Continuous shortwave and microwave diathermy are used most often for a variety of thermal effects, including inducing local relaxation by decreasing muscle guarding and pain; selectively heating joint structures for the purpose of improving joint range of motion by decreasing stiffness and increasing the extensibility of the collagen fibers and the resilience of contracted soft tissues; increasing circulation and improving blood flow to an injured area for the purpose of facilitating resolution of hemorrhage and edema as well as removal of the by-products of the inflammatory process; and in reducing both subacute and chronic pain.[21,24,30]

The majority of recent clinical studies relative to diathermy have focused primarily on the efficacy of pulsed shortwave diathermy in facilitating tissue healing, and to date results have been inconclusive at best.[31] Various claims have been made as to the specific mechanisms that facilitate healing, including an increase in the number and activity of the cells in the area, reduced swelling and inflammation, resorption of hematoma, increased rate of collagen deposition and organization, and increased nerve growth and repair. These claims are based on a limited number of clinical studies and even fewer experimental studies.[20]

There are a number of conditions that may potentially occur in clinical settings that would make diathermy the treatment of choice.

1. If for any reason the skin or some underlying soft tissue is very tender and will not tolerate the loading of a moist heat pack or pressure from an ultrasound transducer, then diathermy should be used.
2. Both continuous shortwave and microwave diathermy are more capable of increasing temperatures to a greater tissue depth than any of the infrared modalities.
3. When the treatment goal is to increase tissue temperatures in a large area (i.e., throughout the entire shoulder girdle, in the low back region), the diathermies should be used.
4. In areas where subcutaneous fat is thick and deep heating is required, the induction technique using either cable or drum electrodes should be used to minimize heating of the subcutaneous fat layer. The capacitance technique with both shortwave diathermy and microwave diathermy is more likely to selectively heat more superficial subcutaneous fat.
5. The therapist should never underestimate the placebo effects that a treatment with any large machine may be capable of producing.

Therapists should take the opportunity to examine several different types of diathermy units, as well as the different applicators available with each unit. They should not only practice using the different applicators on healthy tissue, but they should also experience the sensation themselves. In particular, they should recognize

Indications and Contraindications for Shortwave and Microwave Diathermy

Indications
  Postacute musculoskeletal injuries
  Increased blood flow
  Vasodilation
  Increased metabolism
  Changes in some enzyme reactions
  Increased collagen extensibility
  Decreased joint stiffness
  Muscle relaxation
  Muscle guarding
  Increased pain threshold
  Enhanced recovery from injury
  Joint contractures
  Myofascial trigger points
  Improved joint range of motion
  Increased the extensibility collagen
  Increased circulation
  Reduced subacute and chronic pain
  Resorption of hematoma
  Increased nerve growth and repair

Contraindications
  Acute traumatic musculoskeletal injuries
  Acute inflammatory conditions
  Areas with ischemia
  Areas of reduced sensitivity to temperature or pain
  Fluid filled areas or organs
  Joint effusion
  Synovitis
  Eyes
  Contact lenses
  Moist wound dressings
  Malignancies
  Infection
  Pelvic area during menstruation
  Testes
  Pregnancy
  Epiphyseal plates in adolescents
  Metal implants
  Unshielded cardic pacemakers
  Intrauterine devices
  Watches or jewelry

or experience the difference between the energy flow with an induction-type application as opposed to the capacitor-type application.

DIATHERMY TREATMENT PRECAUTIONS

There are probably more treatment precautions and contraindications for the use of shortwave, and especially microwave, diathermy than for any of the other physical agents used in a clinical setting.

A survey of over 42,000 physical therapists found a modest increase in the risk of miscarriage of pregnant therapists who were regularly exposed to microwave diathermy.[18] Regular exposure to shortwave diathermy during pregnancy, however, did not increase the risk of miscarriage. There are basic differences between microwave and shortwave diathermy that could explain the difference in miscarriage risk. Shortwave diathermy uses high-frequency currents generated at 27.12 MHz and is applied using either a capacitive or inductive applicator, sometimes requiring the patient to become part of the circuit. Microwave diathermy, however, uses higher frequencies of 2450 MHz, and electromagnetic waves are beamed or transmitted into the body by a reflector. Microwave diathermy does not require close contact between the applicator and the therapist, thus allowing some stray emissions.[18] Until further research in this area is performed, it is suggested that the pregnant therapist who treats patients with microwave diathermy first set up the microwave application and then leave the immediate area until the treatment is completed. At this time, however, there is no known risk of miscarriage by pregnant therapists who regularly employ shortwave diathermy.

Diathermy is known to produce a tissue temperature rise and may be contraindicated in any condition where this increased temperature may produce negative or undesired effects, including traumatic musculoskeletal injuries with acute bleeding; acute inflammatory conditions; areas with reduced blood supply (ischemia); and areas with reduced sensitivity to temperature or pain.[11,21,25] It is important to keep in mind that the power meter on the diathermy units does not indicate the energy entering the tissues. Therefore, the therapist must rely on the sensation of pain for a warning that the patient's tolerance levels have been exceeded.[27]

SWD can be continuous or pulsed.

Because diathermy selectively heats tissues that are high in water content, caution must be exercised when using diathermy over fluid-filled areas or organs. Joint effusion may be exacerbated by heating with diathermy. The increase in temperature may cause an increase in synovitis.[25] Because of the high fluid content, it should not be used around the eyes for any prolonged periods of time or for repeated treatments, nor should it be used with contact lenses.[22,38]

In most cases, toweling should be used to absorb perspiration.[13] A single layer of toweling should be used with both the drum and air space plates. However, with other types of applicators, such as pads and cables, the toweling should be more dense and thicker, up to 1 cm or more.[3] Toweling is not necessary with microwave diathermy. There should be no overlapping of skin surfaces. If the buttocks area is to be treated, a towel should be placed in the cleavage between the buttocks. If the shoulder area is to be treated, a towel should be placed between the skin folds in the axilla.

If clothing is permitted in the exposed area, the treatment should be closely monitored. In most cases, however, pulsed shortwave diathermy can be applied over some clothing such as a cotton T-shirt (Fig. 8-19). Be aware that many of the synthetic fabrics worn today allow for no evaporation of moisture, serving as a vapor

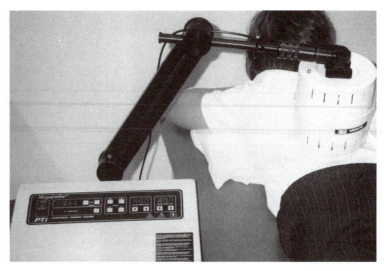

•**Figure 8-19** In most cases pulsed shortwave diathermy can be applied over some clothing such as a cotton T-shirt.

barrier allowing moisture to accumulate. Similarly, moisture can accumulate in patients taped with adhesive tape or wearing compressive wraps or supportive braces. This moisture can create extreme hot spots with diathermy treatments.[34] Diathermy should not be used over moist wound dressings, again because of potential for rapid heating of moisture.[25]

Diathermy should not be applied to the pelvic area of the female who is menstruating, since this can increase blood flow.[25]

Exposure of the gonads to diathermy also should be avoided.[41] The testes are more superficial and thus are more susceptible to injury from microwave treatment than the ovaries. Minimal evidence exists that diathermy may potentially cause damage to the human fetus, and since research in this area is impossible, it is recommended that caution be used in treating the pregnant female.[39]

Caution should be used when using diathermy over bony prominences to avoid burning of the overlying soft tissue.[23] There should be no vigorous heating of the epiphysis in children.[25]

The patient should not come in contact with any of the cables connecting the generator with the air space plates, pad, cable, or drum electrodes. There should be no crossover of the lead cables with any electrode setup. At no time should the antenna within the microwave applicator ever come in contact with skin, since this would cause a buildup of energy sufficient to cause severe burns.

It is very important to use diathermy units at a safe distance from other types of medical electrical devices or equipment that is transistorized. Transcutaneous electrical nerve stimulation units and other low-frequency current units often have transistor-type circuits, and these can be damaged by the reflected or stray radiation that is produced by shortwave and microwave diathermy units.[25] Unshielded cardiac pacemakers may also be damaged by diathermy.[40]

There should be no metal chairs or metal tables used to support the patient during treatment. The area being treated should also be free of metal implants. Women wearing intrauterine devices should not be treated in the low back or lower abdomen. There should be no watches or jewelry in the area because the electromagnetic energy will tend to magnetize the watch, and the electromagnetic energy may heat up the jewelry.[25]

The patient must remain in a reasonably comfortable position for the duration of the treatment so that the field does not change because of movement during treatment.

The skin should be inspected before and after a diathermy treatment. It is recommended that the part being treated either be horizontal or elevated during treatment.

COMPARING SHORTWAVE DIATHERMY AND ULTRASOUND AS THERMAL MODALITIES

The use of therapeutic ultrasound will be discussed in detail in Chapter 10. Ultrasound and pulsed shortwave diathermy are both clinically effective modalities for heating of both superficial and deep tissues; however, ultrasound is used much more frequently than shortwave diathermy. In surveys of physical therapists in both Canada and Australia, only 0.6 and 8 percent of respondents, respectively, used shortwave diathermy daily, yet 94 and 93 percent, respectively, used ultrasound daily.[28,29]

Recent research has demonstrated that shortwave diathermy may be more effective as a heating modality than ultrasound in treating certain conditions.[7,8] A study was done to determine the rate of temperature increase during pulsed shortwave diathermy and the rate of temperature decay postapplication. A 23-gauge thermistor was inserted 3 cm below the skin surface of the anesthetized left medial triceps surae muscle belly of 20 subjects (Fig. 8-20). Diathermy was applied to the muscle belly for 20 minutes at 800 Hz, a pulse duration of 400 μsec, and an intensity of 150 watts. Temperature changes were recorded every 5 minutes during the treatment (Fig. 8-21). The mean baseline temperature was 35.8°C, and the temperature peaked at 39.8°C in 15 minutes, then dropped slightly (0.3°C) during the last

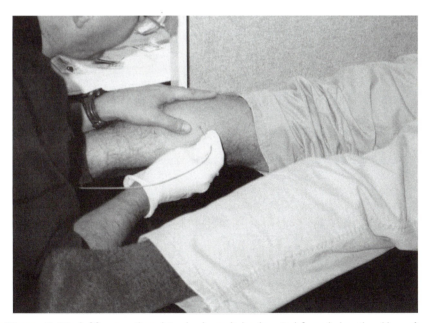

•**Figure 8-20** A 23-gauge thermistor is shown being inserted 3 cm below the skin surface of the anesthetized left medial triceps surae muscle belly.

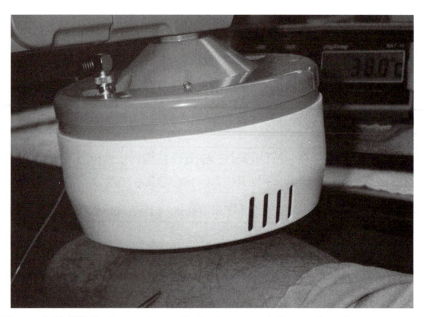

•**Figure 8-21** With the temperature probe in place, muscle temperature changes were measured during shortwave diathermy treatments. (Courtesy, Sportsmedicine research laboratory, Brigham Young University, Provo, Utah.)

5 minutes of treatment. After the treatment terminated, intramuscular temperature dropped 1°C in 5 minutes and 1.8°C by the tenth minute. Based on these findings, it appears that shortwave diathermy compares favorably with heating rates of 1 MHz ultrasound (1W/cm^2 for 12 min = a 4°C temperature increase at 3 cm intramuscularly) (Fig. 8-22).

Shortwave diathermy, however, may be a better modality than ultrasound in some situations, and it appears that there are several advantages of diathermy use over ultrasound.

1. Since the surface of the shortwave applicator drum is 25 times larger than a typical ultrasound treatment area, it heats a much larger area. (A standard drum heating area of the diathermy unit is 200 cm^2, or approximately 25 times that of ultrasound.)

2. Unlike ultrasound that causes a fluctuating tissue heating rate as the transducer is moved, diathermy's applicator is stationary so the heat applied to the area is more constant.

3. The rate of temperature decay is slower following diathermy application. Muscle heated with pulsed shortwave diathermy will retain heat over 60 percent longer than identical muscle depths heated with 1 MHz ultrasound.[9,35] This is important since it provides the clinician more time for stretching, friction massage, and joint mobilization before the temperature drops to an ineffective level.

4. Application of diathermy does not require constant monitoring by the therapist, whereas ultrasound application requires constant monitoring. Thus, a therapist can work with another patient while one is receiving diathermy treatment. This enables the therapist to be more efficient.

GUIDELINES FOR THE SAFE USE OF DIATHERMY

Therapists who are knowledgeable in the physics and biophysics of diathermy, as well as its applications to a variety of cases, tend to achieve good results. Therapists who work with shortwave and microwave diathermy units must spend considerable time experimenting with equipment setup and the application of different types of

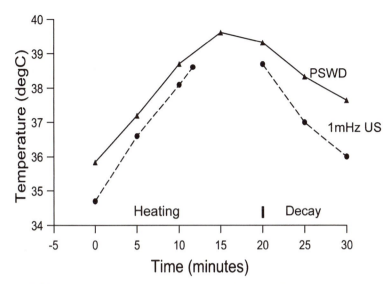

•**Figure 8-22** Intramuscular temperatures during heating and 10 minutes of decay resulting from 20 minutes of shortwave diathermy (PSWD; triangles) and 12 minutes of 1 MHz ultrasound (US; squares) application. This illustrates that shortwave diathermy and 1 MHz ultrasound have similar heating rates, yet muscle heated with shortwave diathermy will retain its heat two to three times longer.

electrodes on a variety of uninjured parts of the body if they are to develop the skills necessary to use diathermy safely and effectively on injured tissue. The following guidelines will help ensure safety.

1. Question patient (contraindications and previous treatments).
2. Position patient (comfort, modesty).
3. Inspect part to be treated (check for rashes, infections, or open wounds).
4. If indicated, drape area with toweling.
5. Place electrode drum on treatment area.
6. Turn unit on.
7. Set pulse duration.
8. Set pulse frequency.
9. Adjust intensity.
10. Set treatment time (15–30 min).
11. Press start button.
12. Periodically ask patient if heating is too vigorous.
13. When timer shuts off, terminating the treatment, turn all dials to zero.
14. Assess treatment efficacy (inspect area; feedback from patient).
15. Record treatment parameters.

SUMMARY

1. Diathermy is the application of high-frequency electromagnetic energy that is primarily used to generate heat in body tissues. Diathermy as a therapeutic agent may be classified as two distinct modalities, shortwave diathermy and microwave diathermy. Shortwave diathermy may be continuous or pulsed.

2. The physiologic effects of continuous shortwave and microwave diathermy are primarily thermal, resulting from high-frequency vibration of molecules. Pulsed

shortwave diathermy has been used for its nonthermal effects in the treatment of soft-tissue injuries and wounds.

3. A shortwave diathermy unit that generates a high-frequency electrical current will produce both an electrical field and a magnetic field in the tissues. The ratio of the electrical field to the magnetic field depends on the characteristics of the different units as well as on the characteristics of electrodes or applicators.

4. The capacitance technique, using capacitor electrodes (air space plates and pad electrodes), creates a strong electrical field that is essentially the lines of force exerted on charged ions by the electrodes that cause charged particles to move from one pole to the other.

5. The inductance technique, using induction electrodes (cable electrodes and drum electrodes), creates a strong magnetic field when current is passed through a coiled cable. It may affect surrounding tissues by inducing localized secondary currents, called eddy currents, within the tissues.

6. Pulsed diathermy is created by simply interrupting the output of continuous shortwave diathermy at consistent intervals. Generators that deliver pulsed shortwave diathermy typically use a drum type of electrode to induce energy in the treatment area via the production of a magnetic field.

7. Microwave diathermy units generate a strong electrical field and relatively little magnetic field through either circular- or rectangular-shaped applicators that beam energy to the treatment area.

8. The diathermies have been used in the treatment of a variety of musculoskeletal conditions, including muscle strains, contusions, ligament sprains, tendinitis, tenosynovitis, bursitis, joint contractures, and myofascial trigger points.

9. There are probably more treatment precautions and contraindications for the use of microwave diathermy than for any of the other physical agents used in a clinical setting.

10. Effective treatments using the diathermies require practice in application and adjustment of techniques to the individual patient.

11. Four advantages for the use of diathermy over ultrasound are larger heating area, more uniform heating, longer stretching window, and more clinician freedom.

REFERENCES

1. Abramson D.I., Burnett C., Bell Y., and Tuck S.: Changes in blood flow, oxygen uptake and tissue temperatures produced by therapeutic physical agents, Am. J. Phys. Med. 47:51–62, 1960.

2. Behrens B.J., Michlovitz S.L.: Physical agents: theory and practice for the physical therapist assistant, Philadelphia, 1996, F.A. Davis Co.

3. Brown M., Baker R.D.: Effect of pulsed shortwave diathermy on skeletal muscle injury in rabbits, Phys. Ther. 67(2):208–213, 1987.

4. Castel J.C., Draper D.O., Knight K., Fujiwara T., and Garrett C.: Rate of temperature decay in human muscle after treatments of pulsed shortwave diathermy, J. Athl. Train. 32: S–34, 1997.

5. DeLateur, B.J., Lehmann, J.F., Stonebridge, J.B., et al: Muscle heating in human subjects with 915 MHz microwave contact applicator, Arch. Phys. Med. 51:147–151, 1970.

6. Delpizzo, V., Joyner, K.H.: On the safe use of microwave and shortwave diathermy units, Aust. J. Physiother. 33(3):152–162, 1987.

7. Draper, D.O.: Current research on therapeutic ultrasound and pulsed short-wave diathermy. presented at Physio Therapy Research Seminars Japan, Nov. 17, Sendai, Japan, 1996.

8. Draper, D.O., Castel, J.C., Knight, K., et al: Temperature rise in human muscle during pulsed short wave diathermy: Does this modality parallel ultrasound? J. Athletic Training 32:S–35, 1997.

9. Draper, D.O., Castel, J.C., and Castel, D.: Rate of temperature increase in human muscle during 1 MHz and 3 MHz continuous ultrasound, J. Orthop. Sports Phys. Ther. 22:142–150, 1995.

10. Fenn, J.E.: Effect of pulsed electromagnetic energy (Diapulse) on experimental haematomas, Can. Med. Assoc. J. 100:251, 1969.

11. Fischer, C., Solomon, S.: Physiologic responses to heat and cold. In Licht, S., editor: Therapeutic Heat and Cold, New Haven, Connecticut, 1965, Elizabeth Licht.

12. Griffin, J.E.: Update on selected physical modalities, Paper presented in Chicago, Dec., 1981.

13. Griffin, J.E., Karselis, T.C.: The diathermies. In Physical agents for physical therapists, ed. 2, Springfield, Illinois, 1982, Charles C Thomas.

14. Griffin, J.E., Santiesleban, A.J., and Kloth, L.: Electrotherapy for instructors, Paper presented in Lacrosse, Wisconsin, Aug., 1982.

15. Guy, A.W., Lehmann, J.F.: On the determination of an optimum microwave diathermy frequency for a direct contact applicator, Inst. Electric. Electron. Eng. Trans. Biomed. Eng. 13:76–87, 1966.

16. Hansen, T.I., Kristensen, J.H.: Effect of massage, shortwave diathermy and ultrasound upon ^{133}Xe disappearance rate from muscle and subcutaneous tissue in the human calf, Scand. J. Rehabil. Med. 5:179–182, 1973.

17. Health devices shortwave diathermy units, Proceedings of the Emergency Care Research Institute, Meeting in Plymouth, Pennsylvania, June, 1979, pp. 175–193.

18. Hellstrom, R.O., Stewart, W.F.: Miscarriages among female physical therapists who report using radio- and microwave-frequency electromagnetic radiation, Am. J. Epidemiol. 138 (10):775–785, 1993.

19. Kitchen, S., Partridge C.: A review of microwave diathermy, Physiotherapy 77(9):647–652, 1991.

20. Kitchen, S., Partridge, C.: Review of shortwave diathermy continuous and pulsed patterns, Physiotherapy 78(4):243–252, 1992.

21. Kloth, L., Ziskin, M.: Diathermy and pulsed electromagnetic fields. In Michlovitz, S.L., editor: Thermal agents in rehabilitation, ed. 2, Philadelphia, 1990, F.A. Davis.

22. Konarska, I., Michneiwicz, L.: Shortwave diathermy of diseases of the anterior portion of the eye, Klin. Oczna. 25:185, 1955.

23. Lehmann, J.F.: Comparison of relative heating patterns produced in tissues by exposure to microwave energy with exposures at 2450 and 900 megacycles, Arch. Phys. Med. Rehab. 46:307, 1965.

24. Lehmann, J.F.: Diathermy. In Krusen, F.H., editor: Handbook of physical medicine and rehabilitation, Philadelphia, 1965, W.B. Saunders.

25. Lehmann, J.F.: Therapeutic heat and cold, ed. 4, Baltimore, 1990, Williams & Wilkins.

26. Lehmann, J.F., deLateur, B.J.: Diathermy and superficial heat and cold. In Krusen, F.H., editor: Krusen's handbook of physical medicine and rehabilitation, ed. 3, Philadelphia, 1982, W.B. Saunders.

27. Lehmann, J.F., Warren, C.G., and Scham, S.M.: Therapeutic heat and cold, Clin. Orthop. 99:207, 1974.

28. Lindsay, D.M., Dearness, J., and McGinley, C.C.: Electrotherapy usage trends in private physiotherapy practice in Alberta, Physiother. Can. 47(1):30–34, 1995.

29. Lindsay, D.M., Dearness, J., Richardson, C., et al: A survey of electromodality usage in private physiotherapy practices, Aust. J. Physiother. 36(4):249–256, 1990.

30. Low, J.L.: The nature and effects of pulsed electromagnetic radiations, NZ Physiother. 6:18, 1978.

31. Low, J.: Dosage of some pulsed shortwave clinical trials. Physiotherapy 81(10):611–616, 1995.

32. Low, J., Reed, A.: Electrotherapy explained: principles and practice, London, 1990, Butterworth-Heinemann.

33. Millard, J.B.: Effect of high frequency currents and infra-red rays on the circulation of the lower limb in man, Ann. Phys. Med. 6:45,1961.

34. Progress Report, American Physical Therapy Association, June, 1980.

35. Rose, S., Draper, D.O., Schulthies, S.S., and Durrant, E.: The stretching window part two: rate of thermal decay in deep muscle following 1 MHz ultrasound, J. Athl. Train. 31:139–143, 1996.

36. Sanseverino, E.G.: Membrane phenomena and cellular processes under the action of pulsating magnetic fields, Presented at the Second International Congress for Magneto Medicine, Rome, 1980.

37. Schliephake, E.: Carrying out treatment. In Thom, H., editor: Introduction to shortwave and microwave diathermy, ed. 3, Springfield, Illinois, 1966, Charles C Thomas.

38. Scott, B.O.: Effect of contact lenses on shortwave field distribution, Br. J. Opthalmol. 40:696, 1956.

39. Smith, D.W., Clarren, S.K., and Harvey, M.A.: Hyperthermia as a possible teratogenic agent, J. Pediatr. 92:878, 1978.

40. Smyth, H.: The pacemaker patient and the electromagnetic environment, JAMA 227:1412, 1974.

41. Van Demark, N.L., Free, M.J.: Temperature effects. In Johnson, A.D., editor: The testis, vol. 3, New York, 1973, Academic Press.

42. Wilson, D.H.: Treatment of soft tissue injuries by pulsed electrical energy, Br. Med. J. 2:269, 1972.

43. Wright, G.G.: Treatment of soft tissue and ligamentous injuries in professional footballers, Physiotherapy 59(12), 1973.

SUGGESTED READINGS

Abramson, D.L., Bell, Y., Rejal, H., et al: Changes in blood flow, oxygen uptake and tissue temperatures produced by therapeutic physical agents, Am. J. Phys. Med. 39:87–95, 1960.

Abramson, D.L., Chu, L.S.W., Tuck, S., et al: Effect of tissue temperature and blood flow on motor nerve conduction velocity, JAMA 198:1082–1088, 1966.

Abramson, D.I: Physiologic basis for the use of physical agents in peripheral vascular disorders, Arch. Phys. Med. Rehabil. 46: 216, 1965.

Adey, W.R.: Electromagnetic field effects on tissue, Physiol. Rev. 61(3):436–514, 1981.

Adey, W.R.: Physiological signaling across cell membranes and co-operative influences of extremely low frequency electromagnetic fields. In Frohlich, H., editor: Biological coherence and response to external stimuli, Heidleberg, 1988, Springer Verlag.

Allberry, J.: Shortwave diathermy for herpes zoster, Physiotherapy 60:386, 1974.

Aronofsky, D.: Reduction of dental post-surgical symptoms using non-thermal pulsed high-peak-power electromagnetic energy, Oral Surg. 32(5)688–696, 1971.

Babbs, C.F., Dewitt, D.P.: Physical principles of local heat therapy for cancer, Med. Instrument. USA 15:367–373, 1981.

Balogun, J., Okonofua, F.: Management of chronic pelvic inflammatory disease with shortwave diathermy: a case report, Phys. Ther. 68(10):1541–1545, 1988.

Bansal, P.S., Sobti, V.K., and Roy, K.S.: Histomorphochemical effects of shortwave diathermy on healing of experimental muscle injury in dogs, Ind. J. Exp. Biol. 28:766–770, 1990.

Barclay, V., Collier, R.J., and Jones, A.: Treatment of various hand injuries by pulsed electromagnetic energy, Physiotherapy 69(6): 186–188, 1983.

Barker, A.T., Barlow, P.S., Porter, J., et al: A double-blind clinical trial of low power pulsed shortwave therapy in the treatment of a soft tissue injury, Physiotherapy 71(12):500–504, 1985.

Barnett, M.: SWD for herpes zoster, Physiotherapy 61:217, 1975.

Bassett, C: The development and application of pulsed electromagnetic fields (PEMFs) for united fractures and arthrodeses, Orthop. Clin. North Am. 15(10):61–89, 1984.

Benson, T.B., Copp, E.P.: The effect of therapeutic forms of heat and ice on the pain threshold of the normal shoulder, Pheumatol. Rehabil. 13:101–104, 1974.

Bentall, R.H., Eckstein, H.B.: A trial involving the use of pulsed electromagnetic therapy on children undergoing orchidopexy, Kinderchirugie 17(4):380–389, 1975.

Brown, M., Baker, R.D.: Effect of pulsed shortwave diathermy on skeletal muscle injury in rabbits, Phys. Ther. 67(2):208–214, 1987.

Brown-Woodnan, P.D.C., Hadley, J.A., Richardson, L., et al: Evaluation of reproductive function of female rats exposed to radio frequency fields (27.12 MHz) near a shortwave diathermy device, Health Phys. 56(4):521–525, 1989.

Burr, B.: Heat as a therapeutic modality against cancer, Report 16, U.S. National Cancer Institute, Bethesda, Maryland, 1974.

Cameron, B.M.: Experimental acceleration of wound healing, Am. J. Orthopaed. 3:336–343, 1961.

Chamberlain, M.A., Care, G., and Gharfield, B.: Physiotherapy in osteo-arthrosis of the knee, Ann. Rheum. Dis. 23:389–391, 1982.

Cole, A., Eagleston, R.: The benefits of deep heat: ultrasound and electromagnetic diathermy, Phys. Sportsmed. 22(2):76–78, 81–82, 84, 1994.

Constable, J.D., Scapicchio, A.P., and Opitz, B.: Studies of the effects of Diapulse treatment on various aspects of wound healing in experimental animals, J. Surg. Res. 11:254–257, 1971.

Coppell, R.: Survey of stray electromagnetic emissions from microwave and shortwave diathermy equipment, NZ J. Physiother. 16(3):9–12, 14, 1988.

Currier, D.P., Nelson, R.M.: Changes in motor conduction velocity induced by exercise and diathermy, Phys. Ther. 49(2):146–152, 1969.

Daels, J.: Microwave heating of the uterine wall during parturition, J. Microwave Power 11:166, 1976.

de la Rosette, J., de Wildt, M., and Alivizatos, G.: Transurethral microwave thermotherapy (TUMT) in benign prostatic hyperplasia: placebo versus TUMT, Urology 44(1):58–63, 1994.

Department of Health: Evaluation Report: Shortwave therapy units, J. Med. Eng. Technol. 11(6):285–298, 1987.

Department of Health and Welfare (Canada): Canada wide survey of non-ionising radiation-emitting medical devices, 80-EHD-52, 1980.

Department of Health and Welfare (Canada): Safety code 25: Shortwave diathermy guidelines for limited radio frequency exposure, 80-EHD-98, 1983.

Doyle, J.R., Smart, B.W.: Stimulation of bone growth by shortwave diathermy, J. Bone Joint Surg. 45A:15, 1963.

Engel, J.P: The effects of microwaves on bone and bone marrow and adjacent tissues, Arch. Phys. Med. Rehabil. 31:453, 1950.

Erdman, W.J.: Peripheral blood flow measurements during application of pulsed high frequency currents, Am. J. Orthopaed. 2:196–197, 1960.

Feibel, H., Fast, H.: Deepheating of joints: a reconsideration, Arch. Phys. Med. Rehabil. 57:513, 1976.

Fenn, J.E.: Effect of pulsed electromagnetic energy (Diapulse) on experimental haematomas, Can. Med. Assoc. J. 100:251–253, 1969.

Foley-Nolan, D., Barry, C., Coughlan, R.J., et al: Pulsed high frequency (27MHz) electromagnetic therapy for persistent neck pain, Orthopaedics 13(4):445–451, 1990.

Foley-Nolan, D., Moore, K., and Codd, M.: Low energy high frequency pulsed electromagnetic therapy for acute whiplash injuries. A double blind randomized controlled study, Scand. J. Rehab. Med. 24(1):51–9, 1992.

Foster, P.: Diathermy burns, Nursing RSA Verpleging 2(10):4–5, 7–9, 1987.

Gibson, T., Grahame, R., Harkness, J., et al: Controlled comparison of shortwave diathermy treatment with osteopathic treatment in non-specific low back pain, Lancet 1:1258–1261, 1985.

Ginsberg, A.J.: Pulsed shortwave in the treatment of bursitis with calcification, Int. Rec. Med. 174(2):71–75, 1961.

Goldin, J.H., Broadbent, N.R.G., Nancarrow, J.D., and Marshall, T.: The effect of diapulse on healing of wounds: a double blind randomized controlled trial in man, Br. J. Plastic Surg. 34: 267–270, 1981.

Grant, A., Sleep, J., McIntosh, J., and Ashurst, H.: Ultrasound and pulsed electromagnetic energy treatment for peroneal trauma:

A randomised placebo-controlled trial, Br. J. Obstet. Gynaecol 96:434–439, 1981.

Guy, A.W.: Biophysics of high frequency currents and electromagnetic radiation, In: Lehmann, J.F., editor: Therapeutic heat and cold, ed 4, Baitimore, 1990, Williams & Wilkins.

Guy, A.W., Lehmann, J.F., and Stonebridge, J.B.: Therapeutic applications of electromagnetic power, Proc. Inst. Electric. Electr. Eng. 62:55–75, 1974.

Guy, A.W., Lehmann, J.F., Stonebridge, J.B., and Sorensen, C.C.: Development of a 915 MHz direct contact applicator for therapeutic heating of tissues, Inst. Electric. Electr. Eng. Microwave Theory Techniques 26:550–556, 1978.

Guy, A.W: Analyses of electromagnetic fields induced in biological tissues by thermographic studies on equivalent phantom models, IEEE Trans. Microwave Theory Tech. Vol MTT 19:205, 1971.

Hall, E.L.: Diathermy generators, Arch. Phys. Med. Rehabil. 33:28, 1952.

Hansen, T.I., Kristensen, J.H.: Effect of massage, shortwave diathermy and ultrasound upon ^{133}Xe disappearance rate from muscle and subcutaneous tissue in the human calf, Scand. J. Rehabil. Med. 5:179–182, 1973.

Harris, R.: Effect of shortwave diathermy on radio-sodium clearance from the knee joint in the normal and in rheumatoid arthritis, Phys. Med. Rehabil. 42:241, 1961.

Hayne, R: Pulsed high frequency energy:Its place in physiotherapy, Physiotherapy 70(12):459–466, 1984.

Herrick, J.F., Krusen, F.H.: Certain physiologic and pathologic effects of microwaves, Elect. Eng. 72:239, 1953.

Herrick, J.F., Jelatis, D.G., and Lee, G.M.: Dielectric properties of tissues important in microwave diathermy, Fed. Proc. 9:60, 1950.

Hoeberlein, T., Katz, J., and Balogun, J.: Does indirect heating using shortwave diathermy over the abdomen and sacrum affect peripheral blood flow in the lower extremities? Phys. Ther. 76(5):S67, 1996.

Hollander, J.L.: Joint temperature measurement in evaluation of antiarthritic agents, J. Clin. Invest. 30:701, 1951.

Hutchinson, W.J., Burdeaux, B.D.: The effects of shortwave diathermy on bone repair, J. Bone Joint Surg. 33A:155, 1951.

Johnson, C.C., Guy, A.W.: Nonionizing electromagnetic wave effects in biological materials and systems, Proc. Inst. Electric. Electr. Eng. 66:692, 1972.

Jones, S.L.: Electromagnetic field interference and cardiac pacemakers, Phys. Ther. 56:1013, 1976.

Kantor, G., Witters, D.M.: The performance of a new 915 MHz direct contact applicator with reduced leakage—a detailed analysis, HHS Publication (FDA) S3-8199, April, 1983.

Kantor, G.: Evaluation and survey of microwave and radio frequency applicators, J. Microwave Power (2)16:135, 1981.

Kaplan, E.G., Weinstock, R.E.: Clinical evaluation of Diapulse as adjunctive therapy following foot surgery, J. Am. Ped. Assoc. 58:218–221, 1968.

Kloth, L.C., Morrison, M., and Ferguson, B.: Therapeutic microwave and shortwave diathermy: a review of thermal effectiveness, safe use, and state-of-the-art-1984, Center for Devices and Radiological Health, DHHS, FDA 85-8237, December, 1984.

Krag, C., Taudorf, U., Siim, E., Bolund, S.: The effect of pulsed electromagnetic energy (Diapulse) on the survival of experimental skin flaps, Scand. J. Plastic and Reconstr. Surg. 13:377–380, 1979.

Lehmann, J.F., McDougall, J.A., Guy, A.W., et al: Heating patterns produced by shortwave diathermy applicators in tissue substitute models, Arch. Phys. Med. Rehabil. 64:575–577, 1983.

Lehmann, J.F., DeLateur, B.J., and Stonebridge, J.B.: Selective muscle heating by shortwave diathermy with a helical coil, Arch. Phys. Med. Rehabil. 50:117, 1969.

Lehmann, J.F: Review of evidence for indications, techniques of application, contraindications, hazards and clinical effectiveness for shortwave diathermy, DHEW/FDA HFA510, Rockville, Maryland, 1974.

Lehmann, J.F., Guy, A.W., deLateur, B.J., et al: Heating patterns produced by shortwave diathermy using helical induction coil applicators, Arch. Phys. Med. 49:193–198, 1968.

Lehmann, J.F.: Microwave therapy: stray radiation, safety and effectiveness, Arch. Phys. Med. Rehabil. 60:578, 1979.

Licht, S., editor: Therapeutic heat and cold, ed. 2, New Haven, Connecticut, 1972, Elizabeth Licht.

Martin, C., McCallum, H., and Strelley, S.: Electromagnetic fields from therapeutic diathermy equipment: a review of hazards and precautions, Physiotherapy 77(1):3–7, 1991.

McDowell, A.D., Lunt, M.J.: Electromagnetlc field strength measurements on Megapulse units, Physiotherapy 77(12):805–809, 1991.

McGill, S.N.: The effect of pulsed shortwave therapy on lateral ligament sprain of the ankle, NZ J Physiother. 10:21–24, 1988.

McNiven, D.R., Wyper, D.J.: Microwave therapy and muscle blood flow in man, J. Microwave Power 11:168–170, 1976.

Martin, C., McCallum, H., and Strelley, S.: Electromagnetic fields from therapeutic diathermy equipment: a review of hazards and precautions, Physiotherapy 77(1):3–7, 1991.

Michaelson, S.M.: Effects of high frequency currents and electromagnetic radiation. In Lehmann, H.F., editor: Therapeutic heat and cold, ed. 4, Baltimore, 1990,Williams & Wilkins.

Millard, J.B.: Effect of high frequency currents and infrared rays on the circulation of the lower limb in man, Ann. Phys. Med. 6(2):45–65, 1961.

Morrissey, L.J.: Effects of pulsed shortwave diathermy upon volume blood flow through the calf of the leg: plethysmography studies, J. Am. Phys. Ther. Assoc. 46:946–952, 1966.

Mosely, H., Davison, M.: Exposure of physiotherapists to microwave radiation during microwave diathermy treatment, Clin. Phys. Physiol. Meas. No. 3. 2:217, 1981.

Nadasdi, M.: Inhibition of experimental arthritis by athermic pulsing shortwave in rats, Am. J. Orthopaed. 2:105–107, 1960.

Nelson, A.J.M., Holt, J.A.G.: Combined microwave therapy, Med. J. Aust. 2:88–90, 1978.

Nicolle, F.V., Bentall, R.M.: The use of radiofrequency pulsed energy in the control of post-operative reaction to blepharoplasty, Anaesth. Plastic Surg. 6:169–171, 1982.

Nielson, N.C., Hansen, R., and Larsen, T.: Heat induction in copper bearing IUDs during shortwave diathermy, Acta Obstetrica et Gynaecologica Scandinavica (Stockh), 58:495, 1972.

Nwuga, G.B.: A study of the value of shortwave diathermy and isometric exercise in back pain management, Proceedings of the IXth International Congress of the WCPT, Legitimerader Sjukgymnasters Riksforbund, Stockholm, Sweden, 1982.

Oliver, D.: Pulsed electromagentic energy—what is it? Physiotherapy 70(12): 458–459, 1984.

Osborne, S.L., Coulter, J.S.: Thermal effects of shortwave diathermy on bone and muscle, Arch. Phys. Ther. 38:281–284, 1938.

Paliwal, B.R.: Heating patterns produced by 434 MHz erbotherm UHF69, Radiology 135:511, 1980.

Pasila, M., Visuri, T., and Sundholm A.: Pulsating shortwave diathermy: Value in treatment of recent ankle and foot sprains, Arch. Phys. Med. Rehabil. 59:383–386, 1978.

Patzold, J.: Physical laws regarding distribution of energy for various high frequency methods applied in heat therapy, Ultrason. Biol. Med. 2:58, 1956.

Quirk, A.S., Newman, R.J., and Newman, K.J.: An evaluation of interferential therapy, shortwave diathermy and exercise in the treatment of osteo-arthrosis of the knee, Physiotherapy 71(2): 55–57, 1985.

Rae, J.W., Herrick, J.F., Wakim, K.G., and Krusen, F.H.: A comparative study of the temperature produced by MWD and SWD, Arch. Phys. Med. Rehabil. 30:199, 1949.

Raji, A.M.: An experimental study of the effects of pulsed electromagnetic field (Diapulse) on nerve repair, J. Hand Surg. 9B(2):105–112, 1984.

Reed, M.W., Bickerstaff, D.R., Hayne, C.R., et al: Pain relief after inguinal herniorrhaphy: ineffectiveness of pulsed electromagnetic energy, Br. J. Clin. Pract. 41(6):782– 784, 1987.

Religo, W., Larson, T.: Microwave thermotherapy: new wave of treatment for benign prostatic hyperplasia, J. Am. Acad. Phys. Assist. 7(4):259–267, 1994.

Richardson, A.W.: The relationship between deep tissue temperature and blood flow during electromagnetic irradiation, Arch. Phys. Med. Rehabil. 31:19, 1950.

Rubin, A., Erdman, W.: Microwave exposure of the human female pelvis during early pregnancy and prior to conception, Am. J. Phys. Med. 38:219, 1959.

Ruggera, P.S.: Measurement of emission levels during microwave and shortwave diathermy treatments, Bureau of Radiological Health Report, HHS Publication (FDA), 80–8119, 1980.

Schwan, H.P.: Interaction of microwave and radio frequency radiation with biological systems. In Cleary, S.F., editor: Biological effects and health implications of microwave radiation, U.S. Department of Health, Education and Welfare, Washington, D.C., 1970.

Schwan, H.P., Piersol, G.M.: The absorption of electromagnetic energy in body tissues. Part I, Am. J. Phys. Med. 33:371, 1954.

Schwan, H.P., Piersol, G.M.: The absorption of electromagnetic energy in body tissues. Part II, Am. J. Phys. Med. 34:425, 1955.

Silverman, D.R., Pendleton, L.A.: A comparison of the effects of continuous and pulsed shortwave diathermy on peripheral circulation, Arch. Phys. Med. Rehabil. 49:429–436, 1968.

Stuchly, M.A., Repacholi, M.H., Lecuyer, D.W., and Mann, R.D.: Exposure to the operator and patient during shortwave diathermy treatments, Health Phys. 42(3):341–366, 1982.

Svarcova, J., Trnavsky, K., and Zvarova, J.: The influence of ultrasound, galvanic currents and shortwave diathermy on pain intensity in patients with osteo-arthritis Scand. J. Rheumatol. supplement 67:83–85, 1988.

Taskinen, H., Kyyronen, P., and Hemminki, K.: The effects of ultrasound, shortwaves and physical exertion on pregnancy outcome in physiotherapists, J. Epidemiol. Commun. Health 44:96–201, 1990.

Thom, H.: Introduction to shortwave and microwave therapy, ed 3, Springfield, Illinois, 1966, Charles C Thomas.

Tzima, E., Martin, C.: An evaluation of safe practices to restrict exposure to electric and magnetic fields from therapeutic and surgical diathermy equipment, Physiol. Measure. 15(2):201–216, 1994.

Van Ummersen, C.A.: The effect of 2450 MHz radiation on the development of the chick embryo. In Peyton, M.F., editor: Biological effects of microwave radiation, vol. 1, New York, 1961, Plenum Press.

Vanharanta, H.: Effect of shortwave diathermy on mobility and radiological stage of the knee in the development of experimental osteo-arthritis, Am. J. Phys. Med. 61(2):59–65, 1982.

Verrier, M., Falconer, K., and Crawford, J.S.: A comparison of tissue temperature following two shortwave diathermy techniques, Physiother. Can. 29(1):21–25, 1977.

Wagstaff, P., Wagstaff, S., and Downie, M.: A pilot study to compare the efficacy of continuous and pulsed magnetic energy (shortwave diathermy) on the relief of low back pain, Physiotherapy 72(11):563–566, 1986.

Ward, A.R.: Electricity fields and waves in therapy, Science Press, Australia, 1980, NSW.

Wilson, D.: Treatment of soft tissue injuries by pulsed electrical energy continuous and pulsed magnetic energy (shortwave diathermy) on the relief of low back pain, Physiotherapy 72(11):563–566, 1986.

Wilson, D.H.: Treatment of soft tissue injuries by pulsed electrical energy, Br. Med. J. 2:269–270, 1972.

Wilson, D.H.: Comparison of shortwave diathermy and pulsed electromagnetic energy in treatment of soft tissue injuries, Physiotherapy 60(10):309–310, 1974.

Wilson, D.H.: The effects of pulsed electromagnetic energy on peripheral nerve regeneration, Ann. NY Acad. Sci. 238:575, 1975.

Wise, C.S.: The effect of diathermy on blood flow, Arch. Phys. Med. Rehabil. 29:17, 1948.

Witters, D.M., Kantor, G.: An evaluation of microwave diathermy applicators using free space electric field mapping, Phys. Med. Biol. 26:1099, 1981.

Worden, R.E.: The heating effects of microwaves with and without ischemia, Arch. Phys. Med. Rehabil. 29:751, 1948.

Wyper, D.J., McNiven, D.R.: Effects of some physiotherapeutic agents on skeletal muscle blood flow, Physiotherapy 63(3): 83–85, 1976.

Glossary

air space plate A capacitor-type electrode in which the plates are separated from the skin by the space in a glass case. Used with shortwave diathermy.

applicator The electrode used to transfer energy in microwave diathermy.

cable electrodes An inductance-type electrode in which the electrodes are coiled around a body part, creating an electromagnetic field.

capacitor electrodes Air space plates or pad electrode that creates a stronger electrical field than a magnetic field.

diathermy The application of high-frequency electrical energy that is used to generate heat in body tissues as a result of the resistance of the tissue to the passage of energy. It may also be used to produce nonthermal effects.

drum electrodes Induction electrodes that produce a strong magnetic field. Primarily used with pulsed shortwave diathermy.

eddy currents Small circular electrical fields induced when a magnetic field is created that results in intermolecular oscillation (vibration) of tissue contents, causing heat generation.

electrical field The lines of force exerted on charged ions in the tissues by the electrodes that cause charged particles to move from one pole to the other.

Federal Communications Commission (FCC) Federal agency charged with assigning frequencies for all radio transmitters, including diathermies.

induction electrodes Cable electrodes or drum electrodes that create a stronger magnetic than electrical field.

intermolecular vibration Movement between molecules that produces friction and thus heat.

magnetic field Created when current is passed through a coiled cable affecting surrounding tissues by inducing localized secondary currents, called eddy currents, within the tissues.

pad electrodes Capacitor-type electrode used with shortwave diathermy to create an electrical field.

pulsed shortwave diathermy Created by simply interrupting the output of continuous shortwave diathermy at consistent intervals, it is used primarily for nonthermal effects.

specific absorption rate (SAR) Represents the rate of energy absorbed per unit area of tissue mass.

LAB ACTIVITY

SHORTWAVE DIATHERMY

DESCRIPTION:

Shortwave diathermy (SWD; *diathermy* means to heat through) utilizes an alternating current (most commonly 27.12 MHz) passed either through a coiled conductor or to a capacitor plate.

With the coil method, the patient is placed in the magnetic field that is generated when the current passes through the coil; the magnetic field then is absorbed by the molecules in the body, increasing the patient's internal energy. This method is referred to as inductive, because the body acts as a secondary coil, and the current in the body is induced by the current in the primary coil; the body never becomes part of the electrical circuit.

With the second method, there are two capacitor plates that are charged, and the body acts as a lower resistance conductor for the discharge of the capacitive current; thus the term capacitive shortwave diathermy. Again, the molecules of the body absorb the energy and have their internal energy increased. In capacitive SWD, the patient becomes part of the electrical circuit.

Because the motion of a molecule is dependent on it's internal energy, when a molecule absorbs any type of energy, it's motion increases. Temperature is a reflection of the average kinetic energy of a system, and the kinetic energy is by definition the random molecular motion. Therefore, when the molecular motion increases, the temperature increases. Although there are increased molecular collisions when the thermal energy of a system increases, these collisions do not produce any energy; they merely transfer the energy from one molecule to another. It is a misconception that the "friction" that occurs between the molecules causes the increased temperature.

Although electrical energy is used in SWD, action potentials are not induced in excitable tissue. At such high frequencies, the phase charge of the current is inadequate to alter the membrane voltage enough for the membrane to reach threshold. The amount of heat generated does follow Joule's law

$$Q = I^2Rt$$

where Q is heat, I is current, R is resistance, and t is time. The heat is generated in the tissue that absorbs the energy, and this varies according to the type of SWD used. Inductive SWD is absorbed mostly by tissues that have a high electrical conductivity, such as muscle. Capacitive SWD is absorbed mostly by tissues that have a low electrical conductivity, such as skin and fat. Because of this, capacitive SWD does not penetrate as deeply as inductive SWD, but does produce a more marked sensation of warmth in the patient. The general guideline for the depth of penetration of capacitive SWD is 1 cm, and 3 to 4 cm for inductive SWD.

PHYSIOLOGIC EFFECTS:

Vasodilation
Decreased pain perception
Increased local metabolism
Increased connective tissue plasticity
Decreased isometric strength (transient)

THERAPEUTIC EFFECTS:

Decreased pain
Increased soft tissue extensibility

INDICATIONS:

Shortwave diathermy is a heating physical agent; therefore, the indications are the same as for any heating agent. However, the depth of penetration, at least for inductive SWD, is greater than for any of the infrared agents. Ultrasound has a deeper penetration than SWD, but SWD can be used to treat a much larger area.

CONTRAINDICATIONS:

- Lack of normal temperature sensibility
- Peripheral vascular disease with compromised circulation
- Over tumors, the testes, open growth plates, acutely inflamed tissue, active hemorrhage, the eyes, or metallic objects
- Pregnancy
- In patients with implanted electrical stimulators (e.g., cardiac pacemakers, phrenic nerve stimulators, etc.)

SHORTWAVE DIATHERMY

PROCEDURE	Evaluation		
	1	2	3
1. Check supplies.			
a. Obtain sheet or towels for draping, timer, signaling device			
b. Check SWD generator for frayed power cords, integrity cables and drum, shields, and so on			
c. Verify that the output control is at zero.			
2. Question patient.			
a. Verify identity of patient (if not already verified).			
b. Verify the absence of contraindications.			
c. Ask about previous thermotherapy treatments; check treatment notes.			
3. Position patient.			
a. Place patient in a well-supported, comfortable position. This is particularly crucial, because the patient should not shift positions after the treatment starts.			
b. Expose body part to be treated; have patient remove all jewelry from the area.			
c. Drape patient to preserve modesty, protect clothing, but allow access to body part.			
4. Inspect body part to be treated.			
a. Check light touch perception.			
b. Check circulatory status (pulses, capillary refill). Assess function of body part (e.g., ROM, irritability).			
5. Apply SWD.			
a. Place a single layer of towel on the treatment area.			
b. Inductive: Position the drum containing the coil parallel to the body part and in contact with the towel. Capacitive: Position the plates parallel to the body part and about 2.5 to 7.5 centimeters away from the body.			
c. Turn on the SWD generator, allow to warm up if necessary.			
d. Inform the patient that he or she should feel only warmth; if it becomes hot, the patient should inform you immediately.			
e. Adjust intensity of SWD to the appropriate level. Set a timer for the appropriate treatment time and give the patient a signaling device. Make sure the patient understands how to use the signaling device.			
f. Check the patient's response after the first 5 minutes by asking how it feels.			

PROCEDURE	Evaluation		
	1	2	3
6. Complete the treatment.			
a. When the treatment time is over, turn the intensity control to zero, and move the generator away from the patient; dry the area with a towel.			
b. Remove material used for draping, assist the patient in dressing as needed.			
c. Have the patient perform appropriate therapeutic exercise as indicated.			
d. Clean the treatment area and equipment according to normal protocol.			
7. Assess treatment efficacy.			
a. Ask the patient how the treated area feels.			
b. Visually inspect the treated area for any adverse reactions.			
c. Perform functional tests as indicated.			

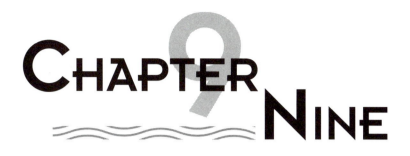

CHAPTER NINE

INFRARED MODALITIES

GERALD W. BELL and
WILLIAM E. PRENTICE

OBJECTIVES

After completion of this chapter, the student therapist will be able to do the following:

✓ Understand how the infrared modalities are classified in the electromagnetic spectrum.
✓ Differentiate between the physiologic effects of therapeutic heat and cold.
✓ Describe the contemporary modalities of the infrared spectrum in thermotherapy and cryotherapy.
✓ Describe the indications and contraindications for each infrared modality discussed.
✓ Select the most effective infrared modalities for a given clinical diagnosis.
✓ Explain how the therapist can use the infrared modalities to reduce pain.

Of the therapeutic modalities discussed in this text, perhaps none are more commonly used than **infrared** modalities. As indicated in Chapter 1, the infrared region of the electromagnetic spectrum falls between the microwave diathermy and the visible light portions of the spectrum in terms of wavelength and frequency. There is a great deal of misunderstanding among therapists regarding which of the modalities used in a clinical setting are actually classified as infrared. Traditionally, the term infrared heating conjures up visions of infrared lamps and bakers. However, it must be emphasized that most of the heat and cold modalities, such as hydrocollator packs, paraffin baths, hot and cold whirlpools, and ice packs, as well as infrared lamps, produce forms of radiant energy that have wavelengths and frequencies that fall into the infrared region. (see Fig. 1-2). This chapter includes a discussion of all the modalities that fall into the infrared portion of the electromagnetic spectrum.

Mechanisms of Infrared Heat Transfer
- Conduction
- Convection
- Radiation

conduction Heat loss or gain through direct contact.

Infrared modalities should be used primarily to provide analgesia and reduce pain.

cryotherapy The use of cold in the treatment of pathology or diseases.

hydrotherapy Cryotherapy and thermotherapy techniques that use water as the medium of heat transfer.

MECHANISMS OF HEAT TRANSFER

Easy application and convenience of use of hot and cold modalities provide the therapist with the necessary tools for primary care of injuries. Heat is defined as the internal vibration of the molecules within a body. The transmission of heat occurs by three mechanisms: **conduction**, **convection**, and **radiation**. A fourth mechanism of heat transfer, **conversion**, is discussed in Chapter 10.

Conduction occurs when the body is in direct contact with the heat or cold source. Convection occurs when particles (air or water) move across the body, creating a temperature variation. Radiation is the transfer of heat from a warmer source to a cooler source through a conducting medium, such as air (e.g., infrared lamps). The body may either gain or lose heat through any of these three processes of heat transfer. The infrared modalities discussed in this chapter use these three methods of heat transfer to effect a tissue temperature increase or decrease.

APPROPRIATE USE OF THE INFRARED MODALITIES

Infrared modalities are often abused by therapists who use a modality randomly without reviewing its benefits. Placing the patient in the whirlpool or a slush bucket of ice simply because these two modalities are available is not an acceptable treatment technique.

Heating techniques used for therapeutic purposes are referred to as **thermotherapy**. Thermotherapy is used when a rise in tissue temperature is the goal of treatment. The use of cold, or **cryotherapy**, is most effective in the acute stages of the healing process immediately following injury, when a loss of tissue temperature is the goal of therapy. Cold applications can be continued into the reconditioning stage of injury management. Thermotherapy and cryotherapy are included in this section on the basis of their classification in the electromagnetic spectrum. The term **hydrotherapy** can be applied to any cryotherapy or thermotherapy technique that uses water as the medium for tissue temperature exchange.

The electromagnetic spectrum has a relatively large region of radiations designated as infrared. The infrared wavelength provides the radiant energy used therapeutically (see Fig. 1-2). Penetration of the energy is dependent on the source but is generally considered to be a superficial form of treatment.

Although this chapter is concerned primarily with application of the infrared modalities and their physiologic effects, several other modalities discussed in this text (e.g., the diathermies and ultrasound) cause similar physiologic responses. Specifically, the effects of heat and cold therapy discussed in this chapter may be applied to any modality that alters tissue temperature.

Heating and cooling agents can be used successfully to treat injuries and trauma.[19] The therapist must know the injury mechanism and specific pathology, as well as the physiologic effects of the heating and cooling agents, to establish a consistent treatment schedule.

PHYSIOLOGIC EFFECTS OF TISSUE HEATING

Local superficial heating (infrared heat) is recommended in subacute conditions for reducing pain and **inflammation** through analgesic effects. Superficial heating produces lower tissue temperatures at the site of the pathology (injury) relative to the higher temperatures in the superficial tissues, resulting in **analgesia**. During the later stages of injury healing, a deeper heating effect is usually desirable; it can be achieved by using the diathermies or ultrasound. Heat dilates blood vessels, causing the patent capillaries to open up and increase circulation. The skin is supplied with sympathetic vasoconstrictor fibers that secrete norepinephrine at their endings (especially evident in feet, hands, lips, nose, and ears). At normal body temperature the sympathetic vasoconstrictor nerves keep vascular anastomoses almost totally closed, but when the superficial tissue is heated, the number of sympathetic impulses is greatly reduced so that the anastomoses dilate and allow large quantities of blood to flow into the venous plexuses. This increases blood flow about twofold, which can promote heat loss from the body.[28]

The **hyperemia** created by heat has a beneficial effect on injury. This is based on increases of blood flow and pooling of blood during the metabolic processes. Recent hematomas (blood clots) should never be treated with heat until resolution of bleeding is completed. Some therapists have advocated never using heat during any therapeutic modality application.[32,34,36,39]

The rate of metabolism of tissues depends partly on temperature. The metabolic rate has increased approximately 13 percent for each 1°C (1.8°F) increase in temperature.[32] A similar decrease in metabolism has been demonstrated when temperatures are lowered.

A primary effect of local heating is an increase in the local metabolic rate with a resulting increase in the production of **metabolites** and additional heat. These two factors lead to an increased intravascular hydrostatic pressure, causing arteriolar **vasodilation** and increased capillary blood flow.[72] However, with increased hydrostatic pressure, there is a tendency toward formation of edema, which may increase the time required for rehabilitation of a particular injury. Increased capillary blood flow is important with many types of injury in which there is mild or moderate inflammation, since it causes an increase in the supply of oxygen, antibodies, leukocytes, and other necessary **nutrients** and enzymes, along with an increased clearing of metabolites. With higher heat intensities, vasodilation and increased blood flow will spread to remote areas, causing increased metabolism in the unheated area. This is known as **consensual heat vasodilation** and may be useful in many conditions where local heating is contraindicated.[23]

The application of heat can produce an analgesic effect, resulting in a reduction in the intensity of pain. The analgesic effect is the most frequent **indication** for the use.[72] Although the mechanisms underlying this phenomenon are not well understood, it is related in some way to the gate control theory of pain modulation.

Heat is applied in musculoskeletal and neuromuscular disorders, such as sprains, strains, articular (joint-related) problems, and muscle spasms, which all describe various types of muscle pain.[23] Heat generally is considered to produce a relaxation effect and a reduction in guarding in skeletal muscle. It also increases the elasticity and decreases the viscosity of connective tissue, which is an important consideration in postacute joint injuries or after long periods of immobilization.

Many therapists empirically believe that heat has little effect on the disease itself but serves rather to facilitate further treatment by producing relaxation in these types of disorders.[23] This is accomplished by relieving pain, lessening hypertonicity of muscles, producing sedation (which decreases spasticity, tenderness, and spasm), and decreasing tightness in muscles and related structures. The physiologic effects of heat are summarized in Table 9-1.

hyperemia Presence of an increased amount of blood in part of the body.

vasodilation Dilation of the blood vessels.

vasoconstriction Narrowing of the blood vessels.

consensual heat vasodilation Vasodilation and increased blood flow will spread to remote areas, causing increased metabolism in the unheated area.

PHYSIOLOGIC EFFECTS OF TISSUE COOLING

The physiologic effects of cold are the opposite of those of heat for the most part; the primary effect being a local decrease in temperature. Cold has its greatest benefit in acute athletic injury.[5,27,33,36,52] There is general agreement that the use of cold is the initial treatment for most conditions in the musculoskeletal system. The primary

TABLE 9-1   **Physiologic Effects of Heat and Cold**

EFFECTS OF HEAT

Increased local temperature superficially
Increased local metabolism
Vasodilation of arterioles and capillaries
Increased blood flow to part heated
Increased leukocytes and phagocytosis
Increased capillary permeability
Increased lymphatic and venous drainage
Increased metabolic wastes
Increased axon reflex activity
Increased elasticity of muscles, ligaments, and capsule fibers
Analgesia
Increased formation of edema
Decreased muscle tone
Decreased muscle spasm

EFFECTS OF COLD

Decreased local temperature, in some cases to a considerable depth
Decreased metabolism
Vasoconstriction of arterioles and capillaries (at first)
Decreased blood flow (at first)
Decreased nerve conduction velocity
Decreased delivery of leukocytes and phagocytes
Decreased lymphatic and venous drainage
Decreased muscle excitability
Decreased muscle spindle depolarization
Decreased formation and accumulation of edema
Extreme anesthetic effects

cryotherapy The use of cold in the treatment of pathology or diseases.

Cold may be better for reducing muscle spasm.

Indications and Contraindications for Cryotherapy

Indications
   During acute or subacute inflammation
   Acute pain
   Chronic pain
   Acute swelling (controlling hemorrhage and edema)
   Myofascial trigger points
   Muscle guarding
   Muscle spasm
   Acute muscle strain
   Acute ligament sprain
   Acute contusion
   Bursitis
   Tenosynovitis
   Tendinitis
   Delayed onset muscle soreness

reason for using cold in acute injury is to lower the temperature in the injured area, thus reducing the metabolic rate with a corresponding decrease in production of metabolites and metabolic heat.[31] This helps the injured tissue survive the hypoxia and limits further tissue injury.[34,36] Cold has been demonstrated to be more effective when applied along with compression than using ice alone for reducing metabolism in injured tissue.[52,53] It is also used immediately after injury to decrease pain and promote local **vasoconstriction**, thus controlling hemorrhage and edema.[51,61] Cold is also used in the acute phase of inflammatory conditions, such as bursitis, tenosynovitis, and tendinitis, in which heat may cause additional pain and swelling.[47]

Cold is also used to reduce pain and the reflex muscle spasm and spastic conditions that accompany it.[52] Its analgesic effect is probably one of its greatest benefits.[18,48,64] One explanation of the analgesic effect is that cold decreases the velocity of nerve conduction, although it does not entirely eliminate it.[15,48,49] It is also possible that cold bombards central pain receptor areas with so many cold impulses that pain impulses are lost through the gate control theory of pain modulation. With ice treatments, the patient usually reports an uncomfortable sensation of cold followed by stinging or burning, then an aching sensation, and finally complete numbness.[37]

Cold also has been demonstrated to be effective in the treatment of **myofascial pain**.[78] This type of pain is referred from active myofascial trigger points with various symptoms, including pain on active movement and decreased range of motion. Trigger points may result from muscle strain or tension, which sensitizes nerves in a localized area. A trigger point may be palpated as a small nodule or as a strip of tense muscle tissue.[79]

It appears that cold is more effective in treating acute muscle pain as opposed to delayed-onset muscle soreness (DOMS), which occurs following exercise.[11] Ultrasound has been shown to be more effective than ice for treating DOMS.[54]

Cold depresses the excitability of free nerve endings and peripheral nerve fibers, and this increases the pain threshold.[42] This is of great value in short-term treatment. Cold applications can also enhance voluntary control in spastic conditions, and in acute traumatic conditions they may decrease painful spasms that result from local muscle irritability.[3]

Reduction in muscle guarding relative to acute trauma has been observed by all active therapists. The literature reviewed indicates various reasons behind reduced muscle guarding, with the common thought of decreased muscle spindle activity.[41]

The initial reaction to cold is local vasoconstriction of all smooth muscle by the central nervous system to conserve heat.[61] Localized vasoconstriction is responsible for the decrease in the tendency toward formation and accumulation of edema, probably as a result of a decrease in local hydrostatic pressure.[72] There is also a decrease in the amount of nutrients and phagocytes delivered to the area, thus reducing phagocytic activity.[72]

It has been hypothesized that when local temperature is lowered considerably for a period of about 30 minutes, intermittent periods of vasodilation occur, lasting 4 to 6 minutes. Then vasoconstriction recurs for a 15- to 30-minute cycle, followed again by vasodilation. This phenomenon is known as the **hunting response** and is necessary to prevent local tissue injury caused by cold.[10,13,46] The hunting response has been accepted for a number of years as fact; in reality, however, these investigations talked about measured temperature changes rather than circulatory changes. Thus, the hunting response is more likely a measurement artifact than an actual change in blood flow in response to cold.[2,37]

If a large area is cooled, the hypothalamus (the temperature-regulating center in the brain) will reflexively induce shivering, which raises the core temperature as a result of increased production of heat. Cooling of a large area might also cause arterial vasoconstriction in other remote parts of the body, resulting in an increased blood pressure.[72] Because of the low thermal conductivity of underlying subcutaneous fat tissue, applications of cold for short periods of time probably are ineffective in cooling deeper tissues. It has been shown also that using cold for too long may be detrimental to the healing process.[27]

The length of treatment time needed to cool tissue effectively depends on differences in subcutaneous tissue thickness. Patients with thick subcutaneous tissue should be treated with cold applications for longer than 5 minutes to produce a significant drop in intramuscular temperature. Grant treated acute and chronic conditions of the musculoskeletal system and found that thin people require shorter icing periods and that response was more successful.[25] McMaster supported these findings.[51] Recommended treatment times range from direct contact of 5 to 45 minutes to obtain adequate cooling.

It is generally believed that cold treatments are more effective in reaching deep tissue than most forms of heat. Cold applied to the skin is capable of significantly lowering the temperature of tissue at a considerable depth. The extent of this lowered tissue temperature is dependent on the type of cold applied to the skin, the duration of its application, the thickness of the subcutaneous fat, and the region of the body on which it is applied.

The application of cold decreases cell permeability, decreases cellular metabolism, and decreases accumulation of edema and should be continued in 5- to 45-minute applications for at least 72 hours after initial trauma.[34] Care should be taken to avoid aggressive cold treatment to prevent disruption of the healing sequence.

If edema continues into the subacute phase, **contrast baths** (hot and cold immersion technique) may be incorporated to facilitate a capillary response for

Contraindications
 Impaired circulation
 Peripheral vascular disease
 Hypersensitivity to cold
 Skin anesthesia
 Open wounds or skin conditions (cold whirlpools and contrast baths)
 Infection

hydrocollator A synthetic hot (170°F) or cold (0°F) gel used as an adjunctive modality to stimulate a rise or fall in tissue temperature.

hunting response A reflex increase in temperature that occurs in response to cold approximately 15 minutes into the treatment.

edema reduction. This consists of alternating hot and cold immersions and is discussed in greater detail in the clinical section.

The physiologic effects of cold are summarized in Table 9-1.

EFFECTS OF TISSUE TEMPERATURE CHANGE ON CIRCULATION

Local application of heat or cold is indicated for **thermal** physiologic effects. The main physiologic effect is on superficial circulation because of the response of the temperature receptors in the skin and the sympathetic nervous system.

Circulation through the skin serves two major functions: nutrition of the skin tissues and conduction of heat from internal structures of the body to the skin so that heat can be removed from the body.[28] The circulatory apparatus is composed of *two major vessel types*: arteries, capillaries, and veins; and vascular structures for heating the skin. Two types of vascular structures are the subcutaneous venous plexus, which holds large quantities of blood that heat the surface of the skin, and the arteriovenous anastomosis, which provides vascular communication between arteries and venous plexuses.[17] The walls of the plexuses have strong muscular coats innervated by sympathetic vasoconstrictor nerve fibers that secrete norepinephrine. When constricted, blood flow is reduced to almost nothing in the venous plexus. When maximally dilated, there is an extremely rapid flow of blood into the plexuses. The arteriovenous anastomoses are found principally in the volar or palmar surfaces of the hands and feet, lips, nose, and ears.

When cold is applied directly to the skin, the skin vessels progressively constrict to a temperature of about 15°C (59°F), at which point they reach their maximum constrictions. This constriction results primarily from increased sensitivity of the vessels to nerve stimulation, but it probably also results at least partly from a reflex that passes to the spinal cord and then back to the vessels. At temperatures below 15°C (59°F), the vessels begin to dilate. This dilation is caused by a direct local effect of the cold on the vessels themselves, producing paralysis of the contractile mechanism of the vessel wall or blockage of the nerve impulses coming to the vessels. At temperatures approaching 0°C (32°F), the skin vessels frequently reach maximum vasodilation.

Skin plexuses are supplied with sympathetic vasoconstrictor innervation. In times of circulatory stress, such as exercise, hemorrhage, or anxiety, sympathetic stimulation of these skin plexuses forces large quantities of blood into internal vessels. Thus, the subcutaneous veins of the skin act as an important blood reservoir, often providing blood to serve other circulatory functions when needed.[28]

Three types of sensory receptors are found in the subepithelial tissue: cold, warm, and pain. The pain receptors are free nerve endings. Temperature and pain are transmitted to the brain via the lateral spinothalamic tract (see Chapter 3). The nerve fibers respond differently at different temperatures. Both cold and warm receptors discharge minimally at 33°C (91.4°F). Cold receptors discharge between 10 and 41°C (50–105.8°F), with a maximum discharge in the 37.5 to 40°C (99.5–104°F) range. Above 45°C (113°F), cold receptors begin to discharge again, and pain receptors are stimulated. Nerve fibers transmitting sensations of pain respond to the temperature extremes. Both warm and cold receptors adapt rapidly to temperature change; the more rapid the temperature change, the more rapid the receptor adaptation. The number of warm and cold receptors in any given small surface area is thought to be few. Therefore, small temperature changes are difficult to perceive in localized areas. Larger surface areas stimulate summation of thermal signals. These larger patterns of excitation activate the vasomotor centers and the

thermotherapy The use of heat in the treatment of pathology or disease.

contrast bath Hot (106°F) and cold (50°F) treatments in a combined sequence to stimulate superficial capillary vasodilation or vasoconstriction.

hypothalamic center.[45,47] Stimulation of the anterior hypothalamus causes cutaneous vasodilation, whereas stimulation of the posterior hypothalamus causes cutaneous vasoconstriction.[28,66]

The cutaneous blood flow depends on the discharge of the sympathetic nervous system. These sympathetic impulses are transmitted simultaneously to the blood vessels for cutaneous vasoconstriction and to the adrenal medulla. Both norepinephrine and epinephrine are secreted into the blood vessels and induce vessel constriction.[28] Most of the sympathetic constriction influences are mediated chemically through these neural transmitters. General exposure to cold elicits cutaneous vasoconstriction, shivering, piloerection, and an increase in epinephrine secretion; therefore, vascular contraction occurs. Simultaneously, metabolism and heat production are increased to maintain the body temperature.[28]

Increased blood flow supplies additional oxygen to the area, explaining the analgesic and relaxation effects on muscle spasm. An increased proprioceptive reflex mechanism may explain these effects. Receptor end organs located in the muscle spindle are inhibited by heat temporarily, whereas sudden cooling tends to excite the receptor end organ.[45,47]

> **Treatment Tip**
> As long as the patient is not complaining of tenderness to touch it is probably safe to switch from cold to some form of heat. When treating deeper tissues it is recommended that either ultrasound or shortwave diathermy be used since the depth of penetration of both is greater than any infrared modality.

EFFECTS OF TISSUE TEMPERATURE CHANGE ON MUSCLE SPASM

Numerous studies deal with the effects of heat and cold in the treatment of many musculoskeletal conditions. Although it is true that the use of heat as a therapeutic modality has long been accepted and documented in the literature, it is apparent that most recent research has been directed toward the use of cold. There seems to be general agreement that the physiologic mechanisms underlying the effectiveness of heat and cold treatments in reducing muscle spasm lie at the level of the muscle spindle, Golgi tendon organs, and the gamma system.[64]

> Cold may be better for reducing muscle spasm.

Heat is believed to have a relaxing effect on skeletal muscle tone.[23] Local application of heat relaxes muscles throughout the skeletal system by simultaneously lessening the stimulus threshold of muscle spindles and decreasing the gamma efferent firing rate. This suggests that the muscle spindles are easily excited. Consequently, the muscles may be electromyographically silent while at rest during the application of heat, but the slightest amount of voluntary or passive movement may cause the efferents to fire, thus increasing muscular resistance to stretch. If this is indeed the case, then it seems logical that decreasing the afferent impulses by raising the threshold of the muscle spindles might be effective in facilitating muscle relaxation, as long as there is no movement.

The rate of firing of both primary and secondary endings is directly proportional to temperature. Local applications of cold decrease local neural activity. Annulospiral, flower-spray (small fibers located in the muscle spindle that detect changes in muscle position), and Golgi tendon organ endings all fire more slowly when cooled. Cooling actually decreases the rate of afferent activity even more, with an increase in the amount of tension on the muscle. Thus, cold appears to raise the threshold stimulus of muscle spindles, and heat tends to lower it.[21] Although firing of the primary spindle afferents increases abruptly with the application of cold, a subsequent decrease in spindle afferent activity occurs and persists as the temperature is lowered.[48]

Simultaneous use of heat and cold in the treatment of muscle spasm has also been studied.[17] Local cooling with ice, although maintaining body temperature to prevent shivering, results in a significant reduction of muscle spasm, greater than that which occurs with the use of heat or cold independently. This effect was attributed to maintenance of body temperature, which decreases efferent activity, whereas local cooling decreases afferent activity. If the core temperature of the body is not maintained, the reflex shivering results in increased muscle tone, thus inhibiting relaxation.

There is a substantial reduction in the frequency of action potential (stimulus intensity necessary for firing muscle fibers) firing of the motor unit when the muscle temperature is reduced. Muscle spindle activity is most significantly reduced when the muscle is cooled, whereas normal body temperature is maintained.

Miglietta[55] presented a slightly different perspective on the effect of cold in reducing muscle spasm. He performed an electromyographic analysis of the effects of cold on the reduction of clonus (increased muscle tone) or spasticity in a group of 15 patients. After immersion of the spastic extremity in a cold whirlpool for 15 minutes, it was observed that electromyographic activity dropped significantly and in some cases disappeared altogether. The cold was thought to induce an afferent bombardment of cold impulses, which modify the cortical excitatory state and block the stream of painful impulses from the muscle. Thus, relaxation of skeletal muscle is assumed to occur with the disappearance of pain.[77] It is not certain whether it is the excitability of the motor neurons or the hyperactivity of the gamma system, which is changed either at the muscle spindle level or at the spinal cord level, that is responsible for the reduction of spasticity. However, it is certain that cold is effective in reducing spasticity by reducing or modifying the highly sensitive stretch-reflex mechanism in muscle.

Another factor that may be important to the reduction of spasticity is reduction in the nerve conduction velocity as a result of the application of cold.[15] These changes may result from a slowing of motor and sensory nerve conduction velocity and a decrease of the afferent discharges from cutaneous receptors.

Several studies investigated the use of cold followed by some type of exercise in the treatment of various injuries to the musculotendinous unit.[25,40] Each of these studies indicated that the use of cold and exercise were extremely effective in the treatment of acute pathologies of the musculoskeletal system that produced restrictions of muscle action. However, if stretching was indicated, it has been stressed that stretching is more important for increasing flexibility than using either heat or cold.[20,73]

paraffin bath A combined paraffin and mineral oil immersion commonly used on the hands and feet for distal temperature gains in blood flow and temperature.

EFFECTS OF TEMPERATURE CHANGE ON PERFORMANCE

Several studies have examined the effects of altering tissue temperature on physical performance capabilities.

Changes in the ability to produce torque during isokinetic testing following the application of heat and cold have been demonstrated, although there appears to be some disagreement relative to the degree of change in concentric and eccentric torque capabilities. One study observed that the strength of an eccentric contraction was improved with the application of ice, whereas another indicated the ice helped to facilitate concentric but not eccentric strength.[14,67] It also appears that higher torque values can be produced following the application of cold packs than hot packs.[12] The use of cryotherapy does not seem to effect peak torque but may increase endurance.[76] Cold appears to have some effect on muscular power; also, it has been shown that performance in vertical jumping is decreased following the application of cold.[24,26]

It seems that heating or cooling of an extremity has minimal or no effects on proprioception, joint position sense, and balance.[8,44,62,65,68,74,75,81] Thus, it follows that tissue temperature changes have no effect on agility or the ability to change direction.[22,38,69]

CLINICAL USE OF THE INFRARED MODALITIES

The physiologic effects of heat and cold discussed previously are rarely the result of direct absorption of infrared energy. There is general agreement that no form of infrared energy can have a depth of penetration greater than 1 cm.[1] Thus, the effects of the infrared modalities are primarily superficial and directly affect the cutaneous blood vessels and the cutaneous nerve receptors.[50]

Absorption of infrared energy cutaneously increases and decreases circulation subcutaneously in both the muscle and fat layers. If the energy is absorbed cutaneously over a long enough period of time to raise the temperature of the circulating blood, the hypothalamus will reflexively increase blood flow to the underlying tissue. Likewise, absorption of cold cutaneously can decrease blood flow via a similar mechanism in the area of treatment.[1]

Thus, if the primary treatment goal is a tissue temperature increase with a corresponding increase in blood flow to the deeper tissues, it is wiser perhaps to choose a modality, such as diathermy or ultrasound, that produces energy that can penetrate the cutaneous tissues and be directly absorbed by the deep tissues. If the primary treatment goal is to reduce tissue temperature and decrease blood flow to an injured area, the superficial application of ice or cold is the only modality capable of producing such a response.

Perhaps the most effective use of the infrared modalities should be to provide analgesia or reduce the sensation of pain associated with injury. The infrared modalities stimulate primarily the cutaneous nerve receptors. Through one of the mechanisms of pain modulation discussed in Chapter 3 (most likely the gate control theory), hyperstimulation of these nerve receptors by heating or cooling reduces pain. Within the philosophy of an aggressive program of rehabilitation, the reduction of pain as a means of facilitating therapeutic exercise is a common practice. As emphasized in the preface to this text, therapeutic modalities are perhaps best used as an adjunct to therapeutic exercise. Certainly, this should be a prime consideration when selecting an infrared modality for use in any treatment program.

Continued investigation and research into the use of heat and cold is warranted to provide useful data for the therapist. Heat and cold applications, when used properly and efficiently, will provide the therapist with the tools to enhance recovery and provide the patient with optimal health care management. Thermotherapy and cryotherapy are only two of the tools available to assist in the well-being and reconditioning of the injured patient.

infrared That portion of the electromagnetic spectrum associated with thermal changes; located adjacent to the red portion of the visible light spectrum.

CRYOTHERAPY TECHNIQUES

Cryotherapy is the use of cold in the treatment of acute trauma and subacute injury and for the decrease of discomfort after reconditioning and rehabilitation.[35] Tools of cryotherapy include ice packs, cold whirlpool, ice whirlpool, ice massage, commercial chemical cold spray, and contrast baths. Application of cryotherapy produces a three- to four-stage sensation. First, there is an uncomfortable sensation of cold followed by a stinging, then a burning or aching feeling, and finally numbness. Each stage is related to the nerve endings as they temporarily cease to function as a result of decreased blood flow. The time required for this sequence varies, but several authors indicate that it occurs within 5 to 15 minutes.[2,4,6,25,29,37,57–59,61] After 12 to

15 minutes the hunting response is sometimes demonstrated with intense cold (10°C [50°F]).[10,39,57,61] Thus, a minimum of 15 minutes are necessary to achieve extreme analgesic effects.

Application of ice is safe, simple, and inexpensive. Cryotherapy is contraindicated in patients with cold allergies (hives, joint pain, nausea), Raynaud's phenomenon (arterial spasm), and some rheumatoid conditions.[2,19,25,28,32]

Depth of penetration depends on the amount of cold and the length of the treatment time because the body is well equipped to maintain skin and subcutaneous tissue viability through the capillary bed by reflex vasodilation of up to four times normal blood flow. The body has the ability to decrease blood flow to the body segment that is supposedly losing too much body heat by shunting the blood flow. Depth of penetration is also related to intensity and duration of cold application and the circulatory response to the body segment exposed. If the person has normal circulatory responses, frostbite should not be a concern. Even so, caution should be exercised when applying intense cold directly to the skin. If deeper penetration is desired, ice therapy is most effective using ice towels, ice packs, ice massage, and ice whirlpools. The patient should be advised of the four stages of cryotherapy and the discomfort he or she will experience. The therapist should explain this sequence and advise the patient of the expected outcome, which may include a rapid decrease in pain.[2,15,25,30]

Ice Massage

Ice massage can be applied by the therapist or the patient if the patient can reach the area of application to administer self-treatment. It is best for the first three treatments to be administered by the therapist to give the patient the full benefit of the treatment. When positioning the patient's body segment to be treated, it should be relaxed, and the patient should be made comfortable. Appropriate seating and positioning should be taken into consideration with the application of ice. Administration must be thorough to get maximal treatment. Ice massage is perhaps best indicated in conditions in which some type of stretching activity is to be used.

Equipment Needed (Figs. 9-1 and 9-2)

1. Styrofoam cups: A regular 6- to 8-ounce styrofoam cup should be filled with water and placed in the freezer. After it is frozen, all the styrofoam on the sides should be removed down to 1 inch from the bottom. A frozen cup of ice with a tongue depressor inserted is preferred because it has a handle with which to hold the block of ice.

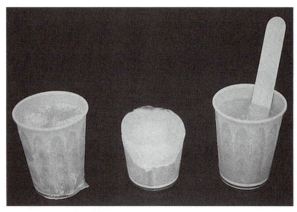

•**Figure 9-1** Water may be frozen in a paper cup, styrofoam cup, or on a Popsicle™ stick for the purpose of ice massage.

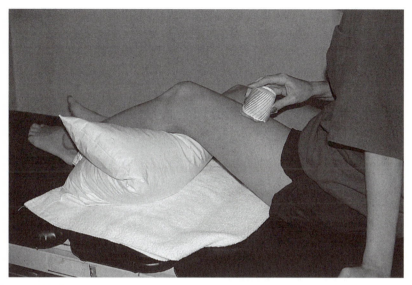

•Figure 9-2 Ice massage may be applied using either circular or longitudinal strokes.

2. Popsicle ice cups: Cups are filled with water, and a wooden Popsicle stick (tongue blade) is placed in each cup. The cups are then placed in the freezer. After it is frozen the paper cup is torn off. A block of ice on a stick is now ready to be used for massage.

3. Paper cups: Utilize same technique as the styrofoam cups, except toweling may be needed to insulate the therapist's hand holding the paper cup.

4. Towels: These are used for positioning and absorbing the melting water in the area of the ice massage application.

Treatment

Preferred positions are side lying, prone, supine, hook lying, or sitting, depending on the area to be treated. Self-treatment should be used when patients can comfortably reach the area to be treated by themselves. Apply ice massage in a circular pattern, with each succeeding stroke covering half the previous stroke, or in a longitudinal motion, with each stroke overlapping half the previous stroke. Ice should be applied for 15 to 20 minutes; consistent patterning of circular and longitudinal strokes includes the sequence described in the clinical uses section.

Physiologic Responses

Cold progression proceeds through the four stages: cold, stinging, burning, and numbness. Reddening of the skin (**erythema**) occurs as a result of blanching or lack of blood in the capillary bed. A common example occurs when one works outside in the cold without gloves or appropriate footwear and returns inside to find the toes beet red. This is an example of the body attempting to pool blood in the area to prevent further temperature loss. Ice applications of 5 to 15 minutes at greater than 10°C (50°F) will not stimulate the hunting response and do not stimulate the reflex vasodilation that creates the body's own physically induced heat or increased blood flow.

erythema Redness of the skin.

Considerations

The time necessary for the surface area to be numbed will depend on the body area to be massaged. Approximate time will depend on how fast the ice melts and what thermopane develops between the skin and ice massage. Patient comfort should be considered at all times. If adequate circulation is present, frostbite should not be a

CASE STUDY 9-1
CRYOTHERAPY

Background: A 35-year-old man sustained a Colles fracture of the right wrist during a fall 13 weeks ago. He was treated with a closed reduction and plaster for 12 weeks; the cast was removed 1 week ago. The fracture is well healed with good position. In addition to active and passive exercise, you begin joint mobilization on an every-other-day schedule. In spite of the fact that the tissues are strong enough to tolerate grade II and III mobilization, the patient experiences so much pain that you are limited to grade I mobilization. To increase the patient's tolerance for mobilization, you decide to perform an ice massage prior to mobilization.

Impression: Limitation of motion secondary to fracture and immobilization.

Treatment Plan: A cup of ice was applied to the anterior and posterior aspects of the wrist until the patient experienced numbness. The duration of the treatment was approximately 9 minutes. Immediately following the ice massage, joint mobilization techniques were used to increase the range of motion of the wrist.

Response: The patient's tolerance for more aggressive mobilization was increased for approximately 5 minutes following the ice massage. As the accessory motions were restored, the active range of motion also improved. After six sessions, joint mobilization was dis-

continued, and the patient continued with active and passive range of motion exercise, and strengthening exercise was added to the program. Ten weeks after removal of the cast, the patient's range of motion in all planes was approximately 90 percent of normal, and the patient was discharged to a home program.

Discussion Questions

- What tissues were injured or affected?
- What symptoms were present?
- What phase of the injury-healing continuum did the patient present for care in?
- What are the therapeutic agent modality's biophysical effects (direct, indirect, depth, and tissue affinity)?
- What are the therapeutic agent modality's indications and contraindications?
- What are the parameters of the therapeutic agent modality's application, dosage, duration, and frequency in this case study?
- What other therapeutic agent modalities could be used to treat this injury or condition? Why? How?

The rehabilitation professional employs therapeutic agent modality to create an optimum environment for tissue healing while minimizing the symptoms associated with the trauma or condition.

---

concern. However, if the patient has diabetes, the extremities, especially the toes, may require reduced temperature and adjustment of the intensity and duration of the cold.

Application

After the type of cold applicator for ice massage is selected, the patient should be positioned comfortably, and clothing should be removed from the area to be treated. The area should be set up before positioning the patient. Remove the top two-thirds of paper from the ice-filled paper or styrofoam cup, leaving 1 inch on the bottom of the cup as a handle for the therapist or patient to use as a handgrip. The therapist should smooth the rough edges of the ice cup by gently rubbing along the edges. Ice should be applied to the patient's exposed skin in circular or longitudinal strokes, with each stroke overlapping the previous stroke. The application should be continued until the patient goes through the cold progression sequence of cold, stinging, burning or aching, and numbness. Once the skin is numb to fine touch, ice application can be terminated. The cold progression is the response of the sensory nerve fibers in the skin. The difference between cold and burning is primarily between the dropping out (sensory deficit) of the cold and warm nerve endings. Standard treatments allow the patient to place cold applications every other 20 minutes, thus facilitating the hunting response. Some thermobarrier is developed during the ice massage in the layer of water directly on the skin, but this allows the ice cup to move smoothly over the skin. The time from application to numbing of the body segment depends on the size of the segment, but progression to numbing should be around 7 to 10 minutes.

COMMERCIAL (COLD) HYDROCOLLATOR PACKS

Cold **hydrocollator** packs (Fig. 9-3) are indicated in any acute injury to a musculoskeletal structure.

Equipment Needed

1. Hydrocollator cold pack: This must be cooled to 8°F (15°C). It needs plastic liners or protective toweling for placement on a body segment. Petroleum distillate gel is the substance contained in the plastic pouch design.
2. Moist cold towels: Towels may be immersed in ice water and molded to the skin surface, or they can be packed in ice and allowed to remain in place. The commercial cold pack should be placed on top of a moist towel.
3. Plastic bag: The hydrocollator should be placed in the bag. Air should be removed from the bag. The plastic bag may then be molded around the body segment.
4. Dry towel: To prevent the cold hydrocollator from losing heat rapidly, the towel is used as a covering to insulate the cold pack.

Treatment

Preferred positions are side lying, prone, supine, hook lying, or sitting, depending on the area to be treated. The patient must remain still during the treatment to maintain appropriate positioning of the cold pack. The cold pack must be molded onto the skin. The pack should be covered with a towel to limit loss of cold. A timer should be set, or time should otherwise be noted. Treatment time should be 20 minutes.

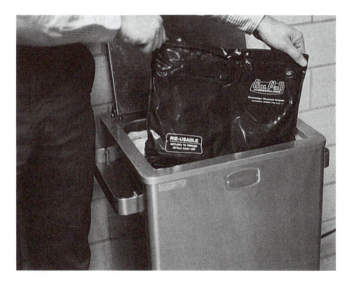

•**Figure 9-3** Commercial cold pack.

Physiologic Responses

Erythema occurs. Cold progression proceeds through the four stages.

Considerations

Body area should be covered to prevent unnecessary exposure.
The physiologic response to cold treatment is immediate.
Patient comfort should be considered at all times.
Frostbite should not be a concern unless circulation is inadequate.

Application

The patient should be positioned with the treatment area exposed and a towel draped to protect clothing. The commercial cold pack should be placed against wet toweling to enhance transfer of cold to the body segment. If the injury is acute or subacute, the body segment should be elevated to reduce gravity-dependent swelling.[80] Pack the cold pack around the joint in a manner designed to remove all air and ensure placement directly against wet toweling. Cold progression will be the same as with ice massage but not as quick because of the toweling between the skin and cold pack. General treatment time required for numbing is about 20 minutes. The importance of a comfortable, properly positioned patient is evident. Checking the sensory area after application is important. Again, frostbite should not be a concern if circulation is intact. If swelling is a concern, a wet compression (elastic) wrap could be applied under the cold pack. A sequence of 20 minutes on and 20 minutes off should be repeated for 2 hours; the same sequence can be used in home treatment. Elevation is a key adjunct therapy during the sleeping hours.

ICE PACKS

Like cold hydrocollator packs, ice packs are indicated in acute stages of injury, as well as for prevention of additional swelling after exercise of the injured part (Fig. 9-4).

Equipment Needed

1. Small plastic bags: Vegetable or bread bags may be used.
2. Ice flaker machine: Flaked or crushed ice is easier to mold than cubed ice.

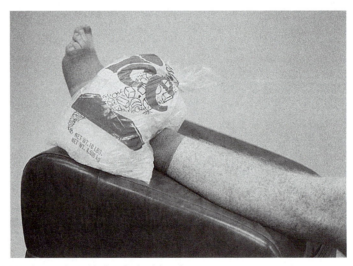

•**Figure 9-4** Ice pack molded to fit the injured part.

3. Moist towels: These are used to facilitate cold transmission and should be placed directly on the skin.

4. Elastic bandaging: Bandaging holds the plastic ice pack in place and applies compression. The body segment to be treated may be elevated.

5. Salt solution: This is used to increase melting temperature. Melting ice has more thermal energy than stable ice and therefore is colder.

Treatment

The patient's position depends on the part to be treated. The patient must remain still during the treatment. A pack must be placed on the skin. The pack should be secured in place with toweling or an elastic bandage. The pack should be covered with a towel to limit cold loss. A timer should be set, or time should otherwise be noted. The treatment time should be 20 minutes.

Physiologic Responses

Cold progression proceeds through the four stages.
Erythema occurs.

Considerations

The body area to be treated should be covered to prevent unnecessary exposure.
The physiologic response to cold is immediate.
Patient comfort should be considered at all times.
Frostbite should not be a concern unless circulation is inadequate.

Application

The application of ice packs is similar to the use of commercial cold hydrocollator packs; the equipment to be set up in the treatment area consists of flaked or cubed ice in a plastic bag large enough for the area to be treated. The plastic bag can be applied directly to the skin and held in place by a moist or dry elastic wrap. Patient comfort is of the utmost importance during this application to facilitate patient relaxation. The therapist may want to add salt to the ice to facilitate melting of the ice to create a colder slush mixture. Melting ice gives off more energy because of its less stable state, and therefore it is colder. A towel should be placed over the ice pack to decrease the warming effect of the environmental air, thus facilitating the cold application. The normal physiologic response progression is cold, stinging, burning, and finally numbness, at which time the setup can be terminated. Because of the pliability of the flaked ice pack, it can be molded to the body segment treated. If cubed ice is used instead of flaked ice, it can still be molded, but it will not readily hold its position and will need to be secured via elastic wrap or toweling.

Treatment Tip
When using ice compression and elevation to control swelling, the ice can be left in place for up to 1 hour as long as the patient does not have any sensitivity reaction to the cold. Because the elastic wrap has been placed underneath the ice bags there is an insulating layer through which the cold must penetrate. The passage of cold can be facilitated if the elastic wrap is wet.

COLD WHIRLPOOL

The cold whirlpool is indicated in acute and subacute conditions in which exercise of the injured part during a cold treatment is desired (Fig. 9-5).

Equipment Needed

1. Whirlpool: The appropriate size whirlpool must be filled with cold water or ice to lower the temperature to 50 to 60°F. The therapist should use flaked ice and make sure the ice melts completely, since pieces of ice could become projectiles if a body segment is in the pool.

2. Ice machine: Flaked ice acts faster than cubed to lower the water temperature.

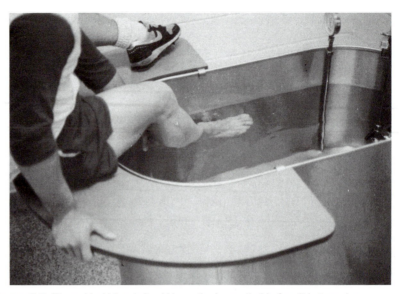

•**Figure 9-5** The cold whirlpool should have the ice melted before it is turned on.

3. Toweling: Sufficient toweling is needed for padding the body segment on the whirlpool and for drying off after treatment.
4. Appropriate setup in area: A chair, whirlpool, and a bench in the whirlpool must be arranged before treatment.

Treatment

The temperature should be set at 50 to 60°F. The body segment to be treated must be immersed. For total body immersion, the water temperature should be set at 65 to 80°F. The treatment time should be 5 to 15 minutes.

Physiologic Responses

Cold progression proceeds through the four stages.
Erythema occurs.

Considerations

Caution: Even though the immediate application of cold will help to control edema if applied immediately following injury, the gravity-dependent positions should be avoided with acute and subacute injuries.[13,16] Cold wet compression or elastic wrap should be put in place before treatment. The body area to be treated should be completely immersed. A cold whirlpool allows exercises to be done during treatment. Patient comfort should be considered at all times. Frostbite should not be a concern unless circulation is inadequate. A toe cap made of neoprene can be used to make the patient more comfortable in the cold whirlpool.[56]

Application

The unit should be turned on after it has been established that the ground fault interrupter (GFI) is functioning. The patient should be positioned in the whirlpool area, and appropriate padding should be provided for the patient's comfort. The timer should be set for the amount of time desired, depending on the size of the body part to be treated. Treatment should continue until the body segment becomes numb (approx 15 min). Numbness is the cutaneous (skin or superficial) response. Frostbite should not be a concern unless the individual has a history of circulatory deficiencies or has diabetes. Treatment time will be between 7 and 15 minutes to allow the complete circulatory response. Caution is indicated in the gravity-dependent position because of the likelihood of additional swelling if the body segment is already swollen.[13] This is the most intense application of cold of the cryotherapy techniques listed. Therefore, the first two or three treatments should be administered with the therapist remaining in the area. One of several reasons for the intensity of cold is that the body cannot develop a **thermopane** (insulating layer of water) on the skin because of the convection effect of the whirlpool. Additional benefits include the massaging and vibrating effect of the water flow. Removal of the part being treated from the whirlpool will necessitate a review of the skin surface and an assessment of edema in the extremities. If total body immersion is used, care should be taken for the intensity and duration of the whirlpool and for protection of the genitals from direct water flow. Applications can be repeated following rewarming of the body segment after sensation has returned. If the cold application is administered before practice, it should be done before the application of preventive strapping. Enough time should also be allowed for sensation to return before taping. Studies have indicated that the reflex vasodilation lasts up to 2 hours. A patient could practice, then return to the training room and receive additional treatment without additional edema created by **congestion** as a result of vascular and capillary insufficiency occurring during the healing process. Increased heart rate and blood pressure are associated with cold application. Conditioned patients should not have a problem with dizziness after cold applications, but care should be taken when transferring the patient from the whirlpool area. Whirlpool cultures of the tank and jet should be taken monthly to keep bacterial growth under control.

thermopane An insulating layer of water next to the skin.

congestion Presence of an abnormal amount of blood in the vessels resulting from an increase in blood flow or obstructed venous return.

Cold Spray

Cold sprays, such as Fluori-Methane or ethyl chloride, do not provide adequate deep penetration, but they do provide adjunctive therapy for acupressure techniques to reduce muscle spasm. Physiologically this is accomplished by stimulating the A fibers involved in the gate control theory. The primary action of a cold spray is reduction of the pain spasm sequence secondary to direct trauma. However, it will not reduce hemorrhage because it works on the superficial nerve endings to reduce the spasm via the stimulation of A fibers to reduce the so-called painful arc. Cold spray is an extremely effective technique in the treatment of myofascial trigger points. Precautions concerning the use of cold spray include protecting the patient's face from the fumes and spraying the skin at an acute rather than a perpendicular angle.[78] Cold spray is indicated when stretching of an injured part is desired along with cold treatment.

Equipment Needed

1. Fluori-Methane.
2. Toweling.
3. Padding.

Treatment

The area to be treated should be sprayed and then stretched.
Spasm should be reduced.
Treatment should be distal to proximal.
A quick jetstream spray or stroking motion should be used.
Cooling should be superficial; no frosting should occur.
Cold sprays may be used in conjunction with acupressure.
Treatment time should be set according to body segment.

Physiologic Responses

Muscle spasm is reduced.

Golgi tendon organ response is facilitated.

Muscle spindle response is inhibited.

Ligament and other musculoskeletal structures may be stimulated.

Considerations

Both the acute and the subacute response should be positive.

The room should be well ventilated to avoid the accumulation of fumes.

Patient comfort should be considered at all times.

Application

The application of Fluori-Methane is typical of the application of other cold sprays (Fig. 9-6). The following application procedures apply specifically to Fluori-Methane, but they provide an outline of the procedures, indications, and precautions applicable to all cold sprays. The therapist should follow the manufacturer's instructions in the use of any cold spray.

Fluori-Methane is a topical vapocoolant that produces a "touch cold sensation," acting as a counterirritant to block pain impulses of muscles in spasm. When used in conjunction with the spray-and-stretch technique, Fluori-Methane can break the pain cycle, allowing the muscle to be stretched to its normal length (pain-free state). The application of spray-and-stretch technique is a therapeutic modality that involves three stages: evaluation, spraying, and stretching. The therapeutic value of spray-and-stretch becomes most effective when the practitioner has mastered all stages and applies them in the proper sequence.

Evaluation

During the evaluation phase the cause of pain is determined as local spasm of an irritated trigger point. The method of applying spray-and-stretch to a muscle spasm

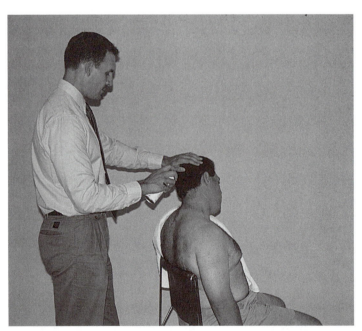

•**Figure 9-6** Spray-and-stretch technique using Fluori-Methane. (Modified with permission of the Gebauer Chemical Company, Cleveland, Ohio, 44104, (800) 321-9348; Ohio (216) 271-5252.)

differs slightly from application to a trigger point. The trigger point is a deep hypersensitive localized spot in a muscle that causes a referred pain pattern. With trigger points the source of pain is seldom the site of the pain. A trigger point may be detected by a snapping palpation over the muscle, causing the muscle in which the irritated trigger point is situated to "jump." In the case of muscle spasm, the source and site of pain are identical.

Spraying

The following steps should be followed to apply Fluori-Methane.

1. The patient should assume a comfortable position.

2. Take precautions to cover the patient's eyes, nose, and mouth if spraying near the face.

3. Hold bottle in an upside-down position 12 to 18 inches away from the treatment surface, allowing the jetstream of vapocoolant to meet the skin at an acute angle to lessen the shock of impact.

4. Apply the spray in one direction only—not back and forth—at a rate of 4 inches (10 cm) per second. Three or four sweeps of the spray in one direction only are sufficient to extinguish the trigger point or to overcome painful muscle spasms. The skin must not be frosted because the intense cold (15°C) of the Fluori-Methane can freeze the skin, cause a first-degree burn similar to frostbite, and result in superficial tissue necrosis. In the case of trigger point, spray should be applied from the trigger point to the area of referred pain. If there is no trigger point, the spray should be applied from the affected muscle to its insertion. The spray should be applied in an even sweep. About two to four parallel, but not overlapping, sweeps of spray should be enough to cover this skin representation of the affected muscle.

Stretching

The stretch should begin as you start spraying from the origin to the insertion (simple muscle spasm pain) or from the trigger point to the referred pain when the trigger point is present. Spray-and-stretch until the muscle reaches its maximal or normal resting length. You will usually feel a gradual increase in range of motion. The spraying and stretching may require two to four spray applications to achieve the therapeutic results in any treatment session. A patient may have multiple treatment sessions in any 1 day.

The spray-and-stretch technique outlined in the preceding must be considered a therapeutic system. The practitioner should spend some time each day practicing until the technique is mastered.

Composition

Fluori-Methane is a combination of two chlorofluorocarbons—15% dichlorodifluoromethane and 85% trichloromonofluoromethane. The combination is not flammable and at room temperature is only volatile enough to expel the contents from the inverted container. Fluori-Methane is supplied in amber Dispenseal bottles that emit a jetstream from a calibrated nozzle.

Indications

Fluori-Methane is a vapocoolant intended for topical application in the management of myofascial pain, restricted motion, and muscle spasm. Clinical conditions that may respond to spray-and-stretch include low back pain (caused by muscle spasm), acute stiff neck, torticollis, acute bursitis of shoulder, muscle spasm associated with osteoarthritis, ankle sprain, tight hamstring, masseter muscle spasm, certain types of headache, and referred pain from trigger points.

Precautions

Federal law prohibits dispensing without a prescription. Although Fluori-Methane is safe for topical application to the skin, care should be taken to minimize inhalation of vapors, especially when it is being applied to the head or neck. Fluori-Methane is not intended for production of local **anesthesia** and should not be applied to the point of frost formation. Freezing can occasionally alter pigmentation.

CONTRAST BATH

Contrast baths are used to treat subacute swelling, gravity-dependent swelling, and vasodilation-vasoconstriction response.

Equipment Needed (Fig. 9-7)

1. Two containers. One container is used to hold cold water (50–60°F), and the other is used to hold warm water (104–106°F). Whirlpools may be used for one or both containers.
2. Ice machine
3. Towels
4. Chair

Treatment

Hot and cold immersions are alternated. Treatment time should be at least 20 minutes. Treatments should consist of five 1-minute cold immersions and five 3-minute

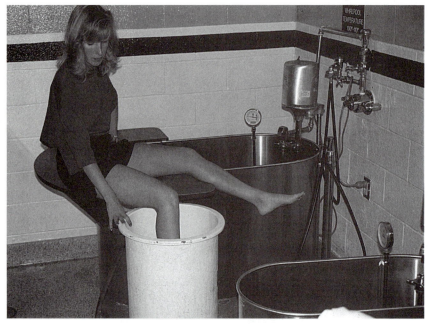

•**Figure 9-7** Contrast bath using a warm whirlpool and ice immersion cylinder.

warm immersions, although the exact ratio of cold to hot treatment is highly variable.

Physiologic Responses

Vasoconstriction and vasodilation occur.
There is a reduction of necrotic cells at the cellular level.
Edema is decreased.

Considerations

The temperatures of the baths must be maintained.
A large area is required for treatment.
Patient comfort must be considered at all times.

Application

After the area is set up, a whirlpool can be used for either hot or cold application, with the opposite method of treatment contained in a bucket or sterile container. The temperatures of these immersion baths must be maintained (cold at 50–60°F, hot at 98–110°F) by adding ice or warm water. It is generally easier to use a large whirlpool for the warm water application and a bucket for the cold water application. There has been considerable controversy regarding the use of contrast baths to control swelling. Contrast baths are most often indicated when changing the treatment modality from cold to hot to facilitate a mild tissue temperature increase. The use of a contrast bath allows for a transitional period during which a slight rise in tissue temperature may be effective for increasing blood flow to an injured area without causing the accumulation of additional edema. The theory that contrast baths induce a type of pumping action by alternating vasoconstriction with vasodilation has little or no credibility. Contrast baths probably cause only a superficial capillary response, resulting from inability of the larger deep blood vessels to constrict and dilate in response to superficial heating.[60,71]

Thus, it is recommended that during the initial stages of contrast bath treatment the ratio of hot to cold treatment begins with a relatively brief period in the hot bath, gradually increasing the length of time in the hot bath during subsequent treatments. Recommendations as to specific lengths of time are extremely variable. However, it would appear that a 3 to 1 ratio (3 min in hot, 1 min in cold) or 4 to 1 ratio for 19 to 20 minutes is fairly well accepted. Whether the treatment is ended with cold or hot depends to some extent on the degree of tissue temperature increase desired. Other therapists prefer to use the same ratios of 3 to 1 or 4 to 1, beginning with cold. The technique may certainly be modified to meet specific needs. Since the extremity is in the gravity-dependent position, once the injured part is removed from the contrast bath, skin sensation and the amount of edema accumulation should be assessed to make sure that the treatment has not actually increased the amount of edema.

ICE IMMERSION

Ice buckets allow ease of application for the therapist. Again, a wet area should be selected (where spilled water is not a concern), with the patient positioned for comfort. The immersion, like the contrast bath, should be maintained until desired results are reached. If cryokinetics are part of the treatment, then the container should be large enough to allow for the movement of the body segment. Ice immersion is similar to cold whirlpool in that the body segment may be subject to gravity-dependent positions.

Treatment Tip
Contrast baths produce little or no "pumping action" and are not very effective in treating swelling. A better alternative is to use cryokinetics, which involves cold followed by active muscle contractions and relaxation to help eliminate swelling.

vasoconstriction Narrowing of the blood vessels.

cryokinetics The use of cold and exercise in the treatment of pathology or disease.

CRYOKINETICS

Cryokinetics is a technique that combines cryotherapy or the application of cold with exercise.[36] The goal of cryokinetics is to numb the injured part to the point of analgesia and then work toward achieving normal range of motion through progressive active exercise.

The technique begins by numbing the body part via ice immersion, cold packs, or ice massage. Most patients will report a feeling of numbness within 12 to 20 minutes. If numbness is not perceived within 20 minutes, the therapist should proceed with exercise regardless. The numbness usually will last for 3 to 5 minutes, at which point ice should be reapplied for an additional 3 to 5 minutes until numbness returns. This sequence should be repeated five times.

Exercises are performed during the periods of numbness. The exercises selected should be pain free and progressive in intensity, concentrating on both flexibility and strength.[63] Changes in the intensity of the activity should be limited by both the nature of the healing process and individual patient differences in perception of pain. However, progression always should be encouraged within the framework of those limiting factors, the ultimate goal being a return to full activity.[34]

edema Excessive fluid in cells.

Indications and Contraindications for Thermotherapy

Indications
   Subacute and chronic inflammatory
      conditions
   Subacute or chronic pain
   Subacute edema removal
   Decreased ROM
   Resolution of swelling
   Myofascial trigger points
   Muscle guarding
   Muscle spasm
   Subacute muscle strain
   Subacute ligament sprain
   Subacute contusion
   Infection

Contraindications
   Acute musculoskeletal conditions
   Impaired circulation
   Peripheral vascular disease
   Skin anesthesia
   Open wounds or skin conditions (cold
      whirlpools and contrast baths)

Treatment Tip
As long as the patient is not complaining of tenderness to touch it is probably safe to switch from cold to some form of heat. When treating deeper tissues it is recommended that either ultrasound or shortwave diathermy be used since the depth of penetration of both is greater than any infrared modality.

THERMOTHERAPY TECHNIQUES

Heat is still used as a universal treatment for pain and discomfort. Much of the benefit is derived from the treatment simply feeling good. However, in the early stages after injury, heat causes increased capillary blood pressure and increased cellular permeability; this results in additional swelling or **edema** accumulation.[2,9,25,37,82] *No patient with edema should be treated with any heat modality until the reasons for the edema are determined.* It is in the best interest of the therapist to use cryotherapy techniques to reduce the edema before applying heat. Superficial heat applications seem to feel more comfortable for complaints of the neck, back, low back, and pelvic areas and may be most appropriate for the patient who exhibits some allergic response to cold applications. However, the tissues in these areas are absolutely no different from those in the extremities. Thus the same physiologic responses to the use of heat or cold will be elicited in all areas of the body.

Primary goals of thermotherapy include increased blood flow and increased muscle temperature to stimulate analgesia, increased nutrition to the cellular level, reduction of edema, and removal of metabolites and other products of the inflammatory process.

WARM WHIRLPOOL

Equipment Needed

1. Whirlpool: The whirlpool must be the correct size for the body segment to be treated.
2. Towels: These are to be used for padding and drying off.
3. Chair.
4. Padding: This is to be placed on the side of the whirlpool.

Treatment

The patient should be positioned comfortably, allowing the injured part to be immersed in the whirlpool. Direct flow should be 6 to 8 inches from the body segment. Temperature should be 98 to 110°F (37–45°C) for treatment of the arm and

CASE STUDY 9-2
THERMOTHERAPY

Background: A 15-year-old boy sustained a non-comminuted, transverse fracture of the left patella during a football game 6 weeks ago. He was treated with plaster immobilization for 6 weeks; the cast was removed yesterday. He has full knee extension (the knee was immobilized in full extension) and has only 20 degrees of flexion. The patella is well healed and non-tender, and patellar mobility is severely limited. As an adjunct to active and passive exercise, you begin joint mobilization of the patellofemoral joint every day. To enhance the response of the connective tissue, you decide to increase the tissue temperature prior to mobilization.

Impression: Limitation of motion secondary to fracture and immobilization.

Treatment Plan: Because the target tissues are immediately subcutaneous, you elect to use a hydrocollator pack. Using a cervical pack, heat was applied to the circumference of the knee for 12 minutes. Immediately after removal of the hot pack, joint mobilization was initiated. Following joint mobilization, active range of motion and strengthening exercises were performed.

Response: The patient was treated 3 days per week for 4 weeks, then discharged to a home program. He had full active and passive range of motion, patellar mobility was normal, and strength was 80 percent of the unaffected limb.

Discussion Questions

- What tissues were injured or affected?
- What symptoms were present?
- What phase of the injury-healing continuum did the patient present for care in?
- What are the therapeutic agent modality's biophysical effects (direct, indirect, depth, and tissue affinity)?
- What are the therapeutic agent modality's indications and contraindications?
- What are the parameters of the therapeutic agent modality's application, dosage, duration, and frequency in this case study?
- What other therapeutic agent modalities could be used to treat this injury or condition? Why?

The rehabilitation professional employs therapeutic agent modality to create an optimum environment for tissue healing while minimizing the symptoms associated with the trauma or condition.

hand. For treatment of the leg, the temperature should be 98 to 104°F (37–40°C), and for full body treatment, the temperature should be 98 to 102°F (37–39°C). Time of application should be 15 to 20 minutes.

Considerations

Patient positioning should allow for exercise of the injured part. The size of the body segment to be treated will determine whether an upper extremity, lower extremity, or full body whirlpool should be used.

Application (Fig. 9-8)

The temperature range of a warm whirlpool is 100 to 110°F (39–45°C). It is similar in setup to a cold whirlpool. The patient must be positioned in the whirlpool with appropriate padding provided for the patient's comfort. The unit should be turned on after it has been ascertained that the GFI is functioning. The timer should be set for the amount of time desired, depending on the size of the body part to be treated (10–30 min). Treatment time should be long enough to stimulate vasodilatation and

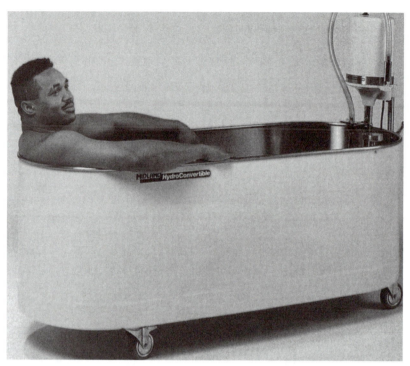

•**Figure 9-8** Warm whirlpool.

reduce muscle spasm (approx 20 min). Again, caution is indicated in the gravity-dependent position in subacute injuries. If some pitting edema exists (i.e., finger pressure on the skin leaves an indentation), cold or contrast baths are better indicated. In addition to increased circulation and reduction of spasm, benefits of the warm whirlpool include the massaging and vibrating effects of the water movement. On removal of the body segment from the whirlpool, it is necessary to review the skin surface and limb girth to see if the warm whirlpool increased swelling; this step is indicated even if the patient is past the subacute stage. After allowing the body segment to cool down, the patient can have appropriate preventive strapping or padding placed on the body segment. If the patient receives the treatment before exercising, it is recommended that he or she gently do range-of-motion exercises to reduce congestion and increase proprioception (sense of position) in all joints. If the patient is complaining of muscle soreness, it would be more appropriate to recommend swimming pool exercises. The whirlpool provides a sedative effect. It is recommended that the patient shower or clean the body surface before using a whirlpool. Random access to the whirlpool is not warranted.

The warm whirlpool is an excellent postsurgical modality to increase systemic blood flow and mobilization of the affected body part. The appropriateness of whirlpool therapy needs to be addressed by the therapist because it is the most commonly abused physical therapy modality. An example of this abuse is the practice of placing an individual in the whirlpool without taking the time to assess the specific physiologic responses desired. However, it is an excellent adjunctive modality when used appropriately in the clinical setting. Whirlpools should be cleaned frequently to prevent bacterial growth. When a patient with any open or infected lesion uses the whirlpool, it must be drained and cleaned immediately. Cleaning should be done using both a disinfecting and antibacterial agent. Particular attention should be paid to cleaning the turbine by placing the intake valves in a bucket containing the disinfecting solution and turning the power on. Bacterial cultures should be monitored periodically from the tank, drain, and jets.

COMMERCIAL (WARM) HYDROCOLLATOR PACKS (FIG. 9-9)

Equipment Needed

1. Unit heat packs: These are canvas pouches of petroleum distillate. A thermostat maintains the high temperature (170°F) and helps prevent burns. Unit heat packs come in three sizes: (1) regular size is 12 × 12 inches for most body segments; (2) double size is 24 × 24 inches for the back, low back, and buttocks; and (3) cervical is 6 × 18 inches for the cervical spine. Packs are removed by tongs or scissor handles.
2. Towels: Regular bath towels and commercial double pad towels are required. Commercial double pad toweling has a pouch for pack placement and 1-inch thick toweling to be placed in cross fashion, tags on the edge of packs folded in, toweling overlapped on one side and four layers on the opposite side. Six layers equal 1 inch of toweling. Additional toweling may be needed depending on total body surface covered.

Treatment

Position six layers of toweling as described in (Fig. 9-10). Sufficient toweling should be provided to protect the patient from burns. Patient position should be comfortable. Treatment time should be 15 to 20 minutes.

Physiologic Responses

Circulation is increased.
Muscle temperature is increased.
Tissue temperature is increased.
Spasms are relaxed.

Considerations

The size of the body segment to be treated should determine how many packs are needed. Patient comfort is always a consideration. Time of application should be 15 to 20 minutes.

Application

Appropriate toweling and positioning of the patient is necessary for a comfortable treatment. The moist heat pack tends to stimulate the circulatory response. Dry heat, as discussed in the infrared section, has a tendency to force blood away from

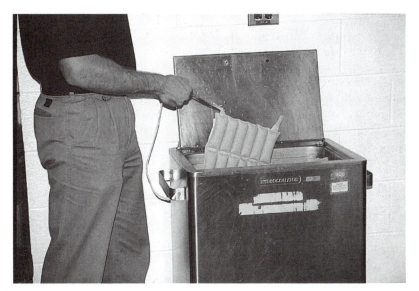

•**Figure 9-9** Hydrocollator packs stored in tank.

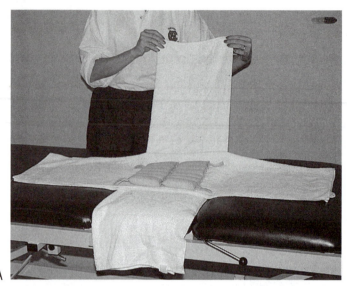

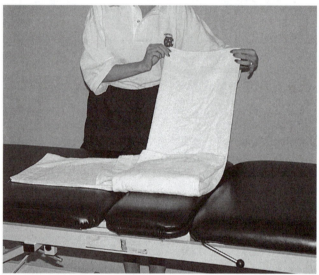

•**Figure 9-10** Techniques of wrapping hydrocollator packs.

the cutaneous capillary bed, thus increasing the possibility of a burn with the skin's inability to dissipate heat.[70] The patient must not be allowed to lie on the packs because this will force the silicate gel out through the seams of the fabric sleeves. If the patient cannot tolerate the weight of the moist heat pack, alternate methods, such as placing the patient side lying with the majority of the weight of the hot pack on the side of the pack and the pack held in place by additional towels or sheets wrapped around the patient, can be used. The most common indications are for muscular spasm, back pain, or as a preliminary treatment to other modalities.

PARAFFIN BATHS

paraffin bath A combined paraffin and mineral oil immersion commonly used on the hands and feet for distal temperature gains in blood flow and temperature.

A **paraffin bath** is a simple and efficient, although somewhat messy, technique for applying a fairly high degree of localized heat. Paraffin treatments provide six times the amount of heat available in water because the mineral oil in the paraffin lowers the melting point of the paraffin. The combination of paraffin and mineral oil has a low specific heat, which enhances the patient's ability to tolerate heat from paraffin better than from water of the same temperature.

The risk of a burn with paraffin is substantial. The therapist should weigh heavily the considerations between a paraffin bath and warm whirlpool bath in the athletic setting. The majority of paraffin baths are used for chronic arthritis in the hands and feet. If the patient has a chronic hand or foot problem, the use of paraffin instead of water usually gives longer lasting pain relief.[7,37]

Equipment Needed

1. Paraffin bath (Fig. 9-11A).
2. Plastic bags and paper towels.
3. Towels.

Treatment

Dipping

The extremity should be dipped into the paraffin for a couple of seconds, then removed to allow the paraffin to harden slightly for a few seconds. This procedure is repeated until six layers have accumulated on the part to be treated.

Wrapping

The paraffin-coated extremity should be wrapped in a plastic bag with several layers of toweling around it to act as insulation (Fig. 9-11B). Treatment time should be 20 to 30 minutes.

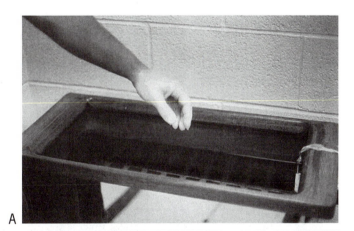

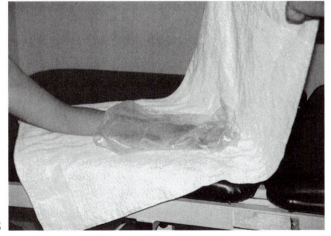

•**Figure 9-11** A. Hand being dipped in paraffin bath. B. After being dipped in paraffin, the hand should be wrapped in plastic bags and toweling.

Physiologic Responses

There is an increase in tissue temperature.
Pain relief occurs.
Thermal hyperthermia occurs.

Considerations

Some units are equipped with thermostats that may elevate the temperature to 212°F, thus killing any bacteria that may grow in the paraffin. Otherwise the temperature should be set at 126°F.

If the paraffin becomes soiled, it should be dumped and replaced at no longer than 6-month intervals.

Application

The purchase of a paraffin bath for the clinic requires that the bath have a built-in thermostat. Before treatment, the patient's body segment should be cleaned thoroughly with soap, water, and finally alcohol to remove any soap residue. This will prevent bacterial buildup in the bottom of the paraffin bath, which is an excellent medium for culture growth.

The mixture ratio of paraffin to mineral oil is 1 gallon of mineral oil to 2 pounds of paraffin. The mineral oil reduces the ambient temperature of the paraffin, which is 126°F (at which temperature a burn could occur). It is important to build six layers of paraffin, with the first layer highest on the body segment and each successive layer lower than the previous one. This is important because when dipping the extremity in the paraffin, if the second layer of paraffin is allowed to get between the skin and the first layer of paraffin, the heat will not dissipate and the patient could be burned. Because heat is retained in the body and is also radiated from the paraffin, there is an increase in capillary dilation and blood supply in the treated segment. The therapist should place the patient in a comfortable position and enclose the paraffin in paper towels, plastic bags, and toweling to maintain the heat. Treatment is applied for approximately 20 to 30 minutes. Removal of the paraffin calls for extra care not to contaminate the used portion so that it does not contaminate the entire bath when it is returned.

Removal of paraffin involves removing towels, plastic bag, and paper towels, then using a tongue depressor to split the paraffin to allow easy removal. If the paraffin has not touched the floor, remove the paraffin cast over the open paraffin bath. It will dissolve on returning to the remaining liquid paraffin. Clean the body segment with soap and water or, if a postsurgical patient is being treated, give a massage, since the mineral oil will make the skin moist and supple. When cleaning the skin, the therapist must examine the surface for burns or mottling. The thermostat will raise the temperature of the paraffin to 212°F, destroy any bacteria, and maintain a sterile contact medium. Paraffin baths require a large amount of supervision to prevent contamination, but they do provide a special type of treatment that is well adapted to the patient with injuries of the hands and feet.

INFRARED LAMPS

When talking about infrared modalities, the therapist most typically thinks of the infrared lamp. The biggest advantage of an infrared lamp is that superficial tissue temperature can be increased, even though the unit does not touch the patient. However, radiant heat is seldom used because it is limited in depth of skin penetration to less than 1 mm. Dry heat from an infrared lamp tends to elevate superficial skin temperatures more than moist heat; however, moist heat probably has a greater depth of penetration.

Superficial skin burns occasionally occur because of intense infrared radiation and the reflector becoming extremely hot (4000°F). It is recommended that a warm moist towel be placed over the body segment to be treated to enhance the heating effects. Dry towels should cover the remainder of the body not being treated. This will allow a greater blood to tissue exchange by trapping the heat buildup in the moist towel and reducing the stagnant air over the body segment. Caution should be used, and the skin should be checked every few minutes for mottling.

Infrared generators may be divided into two categories: luminous and nonluminous. Nonluminous generators consist of a spiral coil of resistant metal wire wound around a cone-shaped piece of nonconducting material. The resistance of the wire to the electric flow produces heat and a dull red glow. A properly shaped reflector then radiates the heat to the body. All incandescent bodies and tungsten and carbon filament lamps are in the category of luminous generators. No nonluminous lamps are currently being manufactured since infrared at a wavelength of 12,000 A will penetrate slightly more deeply than either longer or shorter waves, owing to a certain unique characteristic of human skin. Tungsten filament and special quartz red sources produce significant amounts of infrared heat at 12,000 A. Flare as a result of reflection off the skin can be a serious problem.

Equipment Needed

1. Infrared lamp.
2. Dry toweling: This is to be used for draping the parts of the body not being treated.
3. Moist toweling: Moist towels are used to cover the area to be treated.
4. A GFI should be used with an infrared lamp.

Treatment

The patient should be positioned 20 inches from the source.
Protective toweling should be put in place.
Treatment time should be 15 to 20 minutes.
Skin should be checked every few minutes for mottling.
Areas that are not to be treated must be protected.

Physiologic Responses

A superficial rise in tissue temperature occurs.
There is some decrease in pain.
Moisture and sweat appear on the skin surface.

Considerations

To avoid a generalized temperature rise, only the portion that is injured should be treated. The infrared lamp should be used primarily when a patient cannot tolerate pressure from another type of modality (e.g., hydrocollator packs). Caution must be exercised to avoid burns.

Application (Fig. 9-12)

The patient should be placed in a comfortable position. Moist heat should be used to stimulate blood flow. It is recommended to prevent blood from being forced away from the area as with dry heat. A moist, warm towel should be applied to the area to be treated. A squirt bottle is needed to keep the towel moist. All areas not to be treated should be draped. The distance from the area to be treated to the lamp should be adjusted according to treatment time: The standard formula is 20 inches distance = 20 minutes treatment time. After treatment, the skin surface should be

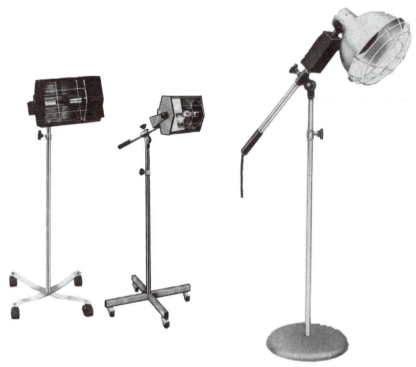

•**Figure 9-12** Infrared baker's or heat lamps.

checked. This type of treatment tends to force the blood away from the capillary bed and should be used only in superficial skin complaints related to dry heat requirements.

FLUIDOTHERAPY

fluidotherapy A modality of dry heat using a finely divided solid suspended in a stream with the properties of liquid.

Fluidotherapy is a unique, multifunctional physical medicine modality. The fluidotherapy unit is a dry heat modality that uses a suspended air stream, which has the properties of a liquid. Its therapeutic effectiveness in rehabilitation and healing is based on its ability to simultaneously apply heat, massage, sensory stimulation for desensitization, levitation, and pressure oscillations. Unlike water, the dry, natural medium does not irritate the skin or produce thermal shocks. This allows for much higher treatment temperatures than with aqueous or paraffin heat transfer. The pressure oscillations may actually minimize edema, even at very high treatment temperatures. Outstanding clinical success has been reported in treatment of pain, range of motion, wounds, acute injuries, swelling, and blood flow insufficiency. Fluidotherapy treatment of the hand at 115°F (46.2°C) results in a sixfold increase in blood flow and a fourfold increase in metabolic rates in a normal adult. These properties will increase blood flow, sedate, decrease blood pressure, and promote healing by accelerating biochemical reactions.[7]

Counterirritation, through mechanoreceptor and thermoreceptor stimulation, reduces pain sensitivity, thus permitting high temperatures without painful heat sensations. Pronounced hyperthermia accelerates the chemical metabolic processes and stimulates the normal healing process. The high temperatures enhance tissue elasticity and reduce tissue viscosity, which improves musculoskeletal mobility. Vascular responses are stimulated by long-lasting hyperthermia and pressure fluctuations, resulting in increased blood flow to the injured area.

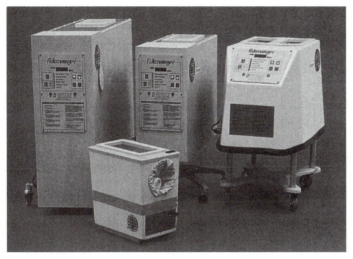

•Figure 9-13 Fluidotherapy treatment units.
(Photo courtesy of Fluidotherapy Corp., 6113 Aletha Lane, Houston, Texas 77081.)

Equipment Needed

1. Fluidotherapy model 104 (Fig. 9-13).
2. Toweling.

Treatment

The patient must be positioned for comfort.

The patient should place the body segment to be treated (hand or foot) in the fluidotherapy unit.

Protective toweling must be placed at the unit interface and body segment.

Treatment time should be 15 to 20 minutes.

Physiologic Responses

Tissue temperature increases.

Pain relief occurs.

Thermal hyperthermia occurs.

Considerations

Fluidotherapy unit must be kept clean.

All knobs must be returned to zero after treatment.

Application

The patient should be positioned comfortably. The treated body segment should be submerged in the medium before the unit is turned on. There is no thermal shock when heat is applied. Treatments are approximately 20 minutes. Recommended temperature varies by body part and patient tolerance, with a range of 110 to 125°F (43–53°C). Maximum temperature rise in the treated part occurs after 15 minutes of treatment. Unless contraindicated, active and passive exercise are encouraged during treatment.

In case of open lesions or infections, a protective dressing is recommended to prevent soiling or contaminating the cloth entry ports. Patients with splints, bandages, tape, orthopedic pins, plastic joint replacement, and artificial tendons may be treated with fluidotherapy. The medium is clean and will not soil clothing. It is not necessary to disrobe to get the full benefit of heat and massage; however, direct contact between skin and the medium is desirable to maximize heat transfer.

In treating the hands, muscles, ankles, and conditions that manifest themselves relatively near the surface of the skin, appreciably higher body temperatures can be achieved using superficial heating modalities.[7] Further, the superficial modalities treat a larger area of the body than ultrasound or microwave diathermies, thus the total amount of heat absorbed will be much higher. Fluidotherapy, hydrotherapy, and paraffin cause about the same amount of temperature increase.[19]

CONCLUSIONS

Infrared sources transmit thermal energy to or from the patient. In most cases, they are simple, efficient, and inexpensive. Therapists who choose to compare modalities and use the most appropriate technique for their patients will be providing quality care for that patient. A haphazard approach to the use of infrared modalities will only reflect a disregard for the health care of the patient.

Questioning, thinking therapists will determine which procedure is best and most appropriate clinically. They will take responsibility for seeing that the most appropriate therapeutic modality is applied to enhance the patient's reconditioning and rehabilitation. Regardless of which infrared modality therapists choose, they should be aware of (1) the physiologic implications relative to circulation; (2) the ease of application; and (3) the short- and long-term benefits of treatment.

Additional areas of concern relate to (1) benefits of the infrared modality application, whether cryotherapy or thermotherapy; (2) economy of modality application; and (3) repeatability of applications. Common sense in the application of these modalities will provide optimum injury management and modality usage for tissue healing of athletic trauma.

SUMMARY

1. Any modality that radiates energy with wavelengths and frequencies that fall into the infrared region of the electromagnetic spectrum are referred to as infrared modalities.

2. When infrared modalities are applied to connective tissue or muscle and soft tissue, they will cause either a tissue temperature decrease or tissue temperature increase.

3. The primary physiologic effect of heat is vasodilatation of capillaries with increased blood flow, increased metabolic activity, and relaxation of muscle spasm.

4. The primary physiologic effects of cold are vasoconstriction of capillaries with decreased blood flow, decreased metabolic activity, and analgesia with reduction of muscle spasm.

5. The infrared energies have a depth of penetration of less than 1 cm, thus the physiologic effects are primarily superficial and directly affect the cutaneous blood vessels and nerve receptors.

6. Examples of thermotherapy are whirlpools, moist heat packs, infrared lamps, heating pads, and fluidotherapy.

7. Examples of cryotherapy are ice packs, ice massage, commercial ice packs, ice whirlpools, and cold sprays.

REFERENCES

1. Abramson, D., Tuck, S., and Lee, S.: Vascular basis for pain due to cold, Arch. Phys. Med. Rehabil. 47:300–305, 1966.
2. Baker, R., Bell, G.: The effect of therapeutic modalities on blood flow in the human calf, JOSPT 13:23, 1991.
3. Basset, S., Lake, B.: Use of cold applications in management of spasticity, Phys. Ther. 38(5):333–334, 1958.
4. Behnke, R.: Cold therapy, Ath. Train. 9(4):178–179, 1974.
5. Bierman, W., Friendiander, M.: The penetrative effect of cold, Arch. Phys. Med. Rehabil. 21:585–592, 1940.
6. Braswell, S., Frazzini, M., and Knuth, A.: Optimal duration of ice massage for skin anesthesia, Phys. Ther. 74(5):S156, 1994.
7. Chambers, R.: Clinical uses of cryotherapy, Phys. Ther. 49(3):145–149, 1969.
8. Clarke, D.: Effect of immersion in hot and cold water upon recovery of muscular strength following fatiguing isometric exercise, Arch. Phys. Med. Rehabil. 44:565–568, 1963.
9. Clarke, D., Stelmach, G.: Muscle fatigue and recovery curve parameters at various temperatures, Res. Quart. 37(4):468–479, 1966.
10. Clarke, R., Hellon, R., and Lind, A.: Vascular reactions of the human forearm to cold, Clin. Sci. 17:165–179, 1958.
11. Clark, R., Lephardt, S., and Baker, C.: Cryotherapy and compression treatment protocols in the prevention of delayed onset muscle soreness, J. Ath. Train. 31(2):S33, 1996.
12. Clemente, F., Frampton, R., and Temoshenka, A.: The effects of hot and cold packs on peak isometric torque generated by the back extensor musculature, Phys. Ther. 74(5):S70, 1994.
13. Cote, D., Prentice, W., and Hooker, D.: A comparison of three treatment procedures for minimizing ankle edema, Phys. Ther. 68(7):1072–1076, 1988.
14. Cutlaw, K., Arnold, B., and Perrin, D.: Effect of cold treatment on concentric and eccentric force velocity relationship of the quads, J. Ath. Train. 30(2):S31, 1995.
15. Dejong, R., Hershey, W., and Wagman, I.: Nerve conduction velocity during hypothermia in man, Anesthesiology 27:805–810, 1966.
16. Dolan, M., Thornton, R., and Mendel, F.: Cold water immersion effects on edema formation following impact injury to hind limbs of rats, J. Ath. Train. 31(2):S48, 1996.
17. Dontigny, R., Sheldon, K.: Simultaneous use of heat and cold in treatment of muscle spasm, Arch. Phys. Med. Rehabil. 43:235–237, 1962.
18. Downer, A.: Physical therapy procedures, ed. 3, Springfield, Illinois, 1978, Charles C Thomas.
19. Downey, J.: Physiological effects of heat and cold, J. Am. Phys. Ther. Assoc. 44(8):713–717, 1964.
20. Dufresne, T., Jarzabski, K., and Simmons, D.: Comparison of superficial and deep heating agents followed by a passive stretch on increasing the flexibility of the hamstring muscle group, Phys. Ther. 74(5):S70, 1994.
21. Eldred, E., Lindsley, D., and Buchwald, J.: The effect of cooling on mammalian muscle spindles, Exp. Neurol. 2:144–157, 1960.
22. Evans, T., Ingersoll, C., and Knight, K.: Agility following the application of cold therapy, J. Ath. Train. 30(3):231–234, 1995.
23. Fischer, E., Soloman, S.: Physiologic responses to heat and cold. In Licht, S., editor: Therapeutic heat, New Haven, Connecticut, 1965, Elizabeth Licht.
24. Gallant, S., Knight, K., and Ingersoll, C.: Cryotherapy effects on leg press and vertical jump force production, J. Ath. Train. 31(2):S18, 1996.
25. Grant, A.: Massage with ice (cryokinetics) in the treatment of painful conditions of the musculoskeletal system, Arch. Phys. Med. Rehabil. 45:233–238, 1964.
26. Grecier, M., Kendrick, Z., and Kimura, I.: Immediate and delayed effects of cryotherapy on functional power and agility, J. Ath. Train. 31(Suppl):S–32, 1996.
27. Griffin, J., Karselis, T.: Physical agents for physical therapists, ed. 2, Springfield, Illinois, 1988, Charles C Thomas.
28. Guyton, A.: Medical physiology, ed. 6, Philadelphia, 1991, W.B. Saunders.
29. Hayden, C.: Cryokinetics in an early treatment program, J. Am. Phys. Ther. Assoc. 44:11, 1964.
30. Hedenberg, L.: Functional improvement of the spastic hemiplegic arm after cooling, Scand. J. Rehab. Med. 2:154–158, 1970.
31. Ho, S., Illgen, R., and Meyer, R.: Comparison of various icing times in decreasing bone metabolism and blood in the knee, Am. J. Sports Med. 23(1):74–76, 1995.
32. Hocutt, J., Jaffe, R., and Rylander, C.: Cryotherapy in ankle sprains, Am. J. Sports Med. 10(3):316–319, 1992.
33. Knight, K.: Effects of hypothermia on inflammation and swelling, Ath. Train. 11:7–10, 1976.
34. Knight, K.: Cryotherapy in sports injury management, Champaign, Illinois, 1995, Human Kinetics.
35. Knight, K.: Ice for immediate care of injuries, Phys. Sports Med. 10(2):137, 1982.
36. Knight, K.: Cryotherapy: theory, technique and physiology, Chattanooga, Tennessee, 1985, Chattanooga Corporation.
37. Knight, K., Aquino, J., and Johannes S.: A reexamination of Lewis' cold induced vasodilation in the finger and the ankle, Ath. Train. 15:248–250, 1980.
38. Knight, K., Ingersoll, C., and Trowbridge, C.: The effects of cooling the ankle, the triceps surae or both on functional agility, J. Ath. Train. 29(2):165, 1994.
39. Knight, K., Londeree, B.: Comparison of blood flow in the ankle of uninjured subjects during therapeutic applications of heat, cold, and exercise, Med. Sci. Sports Exerc. 12(1):76–80, 1980.
40. Knott, M., Barufaldi, D.: Treatment of whiplash injuries, Phys. Ther. 41:8, 1961.
41. Knutsson, E.: Topical cryotherapy in spasticity, Scand. J. Rehab. Med. 2:159–163, 1970.
42. Knutsson, E., Mattson, E.: Effects of local cooling on monosynaptic reflexes in man, Scand. J. Rehab. Med. 1:126–132, 1969.

43. Kolb, P., Denegar, C.: Traumatic edema and the lymphatic system, Ath. Train. 18:339–341, 1983.

44. LaRiviere, J., Osternig, L.: The effect of ice immersion on joint position sense, J. Sport Rehab. 3(1):58–67, 1994.

45. Lehman, J.: Therapeutic heat and cold, ed. 3, Baltimore, 1982, Williams & Wilkins.

46. Lewis, T.: Observations upon the reactions of the vessels of the human skin to cold, Heart 15:177–208, 1930.

47. Licht, S.: Therapeutic heat and cold, New Haven, Connecticut, 1965, Elizabeth Licht.

48. Lippold, O., Nicholls, J., and Redfearn, J.: A study of the afferent discharge produced by cooling a mammalian muscle spindle, J. Physiol. 153:218–231, 1960.

49. Lowden, B., Moore, R.: Determinants and nature of intramuscular temperature changes during cold therapy, Am. J. Phys. Med. 54(5):223–233, 1975.

50. Mancuso, D., Knight, K.: Effects of prior skin surface temperature response of the ankle during and after a 30-minute ice pack application, J. Ath. Train. 27:242–249, 1992.

51. McMaster, W.: A literary review on ice therapy in injuries, Am. J. Sports Med. 5(3):124–126, 1977.

52. Merrick, M., Knight, K., and Ingersoll C.: The effects of ice and compression wraps on intramuscular temperatures at various depths, J. Ath. Train. 28(3):236–245, 1993.

53. Merrick, M., Knight, K., and Ingersoll, C.: The effects of ice and elastic wraps on intratissue temperatures at various depths, J. Ath. Train. 28(2):156, 1993.

54. Mickey, C., Bernier, J., and Perrin, D.: Ice and ice with nonthermal ultrasound effects on delayed onset muscle soreness, J. Ath. Train. 31(2):S19, 1996.

55. Miglietta, O.: Electromyographic characteristics of clonus and influence of cold, Arch. Phys. Med. Rehabil.45:508, 1964.

56. Misasi, S., Morin, G., and Kemler, D.: The effect of a toe cap and bias on perceived pain during cold water immersion, J. Ath. Train. 30(1):149–156, 1995.

57. Moore, R.: Uses of cold therapy in the rehabilitation of athletes: recent advances, Proceedings 19th American Medical Association National Conference on the medical aspects of sports, San Francisco, June 1977.

58. Moore, R., Nicolette, R., and Behnke, R.: The therapeutic use of cold (cryotherapy) in the care of athletic injuries, Ath. Train. 2:613, 1967.

59. Murphy, A.: The physiological effects of cold application, Phys. Ther. 40(2):112–115, 1960.

60. Myrer, J., Draper, D., and Durrant, E.: The effect of contrast therapy on intramuscular temperature in the human lower leg, J. Ath. Train. 29(4):318–322, 1994.

61. Olson, J., Stravino, V.: A review of cryotherapy, Phys. Ther. 62(8):840–853, 1972.

62. Paduano, R., Crothers, J.: The effects of whirlpool treatments and age on a one-leg balance test, Phys. Ther. 74(5):S70, 1994.

63. Pincivero, D., Gieck, J., and Saliba, E.: Rehabilitation of a lateral ankle sprain with cryokinetic and functional progressive exercise, J. Sport Rehab. 2(3):200–207, 1993.

64. Prentice, W: An electromyographic analysis of the effectiveness of heat or cold and stretching for inducing relaxation in injured muscle, J. Orthop. Sports Phys. Ther. 3(3):133–146, 1982.

65. Rivers, D., Kimura, I., and Sitler, M.: The influence of cryotherapy and Aircast bracing on total body balance and proprioception, J. Ath. Train. 30(2):S15, 1995.

66. Rocks, A.: Intrinsic shoulder pain syndrome, Phys. Ther. 59(2):153–159, 1979.

67. Ruiz, D., Myrer, J., and Durrant, E.: Cryotherapy and sequential exercise bouts following cryotherapy on concentric and eccentric strength in the quadriceps, J. Ath. Train. 28(4): 320–323, 1993.

68. Schnatz, A., Kimura, I., and Sitler, M.: Influence of cryotherapy thermotherapy and neoprene ankle sleeve on total body balance and proprioception, J. Ath. Train. 31(2):S32, 1996.

69. Schuler, D., Ingersoll, C., and Knight, K.: Local cold application to foot and ankle, lower leg of both effects on a cutting drill, J. Ath. Train. 31(2):S35, 1996.

70. Smith, K., Draper, D., and Schulthies, S.: The effect of silicate gel hot packs on human muscle temperature, J. Ath. Train. 30(2):S33, 1995.

71. Smith, K., Newton, R.: The immediate effect of contrast baths on edema, temperature and pain in postsurgical hand injuries, Phys. Ther. 74(5):S157, 1994.

72. Stillwell, K.: Therapeutic heat and cold. In Krusen F., Kootke F., and Ellwood P., editors: Handbook of physical medicine and rehabilitation, Philadelphia, 1971, W.B. Saunders.

73. Taylor, B., Waring, C., and Brasher, T.: The effects of therapeutic application of heat or cold followed by static stretch on hamstring muscle length, JOSPT 21(5):283–286, 1995.

74. Thieme, H., Ingersol, C., and Knight, K.: The effect of cooling on proprioception of the knee, J. Ath. Train. 28(2):158, 1993.

75. Thieme, H., Ingersoll, C., and Knight, K.: Cooling does not affect knee proprioception, J. Ath. Train. 31(1):8–11, 1996.

76. Thompson, G., Kimura, I., and Sitler, M.: Effect of cryotherapy on eccentric and peak torque and endurance, J. Ath. Train. 29(2):180, 1994.

77. Travell, J.: Rapid relief of acute "stiff neck" by ethyl chloride spray, Am. Med. Wom. Assoc. 4(3):89–95, 1949.

78. Travell, J.: Ethyl chloride spray for painful muscle spasm, Arch. Phys. Med. Rehabil. 32:291–298, 1952.

79. Travell, J., Simons, D.: Myofascial pain and dysfunction: the trigger point manual, Baltimore, 1983, Williams & Wilkins.

80. Weston, M., Taber, C., and Casagranda, L.: Changes in local blood volume during cold gel pack application to traumatized ankles, J. Orthop. Sports Phys. Ther. 19(4):197–199, 1994.

81. Whittaker, T., Lander, J., and Brubaker, D.: The effect of cryotherapy on selected balance parameters, J. Ath. Train. 29(2):180, 1994.

82. Zankel, H.: Effect of physical agents on motor conduction velocity of the ulnar nerve, Arch. Phys. Med. Rehabil. 47(12): 787–792, 1966.

SUGGESTED READINGS

Abraham, E.: Whirlpool therapy for treatment of soft tissue wounds complicated by extremity fractures, J. Trauma 4:222, 1974.

Abraham, W.: Heat vs. cold therapy for the treatment of muscle injuries, Ath. Train. 9(4):177, 1974.

Abramson, D., Bell, B., and Tuck, S.: Changes in blood flow, oxygen uptake and tissue temperatures produced by therapeutic physical agents: effect of indirect or reflex vasodilation, Am. J. Phys. Med. 40:5–13, 1961.

Abramson, D., Mitchell, R., and Tuck, S.: Changes in blood flow, oxygen uptake and tissue temperatures produced by a topical application of wet heat, Arch. Phys. Med. Rehabil. 42:305, 1961.

Abramson, D., Tuck, S., and Zayas, A.: The effect of altering limb position on blood flow, oxygen uptake and skin temperature, J. App. Physiol. 17:191, 1962.

Abramson, D., Tuck, S., and Chu, L.: Effect of paraffin bath and hot fomentation on local tissue temperature, Arch. Phys. Med. Rehabil. 45:87, 1964.

Abramson, D., Tuck, S., Chu, L.: Indirect vasodilation in thermotherapy, Arch. Phys. Med. Rehabil. 46:412, 1965.

Abramson, D.: Physiologic basis for the use of physical agents in peripheral vascular disorders, Arch. Phys. Med. Rehabil. 46:216, 1965.

Abramson, D., Chu, L., and Tuck, S.: Effect of tissue temperatures and blood flow on motor nerve conduction velocity, JAMA 198:1082, 1966.

Abramson, D., Tuck, S., and Lee, S.: Comparison of wet and dry heat in raising temperature of tissues, Arch. Phys. Med. Rehabil. 48:654, 1967.

Airhihenbuwa, C., St. Pierre, R., and Winchell, D.: Cold vs. heat therapy: a physician's recommendations for first aid treatment of strain, Emergency 19(1):40–43, 1987.

Arnheim, D., Prentice, W.: Principles of athletic training, ed. 9, New York, 1997, McGraw-Hill.

Ascenzi, J.: The need for decontamination and disinfection of hydrotherapy equipment, vol. 1, Surgikos, Inc., 1980, Asepsis Monograph.

Austin, K.: Diseases of immediate type hypersensitivity. In Isselbacher, K., Adams, R., and Braumwald E., editors: Harrison's principles of internal medicine, ed. 9, New York, 1980, McGraw-Hill.

Barnes, L.: Cryotherapy: putting injury on ice, Phys. Sportsmed. 7(6):130–136, 1979.

Basur, R., Shephard, E., and Mouzos G.: A cooling method in the treatment of ankle sprains, Practitioner 216:708, 1976.

Beasley, R., Kester, N.: Principles of medical-surgical rehabilitation of the hand, Med. Clin. North Am. 53:645, 1969.

Belitsky, R., Odam, S., and Humbley-Kozey, C.: Evaluation of the effectiveness of wet ice, dry ice, and cryogen packs in reducing skin temperature, Phys. Ther. 67:1080, 1987.

Benoit, T., Martin, D., and Perrin, D.: Effect of clinical application of heat and cold on knee joint laxity, J. Ath. Train. 30(2):S31, 1995.

Benson, T., Copp, E.: The effects of therapeutic forms of heat and ice on the pain threshold of the normal shoulder, Rheumatol. Rehabil. 13:101, 1974.

Berne, R., Levy, M.: Cardiovascularphysiology, ed. 4, St. Louis, 1981, C.V. Mosby.

Bickle, R.: Swimming pool management, Physiotherapy 57:475, 1971.

Bierman, W.: Therapeutic use of cold, JAMA 157:1189–1192, 1955.

Bocobo, C.: The effect of ice on intra-articular temperature in the knee of the dog, Am. J. Phys. Med. Rehabil. 70:181, 1991.

Boes, M.: Reduction of spasticity by cold, J. Am. Phys. Ther. Assoc. 42(1):29–32, 1962.

Boland, A.: Rehabilitation of the injured athlete. In Strauss, R.A., editor: Physiology, Philadelphia, 1979, W.B. Saunders.

Borrell, R., Henley, E., and Purvis H.: Fluidotherapy: evaluation of a new heat modality, Arch. Phys. Med. Rehabil. 58:69, 1977.

Borrell, R., Parker, R., and Henley, E.: Comparison of in vivo temperatures produced by hydrotherapy, paraffin wax treatment, and fluidotherapy, Phys. Ther. 60(10):1273–1276, 1980.

Boyer, T., Fraser, R., and Doyle, A.: The haemodynamic effects of cold immersion, Clin. Sci. 19:539, 1980.

Boyle, R., Balisteri, F., and Osborne, F.: The value of the Hubbard tank as a diuretic agent, Arch. Phys. Med. Rehabil. 45:505, 1964.

Chastain, P.: The effect of deep heat on isometric strength, Phys. Ther. 58:543, 1978.

Clarke, K., editor: Fundamentals of athletic training: physical therapy procedures, Chicago, 1971, AMA Press.

Claus-Walker, J.: Physiological responses to cold stress in healthy subjects and in subjects with cervical cord injuries, Arch. Phys. Med. Rehabil. 55:485, 1974.

Clendenin, M., Szumski, A.: Influence of cutaneous ice application on single motor units in humans, Phys. Ther. 51(2):166–175, 1971.

Cobb, C., Devries, H., and Urban, R.: Electrical activity in muscle pain, Am. J. Phys. Med. 54:80, 1975.

Cobbold, A., Lewis, O.: Blood flow to the knee joint of the dog: effect of heating, cooling and adrenaline, J. Physiol. 132:379, 1956.

Cohen, A., Martin, G., and Waldin, K.: The effect of whirlpool bath with and without agitation on the circulation in normal and diseased extremities, Arch. Phys. Med. Rehabil. 30:212, 1949.

Conolly, W., Paltos, N., and Tooth, R.: Cold therapy: an improved method, Med. J. Aust. 2:424, 1972.

Cook, D., Georgouras K.: Complications of cutaneous cryotherapy, Med. J. Aust. 161(3):210–213, 1994.

Cordray, Y., Krusen, E.: Use of hydrocollator packs in the treatment of neck and shoulder pains, Arch. Phys. Med. Rehabil. 39:105, 1959.

Covington, D., Bassett, F.: When cryotherapy injures, Phys. Sportsmed. 21(3):78–79, 1993.

Crockford, G., Hellon, R.: Vascular responses of human skin to infrared radiation, J. Physiol. 149:424, 1959.

Crockford, G., Hellon, R., and Parkhouse, J.: Thermal vasomotor response in human skin mediated by local mechanism, J. Physiol. 161:10, 1962.

Culp, R., Taras, J.: The effect of ice application versus controlled cold therapy on skin temperature when used with postoperative bulky hand and wrist dressings: a preliminary study, J. Hand. Ther. 8(4):249–251, 1995.

Currier, D., Kramer, J.: Sensory nerve conduction: heating effects of ultrasound and infrared, Physiother. Can. 34:241, 1982.

Dawson, W., Kottke, P., and Kubicek, W.: Evaluation of cardiac output, cardiac work, and metabolic rate during hydrotherapy exercise in normal subjects, Arch. Phys. Med. Rehabil. 46:605, 1965.

Day, M.: Hypersensitive response to ice massage: report of a case, Phys. Ther. 54:592, 1974.

DeLateur, B., Lehmann, J.: Cryotherapy. In Lehmann, J., editor: Therapeutic heat and cold, ed. 3, Baltimore, 1982, Williams & Wilkins.

Devries, H.: Quantitative electromyographic investigation of the spasm theory of muscle pain, Am. J. Phys. Med. 45:119, 1966.

Draper, D., Schulthies, S., and Sorvisto, P.: Temperature changes in deep muscles of humans during ice and ultrasound therapies: an in vivo study, J. Orthop. Sports Phys. Ther. 21(3):153–157, 1995.

Drez, D.: Therapeutic modalities for sports injuries, Chicago, 1989, Yearbook.

Drez, D., Faust, D., and Evans, J.: Cryotherapy and nerve palsy, Am. J. Sports Med. 9:256, 1981.

Edwards, H., Harris, R., and Hultman, E.: Effect of temperature on muscle energy metabolism and endurance during successive isometric contractions, sustained to fatigue, of the quadriceps muscle in man, J. Physiol. 220:335, 1972.

Epstein, M.: Water immersion: modern researchers discover the secrets of an old folk remedy, Sciences 205:12, 1979.

Eyring, E., Murray, W.: The effect of joint position on the pressure of intraarticular effusion, J. Bone Joint Surg. 46[A](6):1235, 1964.

Farry, P., Prentice, N.: Ice treatment of injured ligaments: an experimental model, NZ Med. J. 9:12, 1950.

Folkow, B., Fox, R., and Krog, J.: Studies on the reactions of the cutaneous vessels to cold exposure, Acta Physiol. Scand. 58:342, 1963.

Fountain, F., Gersten, J., and Senger, O.: Decrease in muscle spasm produced by ultrasound, hot packs and IR, Arch. Phys. Med. Rehabil. 41:293, 1960.

Fox, R.: Local cooling in man, Br. Ed. Bull. 17(1):14–18, 1961.

Fox, R., Wyatt, H.: Cold induced vasodilation in various areas of the body surface in man, J. Physiol. 162:259, 1962.

Gammon, G., Starr, I.: Studies on the relief of pain by counterirritation, J. Clin. Invest. 20:13, 1941.

Gerig, B.: The effects of cryotherapy upon ankle proprioception (abstract), Ath. Train. 25:119, 1990.

Gieck, J.: Precautions for hydrotherapeutic devices, Clin. Manage. 3:44, 1953.

Golland, A.: Basic hydrotherapy, Physiotherapy 67:258, 1951.

Green, G., Zachazewski, J., and Jordan, S.: A case conference: peroneal nerve palsy induced by cryotherapy, Phys. Sportsmed. 17:63, 1989.

Greenberg, R.: The effects of hot packs and exercise on local blood flow, Phys. Ther. 52:273, 1972.

Halkovich, I., Personius, W., and Clamann, H.: Effect of fluorimethane spray on passive hip flexion, Phys. Ther. 61:185, 1981.

Halvorson, G.: Therapeutic heat and cold for athletic injuries, Phys. Sportsmed. 18:87, 1990.

Harb, G.: The effect of paraffin bath submersion on digital blood flow in patients with Raynaud's syndrome, Phys. Ther. 73(6):S9, 1993.

Harrison, R.: Tolerance of pool therapy by ankylosing spondylitis patients with low vital capacity, Physiotherapy 67:296, 1981.

Hayes, K.: Heat and cold in the management of rheumatoid arthritis. Arth. Care Res. 6(3):156–166, 1993.

Head, M., Helms, P.: Paraffin and sustained stretching in the treatment of burn contractures, Burns 4:136, 1977.

Healy, W., Seidman, J., and Pfeifer B.: Cold compressive dressing after total knee arthroplasty, Clin. Orthop. Rel. Res. 299:143–146, 1994.

Hellerbrand, T., Holutz, S., and Eubarik, I.: Measurement of whirlpool temperature, pressure and turbulence, Arch. Phys. Med. Rehabil. 32:17, 1950.

Hendier, E., Crosbie, R., and Hardy, J.: Measurement of heating of the skin during exposure to infrared radiation, J. Appl. Physiol. 12:177, 1958.

Henricksen, A., Fredricksson, K., and Persson, I.: The effect of heat and stretching on the range of hip motion, J. Orthop. Sports Phys. Ther. 6:110, 1984.

Ho, S., Coel, M., and Kagawa, R.: The effects of ice on blood flow and bone metabolism in knees, Am. J. Sports Med. 22(4):537–540, 1994.

Hocutt, J., Jaffe, R., and Rylander, R.: Cryotherapy in ankle sprains, Am. J. Sports Med. 10:316, 1982.

Holcomb, W., Mangus, B., Tandy, R.: The effect of icing with the Pro-Stim Edema Management System on cutaneous cooling, J. Ath. Train. 31(2):126–129, 1996.

Holmes, G.: Hydrotherapy as a means of rehabilitation, Br. J. Phys. Med. 5:93, 1942.

Horton, B., Brown, G., and Roth, G.: Hypersensitiveness to cold with local and systemic manifestations of a histamine-like character: its amenability to treatment, JAMA 107:1263, 1936.

Horvath, S., Hollander, L.: Intra-articular temperature as a measure of joint reaction, J. Clin. Invest. 28:469, 1949.

Hunter, J., Mackin, E.: Edema and bandaging. In Hunter, J., editor: Rehabilitation of the hand, ed. 1, St. Louis, 1978, C.V. Mosby.

Ingersoll, C., Mangus, B.: Sensations of cold reexamined: a study using the McGill pain questionnaire, Ath. Train. 26:240, 1991.

Ingersoll, C., Mangus, B., and Wolf, S.: Cold-induced pain: habituation to cold immersion (abstract), Ath. Train. 25:126, 1990.

Jessup, G.: Muscle soreness: temporary distress of injury? Ath. Train. 15(4):260, 1950.

Jezdirisky, J., Marek, I., and Ochonsky, P.: Effects of local cold and heat therapy on traumatic oedema of the rat hind paw. 1. Effects of cooling on the course of traumatic oedema, Acta Universitatis Palackianae Olomucensis Facultatis Medicae 66:155, 1973.

Johnson, D.: Effect of cold submersion on intramuscular temperature of the gastrocnemius muscle, Phys. Ther. 59:1238, 1979.

Johnson, J., and Leider, F.: Influence of cold bath on maximum handgrip strength, Percept. Mot. Skills 44:323, 1977.

Kaempffe, F.: Skin surface temperature after cryotherapy to a casted extremity, J. Orthop. Sports Phys. Ther. 10(11):448–450, 1989.

Kaul, M., Herring, S.: Superficial heat and cold: how to maximize the benefits, Phys. Sportsmed. 22(12):65–72, 74, 1994.

Kessler, R., Hertling, D.: Management of common musculoskeletal disorders, Philadelphia, 1953, Harper & Row.

Knight, K.: Ankle rehabilitation with cryotherapy, Phys. Sportsmed. 7(11):133, 1979.

Kowal, M.: Review of physiological effects of cryotherapy, J. Orthop. Sports Phys. Ther. 6(2):66–73, 1953.

Kramer, J., Mendryk, S.: Cold in the initial treatment of injuries sustained in physical activity programs, Can. Assoc. Health Phys. Ed. Rec. J. 45(4):27–29, 38–40, 1979.

Krusen, E.: Effects of hot packs on peripheral circulation, Arch. Phys. Med. Rehabil. 31:145, 1950.

Landen, B.: Heat or cold for the relief of low back pain? Phys. Ther. 47:1126, 1967.

Lane, L.: Localized hypothermia for the relief of pain in musculoskeletal injuries, Phys. Ther. 51:182, 1971.

Lee, J., Warren, M., and Mason, S.: Effects of ice on nerve conduction velocity, Physiotherapy 64:2, 1978.

Lehmann, J.: Effect of therapeutic temperatures on tendon extensibility, Arch. Phys. Med. Rehabil. 51:481, 1970.

Lehmann, J., Brurmer, G., and Stow, R.: Pain threshold measurements after therapeutic application of ultrasound, microwaves and infrared, Arch. Phys. Med. Rehabil. 39:560, 1958.

Lehmann, J., Silverman, J., and Baum, B.: Temperature distributions in the human thigh produced by infrared, hot pack and microwave applications, Arch. Phys. Med. Rehabil. 41:291, 1966.

Levine, M., Kabat, H., and Knott, M.: Relaxation of spasticity by physiological techniques, Arch. Phys. Med. Rehabil. 35:214, 1954.

Levy, A., Marmar, E.: The role of cold compression dressings in the postoperative treatment of total knee arthroplasty, Clin. Orthop. Rel. Res. (297):174–178, 1993.

Lundgren, C., Muren, A., and Zederfeldt, B.: Effect of cold vasoconstriction on wound healing in the rabbit, Acta Chir. Scand. 118:1, 1959.

Magness, J., Garrett, T., and Erickson, D.: Swelling of the upper extremity during whirlpool baths, Arch. Phys. Med. Rehabil. 51:297, 1970.

Major, T., Schwingharner, J., and Winston, S.: Cutaneous and skeletal muscle vascular responses to hypothermia, Am J. Physiol. 240 (Heart Circ. Physiol. 9):H868, 1981.

Marek, I., Jezdinsky, J., and Ochonsky, P.: Effects of local cold and heat therapy on traumatic oedema of the rat hind paw. II. Effects of various kinds of compresses on the course of traumatic oedema. Acta Universitatis Palackianae Olomucensis Facultatis Medicae 66:203, 1973.

Matsen, F., Questad, K., and Matsen, A.: The effect of local cooling on post fracture swelling, Clin. Orthop. 109:201, 1975.

McDowell, J., McFarland, E., and Nalli, B.: Use of cryotherapy for orthopaedic patients, Orthop. Nurs. 13(5):21–30, 1994.

McGowen, H.: Effects of cold application on maximal isometric contraction, Phys. Ther. 47:185, 1967.

McGray, R., Patton, N.: Pain relief at trigger points: a comparison of moist heat and shortwave diathermy, J. Orthop. Sports Phys. Ther. 5:175, 1984.

McMaster, W.: Cryotherapy, Phys. Sportsmed. 10(11):112–119, 1982.

McMaster, W., Liddie, S.: Cryotherapy influence on posttraumatic limb edema, Clin. Orthop. 150:283–287, 1980.

McMaster, W., Liddie, S., and Waugh, T.: Laboratory evaluation of various cold therapy modalities, Am. J. Sports Med. 6(5): 291–294, 1978.

Mense, S.: Effects of temperature on the discharges of muscle spindles and tendon organs, Pflugers Arch. 374:159, 1978.

Mermel, J.: The therapeutic use of cold, J. Am. Osteopath. Assoc. 74:1146–1157, 1975.

Michalski, W., Sequin, J.: The effects of muscle cooling and stretch on muscle spindle secondary endings in the cat, J. Physiol. 253:341–356, 1975.

Michlovitz, S.: Thermal agents in rehabilitation, Philadelphia, 1995, F.A. Davis.

Miglietta, O.: Action of cold on spasticity, Am. J. Phys. Med. 52(4):198–205, 1973.

Newton, T., Lchnikuhi, D.: Muscle spindle response to body heating and localized muscle cooling: implications for relief of spasticity, J. Am. Phys. Ther. Assoc. 45(2):91, 105, 1965.

Noonan, T., Best, T., and Seaber, A.: Thermal effects on skeletal muscle tensile behavior, Am. J. Sports Med. 21(4):517–522, 1993.

Nylin, J.: The use of water in therapeutics, Arch. Phys. Med. Rehabil. 13:261, 1932.

Oliver, R., Johnson, D., and Wheelhouse, W.: Isometric muscle contraction response during recovery from reduced intramuscular temperature, Arch. Phys. Med. Rehabil. 60:126–129, 1979.

Panus, P., Carroll, J., and Gilbert, R.: Gender-dependent responses in humans to dry and wet cryotherapy, Phys. Ther. 74(5):S156, 1994.

Perkins, J., Mao-Chih, L., and Nicholas, C.: Cooling and contraction of smooth muscle, Am J. Physiol. 163:14, 1950.

Petajan, H., Watts, N.: Effects of cooling on the triceps surae reflex, Am. J. Phys. Med. 42:240–251, 1962.

Pope, C.: Physiologic action and therapeutic value of general and local whirlpool baths, Arch. Phys. Med. Rehabil. 10:498, 1929.

Preston, D., Irrgang, J., Bullock, A.: Effect of cold and compression on swelling following ACL reconstruction, J. Ath. Train. 28(2):166, 1993.

Price, R.: Influence of muscle cooling on the vasoelastic response of the human ankle to sinusoidal displacement, Arch. Phys. Med. Rehabil. 71(10):745–748, 1990.

Price, R., Lehmann, J., Boswell, S.: Influence of cryotherapy, on spasticity at the human ankle, Arch. Phys. Med. Rehabil. 74(3):300–304, 1993.

Randall, B., Imig, C., and Hines, H.: Effects of some physical therapies on blood flow, Arch. Phys. Med. Rehabil. 33:73, 1952.

Randt, G.: Hot tub folliculitis, Phys. Sports Med. 11:75, 1983.

Ritzmann, S., Levin, W.: Cryopathies: a review, Arch. Intern. Med. 107:186, 1961.

Roberts, P.: Hydrotherapy: its history, theory and practice, Occup. Health 235:5, 1981.

Schaubel, H.: Local use of ice after orthopedic procedures, Am. J. Surg. 72:711, 1946.

Schultz, K.: The effect of active exercise during whirlpool on the band, unpublished thesis. San Jose, California, 1982, San Jose State University.

Shelley, W., Caro, W.: Cold erythema: a new hypersensitivity syndrome, JAMA 180:639, 1962.

Simonetti, A., Miller, R., and Gristina, J.: Efficacy of povidone-iodine in the disinfection of whirlpool baths and hubbard tanks, Phys. Ther. 52:450, 1972.

Steve, L., Goodhart, P., and Alexander, J.: Hydrotherapy burn treatment: use of chloramine-T against resistant microorganisms, Arch. Phys. Med. Rehabil. 60:301, 1979.

Stewart, B., Basmajian, J.: Exercises in water. In Basmaiian, J., editor: Therapeutic exercise, ed. 3, Baltimore, 1978, Williams & Wilkins.

Streator, S., Ingersoll, C., Knight, K.: The effects of sensory information on the perception of cold-induced pain, J. Ath. Train. 29(2):166, 1994.

Strandness, D.: Vascular diseases of the extremities. In Isselbacher, K., Adams, R., and Braunwald, E., editors: Harrison's principles of internal medicine, ed. 9, New York, 1980, McGraw-Hill.

Taber, C., Contryman, K., and Fahrenbach, J.: Measurement of reactive vasodilation during cold gel pack application to non-traumatized ankles, Phys. Ther.72:294, 1992.

Travell, J., Simons, D.: Myofascial pain and dysfunction: the trigger point manual, Baltimore, 1983, Williams & Wilkins.

Urbscheit, N., Johnston, R., and Bishop, B.: Effects of cooling on the ankle jerk and H-response in hemiplegic patients, Phys. Ther. 51:983, 1971.

Wakim, K., Porter, A., and Krusen, K.: Influence of physical agents and of certain drugs on intra-articular temperature, Arch. Phys. Med. Rehabil. 32:714, 1951.

Walsh, M.: Relationship of band edema to upper extremity position and water temperature during whirlpool treatments in normals, Unpublished thesis. Philadelphia, 1983, Temple University.

Warren, G.: The use of heat and cold in the treatment of common musculoskeletal disorders. In Kessler, R., Hertling, D.: Management of common musculoskeletal disorders, Philadelphia, 1983, Harper & Row.

Warren, G., Lehmann, J., and Koblanski, N.: Heat and stretch procedures: an evaluation using rat tail tendon, Arch. Phys. Med. Rehabil. 57:122, 1976.

Watkins, A.: A manual of electrotherapy, ed. 3, Philadelphia, 1972, Lea & Febiger.

Waylonis, G.: The physiological effect of ice massage, Arch. Phys. Med. Rehabil. 48:37–42, 1967.

Weinberger, A., Lev, A.: Temperature elevation of connective tissue by physical modalities, Crit. Rev. Phys. Rehabil. Med. 3:121, 1991.

Wessman, M., Kottke, F.: The effect of indirect heating on peripheral blood flow, pulse rate, blood pressure and temperature, Arch. Phys. Med. Rehabil. 48:567, 1967.

Whitelaw, G., DeMuth, K., and Demos H.: The use of the Cryo/Cuff versus ice and elastic wrap in the postoperative care of knee arthroscopy patients, Am. J. Knee Surg. 8(1):28–30, 1995.

Whitney, S.: Physical agents: heat and cold modalities. In Scully, R., Barnes, M., editors: Physical therapy, Philadelphia, 1987, J.B. Lippincott.

Whyte, H., Reader, S.: Effectiveness of different forms of heating, Ann. Rheum. Dis. 10:449, 1951.

Wickstrom, R., Polk, C.: Effect of whirlpool on the strength endurance of the quadriceps muscle in trained male adolescents, Am. J. Phys. Med. 40:91, 1961.

Wilkerson, G.: Treatment of inversion ankle sprain through synchronous application of focal compression and cold, Ath. Train. 26:220, 1991.

Wolf, S., Basmajian, J.: Intramuscular temperature changes deep to localized cutaneous cold stimulation, Phys. Ther. 53(12):1284–1288, 1973.

Wolf, S., Ledbetter, W.: Effect of skin cooling on spontaneous EMG activity in triceps surae of the decerebrate cat, Brain Res. 91:151–155, 1975.

Wright, V., Johns, R.: Physical factors concerned with the stiffness of normal and diseased joints, Bull. Johns Hopkins Hosp. 106:215, 1960.

Wyper, D., McNiven, D.: Effects of some physiotherapeutic agents on skeletal muscle blood flow, Physiotherapy 62:83, 1976.

Yackzan, L., Adams, C., and Francis, K.: The effects of ice massage in delayed muscle soreness, Am. J. Sports Med. 12(2):159–165, 1984.

Zankel, H.: Effect of physical agents on motor conduction velocity of the ulnar nerve, Arch. Phys. Med. Rehabil. 47:787, 1966.

Zeiter, V.: Clinical application of the paraffin bath, Arch. Phys. Ther. 20:469, 1939.

Zislis, J.: Hydrotherapy. In Krusen, F., editor: Handbook of physical medicine and rehabilitation, ed. 2, Philadelphia, 1971, W.B. Saunders.

GLOSSARY

analgesia Loss of sensibility to pain.

anesthesia Loss of sensation.

conduction Heat loss or gain through direct contact.

congestion Presence of an abnormal amount of blood in the vessels resulting from an increase in blood flow or obstructed venous return.

consensual heat vasodilation Vasodilation and increased blood flow will spread to remote areas, causing increased metabolism in the unheated area.

contrast bath Hot (106°F) and cold (50°F) treatments in a combined sequence to stimulate superficial capillary vasodilation or vasoconstriction.

convection Heat loss or gain through the movement of water molecules across the skin.

conversion Changing from one energy form into another.

cryokinetics The use of cold and exercise in the treatment of pathology or disease.

cryotherapy The use of cold in the treatment of pathology or diseases.

edema Excessive fluid in cells.

erythema Redness of the skin.

fluidotherapy A modality of dry heat using a finely divided solid suspended in a stream with the properties of liquid.

hunting response A reflex vasodilation that occurs in response to cold approximately 15 minutes into the treatment. This has been demonstrated to be only an increase in temperature and not necessarily a change in blood flow.

hydrocollator A synthetic hot (170°F) or cold (0°F) gel used as an adjunctive modality to stimulate a rise or fall in tissue temperature.

hydrotherapy Cryotherapy and thermotherapy techniques that use water as the medium for heat transfer.

hyperemia Presence of an increased amount of blood in part of the body.

inflammation A redness of the skin caused by capillary dilation.

indication The reason to prescribe a remedy or procedure.

infrared That portion of the electromagnetic spectrum associated with thermal changes; located adjacent to the red portion of the visible light spectrum. That part of the electromagnetic spectrum dealing with infrared wavelengths.

metabolites Waste products of metabolism or catabolism.

myofascial pain A type of referred pain associated with trigger points.

nutrients Essential or nonessential food substance.

paraffin bath A combined paraffin and mineral oil immersion technique in which the paraffin substance is heated to 126°F for conductive heat gains; commonly used on the hands and feet for distal temperature gains in blood flow and temperature.

radiation The process of emitting energy from some source, in the form of waves. A method of heat transfer through which heat can either be gained or lost.

thermal Pertaining to heat.

thermopane An insulating layer of water next to the skin.

thermotherapy The use of heat in the treatment of pathology or disease.

vasoconstriction Narrowing of the blood vessels.

vasodilation Dilation of the blood vessels.

LAB ACTIVITY

HOT PACKS

DESCRIPTION:

Commercially available hot packs ("hydrocollator packs") are usually a canvas cover filled with a hydrophilic substance such as bentonite. Hot packs are kept in a commercial water-filled container that maintains a temperature of approximately 71°C. The packs are wrapped in six to eight layers of dry towels to protect the patient from burns; commercial hot pack covers provide approximately four thicknesses of toweling. After use, the hot pack should be returned to the cabinet for at least 30 minutes to insure reheating. Hot packs provide only superficial heating; the maximum depth of therapeutic heating is only about 1 cm, and occurs within 10 minutes of application.

PHYSIOLOGIC EFFECTS:

Vasodilation
Decreased pain perception
Increased local metabolism
Increased connective tissue plasticity
Decreased isometric strength (transient)

THERAPEUTIC EFFECTS:

Decreased pain
Increased soft tissue extensibility

INDICATIONS:

The principal indication for a hot pack is to provide therapeutic warming of superficial tissues. Tissues that are deeper than 1 cm do not reach a therapeutic temperature range of 30 to 40°C. Therefore, if the target tissue is deeper than 1 cm (e.g., the spinal facet joints), a hot pack will not be effective. Other joints, such as the knee, wrist, and ankle, can be effectively heated with a hot pack.

The primary therapeutic effect of superficial heating is to increase the ability of the collagen to remodel. Therefore, heating the tissue is beneficial following a period of reduced mobility if the soft tissue has shortened. In addition, the tissue viscosity is reduced, resulting in a greater ease of motion through the available range of motion. Although generally not a problem, in case of extreme pressure sensitivity, the weight of a hot pack may be more than the patient can tolerate. In these cases, Fluidotherapy or a warm whirlpool may be helpful.

CONTRAINDICATIONS:

- Lack of normal temperature sensibility
- Peripheral vascular disease with compromised circulation
- Over tumors

HOT PACKS

PROCEDURE	Evaluation		
	1	2	3
1. Check supplies.			
a. Obtain dry towels to wrap hot pack in, sheet or towels for draping, timer, signaling device.			
b. Check cabinet for appropriate temperature.			
2. Question patient.			
a. Verify identity of patient (if not already verified).			
b. Verify the absence of contraindications.			
c. Ask about previous thermotherapy treatments, check treatment notes.			
3. Position patient.			
a. Place patient in a well-supported, comfortable position.			
b. Expose body part to be treated.			
c. Drape patient to preserve patient's modesty, protect clothing, but allow access to body part.			
4. Inspect body part to be treated.			
a. Check light touch perception.			
b. Check circulatory status (pulses, capillary refill).			
c. Verify that there are no open wounds or rashes.			
d. Assess function of body part (e.g., ROM, irritability).			
5. Apply hot pack.			
a. Wrap hot pack in towels to provide six to eight layers of towel between the hot pack and the patient. If using a commercial hot pack cover, use at least one layer of towel to keep the cover clean.			
b. Inform the patient that you are going to put the hot pack on the body part to be treated, then do so.			
c. Set a timer for the appropriate treatment time and give the patient a signaling device. Make sure the patient understands how to use the signaling device.			
d. Check the patient's response after the first 5 minutes by asking the patient how it feels as well as visually checking the area under the hot pack. If the area is blotchy, additional toweling may be needed. Recheck verbally about every 5 minutes. A visual inspection every 5 minutes is not inappropriate.			
6. Complete the treatment.			
a. When the treatment time is over, remove the hot pack and dry the area with a towel.			
b. Remove material used for draping, assist the patient in dressing as needed.			
c. Have the patient perform appropriate therapeutic exercise as indicated.			
d. Clean the treatment area and equipment according to normal protocol.			
7. Assess treatment efficacy.			
a. Ask the patient how the treated area feels.			
b. Visually inspect the treated area for any adverse reactions.			
c. Perform functional tests as indicated.			

LAB ACTIVITY

PARAFFIN BATH

DESCRIPTION:

Paraffin baths consist of dipping and removing or immersing the body part in a mixture of wax and mineral oil. The ratio of wax and mineral oil is about 7 to 1, which results in a substance with a melting point of about 47.8°C, a specific heat of about 0.65 cal $\cdot$ g^{-1} $\cdot$ °C^{-1}, and a therapeutic temperature range of 48 to 54°C. Because of the low specific heat, much higher temperatures can be tolerated than if water is used. The paraffin is kept in a thermostatically controlled cabinet.

Paraffin provides a superficial heat, with a depth of therapeutic heating of about 1 cm. However, because paraffin is generally used only for the hands and feet, the depth of penetration is adequate to warm these joints to a therapeutic range.

The two basic techniques of application of paraffin involve repeated dipping of the body part in the mixture, then covering the body part with plastic and toweling. The advantage of this method is that the body part can then be elevated, reducing the potential for swelling. The second method involves dipping the body part in the paraffin once, letting it dry for a few seconds, then immersing the body part for the duration of the treatment. The advantage of this technique is that the source of heat is constant, so the therapeutic temperature can be maintained for a longer period.

PHYSIOLOGIC EFFECTS:

Vasodilation
Decreased pain perception
Increased local metabolism
Increased connective tissue plasticity
Decreased isometric strength (transient)

THERAPEUTIC EFFECTS:

Decreased pain
Increased soft tissue extensibility

INDICATIONS:

The principal indication for a paraffin bath is to provide therapeutic warming of superficial tissues. This is particularly effective in the hands and feet following a period of immobilization. The increased connective tissue plasticity that occurs with warming will enhance the effectiveness of therapeutic exercise.

Paraffin baths are also helpful in alleviation of pain caused by arthritic changes in the hands and feet. Caution should be exercised in using paraffin (or any heating agent) during an acute phase of arthritic pain and swelling.

CONTRAINDICATIONS:

- Lack of normal temperature sensibility
- Peripheral vascular disease with compromised circulation
- Over tumors

PARAFFIN BATH

PROCEDURE	Evaluation		
	1	2	3
1. Check supplies.			
a. Obtain plastic bag and towels to wrap body part in, timer, signaling device.			
b. Check cabinet for appropriate temperature.			
2. Question patient.			
a. Verify identity of patient (if not already verified).			
b. Verify the absence of contraindications.			
c. Ask about previous thermotherapy treatments; check treatment notes.			
3. Prepare patient.			
a. Have patient remove all jewelry from body part, wash well and dry thoroughly.			
b. Explain to the patient that after dipping the body part into the paraffin, there should be no movement of the body part for the duration of the treatment.			
4. Inspect body part to be treated.			
a. Check light touch perception.			
b. Check circulatory status (pulses, capillary refill).			
c. Verify that there are no open wounds or rashes.			
d. Assess function of body part (e.g., ROM, irritability).			
5. Apply paraffin.			
a. Guide the body part into the paraffin, making sure the patient does not contact the bottom of the cabinet or the heating coils.			
b. After 2 or 3 seconds, remove the body part, and keep it above the paraffin so that none of the paraffin drips onto the floor. Reimmerse the body part, and repeat until the appropriate number of dips have been completed, or reimmerse for the duration of the treatment.			
c. Set a timer for the appropriate treatment time and give the patient a signaling device. Make sure the patient understands how to use the signaling device.			
d. Check the patient's response after the first 5 minutes by asking the patient how it feels. Recheck verbally about every 5 minutes.			
6. Complete the treatment.			
a. When the treatment time is over, remove the towel and plastic bag. Help the patient remove the paraffin, and either return the paraffin to the cabinet, or throw away according to local protocol.			
b. Have the patient thoroughly wash and dry the body part.			
c. Have the patient perform appropriate therapeutic exercise as indicated.			
d. Clean the treatment area and equipment according to normal protocol.			
7. Assess treatment efficacy.			
a. Ask the patient how the treated area feels.			
b. Visually inspect the treated area for any adverse reactions.			
c. Perform functional tests as indicated.			

LAB ACTIVITY

INFRARED LAMPS

DESCRIPTION:

Infrared lamps provide superficial (1 ml or less) heating. Because of the extremely limited penetration, they are not capable of elevating connective tissue temperatures to a therapeutic level. Therefore, their primary effect is one of mild analgesia, and their use is very limited.

PHYSIOLOGIC EFFECTS:

Cutaneous vasodilation
Decreased pain perception

THERAPEUTIC EFFECTS:

Decreased pain

INDICATIONS:

The principal indication for infrared lamp heating is localized pain. Elevation of skin temperature may decrease the perception of pain for a short time.

CONTRAINDICATIONS:

- Lack of normal temperature sensibility
- Peripheral vascular disease with compromised circulation
- Over tumors

INFRARED LAMPS			
PROCEDURE	Evaluation		
	1	2	3
1. Check supplies.			
a. Obtain sheet or towels for draping, timer, signaling device.			
b. Check lamp for frayed power cords, integrity of lamp and shields, and so on.			
2. Question patient.			
a. Verify identity of patient (if not already verified).			
b. Verify the absence of contraindications.			
c. Ask about previous thermotherapy treatments, check treatment notes.			
3. Position patient.			
a. Place patient in a well-supported, comfortable position.			
b. Expose body part to be treated, have patient remove all jewelry from the area.			
c. Drape patient to preserve patient's modesty, protect clothing, but allow access to body part.			

PROCEDURE	Evaluation		
	1	2	3
4. Inspect body part to be treated.			
a. Check light touch perception.			
b. Check circulatory status (pulses, capillary refill).			
c. Verify that there are no open wounds or rashes.			
d. Assess function of body part (e.g., ROM, irritability).			
5. Apply infrared light.			
a. Position lamp such that the bulb is parallel to the body part being treated (such that the energy will strike the body at a 90° angle), and is 45 to 60 cm away from the patient. Measure and record the distance from the lamp to the closest part of the body being treated.			
b. Inform the patient that they should feel only a mild warmth; if it is hot, they should inform you. Start the lamp.			
c. Set a timer for the appropriate treatment time and give the patient a signaling device. Make sure the patient understands how to use the signaling device.			
d. Check the patient's response after the first 5 minutes by asking the patient how it feels as well as visually checking the area being treated. Recheck visually and verbally about every 5 minutes.			
6. Complete the treatment.			
a. When the treatment time is over, move the lamp away from the patient; dry the area with a towel. Turn the intensity control to zero.			
b. Remove material used for draping, assist the patient in dressing as needed.			
c. Have the patient perform appropriate therapeutic exercise as indicated.			
d. Clean the treatment area and equipment according to normal protocol.			
7. Assess treatment efficacy.			
a. Ask the patient how the treated area feels.			
b. Visually inspect the treated area for any adverse reactions.			
c. Perform functional tests as indicated.			

LAB ACTIVITY

ICE MASSAGE

DESCRIPTION:

Ice massage is performed by rubbing a small area of the body with a block of ice until superficial anesthesia is achieved. The block of ice is produced by filling and then freezing a cup of water at a temperature of no colder than $-5°C$. Styrofoam cups are often recommended, but the chunks of styrofoam that are removed from the cup during the treatment tend to be messy. Freezing water in empty juice cans, with a tongue depressor for a handle, are sometimes used, but the tongue depressor may abrade the skin during the treatment. The ideal cup is a waxed paper cup; the wax provides some insulation to keep your hand warm, and half the cup can be torn away in a single piece. The bottom of the cup should be removed, not the top. This permits the cup to act as a funnel, and keeps the ice from slipping out of the cup.

PHYSIOLOGIC EFFECTS:

Vasoconstriction
Anesthesia
Decreased local metabolism
Decreased connective tissue elasticity

THERAPEUTIC EFFECTS:

Decreased or prevented swelling
Decreased pain
Decreased inflammation
Minimized secondary tissue damage

INDICATIONS:

The primary indication for ice massage is pain of musculoskeletal origin that is preventing the effective use of therapeutic exercise; for example, an individual with restricted ankle motion who is prevented from applying sufficient force to produce remodeling of the connective tissue owing to pain. Ice massage will decrease the pain enough to permit an effective stretch. However, care must be taken to avoid stressing the connective tissue too much; the anesthesia provided by the ice may allow an overly aggressive individual to produce a sprain or strain.

Ice massage is also useful to help prevent an increase in inflammation and swelling of a joint following a therapeutic exercise session. It is probably no more effective than an ice pack, but often provides a more profound anesthesia.

CONTRAINDICATIONS:

- Lack of normal temperature sensibility
- Cold hypersensitivity (urticaria or hemoglobinuria)
- Vasospastic disorders (e.g., Raynaud's disease)
- Coronary artery disease
- Hypertension

ICE MASSAGE

PROCEDURE	Evaluation		
	1	2	3
1. Check supplies.			
a. Obtain towel to absorb water as it melts, ice cube, sheet or towels for draping.			

PROCEDURE	Evaluation		
	1	2	3
b. Check freezer for appropriate temperature.			
2. Question patient.			
a. Verify identity of patient (if not already verified).			
b. Verify the absence of contraindications.			
c. Ask about previous cryotherapy treatments, check treatment notes.			
3. Position patient.			
a. Place patient in a well-supported, comfortable position.			
b. Expose body part to be treated.			
c. Drape patient to preserve patient's modesty, protect clothing, but allow access to body part.			
4. Inspect body part to be treated.			
a. Check light touch perception.			
b. Check circulatory status (pulses, capillary refill).			
c. Verify that there are no open wounds or rashes.			
d. Assess function of body part (e.g., ROM, irritability).			
5. Apply ice massage.			
a. Expose block of ice.			
b. Rub ice on hand to smooth rough edges.			
c. Warn the patient that you are going to put your cold hand on the body part to be treated, then do so.			
d. Remove your hand after 2 or 3 seconds, and warn the patient that you are going to put the ice on the body part to be treated, then do so.			
e. Begin rubbing the ice block in a circular motion on the body part being treated. Do not put additional pressure on the ice. Move the ice at about 5 to 7 cm per second. Do not let melted water run onto areas of the body that are not being treated.			
f. Check the patient's response verbally about every 2 minutes. Perform a visual check of the area continuously during the treatment. If wheals or welts appear, or if the skin color changes to absolute white within the first 4 minutes of treatment, stop the treatment. Remind the patient to tell you when the area is numb.			
6. Complete the treatment.			
a. When the patient tells you the area is numb, remove the ice and dry the area. Perform a test for light touch sensation to verify anesthesia.			
b. Remove material used for draping, assist the patient in dressing as needed. Place the unused ice in a sink, and the cup in the trash.			
c. Have the patient perform appropriate therapeutic exercise as indicated.			
d. Clean the treatment area and equipment according to normal protocol.			
7. Assess treatment efficacy.			
a. Ask the patient how the treated area feels.			
b. Visually inspect the treated area for any adverse reactions (e.g., wheals, welts).			
c. Perform functional tests as indicated.			

LAB ACTIVITY

ICE PACKS

DESCRIPTION:

An ice pack uses crushed ice at a temperature of 0 to −5°C. The ice may be placed in a plastic bag and wrapped in a wet towel or may be placed directly in a wet towel. The use of a plastic bag will minimize the potential mess from water dripping, but it may also decrease the conduction of thermal energy from the patient. A major advantage of an ice pack over a cold pack is that the ice pack can be almost any size and shape; therefore, an ice pack is useful for treating any body part.

PHYSIOLOGIC EFFECTS:

Vasoconstriction
Superficial anesthesia
Decreased local metabolism
Decreased connective tissue elasticity

THERAPEUTIC EFFECTS:

Decreased or prevented swelling
Decreased pain
Decreased inflammation
Decreased secondary tissue damage

INDICATIONS:

The primary indication for the use of an ice pack is in the acute phase of a soft tissue injury. The cooling of the injured area will help prevent the development of swelling and may assist in the resolution of swelling by altering the Starling-Landis forces at the capillary bed.

An ice pack is also useful to minimize or prevent increased inflammation or pain following a session of therapeutic exercise. The depth of anesthesia achieved with an ice pack is generally considerably less than with an ice massage.

CONTRAINDICATIONS:

- Lack of normal temperature sensibility
- Cold hypersensitivity (urticaria or hemoglobinuria)
- Vasospastic disorders (e.g., Raynaud's disease)
- Coronary artery disease
- Hypertension

ICE PACKS			
PROCEDURE	Evaluation		
	1	2	3
1. Check supplies.			
a. Obtain wet towel to wrap ice in, an appropriate amount of crushed ice, sheet, or towels for draping.			
b. Check freezer for appropriate temperature.			

PROCEDURE	Evaluation		
	1	2	3
2. Question patient.			
a. Verify identity of patient (if not already verified).			
b. Verify the absence of contraindications.			
c. Ask about previous cryotherapy treatments, check treatment notes.			
3. Position patient.			
a. Place patient in a well-supported, comfortable position.			
b. Expose body part to be treated.			
c. Drape patient to preserve patient's modesty, protect clothing, but allow access to body part.			
4. Inspect body part to be treated.			
a. Check light touch perception.			
b. Check circulatory status (pulses, capillary refill).			
c. Verify that there are no open wounds or rashes.			
d. Assess function of body part (e.g., ROM, irritability).			
5. Apply ice pack.			
a. Warn the patient that you are going to put the ice pack on the body part to be treated, then do so. Make sure the draping will catch any water that melts from the ice pack.			
b. Set a timer for the appropriate treatment time (generally about 20 minutes), and give the patient a signaling device. Make sure the patient understands how to use the signaling device.			
c. Check the patient's response verbally after the first 2 minutes, then about every 5 minutes. Perform a visual check of the area if the patient reports any unusual sensation. If wheals or welts appear, or if the skin color changes to absolute white within the first 4 minutes of treatment, stop the treatment.			
6. Complete the treatment.			
a. When the treatment time is over, remove the ice pack and dry the area with a towel.			
b. Remove material used for draping, assist the patient in dressing as needed.			
c. Dispose of the unmelted ice in a sink.			
d. Have the patient perform appropriate therapeutic exercise or apply tape or compression wrap as indicated.			
e. Clean the treatment area and equipment according to normal protocol.			
7. Assess treatment efficacy.			
a. Ask the patient how the treated area feels.			
b. Visually inspect the treated area for any adverse reactions (e.g., wheals, welts).			
c. Perform functional tests as indicated.			

LAB ACTIVITY

COLD PACKS

DESCRIPTION:

Commercially available cold packs are usually a vinyl cover filled with a gel that does not solidify at low temperatures. Cooling units designed specifically for the cold packs are available, but they may be kept in a household-type freezer. The temperature of the freezer should be 0 to −5°C. Packs are available in various sizes, including one designed to encircle the cervical region. The packs are generally wrapped in a wet towel to increase the thermal conductivity from the patient.

PHYSIOLOGIC EFFECTS:

Vasoconstriction
Superficial anesthesia
Decreased local metabolism
Decreased connective tissue elasticity

THERAPEUTIC EFFECTS:

Decreased or prevented swelling
Decreased pain
Decreased inflammation
Decreased secondary tissue damage

INDICATIONS:

The primary indication for the use of a cold pack is in the acute phase of a soft tissue injury. The cooling of the injured area will help prevent the development of swelling and may assist in the resolution of swelling by altering the Starling-Landis forces at the capillary bed.

A cold pack is also useful to minimize or prevent increased inflammation or pain following a session of therapeutic exercise. The depth of anesthesia achieved with a cold pack is generally considerably less than with an ice massage.

CONTRAINDICATIONS:

- Lack of normal temperature sensibility
- Cold hypersensitivity (urticaria or hemoglobinuria)
- Vasospastic disorders (e.g., Raynaud's disease)
- Coronary artery disease
- Hypertension

COLD PACKS

PROCEDURE	Evaluation		
	1	2	3
1. Check supplies.			
a. Obtain wet towel to wrap cold pack in, cold pack, sheet or towels for draping.			
b. Check freezer for appropriate temperature.			

PROCEDURE	Evaluation		
	1	2	3
2. Question patient.			
a. Verify identity of patient (if not already verified).			
b. Verify the absence of contraindications.			
c. Ask about previous cryotherapy treatments and check treatment notes.			
3. Position patient.			
a. Place patient in a well-supported, comfortable position.			
b. Expose body part to be treated.			
c. Drape patient to preserve patient's modesty, protect clothing, but allow access to body part.			
4. Inspect body part to be treated.			
a. Check light touch perception.			
b. Check circulatory status (pulses, capillary refill).			
c. Verify that there are no open wounds or rashes.			
d. Assess function of body part (e.g., ROM, irritability).			
5. Apply cold pack.			
a. Wrap cold pack in wet towel.			
b. Warn the patient that you are going to put the cold pack on the body part to be treated, then do so.			
c. Set a timer for the appropriate treatment time (generally about 20 minutes), and give the patient a signaling device. Make sure the patient understands how to use the signaling device.			
d. Check the patient's response verbally after the first 2 minutes, then about every 5 minutes. Perform a visual check of the area if the patient reports any unusual sensation. If wheals or welts appear, or if the skin color changes to absolute white within the first 4 minutes of treatment, stop the treatment.			
6. Complete the treatment.			
a. When the treatment time is over, remove the cold pack and dry the area with a towel.			
b. Remove material used for draping, assist the patient in dressing as needed.			
c. Have the patient perform appropriate therapeutic exercise or apply tape or compression wrap as indicated.			
d. Clean the treatment area and equipment according to normal protocol.			
7. Assess treatment efficacy.			
a. Ask the patient how the treated area feels.			
b. Visually inspect the treated area for any adverse reactions (e.g., wheals, welts).			
c. Perform functional tests as indicated.			

LAB ACTIVITY

VAPOCOOLANT SPRAY

DESCRIPTION:

Vapocoolant sprays, such as Fluori-Methane and ethyl chloride, are liquids that are sprayed on the skin. Thermal energy from the body is absorbed by the liquids, which have low boiling points; therefore, the liquid almost immediately evaporates. As it evaporates, thermal energy is removed from the body, resulting in a superficial cooling.

Fluori-Methane, a mixture of 85% trichloromonofluoromethane and 15% dichlorodifluoromethane, is not flammable and is nontoxic. Ethyl chloride is flammable, and therefore is not recommended for use.

PHYSIOLOGIC EFFECTS:

Superficial anesthesia

THERAPEUTIC EFFECTS:

Inhibition of painful trigger points
Decrease in pain with stretching musculotendinous tissue

INDICATIONS:

Vapocoolant sprays are used mostly for the treatment of trigger points and for stretching of tight musculotendinous tissue. Trigger points are a poorly understood phenomenon, but many pain syndromes are ascribed to active trigger points. Two relatively common treatments for trigger points are deep friction massage (similar to vigorous acupressure) and stretching of the muscle the trigger point is located within. Because direct pressure on and stretching of the trigger points is painful, the area can be sprayed with a vapocoolant to decrease the pain during the treatment.

In a similar manner, if a musculotendinous strain has resulted in a loss of range of motion, spraying the skin over the injured muscle may decrease the pain perception while the therapist stretches the body part. Care must be taken to not overstretch the tissue and produce further injury.

CONTRAINDICATIONS:

- Lack of normal temperature sensibility
- Cold hypersensitivity (urticaria or hemoglobinuria)
- Vasospastic disorders (e.g., Raynaud's disease)

VAPOCOOLANT SPRAY

PROCEDURE	Evaluation		
	1	2	3
1. Check supplies.			
a. Obtain vapocoolant.			
b. Obtain toweling or other draping materials needed.			
2. Question patient.			
a. Verify identity of patient (if not already verified).			
b. Verify the absence of contraindications.			
c. Ask about previous cryotherapy treatments, check treatment notes.			

PROCEDURE	Evaluation		
	1	2	3
3. Position patient.			
a. Place patient in a well-supported, comfortable position.			
b. Expose body part to be treated.			
c. Drape patient to preserve patient's modesty, protect clothing, but allow access to body part.			
4. Inspect body part to be treated.			
a. Check light touch perception.			
b. Check circulatory status (pulses, capillary refill).			
c. Verify that there are no open wounds or rashes.			
d. Assess function of body part (e.g., ROM, irritability).			
5. Apply vapocoolant.			
a. Position body part such that the area to be treated is on a stretch.			
b. Protect the patient's eyes and insure the patient does not inhale fumes.			
c. Holding the vapocoolant upside down, with the nozzle at about a 30° angle from the perpendicular with the skin, and about 45 cm from the skin, spray the skin from distal to proximal.			
d. Spray in one direction only 3 to 4 times, then apply direct pressure or increased stretch as indicated and tolerated by the patient. Repeat the procedure as needed after the skin has rewarmed.			
e. Check the patient's response frequently during the treatment.			
6. Complete treatment.			
a. On attainment of the desired therapeutic effect (or up to 4 repetitions of spray-and-stretch or pressure or to patient tolerance), inspect the treated body part for adverse reactions.			
b. Remove draping materials, assist the patient in dressing as needed.			
c. If further therapeutic exercise is indicated, instruct the patient to perform it.			
d. Clean the treatment area and equipment according to normal protocol.			
7. Assess treatment efficacy.			
a. Ask the patient how the treated area feels.			
b. Visually inspect the treated area for any adverse reactions (e.g., wheals, welts).			
c. Perform functional tests as indicated.			

LAB ACTIVITY

WARM WHIRLPOOL

DESCRIPTION:

A whirlpool is a tank filled with water of a particular temperature, depending on the desired therapeutic effect. The tank also contains a turbine or pump that creates convection currents in the water. Although water that is any temperature above the temperature of the body surface could be considered "warm," generally water at 35 to 43°C is used. If the entire body is to be immersed, temperatures above 38°C should not be used to avoid interference with thermoregulation. The use of the turbine avoids the development of a layer of cooler water adjacent to the body part, thus producing more uniform warming. Because of the dependent position of the body part in the whirlpool and the increased temperature of the body part, a warm whirlpool may increase soft tissue swelling; even in noninjured limbs, there may be a considerable increase in interstitial fluid following a warm whirlpool.

Because the turbine is powered by electricity, it is generally prudent to not let the patient touch any part of the turbine. Also, patients should not be left in the whirlpool unattended; this is true whether the entire body or only a limb is immersed.

PHYSIOLOGIC EFFECTS:

Vasodilation
Decreased pain perception
Increased local metabolism
Increased connective tissue plasticity
Decreased isometric strength (transient)

THERAPEUTIC EFFECTS:

Decreased pain
Increased soft tissue extensibility
Sedative

INDICATIONS:

The principal indication for a warm whirlpool is to provide therapeutic warming of a larger area of the body than can be achieved readily with a hot pack. The effective depth of therapeutic heating is the same at approximately 1 cm. In addition, the patient can perform active exercise during the application, or the therapist can perform joint mobilization on the injured limb while immersed in the water. Some therapists use whirlpool for cleaning a limb after removal of a cast; equally effective and at less cost is a shower.

The primary therapeutic effect of superficial heating is to increase the ability of the collagen to remodel. Therefore, heating the tissue is beneficial following a period of reduced mobility if the soft tissue has shortened. In addition, the tissue viscosity is reduced, resulting in a greater ease of motion through the available range of motion.

CONTRAINDICATIONS:

- Lack of normal temperature sensibility
- Peripheral vascular disease with compromised circulation
- Over tumors
- Coronary artery disease

WARM WHIRLPOOL

PROCEDURE	Evaluation		
	1	2	3
1. Check supplies and equipment.			
a. Obtain towels for padding the edge of the whirlpool tank, as well as for drying the treated part.			
b. Check temperature of tank before applying treatment.			
c. Position chair of correct height next to whirlpool.			
2. Question patient.			
a. Verify identity of patient (if not already verified).			
b. Verify the absence of contraindications.			
c. Ask about previous thermotherapy or whirlpool treatments, check treatment notes.			
3. Position patient.			
a. Have patient sit on chair with body part out of water.			
b. Expose body part to be treated.			
c. Drape patient to preserve patient's modesty, protect clothing, but allow access to body part.			
4. Inspect body part to be treated.			
a. Check light touch perception.			
b. Check circulatory status (pulses, capillary refill).			
c. Verify that there are no open wounds or rashes.			
d. Assess function of body part (e.g., ROM, irritability).			
5. Administer warm whirlpool.			
a. Pad edge of tank with toweling; ask patient to tell you if the water is too hot, then place body part in water.			
b. Instruct patient to keep away from all parts of the turbine.			
c. Turn on the turbine, adjust the aeration, agitation, and direction of the water being pumped.			
d. Check the patient's response verbally and visually about every 2 minutes. Remind the patient to tell you if the area starts hurting or if sensation is lost.			
6. Complete the treatment.			
a. Turn off the turbine at the completion of the treatment time.			
b. Remove the body part from the water and dry it off.			
c. Assist the patient in dressing as needed and instruct in therapeutic exercise as indicated.			
d. Clean the treatment area and equipment according to normal protocol.			
7. Assess treatment efficacy.			
a. Ask the patient how the treated area feels.			
b. Visually inspect the treated area for any adverse reactions (e.g., wheals, welts).			
c. Perform functional tests as indicated.			

LAB ACTIVITY

COLD WHIRLPOOL

DESCRIPTION:

A whirlpool is a tank filled with water of a particular temperature, depending on the desired therapeutic effect. The tank also contains a turbine or pump that creates convection currents in the water. Although water that is any temperature below the temperature of the body surface could be considered "cold," generally water at 10 to 16°C is used. Because water from the tap is rarely this cold, ice must be added to the tank. Crushed ice results in the most rapid cooling of the water, and all ice must be melted before the turbine is turned on. Using the turbine insures that a layer of warm water does not develop adjacent to the skin, thus providing a more effective cooling of the tissues. Because the limb is in a dependent position, any effect of the cooling on decreasing soft tissue swelling may be negated; using a compression bandage during the treatment may help in reducing the effects of dependency. As with a warm whirlpool, the patient should not be left unattended and should be warned against touching any part of the turbine.

PHYSIOLOGIC EFFECTS:

Vasoconstriction
Superficial anesthesia
Decreased local metabolism
Decreased connective tissue elasticity

THERAPEUTIC EFFECTS:

Decreased or prevented swelling
Decreased pain
Decreased inflammation
Decreased secondary tissue damage

INDICATIONS:

The principal indication for a cold whirlpool is to provide therapeutic cooling of a larger area of the body than can be achieved readily with an ice or cold pack. Also, irregularly shaped areas of the body can be treated with total contact. In addition, the patient can perform active exercise during the application, or the therapist can perform joint mobilization on the injured limb while immersed in the water.

In addition, use of a cold whirlpool may minimize inflammation and swelling following a therapeutic exercise session. The advantage of a cold whirlpool over an ice or cold pack is the greater area that can be treated; a disadvantage is the possibility of increased swelling when the limb is in a dependent position.

CONTRAINDICATIONS:

- Lack of normal temperature sensibility
- Cold hypersensitivity (urticaria or hemoglobinuria)
- Vasospastic disorders (e.g., Raynaud's disease)
- Coronary artery disease
- Hypertension

COLD WHIRPOOL

PROCEDURE	Evaluation		
	1	2	3
1. Check supplies and equipment.			
a. Obtain towels for padding the edge of the whirlpool tank, as well as for drying the treated part.			
b. Check temperature of tank, insure all ice is melted before applying treatment.			
c. Position chair of correct height next to whirlpool.			
2. Question patient.			
a. Verify identity of patient (if not already verified).			
b. Verify the absence of contraindications.			
c. Ask about previous cryotherapy or whirlpool treatments, check treatment notes.			
3. Position patient.			
a. Have patient sit on chair with body part out of water.			
b. Expose body part to be treated.			
c. Drape patient to preserve patient's modesty, protect clothing, but allow access to body part.			
4. Inspect body part to be treated.			
a. Check light touch perception.			
b. Check circulatory status (pulses, capillary refill).			
c. Verify that there are no open wounds or rashes.			
d. Assess function of body part (e.g., ROM, irritability).			
5. Administer cold whirlpool.			
a. Pad edge of tank with toweling, warn patient that the water is cold, then place body part in water.			
b. Instruct patient to keep away from all parts of the turbine.			
c. Turn on the turbine, adjust the aeration, agitation, and direction of the water being pumped.			
d. Check the patient's response verbally and visually about every 2 minutes. Remind the patient to tell you if the area starts hurting or if sensation is lost.			
6. Complete the treatment.			
a. Turn off the turbine at the completion of the treatment time.			
b. Remove the body part from the water and dry it off.			
c. Assist the patient in dressing as needed and instruct in therapeutic exercise as indicated.			
d. Clean the treatment area and equipment according to normal protocol.			
7. Assess treatment efficacy.			
a. Ask the patient how the treated area feels.			
b. Visually inspect the treated area for any adverse reactions (e.g., wheals, welts).			
c. Perform functional tests as indicated.			

LAB ACTIVITY

CONTRAST BATH

DESCRIPTION:

A contrast bath involves the alternating immersion of the involved body part in warm water and cold water. Usually, the wrist and hand or foot and ankle are treated, though the entire upper or lower member could be treated using two whirlpool tanks. The duration of immersion in each temperature water is variable, as is the number of times immersed during a single treatment session. A suggested sequence is to start with 3 minutes in warm, followed by 1 minute in cold, with the sequence repeated five times (e.g., 3W-1C-3W-1C-3W-1C-3W-1C-3W-1C); however, some therapists recommend starting and ending with warm water. The warm water should be 40 to 41°C, and the cold water 10 to 16°C.

PHYSIOLOGIC EFFECTS:

Alternating vasodilation and vasoconstriction

THERAPEUTIC EFFECTS:

Variable effects on swelling
Decreased pain

INDICATIONS:

Contrast baths are often used in the subacute and chronic stages of recovery. Most of the information regarding benefits of contrast baths is anecdotal; there is little research documenting the efficacy of this treatment.

CONTRAINDICATIONS:

- Lack of normal temperature sensibility
- Cold hypersensitivity (urticaria or hemoglobinuria)
- Vasospastic disorders (e.g., Raynaud's disease)

CONTRAST BATH

PROCEDURE	Evaluation		
	1	2	3
1. Check supplies and equipment.			
a. Obtain towels, containers, ice, timer, and so on.			
b. Check temperature of water in each container.			
2. Question patient.			
a. Verify identity of patient (if not already verified).			
b. Verify the absence of contraindications.			
c. Ask about previous cryotherapy or thermotherapy, treatments, check treatment notes.			
3. Position patient.			
a. Have patient sit in a comfortable position.			
b. Expose body part to be treated.			
c. Drape patient to preserve patient's modesty, protect clothing, but allow access to body part.			

PROCEDURE	Evaluation		
	1	2	3
4. Inspect body part to be treated.			
a. Check light touch perception.			
b. Check circulatory status (pulses, capillary refill).			
c. Verify that there are no open wounds or rashes.			
d. Assess function of body part (e.g., ROM, irritability).			
5. Administer contrast bath.			
a. Set timer for appropriate interval, help patient immerse body part fully into warm water; start timer.			
b. After the timer goes off, set it for the next interval. Warn patient that the cold water will feel very cold; help patient immerse body part fully into cold water; start timer.			
c. Continue the cycles until the treatment is complete. Usually, the patients can time each immersion themselves.			
d. Check the patient's response verbally and visually about every 2 minutes. Remind the patient to tell you if the area starts hurting or if sensation is lost.			
6. Complete the treatment.			
a. Remove the body part from the water and dry it off.			
b. Assist the patient in dressing as needed and instruct in therapeutic exercise as indicated.			
c. Clean the treatment area and equipment according to normal protocol.			
7. Assess treatment efficacy.			
a. Ask the patient how the treated area feels.			
b. Visually inspect the treated area for any adverse reactions (e.g., wheals, welts).			
c. Perform functional tests as indicated.			

LAB ACTIVITY

FLUIDOTHERAPY

DESCRIPTION:

Fluidotherapy is a device manufactured by Henley International of Sugarland, Texas. Heated air is forced through a container filled with cellulose particles; when heated, the cellulose takes on fluidlike characteristics. The body part to be treated is immersed in the cellulose particles, and the particles are circulated in the container, thus providing elevation of tissue temperature and a mechanical stimulation of the skin. The temperature of the unit is adjustable within a range of about 39 to 48°C.

There are several advantages to using Fluidotherapy to treat affected hands or feet. The source of heat is constant, so the tissue temperature can be maintained at a therapeutic level for the duration of the treatment. The body part can be exercised during the treatment, either actively or passively by the therapist. The mechanical stimulation of the skin with the cellulose particles may provide some analgesic effect and may help desensitize the injured area.

PHYSIOLOGIC EFFECTS:

Vasodilation
Decreased pain perception
Increased local metabolism
Increased connective tissue plasticity
Decreased isometric strength (transient)

THERAPEUTIC EFFECTS:

Decreased pain
Increased soft tissue extensibility

INDICATIONS:

The principal indication for Fluidotherapy is to provide therapeutic warming of a larger area of the body than can be achieved readily with a hot pack. In addition, the patient can perform active exercise during the application, or the therapist can perform joint mobilization on the injured limb while in the unit.

The primary therapeutic effect of superficial heating is to increase the ability of the collagen to remodel. Therefore, heating the tissue is beneficial following a period of reduced mobility if the soft tissue has shortened. In addition, the tissue viscosity is reduced, resulting in a greater ease of motion through the available range of motion.

CONTRAINDICATIONS:

- Lack of normal temperature sensibility
- Peripheral vascular disease with compromised circulation
- Over tumors
- Coronary artery disease

FLUIDOTHERAPY			
PROCEDURE	Evaluation		
	1	2	3
1. Check supplies and equipment.			
a. Obtain timer, signaling device, and so on.			
b. Check temperature of Fluidotherapy unit before applying treatment.			

PROCEDURE	Evaluation		
	1	2	3
c. Position chair of correct height next to unit.			
2. Question patient.			
a. Verify identity of patient (if not already verified).			
b. Verify the absence of contraindications.			
c. Ask about previous thermotherapy treatments, check treatment notes.			
3. Position patient.			
a. Have patient remove jewelry from area to be treated and thoroughly wash and dry area.			
b. Have patient sit on chair next to unit.			
c. Expose body part to be treated.			
d. Drape patient to preserve patient's modesty, protect clothing, but allow access to body part.			
4. Inspect body part to be treated.			
a. Check light touch perception.			
b. Check circulatory status (pulses, capillary refill).			
c. Verify that there are no open wounds or rashes.			
d. Assess function of body part (e.g., ROM, irritability).			
5. Administer Fluidotherapy.			
a. With the agitation off, open the sleeved portion of the unit.			
b. Instruct patient to insert body part into cellulose particles, reminding them to tell you if the temperature is too hot.			
c. Fasten the sleeve around the body part to prevent the cellulose particles from being blown out of the unit, and start the agitation.			
d. Check the patient's response verbally after about 5 minutes. Remind the patient to tell you if the heating sensation becomes uncomfortable.			
e. Instruct the patient in any indicated therapeutic exercise to be performed during the treatment.			
6. Complete the treatment.			
a. Turn off the agitation at the completion of the treatment time.			
b. Remove the body part from the unit, having the patient brush or shake off as much of the cellulose as possible.			
c. Assist the patient in dressing as needed and instruct in therapeutic exercise as indicated.			
d. Clean the treatment area and equipment according to normal protocol.			
7. Assess treatment efficacy.			
a. Ask the patient how the treated area feels.			
b. Visually inspect the treated area for any adverse reactions (e.g., wheals, welts).			
c. Perform functional tests as indicated.			

LAB ACTIVITY

PATIENT POSITIONING

DESCRIPTION:

The positioning of a patient prior to the application of a physical agent modality is one of the most important aspects contributing to a successful treatment. Placing the patient in an aligned and supported position insures muscular relaxation and facilitates venous flow of blood. Proper positioning allows the use of optimal body mechanics by the therapist in the application of the selected treatment.

THERAPEUTIC EFFECTS:

Muscular relaxation
Facilitated venous blood flow

PATIENT POSITIONING

PROCEDURE	Evaluation		
	1	2	3
1. Check supplies.			
a. Pillows			
b. Towels			
c. Sheets			
2. Question patient.			
a. Verify identity.			
b. Verify treatment area.			
3. Position patient.			
a. Prone on table.			
i. Place pillow under abdomen; lumbar spine should be flat.			
ii. Place pillow under ankles.			
iii. Insure proper body alignment.			
iv. Drape patient to maintain modesty.			
b. Supine.			
i. Place pillow under head and knees.			
ii. Insure proper body alignment.			
iii. Drape patient to maintain modesty.			
c. Sitting.			
i. Seat patient on chair or stool leaning forward.			
ii. Support head and shoulders with pillows.			
iii. Rest forearms and hands on table.			
iv. Insure proper body alignment.			
v. Drape patient to maintain modesty.			
4. Administer the treatment.			
5. Complete the treatment.			
6. Return equipment to storage after cleaning.			

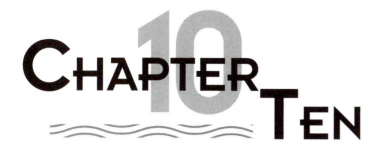

Chapter Ten

Therapeutic Ultrasound

DAVID O. DRAPER and
WILLIAM E. PRENTICE

OBJECTIVES

Following completion of this chapter the student therapist will be able to:

- ✓ Describe the transmission of acoustic energy in biologic tissues relative to waveforms, frequency, velocity, and attenuation.
- ✓ Discuss the basic physics involved in the production of a beam of therapeutic ultrasound.
- ✓ Discuss both the thermal and nonthermal physiologic effects of therapeutic ultrasound.
- ✓ Discuss specific techniques of application of therapeutic ultrasound and how they may be modified to achieve treatment goals.
- ✓ Identify the most appropriate and clinically effective uses for therapeutic ultrasound.
- ✓ Discuss the technique and clinical application of phonophoresis.
- ✓ Describe the contraindications and precautions that should be observed with therapeutic ultrasound.

In the medical community, ultrasound is a modality that is used for a number of different purposes, including diagnosis, destruction of tissue, and as a therapeutic agent. Diagnostic ultrasound has been used for more than 30 years for the purpose of imaging internal structures. Most typically, diagnostic ultrasound is used to image the fetus during pregnancy. Ultrasound has also been used to produce extreme tissue hyperthermia that has been demonstrated to have tumoricidal effects in cancer patients.

In clinical practice, ultrasound is one of the most widely used therapeutic modalities in addition to superficial heat and cold and electrical stimulating currents. It has been used for therapeutic purposes as a valuable tool in the rehabilitation of many different injuries primarily for the purpose of stimulating the repair of soft tissue injuries and for relief of pain.[30]

Ultrasound is one of the most widely used modalities in sports medicine

As discussed in Chapter 1, ultrasound is a form of acoustic rather than electromagnetic energy. Ultrasound is defined as inaudible, acoustic vibrations of high frequency that may produce either thermal or nonthermal physiologic effects.[43] The use of ultrasound as a therapeutic agent may be extremely effective if the therapist has an adequate understanding of its effects on biologic tissues and of the physical mechanisms by which these effects are produced.[30]

ULTRASOUND AS A THERMAL MODALITY

Ultrasound and diathermy = deep heating modalities

Ultrasound = acoustic energy

In Chapters 8 and 9, heat is discussed as a treatment modality. Warm whirlpools, paraffin baths, and hot packs, to name a few, all produce therapeutic heat. However, the depth of penetration of these modalities is superficial and at best only 1 to 2 cm.[72] Ultrasound, along with diathermy, has traditionally been classified as a "deep heating modality" and has been used primarily for the purpose of elevating tissue temperatures.

Suppose a patient is lacking dorsiflexion. It is determined through evaluation that a tight soleus is the problem, and as a therapist your desire is to use thermotherapy followed by stretching. Will superficial heat adequately prepare this muscle to be stretched? Since the soleus lies deep under the gastrocnemius muscle, it is beyond the reach of superficial heat.

One of the advantages of using ultrasound over other thermal modalities is that it can provide deep heating.[72] The heating effects of silicate gel hot packs and warm whirlpools have been compared with ultrasound. At an intramuscular depth of 3 cm, a 10-minute hot pack treatment yielded an increase of 0.8°C, whereas at this same depth, 1 MHz ultrasound has raised muscle temperature nearly 4°C in 10 minutes.[25,90] At 1 cm below the fat surface, a 4-minute warm whirlpool (40.6°C) raised the temperature 1.1°C; however, at this same depth, 3 MHz ultrasound raised the temperature 4°C in 4 minutes.[25,26,77]

TRANSMISSION OF ACOUSTIC ENERGY IN BIOLOGIC TISSUES

Unlike electromagnetic energy, which travels most effectively through a vacuum, acoustic energy relies on molecular collision for transmission. Molecules in a conducting medium will cause vibration and minimal displacement of other surrounding molecules when set into vibration, so that eventually this "wave" of vibration has propagated through the entire medium. Sound waves travel in a manner similar to waves created by a stone thrown into a pool of water. Ultrasound is a mechanical wave in which energy is transmitted by the vibrations of the molecules of the biologic medium through which the wave is traveling.[94]

TRANSVERSE VERSUS LONGITUDINAL WAVES

longitudinal wave The primary waveform in which ultrasound energy travels in soft tissue with the molecular displacement along the direction in which the wave travels.

transverse wave Occurring only in bone, the molecules are displaced in a direction perpendicular to the direction in which the ultrasound wave is moving.

There are two types of waves that can travel through a solid medium, **longitudinal** and **transverse waves.** In a longitudinal wave, the molecular displacement is along the direction in which the wave travels. Within this longitudinal wave pathway are regions of high molecular density referred to as **compressions** (the molecules are squeezed together) and regions of lower molecular density called **rarefactions** (the molecules spread out) (Fig. 10-1). This is much like the squeezing and spreading action when using a child's toy "slinky." In a transverse wave, the molecules are dis-

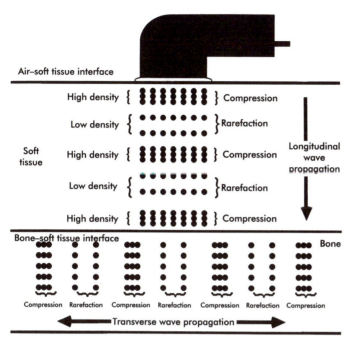

• **Figure 10-1** Ultrasound travels through soft tissue as a longitudinal wave alternating regions of high molecular density (compressions) and areas of low molecular density (rarefactions). Transverse waves are found primarily in bone.

placed in a direction perpendicular to the direction in which the wave is moving. Although longitudinal waves travel both in solids and liquids, transverse waves can travel only in solids. Since soft tissues are more like liquids, ultrasound travels primarily as a longitudinal wave; however, when it contacts bone a transverse wave results.[94]

rarefactions Regions of lower molecular density (i.e., a small amount of ultrasound energy) within a longitudinal wave.

FREQUENCY OF WAVE TRANSMISSION

The *frequency* of audible sound ranges between 16 KHz and 20 KHz (kilohertz = 1000 cycles per second). Ultrasound has a frequency above 20 KHz. The frequency range for therapeutic ultrasound is between 0.75 and 3 MHz (megahertz = 1,000,000 cycles per second). The higher the frequency of the sound waves emitted from a sound source, the less the sound will diverge and thus a more focused beam of sound is produced. In biologic tissues, the lower the frequency of the sound waves the greater the depth of penetration. Higher frequency sound waves are absorbed in the more superficial tissues.

VELOCITY

The *velocity* at which this vibration or sound wave is propagated through the conducting medium is directly related to the density. Denser and more rigid materials will have a higher velocity of transmission. At a frequency of 1 MHz, sound travels through soft tissue at 1540 m/sec and through compact bone at 4000 m/sec.[104]

ATTENUATION

As the ultrasound wave is transmitted through the various tissues, there will be **attenuation** or a decrease in energy intensity. This decrease is owing to either

attenuation A decrease in energy intensity as the ultrasound wave is transmitted through various tissues owing to scattering and dispersion.

TABLE 10-1   Relationship between Penetration and Absorption (1 MHz)

Medium	Absorption	Penetration
Water	1	1200
Blood plasma	23	52
Whole blood	60	20
Fat	390	4
Skeletal muscle	663	2
Peripheral nerve	1193	1

From Griffin, J.E.: J. Am. Phys. Ther. 46(1):18–26, 1966. Reprinted with permission of the American Physical Therapy Association.

Penetration and absorption are inversely related.

absorption of energy by the tissues or *dispersion* and *scattering* of the sound wave that results from reflection or refraction.[94]

Ultrasound penetrates through tissue high in water content and is absorbed in dense tissues high in protein where it will have its greatest heating potential.[48] The capability of acoustic energy to penetrate or be transmitted to deeper tissues is determined by the frequency of the ultrasound as well as the characteristics of the tissues through which ultrasound is traveling. Penetration and absorption are inversely related. Absorption increases as the frequency increases, thus less energy is transmitted to the deeper tissues.[60] Tissues that are high in water content have a low rate of absorption, whereas tissues high in protein have a high absorption rate.[31] Fat has a relatively low absorption rate, and muscle absorbs considerably more. Peripheral nerve absorbs at a rate twice that of muscle. Bone, which is relatively superficial, absorbs more ultrasonic energy than any of the other tissues (Table 10-1).

When a sound wave encounters a boundary or an interface between different tissues, some of the energy will scatter owing to reflection or refraction. The amount of energy reflected, and conversely the amount of energy that will be transmitted to deeper tissues, is determined by the relative magnitude of the **acoustic impedances** of the two materials on either side of the interface. Acoustic impedance may be determined by multiplying the density of the material by the speed at which sound travels inside it. If the acoustic impedance of the two materials forming the interface is the same, all of the sound will be transmitted and none will be reflected. The larger the difference between the two acoustic impedances, the more energy is reflected and the less that can enter a second medium (Table 10-2).[99]

Sound passing from the transducer to air will be almost completely reflected. Ultrasound is transmitted through fat. It is both reflected and refracted at the muscular interface. At the soft tissue–bone interface virtually all of the sound is reflected. As the ultrasound energy is reflected at tissue interfaces with different acoustic impedances, the intensity of the energy is increased as the reflected energy meets new energy being transmitted, creating what is referred to as a **standing wave** or a **"hot spot."** This increased level of energy has the potential to produce tissue damage. Moving the sound transducer or using pulsed wave ultrasound can help to minimize the development of hot spots.[31]

TABLE 10-2 The Percentage of the Incident Energy Reflect at Tissue Interfaces[98]

Interface	Percent Reflection
Soft tissue/air	99.9
Water/soft tissue	0.2
Soft tissue/fat	1.0
Soft tissue/bone	15–40

BASIC PHYSICS OF THERAPEUTIC ULTRASOUND

COMPONENTS OF A THERAPEUTIC ULTRASOUND GENERATOR

An ultrasound generator consists of a high frequency electrical generator connected through an oscillator circuit and a transformer via a coaxial cable to a transducer housed in a type of insulated applicator (Fig. 10-2). The oscillator circuit produces a sound beam at a specific frequency that is adjusted by the manufacturer to the frequency requirements of the transducer. The control panel of an ultrasound unit usually has a timer that can be preset, a power meter, an intensity control, a duty cycle control switch, a selector for continuous or pulsed modes, and possibly output power in response to tissue loading, and automatic shut-off in case of overheating of the transducer. Recently dual soundheads and dual frequency choices have become standard equipment on ultrasound units (Fig. 10-3). Table 10-3 provides a list of the most desirable features in an ultrasound generator.

TRANSDUCER

The transducer, also referred to as an applicator or a soundhead, must be matched to particular units and are generally not interchangeable.[18] The transducer consists of some piezoelectric crystal, such as quartz, or synthetic ceramic crystals made of lead zirconate or titanate, barium titanate, or nickel-cobalt ferrite of approximately 2 to

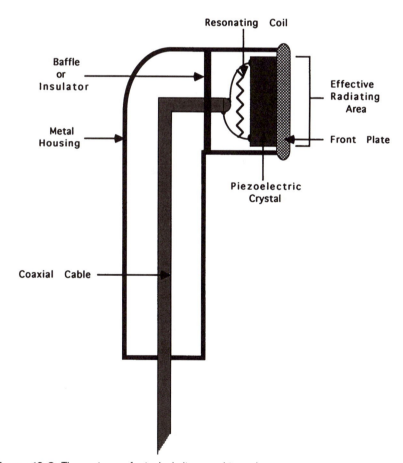

•**Figure 10-2** The anatomy of a typical ultrasound transducer.

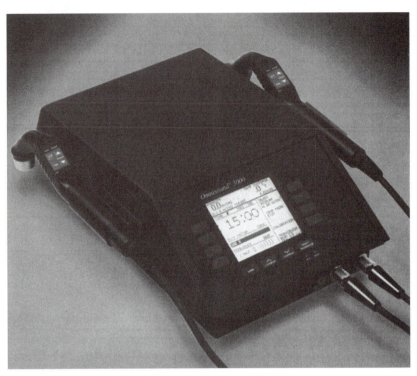

•**Figure 10-3** State of the art ultrasound unit with dual soundheads, dual frequencies, intensity, and frequency controls located on transducers and preprogrammed temperature increase settings (manufactured by Physio Technology, Inc., Topeka, Kansas).

3 mm in thickness. It is the crystal within the transducer that converts electrical energy to acoustic energy through mechanical deformation of the piezoelectric crystal.

Piezoelectric Effect

When an alternating electrical current generated at the same frequency as the crystal resonance is passed through the piezoelectric crystal, the crystal will expand and contract, creating what is referred to as the **piezoelectric effect.** There are two forms of this piezoelectric effect (Fig. 10-4). A *direct* piezoelectric effect is the generation

piezoelectric effect When an alternating electrical current generated at the same frequency as the crystal resonance is passed through the piezoelectric crystal, the crystal will expand and contract or vibrate at the frequency of the electrical oscillation thus generating ultrasound at a desired frequency.

TABLE 10-3 The State of the Art "Ultimate" Ultrasound Machine Would Contain the Following:

Low BNR (,4:1)
High ERA (nearly matches the size of the soundhead)
Multiple frequencies (1 and 3 MHz)
Multiple sized soundheads
Sensing device that shuts off the unit when overheating
Well insulated to be used underwater
Output jack for combination therapy
Several pulsed duty cycles
High quality synthetic crystal
Transducer handle that maintains the operators wrist in a natural, relaxed position
Durable transducer face that will protect the crystal if dropped
Computer controlled timer that makes adjustments in treatment duration as the intensity is adjusted (much like iontophoresis where the treatment time adjusts according to the dose applied)

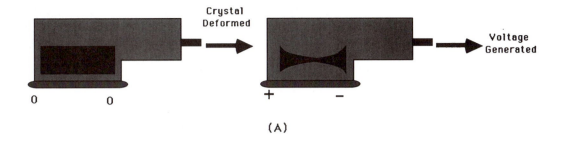

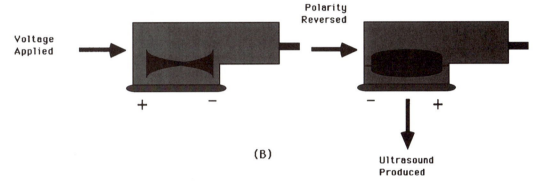

•**Figure 10-4** Piezoelectric effect. A. In a direct piezoelectric effect, a mechanical deformation of the crystal generates a voltage. B. In the reverse piezoelectric effect, as the alternating current reverses polarity, the crystal expands and contracts, producing ultrasound energy.

of an electrical voltage across the crystal when it is compressed or expanded. An *indirect* or *reverse* piezoelectric effect is created when an alternating current moves through the crystal, producing compression or expansion. It is this change in voltage polarity that causes the crystal to expand and contract and thus vibrate at the frequency of the electrical oscillation. Thus, the reverse piezoelectric effect is used to generate ultrasound at a desired frequency.

Effective Radiating Area (ERA)

That portion of the surface of the transducer that actually produces the sound wave is referred to as the **effective radiating area (ERA).** ERA is dependent on the surface area of the crystal and ideally nearly matches the diameter of the transducer faceplate (Fig. 10-5).[30] The ERA is determined by scanning the transducer at a distance of 5 mm from the radiating surface and recording all areas in excess of 5 percent of the maximum power output found at any location on the surface of the transducer. The acoustic energy is contained with a focused cylindrical beam that is roughly the same diameter as the soundhead.[99]

Since the effective radiating area is always smaller than the transducer surface, the size of the transducer is not indicative of the actual radiating surface. A very common mistake is to assume that because you have a large transducer surface the entire surface radiates ultrasound output. This is generally not true, particularly with larger 10-cm² transducers. There is really no point in having a large transducer with a small radiating surface as it only mechanically limits the coupling in smaller areas (see Fig. 10-5). The transducer ERA should match the total size of the soundhead as closely as possible for ease of application to various body surfaces, in order to maintain the most effective coupling.

effective radiating area The total area of the surface of the transducer that actually produces the soundwave.

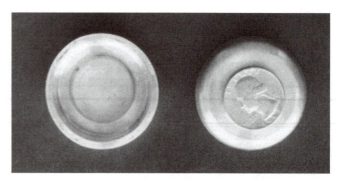

•**Figure 10-5** (left) Photo of a quarter-sized crystal mounted to the inside of the transducer faceplate. A quarter (right) is placed on the transducer face to illustrate that this crystal is smaller than the faceplate. Ideally, they should be closer to the same size.

The appropriate size of the area to be treated using ultrasound is two to three times the size of the ERA of the crystal.[11,86] To support this premise, peak temperature in human muscle was measured during 10 minutes of 1 MHz ultrasound delivered at 1.5W/cm^2 (Fig. 10-6). The treatment size for 10 subjects was two ERA, and for the other 10 it was six ERA. The two ERA group's temperature increased 3.6°C (moderate to vigorous heating); whereas subjects' temperature in the six ERA group only increased 1.1°C (mild heating). Thus, ultrasound is most effectively used for treating small areas.[23] Hot packs, whirlpools, and shortwave diathermy have an advantage over ultrasound in that they can be used to heat much larger areas.

FREQUENCY OF THERAPEUTIC ULTRASOUND

Therapeutic ultrasound produced by a piezoelectric transducer has a frequency range between 0.75 and 3.0 MHz. Frequency is the number of wave cycles completed each second. The majority of the older ultrasound generators are set at a frequency of 1 MHz (meaning the crystal is deforming 1 million times per second), whereas some of the newer models also contain the 3 MHz frequency (the crystal is deforming 3 million times per second). Certainly, a generator that can be set between 1 and 3 MHz affords the therapist the greatest treatment flexibility.

A common misconception is that intensity determines the depth of ultrasonic penetration, thus high intensities (1.5 or 2 W/cm^2) are used for deep heating, and low intensities (<1 W/cm^2) are used for superficial heating. However, depth of tissue penetration is determined by ultrasound frequency and not by intensity.[41] Ultrasound energy generated at 1 MHz is transmitted through the more superficial tissues and absorbed primarily in the deeper tissues at depths of 2 to 5 cm (Fig. 10-7).[25] A 1 MHz frequency is most useful in patients with high percent body fat cutaneously and whenever desired effects are in the deeper structures, such as the soleus or piriformis muscles.[43] At 3 MHz the energy is absorbed in the more superficial tissues with a depth of penetration between 1 and 2 cm, making it ideal for treating superficial conditions such as plantar fasciitis, patellar tendinitis, and epicondylitis.[104]

As previously mentioned, attenuation is the decrease in the energy of ultrasound as the distance it travels through tissue increases. The rate of absorption, and therefore attenuation, increases as the frequency of the ultrasound increases.[56] The 3 MHz frequency is not only absorbed more superficially, it is also absorbed three times faster than 1 MHz ultrasound. This faster rate of absorption results in faster peak heating in tissues. It has been demonstrated that 3 MHz ultrasound heats human muscle three times faster than 1 MHz ultrasound.[25]

Treatment Tip
The lower the frequency of ultrasound the less the energy is absorbed in the superficial tissues, and thus the deeper it penetrates. The majority of the sound waves generated from the 3 MHz treatment would be absorbed in the muscle or tendon. Also, when treating subcutaneous structures 3 MHz heats more rapidly, and is more comfortable than 1 MHz.

3 MHz = superficial heat
1 MHz = deep heat

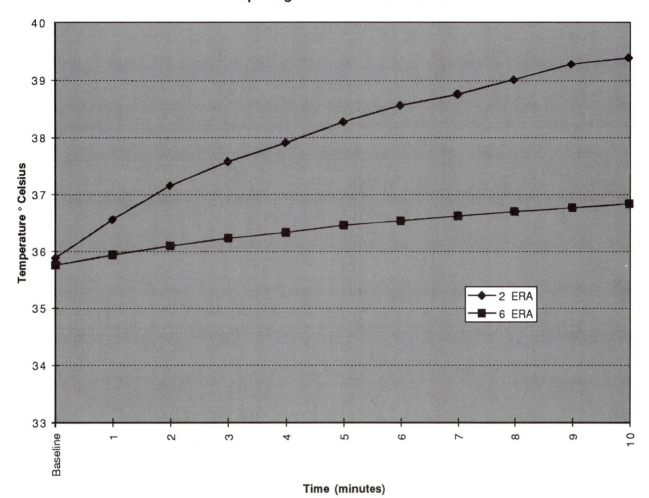

**Temperature During 1 MHz Ultrasound Treatment
Comparing 2 & 6 ERA at 1.5w/cm2**

•**Figure 10-6** This graph illustrates that ultrasound is ineffective in heating areas much larger than twice the size of the transducer face. Mean temperature increase for 2 ERA was 3.4°C and only 1.1°C for an area 6 times the effective radiating area ERA. (From: Chudliegh, D., Schulthies, S.S., Draper, D.O., and Myrer, J.W.: Muscle temperature rise with 1 MHz ultrasound in treatment sizes of 2 and 6 times the effective radiating area of the transducer, master's thesis, Brigham Young University, July, 1997.)

THE ULTRASOUND BEAM

If the wavelength of the sound is larger than the source that produced it, then the sound will spread in all directions.[99] Such is the case with audible sound, thus explaining why it is possible for a person behind you to hear your voice almost as well as a person in front of you. In the case of therapeutic ultrasound, the sound is less divergent, thus concentrating energy in a limited area (1 MHz at a velocity 1540 m/sec in soft tissue and a wavelength of 1.5 mm, emitted from a transducer that is larger than the wavelength at approximately 25 mm in diameter).

The larger the diameter of the soundhead, the more focused or **collimated** the beam. Smaller soundheads produce a more divergent beam. Also, the beam from ultrasound generated at a frequency of 1 MHz is more divergent than ultrasound generated at 3 MHz (see Fig. 10-7).

collimated beam A focused, less divergent beam of ultrasound energy produced by a large diameter transducer.

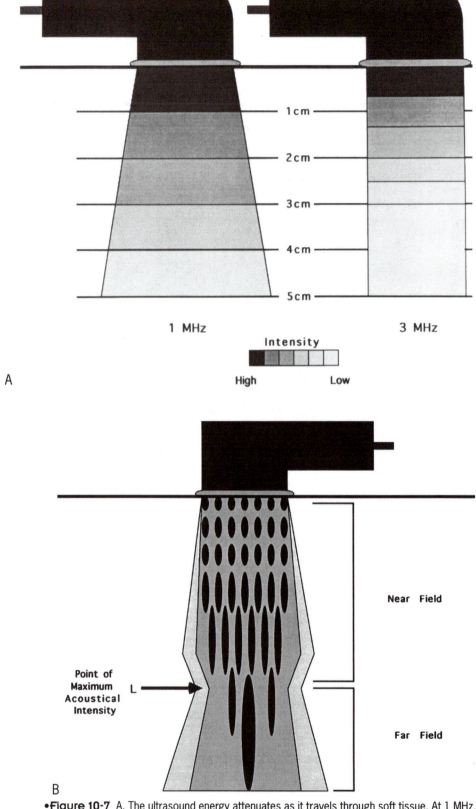

•**Figure 10-7** A. The ultrasound energy attenuates as it travels through soft tissue. At 1 MHz, the energy can penetrate to the deeper tissues although the beam diverges slightly. At 3 MHz the effects are primarily in the superficial tissues and the beam is less divergent. B. In the near field the distribution of energy is nonuniform. In the far field energy distribution is more uniform but the beam is more divergent. L represents the point of highest acoustic intensity.

CASE STUDY 10-1
ULTRASOUND

Background: An 18-year-old college freshman sustained a fracture of the fifth metacarpal of the left hand during a prank in the dormitory. The fracture required gauntlet cast immobilization for 6 weeks. At the time of cast removal the patient noted significant restriction of motion and weakness in the left wrist. A referral was initiated. Physical examination revealed flexion 0 to 45°, extension 0 to 30° with radial and ulnar deviation unaffected. There was point tenderness at the callus site on the shaft of the fifth metacarpal. Finger motion was grossly within normal limits at all constituent joints.

Impression: Wrist capsule motion restriction secondary to immobilization, muscular weakness secondary to immobilization.

Treatment Plan: A course of therapeutic ultrasound was initiated to decrease joint stiffness through increased collagen-connective tissue extensibility. Given the small and irregular surface of the wrist joint, underwater coupling was chosen as the mode of ultrasound delivery. After checking the left wrist and hand for any rashes or open wounds and verifying that sensation and circulation were normal in the distal portion of the extremity; the left forearm, wrist, and hand were immersed in a plastic basin filled with warm water. An ultrasound treatment of 1.5 W/cm² for 6 minutes was applied to the dorsal aspect of the left wrist. Patient reported a mild sensation of warmth. At the conclusion of the treatment the patient was instructed in active and active-assistive wrist mobilization exercises.

Response: Following initial ultrasound treatment and exercise patient experienced a 10° improvement in both flexion and extension range of motion. At the completion of the sixth treatment wrist range of motion was within normal limits and the patient was aggressively pursuing a wrist curl strengthening regimen. Ultrasound treatments were discontinued at that time with efforts focused on strengthening and functional use of the left upper extremity.

The rehabilitation professional employs therapeutic agent modalities to create an optimum environment for tissue healing while minimizing the symptoms associated with the trauma or condition.

Discussion Questions

- What tissues were injured or affected?
- What symptoms were present?
- What phase of the injury healing continuum did the patient present for care in?
- What are the therapeutic agent modality's biophysical effects (direct, indirect, depth, and tissue affinity)?
- What are the therapeutic agent modality's indications and contraindications?
- What are the parameters of the therapeutic agent modality's application, dosage, duration, and frequency in this case study?
- What other therapeutic agent modalities could be utilized to treat this injury or condition? Why? How?

Within this cylindrical beam the distribution of sound energy is highly nonuniform, particularly in an area close to the transducer referred to as the near field or near zone (Fig. 10-7B). The near field is a zone of spatially fluctuating ultrasound strength. The fluctuation occurs because of differences in pressure created by the waves emitted from the transducer. As the beam moves away from the transducer, the waves eventually become indistinguishable, arriving at a certain point simultaneously, creating a point of highest acoustic intensity.[99] The point of maximum acoustic intensity can be determined by calculating the distance (L) from the surface of the transducer:

$$L = \frac{D^2}{4W}$$

where D is the diameter of the transducer and W is the wavelength.[60] From this point the beam moves into the far field or far zone where the distribution of energy is much more uniform but the beam becomes more divergent.

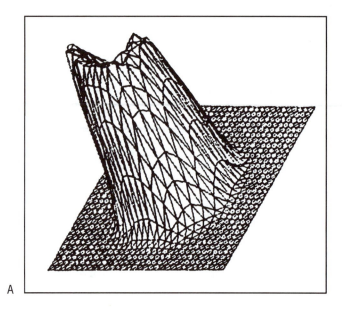

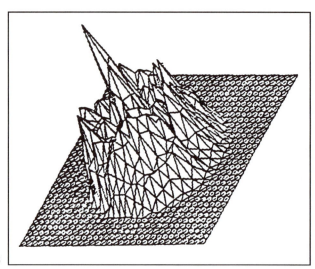

•**Figure 10-8** A. Graphic representation of a low BNR of 2 to 1. B. Graphic representation of a high BNR of 6 to 1.

Treatment area = 2–3 ERA

Beam Nonuniformity Ratio

Ultrasound beams are not homogeneous along their longitudinal axis; some points are of higher intensity than others away from the transducer surface. The amount of variability of intensity within the ultrasound beam is indicated by the **beam nonuniformity ratio (BNR).** This ratio is determined by using an underwater microphone (acoustic hydrophone) to measure the maximal point intensity of the transducer to the average intensity across the transducer surface. For example, a BNR of 2 to 1 means when the average output intensity is 1 W/cm^2, the peak or maximal point intensity of the beam is 2 W/cm^2. Optimally the BNR would be 1 to 1; however, since this is not possible, the BNR should fall between 2 and 6. Some ultrasound units have BNRs as high as 8 to 1. Peak intensities of 8 W/cm^2 have been shown to damage tissue; therefore, the patient runs a risk of tissue damage if intensities greater than 1 W/cm^2 are used on a machine with an 8 to 1 BNR. The lower the BNR the more uniform the output and therefore the lower the chance of developing "hot spots" of concentrated energy. The Food and Drug Administration requires all ultrasound units to list the BNR and the therapist should be aware of the BNR for that particular unit.[38]

The high peak intensities associated with high BNRs are responsible for much of the discomfort or periosteal pain often associated with ultrasound treatment.[51] Therefore, the higher the BNR the more important it is to move the transducer faster during treatment to avoid hot spots and areas of tissue damage or cavitation. Figure 10-8 shows the high beam homogeneity of a low BNR transducer and the typical beam profile of a high BNR transducer at 3 MHz output frequency.

Some researchers give little credence to BNR as a factor in good ultrasound equipment and say that it has little effect in treatment quality. However, most would agree that a continuous thermal ultrasound treatment is effective only if it is tolerated by the patient, and if it produces uniform heating through the tissues. Some have speculated that a beam flowing from a poor quality ultrasound crystal might be a reason patients experience pain and might cause uneven heating of tissue. Patient compliance should be better when thermal ultrasound is delivered via an ultrasound device with a low beam nonuniformity ratio. This will encourage patients to return for needed ultrasound treatments and allow the therapist to increase the intensity to the point where the patient feels local heat. When a heat modality is applied to tissue, it only makes sense that the patient should feel heat. If warmth is not felt, either the therapist is moving the soundhead too fast, or the intensity is too low.

> Ultrasound may be continuous or pulsed.

Pulsed versus Continuous Wave Ultrasound

Virtually all therapeutic ultrasound generators can emit either continuous or pulsed ultrasound waves. If **continuous wave ultrasound** is used, the sound intensity remains constant throughout the treatment, and the ultrasound energy is being produced 100 percent of the time (Fig. 10-9).

With **pulsed ultrasound** the intensity is periodically interrupted, with no ultrasound energy being produced during the off period (Fig. 10-10). When using pulsed

> **continuous wave ultrasound** The sound intensity remains constant throughout the treatment and the ultrasound energy is being produced 100 percent of the time.

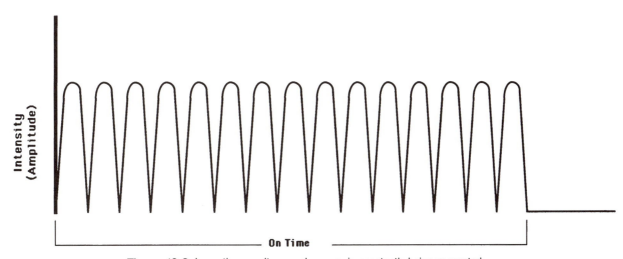

•**Figure 10-9** In continuous ultrasound, energy is constantly being generated.

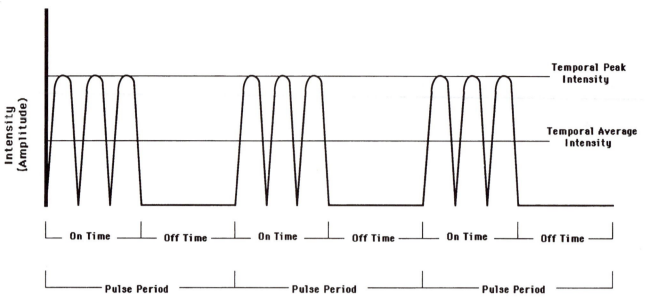

•Figure 10-10 In pulsed ultrasound, energy is generated only during the on time. Duty cycle is determined by the ratio of on time to pulse period.

ultrasound, the average intensity of the output over time is reduced. The percentage of time that ultrasound is being generated (pulse duration) over one pulse period is referred to as the **duty cycle.**

$$\text{Duty cycle} = \frac{\text{Duration of pulse (on time)} \times 100}{\text{Pulse period (on time + off time)}}$$

Thus, if the pulse duration is 1 msec and the total pulse period is 5 msec, the duty cycle would be 20 percent. Therefore, the total amount of energy being delivered to the tissues would be only 20 percent of the energy delivered if a continuous wave was being used. The majority of ultrasound generators have duty cycles that are preset at either 20 or 50 percent; however, some provide several optional duty cycles. Occasionally the duty cycle is also referred to as the *mark:space* ratio.

Continuous ultrasound is most commonly used when thermal effects are desired. The use of pulsed ultrasound results in a reduced average heating of the tissues. Pulsed ultrasound or continuous ultrasound at a low intensity will produce nonthermal or mechanical effects that may be associated with soft tissue healing.

AMPLITUDE, POWER, AND INTENSITY

Amplitude is a term used to describe the magnitude of the vibration in a wave. It is the maximum distance from equilibrium that any particle reaches. Amplitude is used to describe either the movement of particles in the medium through which it travels in units of distance (centimeters or meters), or the variation in pressure found along the path of the wave in units of pressure (Newtons/meter^2).[18]

Power is the total amount of ultrasound energy in the beam and is expressed in watts. **Intensity** is a measure of the rate at which energy is being delivered per unit area. Since power and intensity are unevenly distributed in the beam, several varying types of intensities must be defined.

pulsed ultrasound The intensity is periodically interrupted with no ultrasound energy being produced during the off period. When using pulsed ultrasound, the average intensity of the output over time is reduced.

Spatial-averaged intensity is the intensity of the ultrasound beam averaged over the area of the transducer. It may be calculated by dividing the power output in watts by the total effective radiating area of the soundhead in cm^2 and is indicated in watts per square centimeter (W/cm^2). If ultrasound is being produced at a power of 6 watts and the effective radiating area of the transducer is 4 cm^2, the spatial-averaged intensity would be 1.5 W/cm^2. On many ultrasound units, both the power in watts and the spatial-average intensity in W/cm^2 may be displayed. If the power output is constant, increasing the size of the transducer will decrease the spatial-averaged intensity.

Spatial peak intensity is the highest value occurring within the beam over time. With therapeutic ultrasound, maximum intensities can range between 0.25 and 3.0 W/cm^2.

Temporal peak intensity, sometimes also referred to as *pulse-averaged intensity,* is the maximum intensity during the on period with pulsed ultrasound, indicated in W/cm^2 (see Fig. 10-10).

Temporal-averaged intensity is important only with pulsed ultrasound and is calculated by averaging the power during both the on and off periods. For a pulsed sound beam with a duty cycle of 20 percent with a temporal peak intensity of 2.0 W/cm^2, temporal-averaged intensity would be 0.4 W/cm^2. It should be pointed out that on some machines, the intensity setting indicates the temporal peak intensity or on time, whereas on others it shows the temporal-averaged intensity or the mean of the on-off intensity (see Fig. 10-10).[73]

Spatial-averaged temporal peak (SATP) intensity is the maximum intensity occurring in time of the spatially averaged intensity. The SATP intensity is simply the spatial average during a single pulse.

There are no definitive rules that govern selection of specific ultrasound intensities during treatment, yet using too much may likely damage tissues and exacerbate the condition.[99] One recommendation is that the lowest intensity of ultrasound energy at the highest frequency that will transmit the energy to a specific tissue should be used to achieve a desired therapeutic effect.[73] Some guidance for selecting intensities has come from published reports from those who have obtained successful, yet subjective clinical outcomes. Table 10-4 provides a summary of various studies from the literature that have made recommendations regarding intensities, frequencies, and treatment mode.[73]

It is important to remember that everyone's tolerance to heat is different, and thus ultrasound intensity should always be adjusted to patient tolerance.[51] At the beginning of the treatment, turn the intensity to the point where the patient feels deep warmth, and then back the intensity down slightly until gentle heating is felt.[21,22] During the treatment ask the patient for feedback, and make the necessary intensity adjustments. This idea only applies to continuous mode ultrasound since pulsed ultrasound generally does not produce heat. Regardless, the treatment should never produce reports of pain. If the patient reports that the transducer feels hot at the skin surface, it is likely that the coupling medium is inadequate, and possible that the piezoelectric crystal has been damaged and the transducer is overheating.

Ultrasound treatments should be temperature dependent, not time dependent. Thermal ultrasound is used in order to bring about certain desired effects, and tissues respond according to the amount of heat they receive.[63,64] Any significant adjustment in the intensity must be countered with an adjustment in the treatment time. It is possible that ultrasound treatments of the future will be like iontophoresis, where the treatment time is dependent on the dosage delivered. For this reason, it is likely that the new generation of ultrasound generators will have the capability of automatically decreasing treatment time as the intensity is increased and increasing treatment time as the intensity is decreased (see Fig. 10-3).

amplitude Describes the magnitude of the vibration in a wave. It is the maximum distance from equilibrium that any particle reaches.

power The total amount of ultrasound energy in the beam and is expressed in watts.

intensity A measure of the rate at which energy is being delivered per unit area.

TABLE 10-4   **Summary of Research Relating to Ultrasound**

Application	Authors	Frequency
SOFT TISSUE LESIONS		
Acute injuries		
Sports injuries	Patrick (1978)	*
Minor fractures		
Recent occupational soft tissue injuries	Middlemast and Chatterjee (1978)	1.5
Subacute		
Acute subacromial bursitis	Bearzy (1953)	1.0
Bursitis shoulder	Newman et al. (1958)	1.0
Painful shoulder	Downing and Weinstein (1986)	1.0
Subacromial bursitis	Munting (1978)	1.5
Chronic arthritis	Griffin et al (1970)	0.89/1.0
Plantar fasciitis	Clarke and Stenner (1976)	0.75/1.5
Rheumatoid nodules		3.0
Phonophoresis		
Arthritis	Griffin et al. (1967)	1.0
Epicondylitis/bursitis	Kleinkort and Wood (1975)	1.0
Wounds		
Episiotomies	Fieldhouse (1979)	*
Episiotomies and surgical wounds	Ferguson (1981)	1.0
Episiotomies	McLaren (1984)	*
Scars		
Contracture after hip fixation	Lehmann et al. (1961)	*
Hand scars	Bierman (1954)	1.0
Dupuytren's contracture	Markham et al. (1980)	1.0/3.0
PAIN		
Low back pain		
Nerve root pain	Patrick (1966)	*
Prolapsed intervertebral disc	Nwuga (1983)	*

PHYSIOLOGIC EFFECTS OF ULTRASOUND

Therapeutic ultrasound may induce clinically significant responses in cells, tissues, and organs through both thermal effects and nonthermal biophysical effects.[7,30–32,41,56,80,94,99,104] Ultrasound will affect both normal and damaged biologic tissues. It has been suggested that damaged tissue may be more responsive to ultrasound than normal tissue.[34] When ultrasound is applied for its thermal effects, nonthermal biophysical effects will also occur that may damage normal tissues.[56] If appropriate, treatment parameters are selected; however, nonthermal effects can occur with minimal thermal effects.

THERMAL EFFECTS

The ultrasound wave attenuates as it travels through the tissue. Attenuation is caused primarily by the conversion of ultrasound energy into heat through absorption and to some extent by scattering and beam deflection. Traditionally, ultrasound

SATP Intensity	Mode	Regimen	Outcome
*	P	*	
0.5-2.0	P	5 times a week	Significant improvement
2.0-4.0	*	up to 5 min daily × 3 then alternate days	Success with acute only
0.8-3.0	*	5-10 min × 12	Improvement
1.2-1.3	CW	6 min 3 times a week × 4	No significant difference
0.5	CW	3-5 min × 10	Improvement
2.0	*	3 times a week × 3	0.89 MHz more successful
1.0-2.5	CW	5 min × 8-10	Decreased pain
1.05-2.5	CW	5 min × 8-10	Size unchanged; pain decreased
1.5 max	CW	1 time a week × 9 max	Successful
2.0 max	CW	6-9 min	Improvement
0.5-0.8	*	5 min 3 times a week × 6	Improvement
0.5	P1:5	3 min daily × 2-4	Improvement
0.5	*	5 min	Improvement
1.0-2.5	*	5 min daily up to 3 weeks	Significant improvement
1.0-2.0	*	6-8 min, alternate days	Improvement
0.25-0.75	CW	4-10 min 1 time a week	Improvement
	*		
1.0-1.5	P	5 min daily × 10 max	Improvement
1.0-2.0	*	10 min 3 times a week × 4	Significant improvement

p = Pulsed; *cw* = Continuous wave.

has been used primarily to produce a tissue temperature increase.[6,40,66,69,89,98] The clinical effects of using ultrasound to heat tissues are similar to other forms of heat that may be applied, including:[63]

1. An increase in the extensibility of collagen fibers found in tendons and joint capsules
2. Decrease in joint stiffness
3. Reduction of muscle spasm
4. Modulation of pain
5. Increased blood flow
6. Mild inflammatory response that may help in the resolution of chronic inflammation

It has been suggested that for the majority of these effects to occur the tissues must be raised to a level of 40 to 45°C for a minimum of 5 minutes.[31] Others are of the opinion that absolute temperatures are not the key, but rather how much the temperature rises above baseline.[63–65] They report that tissue temperature increases of 1°C increase metabolism and healing, increases of 2 to 3°C decrease pain and muscle spasm, and increases of 4°C or greater increase extensibility of collagen and decrease joint stiffness.[10,11,63] It has been shown that temperatures above 45°C may be potentially damaging to tissues, yet patients usually experience pain prior to these extreme temperatures.[25]

Ultrasound at 1 MHz with an intensity of 1 W/cm^2 has been reported to raise soft tissue temperature by as much as 0.86°C per minute in tissues with a poor vascular supply.[99] It has been shown that 3 MHz ultrasound at 1 W/cm^2 to raise human patellar tendon temperatures 2°C per minute.[12] In muscle, which is quite vascular, 1 and 3 MHz ultrasound at 1 W/cm^2 increase the temperature 0.2 and 0.6°C per minute, respectively.[25]

The primary advantage of ultrasound over other nonacoustic heating modalities is that tissues high in collagen, such tendons, muscles, ligaments, joint capsules, joint menisci, intermuscular interfaces, nerve roots, periosteum, cortical bone, and other deep tissues, may be selectively heated to the therapeutic range without causing a significant tissue temperature increase in skin or fat.[66,95] Ultrasound will penetrate skin and fat with little attenuation.[29]

The thermal effects of ultrasound are related to frequency. As indicated earlier, an inverse relationship exists between depth of penetration and frequency. Most of the energy in a sound wave at 3 MHz will be absorbed in the superficial tissues. At 1 MHz there will be less attenuation, and the energy will penetrate to the deeper tissues, selectively heating them.

Heating will occur with both continuous and pulsed ultrasound, depending on the intensity of the total current being delivered to the patient. Significant thermal effects will be induced whenever the upper end of the available intensity range is used. Regardless of whether ultrasound is pulsed or continuous, if the spatial-averaged temporal-averaged intensity is in the 0.1 to 0.2 W/cm^2 range, the intensity is too low to produce a tissue temperature increase and only nonthermal effects will occur.[31]

Unlike the other heating modalities discussed in this text, whenever ultrasound is used to produce thermal changes, nonthermal changes also simultaneously occur.[32] An understanding of these nonthermal changes, therefore, is essential.

NONTHERMAL EFFECTS

acoustic microstreaming The unidirectional movement of fluids along the boundaries of cell membranes resulting from the mechanical pressure wave in an ultrasonic field.

The nonthermal effects of therapeutic ultrasound include **cavitation** and **acoustic microstreaming** (Fig. 10-11). Cavitation is the formation of gas-filled bubbles that expand and compress owing to ultrasonically induced pressure changes in tissue fluids.[31,94] Cavitation may be classified as being either *stable* or *unstable*. In stable cavitation, the bubbles expand and contract in response to regularly repeated pressure changes over many acoustic cycles. In unstable or transient cavitation, there are violent large excursions in bubble volume before implosion and collapse occurs after only a few cycles. Therapeutic benefits are derived only from stable cavitation, whereas the collapse of bubbles is thought to create increased pressure and high temperatures that may cause local tissue damage. Unstable cavitation clearly should be avoided. It is likely that high intensity, low frequency ultrasound may produce unstable cavitation, particularly if standing waves develop at tissue interfaces.[31]

cavitation The formation of gas-filled bubbles that expand and compress because of ultrasonically induced pressure changes in tissue fluids.

Cavitation results in an increased flow in the fluid around these vibrating bubbles. Microstreaming is the unidirectional movement of fluids along the boundaries of cell membranes resulting from the mechanical pressure wave in an ultrasonic field.[31,94] Microstreaming produces high viscous stresses, which can alter cell membrane structure and function due to changes in cell membrane permeability to sodium and calcium ions important in the healing process. As long as the cell membrane is not damaged, microstreaming can be of therapeutic value in accelerating the healing process.[31]

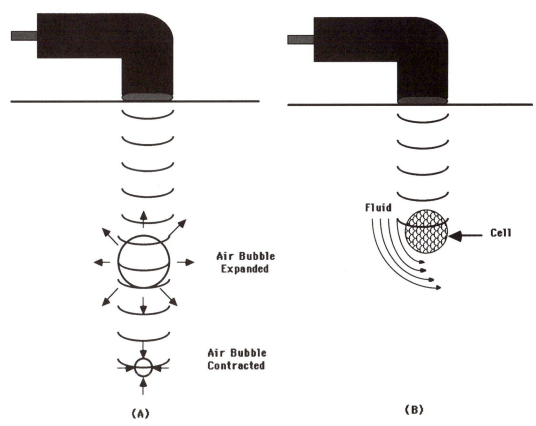

•**Figure 10-11** Nonthermal effects of ultrasound. A. Cavitation is the formation of gas-filled bubbles that expand and compress owing to ultrasonically induced pressure changes in tissue fluids. B. Microstreaming is the unidirectional movement of fluids along the boundaries of cell membranes resulting from the mechanical pressure wave in an ultrasonic field.

It has been well documented that the nonthermal effects of therapeutic ultrasound in the treatment of injured tissues may be as important if not more important than the thermal effects. Therapeutically significant nonthermal effects have been identified in soft tissue repair via stimulation of fibroblast activity, which produces an increase in protein synthesis, tissue regeneration, increased blood flow in chronically ischemic tissues, bone healing and repair of nonunion fractures, and in phonophoresis.[34,52,83]

The nonthermal effects of cavitation and microstreaming can be maximized while minimizing the thermal effects by using a spatial-averaged temporal-averaged intensity of 0.1 to 0.2 W/cm^2 with continuous ultrasound. This range may also be achieved using a low temporal-averaged intensity by pulsing a higher temporal-peak intensity of 1.0 W/cm^2 at a duty cycle of 20 percent, to give a temporal average intensity of 0.2 W/cm^2.

Treatment Tip

The nonthermal effects of cavitation and microstreaming can be maximized while minimizing the thermal effects by using a spatial-averaged temporal-averaged intensity of 0.1 to 0.2 W/cm^2 with continuous ultrasound. This range may also be achieved using a low temporal-averaged intensity by pulsing a higher temporal-peak intensity of 1.0 W/cm^2 at a duty cycle of 20 percent, to give a temporal average intensity of 0.2 W/cm^2.

TECHNIQUES OF APPLICATION

The principles and theories of therapeutic ultrasound are well understood and documented. However, specific practical recommendations as to how ultrasound may best be applied to a patient therapeutically are quite controversial and are based primarily on the experience of the clinicians who have used it. Even though there are numerous laboratory and clinically based reports in the literature, treatment procedures and parameters are highly variable and many contradictory results and conclusions have been presented in the literature.[73]

FREQUENCY OF TREATMENT

It is generally accepted that acute conditions require more frequent treatments over a shorter period of time, whereas more chronic conditions require fewer treatments over a longer period of time.[73] Ultrasound treatments should begin as soon as possible following injury, ideally within hours but definitely within 48 hours to maximize effects on the healing process.[42,79,81] Acute conditions may be treated using low intensity or pulsed ultrasound once or even twice daily for 6 to 8 days until acute symptoms such as pain and swelling subside. In chronic conditions, when acute symptoms have subsided, treatment may be done on alternating days.[93] Ultrasound treatment should continue as long as there is improvement. Assuming that appropriate treatment parameters are chosen and the ultrasound generator is functioning properly, if no improvement is noted following three or four treatments, ultrasound should be discontinued, or different parameters (i.e., duty cycle, frequency) employed.

The question is often asked, "How many ultrasound treatments can be given?" It must be pointed out that most of the research regarding treatment longevity has been performed on animals, and it takes quite a leap of logic to assume that the same negative effects would occur in humans. If the correct parameters are followed using a high-quality, recently calibrated ultrasound machine, treatments could occur daily for several weeks. In the past, it has been recommended that ultrasound be limited to 14 treatments in the majority of conditions, although this has not been documented scientifically. More than 14 treatments can reduce both red and white blood cell counts. After these 14 treatments some authors advise avoiding ultrasound use for 2 weeks.[43]

DURATION OF TREATMENT

In the past, modality textbooks have been quite vague with respect to treatment time, and generally the suggested duration has been too short.[51,92] Typically recommended treatment times have ranged between 5 and 10 minutes in length; however, these times may be insufficient. The length of the treatment is dependent on several factors: the size of the area to be treated; the intensity in W/cm^2; the frequency; and the desired temperature increase. As stated previously, specific temperature increases are required to achieve beneficial effects in tissue. The therapist must determine what the desired effects of the treatment are before a treatment duration is set (Fig. 10-12).

An accepted recommendation is that ultrasound be administered in an area two times the ERA (roughly twice the size of the soundhead). If thermal effects are desired in an area larger than this, obviously the treatment time needs to be increased.

The higher the intensity applied in W/cm^2, the shorter the treatment time, and vice versa. It just does not make clinical sense to treat one patient at 1 W/cm^2 and another at 2 W/cm^2 at identical treatment durations when both patients require vigorous heating. Based on this scenario, patient two will produce tissue temperature increases of twice that of patient one.

Ultrasound frequency (MHz) not only determines the depth of penetration, it also determines the rate of heating. The energy produced with 3 MHz ultrasound is absorbed three times faster than that produced from 1 MHz ultrasound, the result of

Ideal BNR = 1:1

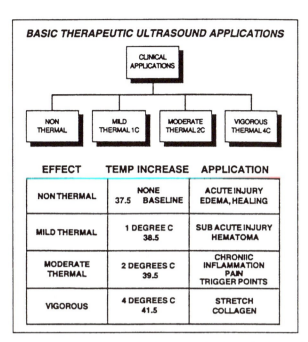

•Figure 10-12 It is important to have a treatment goal and to adjust the ultrasound treatment time accordingly.

which is faster heating. Ultrasound at 3 MHz consistently heats tissues three times faster than 1 MHz, thus reducing the required treatment duration by one-third.[23,25]

The desired temperature increase is also a factor in determining the duration of an ultrasound treatment. Table 10-5 displays the rate of muscle temperature increase per minute, per W/cm^2, at various intensities and frequencies.[25] Based on this information, the therapist can determine the appropriate duration of an ultrasound treatment. For example, a patient has limited range of motion because of scar tissue buildup from a chronic hamstring strain at the musculotendinous junction. An appropriate goal would be to vigorously heat the muscle (an increase of 4°C) and immediately perform passive hamstring stretching. If 1 MHz ultrasound were used at an intensity of 2 W/cm^2, the 4°C increase would take about 10 minutes. At 2 minutes into the treatment, however, the patient complains that the treatment is too hot. Most of us would respond by decreasing the intensity, but we may forget to increase the treatment time. In this case if we decreased the intensity to 1.5 W/cm^2, we would need to add 2 minutes to the treatment time in order to ensure a 4°C increase in muscle temperature. It is important to note that this chart requires a treatment size of two to three ERA, and these temperatures were reported in muscle. It has also been suggested that tendon heats over three times faster than muscle.[12]

TABLE 10-5   Ultrasound Rate of Heating per Minute[25]

Intensity (W/cm^2)	1 MHz	3 MHz
0.5	0.04°C	0.3°C
1.0	0.2°C	0.6°C
1.5	0.3°C	0.9°C
2.0	0.4°C	1.4°C

COUPLING METHODS

The greatest amount of reflection of ultrasonic energy occurs at the air-tissue interface. To ensure that maximal energy will be transmitted to the patient the face of the transducer should be parallel with the surface of the skin so that the ultrasound will strike the surface at a 90° angle. If the angle between the transducer face and the skin is greater than 15° a large percentage of the energy will be reflected and the treatment effects will be minimal.[93]

Reflection at the air-tissue interface can be further reduced by applying the ultrasound via the use of some coupling agent. The purpose of the **coupling medium** is to exclude air from the region between the patient and the transducer so that ultrasound can get to the area to be treated.[99] The acoustical impedance of the coupling medium should match the impedance of the transducer and should be slightly higher than the skin. Also, the medium should have a low coefficient of absorption to minimize attenuation in the coupling medium. It is important that the medium remains free of air bubbles during treatment. The coupling agent should be viscous enough to act as a lubricant as the transducer is moved over the surface of the skin.[73]

The coupling medium should be applied to the skin surface and the ultrasound transducer should be in contact with the coupling medium before the power is turned on. If the transducer is not in contact with the skin via the coupling medium, or if for some reason the transducer is lifted away from the treatment area, the piezoelectric crystal may be damaged and the transducer can overheat.

A number of studies have looked at the efficacy of different coupling media in transmitting ultrasound.[2,28,31,86] Water, light oils, and various brands of ultrasonic gel have been recommended as coupling agents. The recommendations of these studies have proven to be somewhat contradictory. Essentially it appears that all of these agents have very similar acoustic properties and are effective as coupling agents.[19]

Water is an effective coupling medium but its low viscosity reduces its suitability in surface application. Light oils, such as mineral oil and glycerol, have relatively higher absorption coefficients and are somewhat difficult to clean up following treatment. Water-soluble gels seem to have the most desirable properties necessary for a good coupling medium.[19,28] Perhaps the only disadvantage is that the salts in the gel may damage the metal face of the transducer with improper cleaning. Out of convenience, some therapists have used massage lotion instead of ultrasound gel; however, experience has revealed that massage lotion is not an adequate ultrasound conducting medium. Table 10-6 describes a technique that can be used to check the relative transmission capability of a medium.

coupling medium A substance used to decrease the acoustical impedance at the airskin interface and thus facilitate the passage of ultrasound energy.

TABLE 10-6 Technique That Can Be Used to Check the Relative Transmission Capability of a Medium

Encircle the transducer with tape while leaving about 2 cms of tape exposed (making a tape tube).

Fill the tape tube with 1 cm thickness of ultrasound gel medium.

Fill the tube to the top with water.

Adjust the intensity and watch the water bubble.

Repeat the procedure yet substitute the gel with the medium you are testing.

If the water has little or no bubbles, your desired medium is not a good couplant after all.

EXPOSURE TECHNIQUES

Direct Contact

Direct application of ultrasound involves actual contact between the applicator and the skin, with a thin film of couplant between. A layer of gel should be applied to the treatment area in sufficient amounts to maintain good contact and lubrication between the transducer and the skin, but not so much that air pockets may form from movement of the transducer. A thin film of gel should be applied directly to the transducer face before transmission begins (Fig. 10-13).[73] A direct technique of exposure may be used as long as the surface being treated is larger than the diameter of the transducer. If a smaller surface area is to be treated, a smaller transducer should be used so that direct application can still be performed.

Heating of the ultrasound gel prior to treatment has been recommended to improve the thermal effects of ultrasound in deeper tissues; however, this is not the case. Since ultrasound heats only through conversion of mechanical vibration to heat and not through conduction, heating of the gel will have no effect in the deeper tissues.[43] The only rationale for heating cold ultrasound gel is strictly for patient comfort and compliance.

Recently several manufacturers of analgesic creams have been promoting their use as ultrasound couplants. Patients are treated with ultrasound via a conducting medium of gel mixed with their product. One company recommended a mixture of two parts gel to one part analgesic cream (this has recently been changed to 80% gel to 20% cream), whereas another recommended a 50/50 ratio of ultrasound gel and their analgesic cream. Small mixtures of analgesic creams with 80 or 90 percent gel may produce significant heating, but as yet have not been tested. Some of these products have been shown to actually impede the transmission of ultrasound. Many of these over-the-counter medications presently used are only minimally effective as ultrasound couplants.[24] If a patient wants the added benefits of heat and analgesia, first massage the balm into the area, then apply 100 percent ultrasound gel followed by ultrasound. Until further research is performed in this area, it is suggested that the practice of using analgesic creams mixed with ultrasound gel be discontinued when vigorous heating is desired. Figure 10-14 displays the results of research involving two such products and their effect on muscle temperature increase via ultrasound.

Water soluble gels = best coupling medium

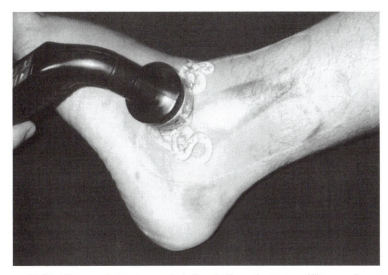

•**Figure 10-13** Ultrasound may be applied directly through some gel-like coupling medium.

FLEX-ALL V.S. BIOFREEZE

Depth	50/50 flex-all; gel	50/50 biofreeze; gel	100%Gel
3cm	2.8°C	1.8°C	3.4°C
5cm	1.8°C	1.3°C	2.5°C

**Muscle temperature increase from continuous
1 MHz ultrasound at 1.5 W/cm² for 10 minutes.**

•**Figure 10-14** Two popular analgesic creams were mixed with ultrasound gel and used as coupling media. Only the treatments that used 100 percent ultrasound gel as the couplant yielded temperatures consistent with vigorous heating. We conclude that these creams, although they might decrease pain perception, actually impede ultrasound transmission. *Note:* These manufacturers are now recommending mixtures of 80 percent ultrasound gel with 20 percent of their product. At press time, this had not been tested.

Immersion

Although direct application with gel has been shown to be the most effective application technique, there are some instances where water immersion is warranted. The immersion technique is recommended if the area to be treated is smaller than the diameter of the available transducer or if the treatment area is irregular with bony prominences (Fig. 10-15). A plastic, ceramic, or rubber basin should be used, since a metal basin or whirlpool will reflect some of the ultrasound, increasing the intensity near the basin walls. Tap water seems to be just as effective as degassed water as a

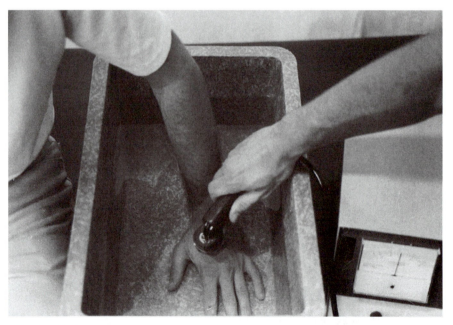

•**Figure 10-15** The immersion technique is recommended when using ultrasound over irregular surfaces.

coupling medium for the immersion technique and less likely to produce surface heating than mineral oil or glycerin.[42,86] The transducer should be moved parallel to the surface being treated at a distance of 0.5 to 1 cm.[104] If air bubbles accumulate on the transducer or over the treatment area, they may be wiped away quickly during the treatment. In order to ensure adequate heating, the intensity should be increased, possibly as much as 50 percent.[28]

Bladder Technique

If for some reason the treatment area cannot be immersed in water, a bladder technique can be used in which a balloon is filled with water and the ultrasound energy is transmitted from the transducer to the treatment surface through this bladder (Fig. 10-16). Both sides of the balloon should be coated with gel to assure better contact. Treatments using a bladder filled with either gel or silicone have also been recommended as effective at higher ultrasound intensities.[2]

MOVING THE TRANSDUCER

In the past, treatment techniques that involve both moving the transducer and holding the transducer stationary have been recommended. The stationary technique was most often used when the treatment area was small or when pulsed ultrasound was used at a low temporal-averaged intensity. However, because of the nonuniformity of the ultrasound beam, the energy distribution in the tissue is uneven, thus creating potential tissue-damaging "hot spots."[104] If the ultrasound beam is stationary, the spatial-peak intensity determines the point of maximal temperature increase. With the moving technique, the spatial-averaged intensity gives the most reasonable measure of the average rate of heating within the treatment area.[99] This stationary technique has been demonstrated to produce disruption of blood flow, platelet aggregation, and damage to the venous system, therefore the stationary technique is no longer recommended.[103]

Treatment Tip
When using a large soundhead to treat over bony prominences the immersion technique done in a plastic or rubber tub can be effective. Also the bladder technique could be used to make certain that there is consistent contact between the soundhead and the coupling medium.

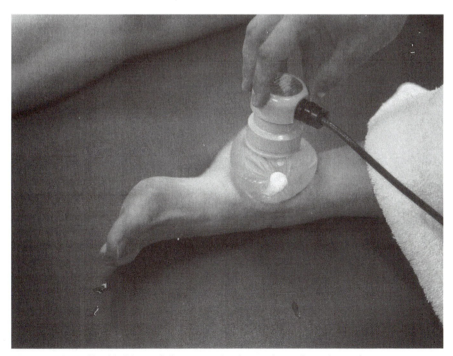

•**Figure 10-16** The bladder technique may also be used over irregular surfaces.

Moving the transducer during treatment leads to a more even distribution of energy within the treatment area, especially if the unit has a low BNR.[10] This can reduce the damaging effects of standing waves, particularly those which are most likely to occur at bone-tissue interfaces. Overlapping circular motions or a longitudinal stroking pattern can be used. The transducer should be moved slowly at approximately 4 cm per second, covering a treatment area that is two to three times larger than the ERA of the transducer.[59,72] Movement speed of the transducer is BNR-dependent, and the higher the BNR the more important it is to move the transducer faster during treatment to avoid periosteal irritation and transient cavitation.[51,92] However, moving the transducer too rapidly decreases the total amount of energy absorbed per unit area. Rapid movement of the soundhead causes the therapist to slip into treating a larger area, thus the desired temperatures may not be attained.

Equipment with a low BNR usually allows for a slower stroking movement of the ultrasound transducer. Slow strokes are more controlled and can easily be contained to a small area (2 ERA). Slow movement of the applicator results in evenly distributed sound waves throughout the area, whereas a fast moving transducer will not allow for adequate absorption of the sound waves, and sufficient heating will not occur. If the patient complains of pain, decrease the output intensity, while making the appropriate adjustments in treatment duration. The transducer should be kept in maximum contact with the skin via some coupling agent.

RECORDING ULTRASOUND TREATMENTS

It is recommended that the therapist report or record the specific parameters used in an ultrasound treatment when completing treatment records or progress notes so that the treatment may be reproduced or altered. The parameters which should be recorded include frequency, spatial-averaged temporal peak intensity, whether the beam is pulsed or continuous, the duty factor (if pulsed), effective radiating surface area of the transducer, duration of the treatment, and the number of treatments per week.[73]

A typical treatment might be recorded as 3 MHz, at 1.0 W/cm^2, pulsed at 20 percent (0.2) duty factor, 5-cm transducer head, 5 minutes, four times per week.

CLINICAL USES OF THERAPEUTIC ULTRASOUND

Ultrasound is generally recognized clinically as one of the most effective and widely used modalities in the treatment of many soft tissue and bony lesions. Considering the extensive use of ultrasound in treating soft tissue injuries, until the past decade there has been relatively little documented evidence from the medical community concerning the efficacy of this modality (however, research in this area is increasing). Many of the decisions as to how ultrasound should be used are empirically based on personal opinion and experience. This section summarizes the various clinical applications of therapeutic ultrasound used in a clinical setting.

SOFT TISSUE HEALING AND REPAIR

Soft tissue repair may be accelerated by both thermal and nonthermal ultrasound.[30,35] Repair of soft tissues involves three phases of healing; inflammation, proliferation, and remodeling. Ultrasound does not seem to have any anti-inflammatory effects, rather it is thought to accelerate the inflammatory phase of healing.

It has been shown that a single treatment with ultrasound can stimulate the release of histamine from mast cells.[50] The mechanism for this may be attributed primarily to nonthermal effects involving cavitation and streaming that increase the transport of calcium ions across the cell membrane thus stimulating release of histamine by the mast cells.[31] Histamine attracts polymorphonuclear leukocytes that "clean up" debris from the injured area, along with monocytes whose primary function is to release chemotactic agents and growth factors that stimulate fibroblasts and endothelial cells to form a collagen-rich, well vascularized tissue used for the development of new connective tissue that is essential for rapid repair. Thus, ultrasound can be effective in facilitating the process of inflammation and therefore healing, if applied after bleeding has stopped but still within the first few hours after injury during the early stages of inflammation.[31] It has been suggested that this response occurs using pulsed ultrasound at 0.5 W/cm^2 with a duty cycle of 20 percent for 5 minutes or continuous ultrasound at 0.1 W/cm^2.[32]

These treatments have been described as being "pro-inflammatory" and are of value in accelerating repair in short-term or acute inflammation.[91] However, in chronic inflammatory conditions, the pro-inflammatory effects are of questionable value.[50] If an inflammatory stimulus such as overuse remains, the response to therapeutic ultrasound is of questionable value.[5]

Pitting edema is a condition that sometimes provides a challenge for therapists. Pitting edema may be treated with continuous 3 MHz ultrasound at intensities of 1 to 1.5 W/cm^2. The heat seems to liquefy the "gel like" cellular debris. The limb is then elevated, massaged or EMS used to pump the fluid and promote lymphatic drainage.

During the proliferative phase of healing, a connective tissue matrix is produced into which new blood vessels will grow. Fibroblasts are mainly responsible for producing this connective tissue. Fibroblasts exposed to therapeutic ultrasound are stimulated to produce more collagen that gives connective tissue most of its strength.[49] Again, cavitation and streaming alter cell membrane permeability to calcium ions that facilitate increases in collagen synthesis and in tensile strength. The intensity levels of therapeutic ultrasound that produce these changes during the proliferative phase are too low to be entirely thermal.

> Ultrasound accelerates the inflammatory process.

SCAR TISSUE AND JOINT CONTRACTURE

During remodeling, collagen fibers are realigned along lines of tensile stresses and strains, forming scar tissue. This process may continue for months or even years. In scar tissue, collagen never attains the same pattern and remains weaker and less elastic than normal tissue prior to injury. Scar tissue in tendons, ligaments, and capsules surrounding joints can produce joint contractures that limit range of motion. Increased tissue temperatures increase the elasticity and decrease the viscosity of collagen fibers. Since the deeper tissues surrounding joints which most often restrict range are rich in collagen, ultrasound is the treatment modality of choice.[61,104]

A number of studies have investigated the effects of ultrasound treatment on scar tissue and joint contracture. Ultrasound has been demonstrated to increase mobility in mature scar.[4] A greater residual increase in tissue length with less potential damage is produced through preheating with ultrasound prior to stretching, or by putting the joint on stretch while insonating.[26,62,88] Tissue extensibility increases when continuous ultrasound is applied at higher intensities causing vigorous heating of tissues.[44] Thigh, periarticular structures, and scar tissues become significantly more extensible following treatment with ultrasound involving thermal effects at intensities of 1.2 to 2.0 W/cm^2.[62] Scar tissue can be softened if treated with ultrasound at an early stage.[81] Dupuytren's contracture shows a beneficial effect on long standing contracted bands of scar and a decrease in pain when treated early on with ultrasound.[71]

Treatment Tip
To heat a large area in the low back the best treatment choice is to use either hydrocollator packs or diathermy rather than ultrasound. If depth of penetration is a concern, then shortwave diathermy is the treatment modality of choice.

The majority of the earlier studies attributed the effectiveness of ultrasound to thermal effects and used continuous moderate intensities between 0.5 and 2.0 W/cm².

STRETCHING OF CONNECTIVE TISSUE

Collagenous tissue when stressed is fairly rigid, yet when heated it becomes much more yielding.[44,62] However, the combination of heat and stretching produces a residual lengthening of connective tissue, which increases according to the force applied.

The time period of vigorous heating when tissues will undergo the greatest extensibility and elongation, is referred to as the **"stretching window."**[26,88] To explain this concept, I refer to the analogy of the plastic spoon.[10] When a plastic spoon is dipped in hot water it softens, and by pulling on the ends, we are able to stretch it. As the plastic cools, however, it hardens and is no longer able to be stretched. Likewise, if we vigorously heat tissue it becomes more pliable and less resistant to stretch, yet as the tissue cools it withstands stretching, and can actually be damaged if too great of a force is applied.

The rate of tissue cooling following continuous ultrasound at both 1 MHz and 3 MHz frequencies has been determined (Fig. 10-17).[26,88] Thermistor probes were inserted 1.2 cm below the skins surface and ultrasound was applied. The treatment raised the tissue temperature 5.3°C for the 3 MHz frequency. The average time it took for the temperature to drop each degree as expressed in minutes and seconds was: 1°C = 1:20; 2°C = 3:22; 3°C = 5:50; 4°C = 9:13; 5°C = 14:55. In this case the temperature remained in the vigorous heating phase for only 3.3 minutes following an ultrasound treatment.

The same methods were used to determine the stretching window at 1 MHz. The temperature was recorded 4 cm deep in the muscle. It took 2 minutes for the temperature to drop 1°C, and a total of 5.5 minutes to drop 2°C. The deeper muscle cools at a slower rate than superficial muscle since the added tissue serves as a barrier to escaping heat. Regardless, tissue heated by ultrasound loses its heat at a fairly rapid rate; therefore, stretching, friction massage, or joint mobilization should be performed immediately postultrasound. To increase the duration of the stretching window, it is recommended that stretching be done during and immediately after ultrasound application.

CHRONIC INFLAMMATION

There are few clinical or experimental studies that discuss the effects of therapeutic ultrasound on the chronic inflammations (i.e., tendinitis, bursitis, epicondylitis). Treatment of bicipital tendinitis with ultrasound decreases pain and tenderness, and increases range of motion.[36] Although earlier studies have shown ultrasound to be effective in treating pain and increasing range of motion in subacromial bursitis, a more recent study shows no improvement in the general condition of the shoulder when using continuous ultrasound at 1.0 to 2.0 W/cm².[20] Ultrasound applied at an intensity of 1.0 to 2.0 W/cm² at a 20 percent duty cycle significantly enhanced recovery in patients with epicondylitis.[5]

In these chronic inflammatory conditions, ultrasound seems to be effective in increasing blood flow for healing, and for pain reduction through heating.[104]

BONE HEALING

Since bone is a type of connective tissue, damaged bone progresses through the same stages of healing as other soft tissues, the major difference being the deposition of

Indications
Acute and postacute conditions (ultrasound with nonthermal effects)
Soft tissue healing and repair
Scar tissue
Joint contracture
Chronic inflammation
Increase extensibility of collagen
Reduction of muscle spasm
Pain modulation
Increase blood flow
Soft tissue repair
Increase in protein synthesis
Tissue regeneration
Bone healing
Repair of nonunion fractures
Inflammation associated with myositis ossificans
Plantar warts
Myofascial trigger points

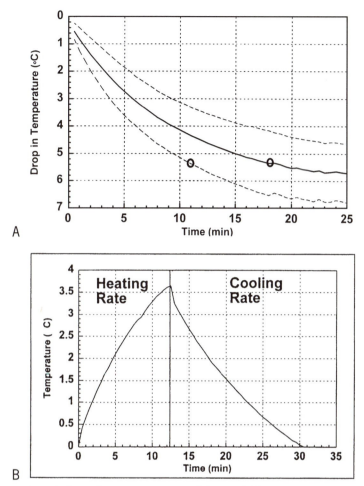

•**Figure 10-17** A. Rate of temperature decay following 3 MHz ultrasound treatments. Solid line = mean temperature decay. Hatched lines = 1 standard deviation above and below the mean. Oval = time to preultrasound baseline. B. Rate of temperature increase during 1 MHz ultrasound applied at 1.5 W/cm², followed by the rate of temperature decay at termination of insonation. The thermistor was 4 cm deep in the triceps surae muscle.[27,87]

bone salts.[102] Several researchers have observed acceleration of fracture repair following treatment with ultrasound.[83] It has been shown that the application of ultrasound within the first 2 weeks post–fibular fracture during the inflammatory and proliferative stages increases the rate of healing. Treatment parameters were 0.5 W/cm² at a duty cycle of 20 percent for 5 minutes, four times per week.[33] Ultrasound was effectively used to stimulate bone repair following osteotomy and fixation of the tibia in rabbits.[8]

Treatment given during the first 2 weeks after injury is sufficient to accelerate bony union. However, ultrasound given to an unstable fracture during the phase of cartilage formation may cause proliferation of cartilage and consequent delayed bony union.[30] It appears that nonthermal mechanisms are most responsible for the accelerated bone healing.[73]

Several researchers have looked at the use of ultrasound over growing epiphyses.[16,48,97] Although results have been somewhat inconsistent, some form of damage was observed in each study, including premature closure of the epiphysis, epiphyseal displacement, widening of the epiphyseal, fractures, condyle erosion, and shortening of the bones. The degree of destruction appears to be unpredictable; therefore, it is not recommended that ultrasound be applied to growing bone.[43]

No documented evidence exists that ultrasound treatment can cause reabsorption of calcium deposits. However, it has been suggested that ultrasound may help to reduce inflammation surrounding a calcium deposit, thus reducing pain and improving function.[104]

Myositis ossificans is calcification within the muscle following acute or repeated trauma. This condition may be exacerbated by applying heat or massaging the area. Thus ultrasound is contraindicated in acute hematomas, and it is a large leap of logic to assume it capable of reducing the size of the mature calcification.

Ultrasound in Assessing Stress Fractures

The use of ultrasound as a reliable technique for identifying stress fractures has been recommended.[67] Using a continuous beam at 1 MHz with a small transducer and a water-based coupling medium, the therapist moves the transducer slowly over the injured area while gradually increasing the intensity from 0 to 2.0 W/cm^2 until the patient indicates that he or she feels uncomfortable (periosteal irritation), at which point the ultrasound is turned off. If the patient reports a feeling of pressure, bruising, or aching, then a stress fracture may be present. Another technique is to first apply 1 MHz continuous ultrasound in the stationary mode to the contralateral limb. The intensity is slowly increased until the individual reports pain. This is then repeated on the affected area. Typically with a stress fracture, pain will be reported at a lower intensity than on the opposite site. Either a radiograph or a bone scan is then necessary to confirm this diagnosis.

PAIN REDUCTION

Many of the studies discussed previously have noted that reduction in pain occurs with ultrasound treatment, even though the treatment was given for other purposes. Several mechanisms have been proposed that might explain this pain reduction. Ultrasound is thought to elevate the threshold for activation of free nerve endings through thermal effects.[100] Heat produced by ultrasound in large-diameter myelinated nerve fibers may reduce pain through the gating mechanism.[15,73] Ultrasound may also increase nerve conduction velocity in normal nerves, creating a counterirritant effect through thermal mechanisms.[57] There is no consensus of opinion in the literature as to the exact mechanism of pain reduction.

Pain reduction following application of ultrasound has been reported in patients with lateral epicondylitis,[4] shoulder pain, plantar fasciitis, surgical wounds, bursitis, prolapsed intervertebral disks, ankle sprains, in reflex sympathetic dystrophy, and in various other soft tissue injuries.[4,14,39,46,70,74,76,78,84]

PLANTAR WARTS

Plantar warts are occasionally seen on the weightbearing areas of the feet owing to either a virus or trauma. These lesions contain thrombosed capillaries in a whitish-colored soft core covered by hyperkeratotic epithelial tissue. Among other more conventional techniques, several studies have recommended ultrasound as being an effective painless method for eliminating plantar warts.[55,85,96] Intensities average 0.6 W/cm^2 for 7 to 15 minutes.[17]

PLACEBO EFFECTS

Whereas the physiologic effects of ultrasound have been discussed in detail, it should also be mentioned that ultrasound can have significant therapeutic psychologic effects.[31] A number of studies have demonstrated a placebo effect in patients receiving sham ultrasound.[37,50,68]

PHONOPHORESIS

Phonophoresis is a technique in which ultrasound is used to drive a topical application of a selected medication into the tissues. Perhaps the greatest advantage of phonophoresis is that medication can be delivered via a safe, painless, noninvasive technique, as was the case with iontophoresis, discussed in Chapter 6. It is thought that active transport occurs as a result of increased membrane permeability during sonation.

Medications commonly applied through phonophoresis most often are either anti-inflammatories, such as cortisol, salicylates, or dexamethasone, or anagelsics, such as lidocaine. When applying phonophoresis it is important to select the appropriate drug for the pathology. Since phonophoresis may increase drug penetration, it may also increase the clinical benefits as well as the risks of topical drug application.[9]

The thermal effects of ultrasound increases tissue permeability, and the acoustic pressure created by the ultrasound beam drives the medication into the tissues.[48] Thus, the medication follows the path of the beam. Both pulsed and continuous ultrasound have been used in phonophoresis. Continuous ultrasound at an intensity great enough to produce thermal effects may induce a pro-inflammatory response.[32] If the goal is to decrease inflammation, pulsed ultrasound with low spatial-averaged temporal peak intensity may be the best choice.[43]

Unlike iontophoresis discussed earlier, phonophoresis drives whole molecules into the tissues as opposed to ions.[1] Consequently phonophoresis is not as likely to damage or burn skin. Also the potential depth of penetration with phonophoresis is substantially greater than with iontophoresis.

The most widespread use of the phonophoresis technique in the clinical setting has been to deliver hydrocortisone which has anti-inflammatory effects. Typically, either 1 or 10% hydrocortisone cream is used in treatment. The 10% hydrocortisone preparation appears to be superior to the 1% preparation.[58] Several studies have looked at the efficacy of this technique.[53] Using phonophoresis with hydrocortisone was shown to be superior to ultrasound alone in alleviating pain and reducing inflammation in patients with arthritic disorders.[47] It has been used in treating patients with various inflammatory disorders including bursitis, tendinitis, and neuritis.[58] It has also been used to treat temporomandibular joint dysfunction.[54,101] Griffin and Kleinkhort have demonstrated the effective penetration of corticosteroids into tissue with ultrasound.[47,58] However, Benson and colleagues have shown that many phonophoresis treatments are ineffective.[3]

Salicylates are compounds that evoke a number of pharmocologic effects including analgesia and decreased inflammation owing to a reduction in prostaglandins. There are few reports that suggest that phonophoresis using salicylates enhances analgesic or anti-inflammatory effects. However, it has been reported that salicylate phonophoresis may be used to decrease delayed onset muscle soreness without promoting cellular changes that m imic an inflammatory response.[13]

Lidocaine is a commonly used local anesthetic drug. The use of phonophoresis with lidocaine was found to be effective in treating a series of trigger points.[75]

The efficacy of various coupling media has been discussed previously. The addition of an active ingredient into the coupling medium is common practice. However, topical pharmacologic products are usually not formulated to optimize their efficiency as ultrasound coupling media.[3] For example, 1 or 10% hydrocortisone usually comes in a thick white cream base that has been demonstrated to be a poor

phonophoresis A technique in which ultrasound is used to drive a topical application of a selected medication into the tissues.

conductor of ultrasound. Clinicians have tried mixing this preparation with ultrasound gel (which is known to be a good transmitter) without improvement in transmission capabilities. The use of topical preparations with poor transmission capabilities may negate the effectiveness of ultrasound therapy. Unfortunately there are few suitable products available and there is clearly a need for appropriate active ingredients in gel form. Table 10-7 provides a list of transmission capabilities of various commercially available phonophoresis media.[9]

Since research has shown some of these medications to impede the sound, one suggestion is to apply the medication and gel separately.[24] This is accomplished by

TABLE 10-7	Ultrasound Transmission by Phonophoresis Media
Product	**Transmission Relative to Water (%)**
MEDIA THAT TRANSMIT ULTRASOUND WELL	
Lidex® gel, fluocinonide 0.05%[a]	97
Thera-Gesic® cream, methyl salicylate 15%[b]	97
Mineral oil[c]	97
US gel[d]	96
US lotion[e]	90
Betamethasone 0.05% in US gel[d]	88
MEDIA THAT TRANSMIT ULTRASOUND POORLY	
Diprolene® ointment, betamethasone 0.05%[g]	36
Hydrocortisone (HC) powder 1%[b] in US gel[d]	29
HC powder 10%[b] in US gel[d]	7
Cortril® ointment, HC 1%[i]	0
Eucerin® cream[f]	0
HC cream 1%[k]	0
HC cream 10%[k]	0
HC cream 10%[k] mixed with equal weight US gel[d]	0
Myoflex® cream, trolamine salicylate 10%[l]	0
Triamcinolone acetonide cream 0.1%[k]	0
Velva HC cream 10%[b]	0
Velva HC cream 10%[b] with equal weight US gel[d]	0
White petrolatum[m]	0
OTHER	
Chempad-L®[n]	68
Polyethylene wrap[o]	98

[a]Syntex Laboratories Inc, 3401 Hillview Ave, PO Box 10850, Palo Alto, CA 94303.
[b]Missions Pharmacal Co, 1325 E Durango, San Antonio, TX 78210.
[c]Pennex Corp, Eastern Ave at Pennex Dr, Verona, PA 15147.
[d]Ultraphonic®, Pharmaceutical Innovations Inc, 897 Frelinghuysen Dr, Newark, NJ 07114.
[e]Polysonic, Parker Laboratories Inc, 307 Washington St, Orange NJ 07050.
[f]Pharmfair Inc, 110 Kennedy Dr, Hauppauge, NY 11788.
[g]Schering Corp, Galloping Hill Rd, Kenilworth, NJ 07033.
[h]Purepace Pharmaceutical Co, 200 Elmora Ave, Elizabeth, NJ 07207.
[i]Pfizer Labs Division, Pfizer Inc, 253 E 42nd St, New York, NY 10017.
[j]Beiersdorf Inc, PO Box 5529, Norwalk, CT 06856-5529.
[k]E Fougera & Co, 60 Baylis Rd, Melville, NY 11747.
[l]Rorer Consumer Pharmaceuticals, Div of Rhône-Poulenc Rorer Pharmaceuticals Inc, 500 Virginia Dr, Fort Washington, PA 19034.
[m]Universal Cooperatives Inc, 7801 Metro Pkwy, Minneapolis, MN 55420.
[n]Henley International, 104 Industrial Blvd, Sugar Land, TX 77478.
[o]Saran Wrap®, Dow Brands Inc, 9550 Zionsville Rd, Indianapolis, IN 46268.
From Cameron M, Monroe, L: Relative transmission of ultrasound by media customarily used for phonophoresis, *Phys Ther* 72(2): 142-148, 1992. Reprinted with permission from the American Physical Therapy Association.

rubbing the medication directly onto the surface of the treatment area, then applying gel couplant followed by insonation. With the direct technique transmission gel should be applied, and with immersion the treatment area with the preparation applied is simply treated underwater.

USING ULTRASOUND IN COMBINATION WITH OTHER MODALITIES

In a clinical setting, it is not uncommon to combine modalities to accomplish a specific treatment goal. Ultrasound is frequently used with other modalities including hot packs, cold packs, and electrical stimulating currents. Unfortunately, there is very little documented evidence in the literature to substantiate the effectiveness of ultrasound and electrical currents; however, recent studies of cooling or heating the area prior to ultrasound application have produced interesting results.[22,27,87]

Hot packs, like continuous or high intensity ultrasound, are used primarily for their thermal effects. Heat is effective in reducing muscle spasm and muscle guarding and is useful in pain reduction. For these reasons heat and ultrasound used in combination can be effective for accomplishing these treatment goals. In one study, a 15-minute hot pack application prior to ultrasound had an additive heating effect. It was suggested that the ultrasound treatment duration can be decreased 3 to 5 minutes when tissues are preheated with hot packs.[22] However, it should be pointed out that since hot packs produce an increase in blood flow particularly to the superficial tissues creating a less dense medium for transmission of ultrasound, attenuation may be increased and the depth of penetration of ultrasound reduced.

Some authors have provided a rationale for ultrasound use immediately after ice. According to this premise, the application of a cold pack to human tissues initiates physiologic responses such as vasoconstriction and decreased blood flow. Thus cooling the area not only results in decreased local temperature, but it may assist in temporarily increasing the density of the tissue to be heated. This occurs by decreasing superficial attenuation and facilitating transmission to deeper tissues and consequently improving the thermal effects of ultrasound.[27,63,87] Although this theory sounds good, two recent studies appear to refute such claims.[27,87] Whether an ice pack was applied for 5 minutes or 15 minutes, significant cooling took place in the muscle reducing the rate and intensity of muscle temperature rise via ultrasound (Fig. 10-18). It just does not make sense to cool something that you immediately want to heat.

When treating acute and postacute injuries, however, the combination of cold to reduce blood flow (i.e., swelling) and produce analgesia, and low intensity ultrasound for its nonthermal effects that promote soft tissue healing, may be the treatment of choice. Cold packs are most often used for analgesia and to decrease blood flow acutely following injury. Because cold is such an effective analgesic, caution must be exercised when using ultrasound at higher intensities that produce thermal effects, since the patient's perception of temperature and pain are diminished. Pulsed ultrasound, however, could be used after ice application if the goal is pain reduction and healing in the acute stage.[10,11]

Ultrasound and electrical stimulating currents are frequently used in combination (Fig. 10-19). Electrical stimulating currents are used for analgesia or producing muscle contraction. Ultrasound and electrical stimulating currents in combination have been recommended in the treatment of myofascial trigger points.[45] Both modalities provide analgesic effects, and both have been shown to be effective in reducing the pain-spasm-pain cycle, although the mechanisms responsible are not clearly understood.

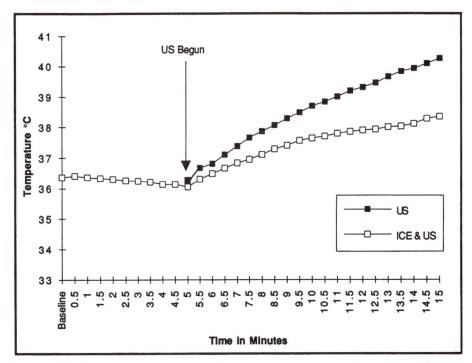

•**Figure 10-18** When an ice pack was applied for 5 minutes, it impeded the heat produced from ultra-sound. The increase in muscle temperature was greater and faster during the ultrasound treatment (increase of 4°C) than during the ice/ultrasound treatment (increase of 1.8°C). (From: Draper, D.O., Schulthies, S., Sorvisto, P., Hautala, A.: Temperature changes in deep muscles of humans during ice and ultrasound therapies: An in-vivo study, J. Orthop. Sports Phys. Ther. 21:153–157, 1995.

TREATMENT PRECAUTIONS

There are a number of treatment precautions to the use of therapeutic ultrasound.

The use of continuous ultrasound with a high spatial-averaged temporal peak intensity should be avoided in acute and postacute conditions because of the associated thermal effects.

Caution should be used when treating areas of decreased sensation, particularly when there is a problem in perceiving pain and temperature.

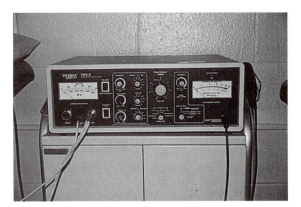

•**Figure 10-19** Ultrasound is frequently used in combination with electrical stimulating currents.

In areas of decreased circulation caution must be exercised owing to excessive heat build up that can potentially damage tissues.

Individuals with vascular problems involving thrombophlebitis should not receive ultrasound because of the possibility of dislodging a clot and creating an embolus.

Ultrasound should not be applied around the eye since heat is not dissipated well and both the lens and the retina may be damaged.

Ultrasound should not be applied over reproductive organs, especially the testes since temporary sterility may result. Caution should be used in treating the abdominal region of the female during the reproductive years or immediately following menses.

The use of ultrasound is contraindicated during pregnancy because of potential damage to the fetus.

Some precaution should be used when treating areas around the heart due to potential changes in ECG activity. Ultrasound can certainly interfere with normal function of a pacemaker.

Therapeutic ultrasound should not be used over malignant tissue since it has been suggested that this may cause cell detachment and metastasis.

As previously mentioned, ultrasound should never be used over epiphyseal areas in young children.

Ultrasound may be used safely over metal implants since it has been shown that there is no increase in temperature of tissue adjacent to the implant because metal has high thermal conductivity and thus heat is removed from the area faster than it can be absorbed. However, in cases of total joint replacement, the cement used (methyl methacrylate) absorbs heat rapidly and may be overheated, damaging surrounding soft tissues.

Contraindications
Acute and postacute conditions (ultrasound with thermal effects)
Areas of decreased temperature sensation
Areas of decreased circulation
Vascular insufficiency
Thrombophlebitis
Eyes
Reproductive organs
Pelvis immediately following menses
Pregnancy
Pacemaker
Malignancy
Epiphyseal areas in young children
Total joint replacements
Infection

GUIDELINES FOR THE SAFE USE OF ULTRASOUND EQUIPMENT

Currently, ultrasound units are the only therapeutic modality for which Federal Performance Standards exist.[82] Ultrasound units produced since 1979 are required to indicate the magnitudes of ultrasound power and intensity with an accuracy of ±20 percent and accurately control treatment time. It is recommended that intensity output, pulse regime accuracy, and timer accuracy be checked at regular intervals by qualified personnel who have access to the appropriate testing equipment. The effective radiating area and the beam nonuniformity ratio of the transducer should be accurately provided by the manufacturer. The following treatment guidelines will help to ensure patient safety:

1. Question patient (contraindications/previous treatments).
2. Position patient (comfort, modesty).
3. Inspect part to be treated (check for rashes, infections, or open wounds).
4. Obtain appropriate soundhead size.
5. Determine ultrasound frequency (1 MHz for deep, 3 MHz for superficial).
6. Set duty cycle (choose either continuous or pulsed setting).
7. Apply couplant to area.
8. Set treatment duration (vigorous heat = 10–12 min at 1 MHz and 3–4 min at 3 MHz).
9. Maintain contact between the skin and the applicator (move at a rate of 4 cm/sec, for 2 ERA).
10. Adjust intensity to perception of heat. (If this gets too hot, turn down the intensity or move applicator slightly faster.)

11. If goal is increased joint ROM, put part on stretch. (For the last 2–3 min of insonation, and maintain stretch or friction massage 2–5 min after termination of treatment.)

12. Terminate treatment. (Turn all dials to zero, clean gel from unit.)

13. Assess treatment efficacy. (Inspect area, feedback from client.)

14. Record treatment parameters.

Note: Ultrasound units should be recalibrated every 6 to 12 months, depending on the frequency of use.

SUMMARY

1. Ultrasound is defined as inaudible, acoustic vibrations of high frequency that may produce either thermal or nonthermal physiologic effects.

2. Ultrasound travels through soft tissue as a longitudinal wave at a therapeutic frequency of either 1 or 3 MHz.

3. As the ultrasound wave is transmitted through the various tissues, there will be attenuation or a decrease in energy intensity owing to either absorption of energy by the tissues or dispersion and scattering of the sound wave.

4. Ultrasound is produced by a piezoelectric crystal within the transducer that converts electrical energy to acoustic energy through mechanical deformation via the piezoelectric effect.

5. Ultrasound energy travels within the tissues as a highly focused collimated beam with a nonuniform intensity distribution.

6. Although continuous ultrasound is most commonly used when the desired effect is to produce thermal effects, pulsed ultrasound or continuous ultrasound at a low intensity will produce nonthermal or mechanical effects.

7. Therapeutic ultrasound when applied to biologic tissue may induce clinically significant responses in cells, tissues, and organs through both thermal effects, which produce a tissue temperature increase, and nonthermal effects, which include cavitation and microstreaming.

8. Recent research has provided answers to many of the contradictory results and conclusions of previous, numerous laboratory and clinically based reports in the literature.

9. Therapeutic ultrasound is most effective when an appropriate coupling medium and technique using either direct contact, immersion, or a bladder is combined with a moving transducer.

10. Even though there is relatively little documented evidence from the clinical community concerning the efficacy of ultrasound, it is most often used for soft tissue healing and repair; with scar tissue and joint contracture; for chronic inflammation; for bone healing; with plantar warts; and for placebo effects.

11. Phonophoresis is a technique in which ultrasound is used to drive molecules of a topically applied medication, usually either anti-inflammatories or analgesics, into the tissues.

12. In a clinical setting, ultrasound is frequently used in combination with other modalities, including hot packs, cold packs, and electrical stimulating currents, to produce specific treatment effects.

13. Although ultrasound is a relatively safe modality if used appropriately, the therapist must be aware of the various contraindications and precautions.

14. For ultrasound to be effective, the therapist must pay particular attention to correct parameters such as intensity, frequency, duration, and treatment size.

REFERENCES

1. Antich, T.J.: Phonophoresis: the principles of the ultrasonic driving force and efficacy in treatment of common orthopedic diagnosis, J. Orthop. Sport Phys. Ther. 4(2):99–103, 1982.

2. Balmaseda, M.T., Fatehi, M.T., and Koozekanani, S.H.: Ultrasound therapy: A comparative study of different coupling medium, Arch. Phys. Med. Rehabil. 67:147, 1986.

3. Benson, H.A.E., McElnay, I.C.: Transmission of ultrasound energy through topical pharmaceutical products, Physiotherapy 74:587, 1988.

4. Bierman, W.: Ultrasound in the treatment of scars, Arch. Phys. Med. Rehabil. 35:209, 1954.

5. Binder, A., Hodge, J., and Greenwood, T.: Is therapeutic ultrasound effective in treating soft tissue lesions? Br. Med. J. 290:512, 1985.

6. Black, K., Halverson, J.L., Maierus, K., and Soderbere, G.L.: Alterations in ankle dorsiflexion torque as a result of continuous ultrasound to the anterior tibial compartment, Phys. Ther. 64(6):910–913, 1984.

7. Bly, N., McKenzie, A., West, J., and Whitney, J.: Low dose ultrasound effects on wound healing: a controlled study with Yucatan pigs, Arch. Phys. Med. Rehabil. 73:656–664, 1992.

8. Brueton, R.N., Campbell, B.: The use of geliperm as a sterile coupling agent for therapeutic ultrasound. Physiotherapy 73: 653, 1987.

9. Cameron, M., Monroe, L.: Relative transmission of ultrasound by media customarily used for phonophoresis, Phys. Ther. 72(2):142–148, 1992.

10. Castel, J.C.: Electrotherapy application in clinical for neuromuscular stimulation and tissue repair. Presented at the 46th Annual Clinical Symposium of the National Athletic Trainer's Association; June 16, 1995, Indianapolis.

11. Castel, J.C.: Therapeutic ultrasound. Rehab and Therapy Products Review. 1993; Jan/Feb: 22–32.

12. Chan, A., Myrer, J.W., Measom, G., and Draper, D.O.: Temperature change in human patellar tendon in response to therapeutic ultrasound. Presented at the American College of Clinical Annual Symposium; June 1997, Denver, Colorado.

13. Ciccone, C., Leggin, B., and Callamaro, J.: Effects of ultrasound and trolamine salicylate phonophoresis on delayed-onset muscle soreness, Phys. Ther. 71(9): 666–675, 1991.

14. Clarke, G.R., and Stenner, L.: Use of therapeutic ultrasound, Physiotherapy 62(6):85–190, 1976.

15. Currier, D.P., Kramer, I.F.: Sensory nerve conduction: heating effects of ultrasound and infrared, Physiother. Can. 34:241, 1982.

16. DeForest, R.E., Henick, J.F., and Janes J.M.: Effects of ultrasound on growing bone: an experimental study. Arch. Phys. Med. Rehabil. 34:21, 1953.

17. Delacerda, F.G.: Ultrasonic techniques for treatment of plantar warts in patients. J. Orthop. Sports Phys. Ther. 1:100, 1979.

18. Docker, M.F.: A review of instrumentation available for therapeutic ultrasound. Physiotherapy 73(4):154, 1987.

19. Docker, M.F., Foulkes, D.J., and Patrick, M.K.: Ultrasound couplants for physiotherapy, Physiotherapy. 68(4):124–125, 1982.

20. Downing, D.S., Weinstein, A.: Ultrasound therapy of subacromial bursitis (abstr). Phys. Ther. 66:194, 1986.

21. Draper, D.O.: Ten mistakes commonly made with ultrasound use: Current research sheds light on myths. Ath. Train. Sports Health Care Perspect. 2:95–107, 1996.

22. Draper, D.O.: The latest research on therapeutic ultrasound: clinical habits may need to be changed. Presented at the 46th Annual Meeting and Clinical Symposium of the National Athletic Trainer's Association; June 16, 1995, Indianapolis, Indiana.

23. Draper, D.O.: Current research on therapeutic ultrasound and pulsed short-wave diathermy. Presented at Physio Therapy Research Seminars Japan, Nov. 17, 1996, Sendai, Japan.

24. Draper, D.O., Ashton, D., Cosgrove, C., et al: Comparison of Flex-all 454 and Biofreeze as ultrasound couplants. Presented at the Annual Symposium of the National Athletic Trainer's Association, June 14, 1996, Orlando, Florida.

25. Draper, D.O., Castel, J.C., and Castel, D.: Rate of temperature increase in human muscle during 1 MHz and 3 MHz continuous ultrasound, J. Orthop. Sports Phys. Ther. 22:142–150, 1995.

26. Draper, D.O., Ricard, M.D.: Rate of temperature decay in human muscle following 3 MHz ultrasound: the stretching window revealed, J. Ath. Train. 30:304–307, 1995.

27. Draper, D.O., Schulthies, S., Sorvisto, P., and Hautala, A.: Temperature changes in deep muscles of humans during ice and ultrasound therapies: An in-vivo study, J. Orthop. Sports Phys. Ther. 21:153–157, 1995.

28. Draper, D.O., Sunderland, S., Kirkendall, D.T., and Ricard, M.D.: A comparison of temperature rise in the human calf muscles following applications of underwater and topical gel ultrasound, J. Orthop. Sports Phys. Ther. 17:247–251, 1993.

29. Draper, D.O., Sunderland, S.: Examination of the law of Grotthus-Draper: does ultrasound penetrate subcutaneous fat in humans? J. Ath. Train. 28:246–250, 1993.

30. Dyson, M.: The use of ultrasound in sports physiotherapy. In: Grisogono, V., editor: Sports injuries (international perspectives in physiotherapy), Edinburgh, 1989, Churchill Livingstone.

31. Dyson, M.: Mechanisms involved in therapeutic ultrasound, Physiotherapy 73(3):116–120, 1987.

32. Dyson, M.: Therapeutic application of ultrasound. In Nyborg, W.L., Ziskin, M.C., editors: Biological effects of ultrasound, Edinburgh, 1985, Churchill-Livingstone.

33. Dyson, M., Brookes, M.: Stimulation of bone repair by ultrasound (abstr). Ultrasound Med. Biol. 8(Suppl 50):50, 1982.

34. Dyson, M., Luke, D.A.: Induction of mast cell degranulation in skin by ultrasound, IEEE Trans. Ultrasonics. Ferroelectrics Freq. Control UFFC-33:194, 1986.

35. Dyson, M., Pond, J.B.: The effect of pulsed ultrasound on tissue regeneration, J. Physiother. 105–108, 1970.

36. Echternach, J.L.: Ultrasound: an adjunct treatment for shoulder disability, Phys. Ther. 45:565, 1965.

37. El Hag, M., Coghlan, K., and Christmas, P.: The anti-inflammatory effects of dexamethasone and therapeutic ultrasound in oral surgery, Br. J. Oral Maxillofacial Surg. 23:17, 1985.

38. Ferguson, B.A.: A practitioner's guide to ultrasonic therapy equipment standard, U.S. Dept. of Health and Human Services, Public Health Service, Food and Drug Administration, Rockville, Maryland, 1985.

39. Ferguson, H.N.: Ultrasound in the treatment of surgical wounds, Physiotherapy 67:12, 1981.

40. Frizell, L.A., Dunn, F.: Biophysics of ultrasound; bioeffects of ultrasound. In: Lehmann, J.F., editor: Therapeutic heat and cold, ed. 3. Baltimore, 1982, Williams & Wilkins.

41. Fyfe, M.C., Bullock, M.: Therapeutic ultrasound: some historical background and development in knowledge of its effects on healing, Aust. J. Physiother. 31(6):220–224, 1985.

42. Fyfe, M.C., Chahl, L.A.: The effect of single or repeated applications of "therapeutic" ultrasound on plasma extravasation during silver nitrate induced inflammation of the rat hindpaw ankle joint, Ultrasound Med. Biol. 11:273, 1985.

43. Gann, N.: Ultrasound: current concepts, Clin. Manage. 11(4):64–69, 1991.

44. Gersten J.W.: Effect of ultrasound on tendon extensibility, Am. J. Phys. Med. 34:662, 1955.

45. Girardi, C.Q., Seaborne, D., and Savard-Goulet, F.: The analgesic effect of high voltage galvanic stimulation combined with ultrasound in the treatment of low back pain: a one group pretest/posttest study, Physiother. Can. 36(6):327–333, 1984.

46. Gorkiewicz, R.: Ultrasound for subacromial bursitis, Phys. Ther. 64:46, 1984.

47. Griffin, J.E., Echternach, J.L., and Price, R.E.: Patients treated with ultrasonic-driven hydrocortisone and ultrasound alone, Phys. Ther. 47:594–601, 1967.

48. Griffin, J.E., Karsalis, T.C.: Physical agents for physical therapists, Springfield, Illinois, 1978, Charles C. Thomas.

49. Harvey, W., Dyson, M., and Pond, J.B.: The simulation of protein synthesis in human fibroblasts by therapeutic ultrasound, Rheumat. Rehabil. 14:237, 1975.

50. Hashish, I., Harvey, W., and Harris, M.: Antiinflammatory effects of ultrasound therapy: evidence for a major placebo effect, Br. J. Rheumatol. 25:77, 1986.

51. Hecox, B., Mehreteab, T.A., and Weisbergm, J.: Physical agents: a comprehensive text for physical therapists, Norwalk, Connecticut, 1994, Appleton & Lange.

52. Hogan, R.D., Burke, K.M., and Franklin, T.D.: The effect of ultrasound on microvascular hemodynamics in skeletal muscle: effects during ischemia, Microvasc. Res. 23:370, 1982.

53. Holdsworth, L.K., Anderson, D.M.: Effectiveness of ultrasound used with hydrocortisone coupling medium or epicondylitis clasp to treat lateral eoicondylitis: pilot study, Physiotherapy 79(1):19–25, 1993.

54. Kahn J: Iontophoresis and ultrasound for post-surgical temporomandibular trismus and paresthesia, Phys. Ther. 60(3):307–308, 1980.

55. Kent, H.: Plantar wart treatment with ultrasound, Arch. Phys. Med. Rehabil. 40:15, 1959.

56. Kitchen, S., Partridge, C.: A review of therapeutic ultrasound: Part 1, Background and physiological effects, Physiotherapy 76(10):593–595, 1990.

57. Kitchen S, Partridge C: A review of therapeutic ultrasound: Part 2, The efficacy of ultrasound, Physiotherapy 76(10): 595–599, 1990.

58. Kleinkort, I.A., Wood, F.: Phonophoresis with 1 percent versus 10 percent hydrocortisone, Phys. Ther. 55:1320, 1975.

59. Kramer, J.F.: Ultrasound: evaluation of its mechanical and thermal effects, Arch. Phys. Med. Rehabil. 65:223, 1984.

60. Kremkau, F.: Physical conditioning, in Nyborg, W.L., Ziskin, M.C., editors: Biological effects of ultrasound, Edinburgh, 1985, Churchill Livingstone.

61. Lehmann, J.F.: Clinical evaluation of a new approach in the treatment of contracture associated with hip fracture after internal fixation, Arch. Phys. Med. Rehabil. 42:95, 1961.

62. Lehmann, J.F.: Effect of therapeutic temperatures on tendon extensibility, Arch. Phys. Med. Rehabil. 51:481, 1970.

63. Lehmann, J.F., de Lateur, B.J.: Therapeutic heat. In Lehmann, J.F., editor: Therapeutic heat and cold,. ed. 4. Baltimore, 1990, Williams & Wilkins.

64. Lehmann, J.F., de Lateur, B.J., and Silverman, D.R.: Selective heating effects of ultrasound in human beings,. Arch. Phys. Med. Rehabil. 46:331, 1966.

65. Lehman, J.F., DeLateur, B.J., Stonebridge, J.B., and Warren, G.: Therapeutic temperature distribution produced by ultrasound as modified by dosage and volume of tissue exposed, Arch. Phys. Med. Rehabil. 48:662–666, 1967.

66. Lehmann, J.F., Guy, A.W.: Ultrasound therapy. In Reid, J., Sikov, M.R., editors: Interaction of ultrasound and biological tissues, DHEW Pub. (FDA) 73-8008, Session 3(8):141, 1971.

67. Lowden, A.: Application of ultrasound to assess stress fractures, Physiotherapy 72(3):160–161, 1986.

68. Lundeberg, T., Abrahamsson, P., and Haker, E.: A comparative study of continuous ultrasound, placebo ultrasound and rest in epicondylalgia, Scand. Rehabil. Med. 20:99, 1988.

69. MacDonald, B. L., and Shipster, S.B.: Temperature changes induced by continuous ultrasound, South African J. Physiother. 37(1):13–15, 1981.

70. Makuloluwe, R.T., Mouzas, G.L.: Ultrasound in the treatment of sprained ankles, Practitioner 218:586–588, 1977.

71. Markham, D. E., and Wood, M.R.: Ultrasound for Dupytren's Contracture, Physiotherapy 66(2):55–58, 1980.

72. Michlovitz, S.: Thermal agents in rehabilitation, Philadelphia, 1996, F.A. Davis 1996.

73. McDiarmid, T., Burns, P.N.: Clinical applications of therapeutic ultrasound, Physiotherapy 73:155, 1987.

74. Middlemast, S., Chatterjee, D.S.: Comparison of ultrasound and thermotherapy for soft tissue injuries, Physiotherapy 64:331, 1978.

75. Moll, M.J.: A new approach to pain: Lidocaine and decadron with ultrasound, USAF Medical Service Digest, May–June 8, 1977.

76. Munting, E.: Ultrasonic therapy for painful shoulders, Physiotherapy 64:180, 1978.

77. Myrer, J.W., Draper, D.O., and Durrant, E.: Contrast therapy and intramuscular temperature in the human leg, J. Ath. Train. 29:318–322, 1994.

78. Nwuga, V.C.B.: Ultrasound in treatment of back pain resulting from prolapsed intervertebral disc, Arch. Phys. Med. Rehabil. 64:88, 1983.

79. Oakley, E.M.: Application of continuous beam ultrasound at therapeutic levels, Physiotherapy 64(4):103–104, 1978.

80. Partridge, C.J.: Evaluation of the efficacy of ultrasound, Physiotherapy 73(4):166–168, 1987.

81. Patrick, M.K.: Applications of pulsed therapeutic ultrasound, Physiotherapy 64(4):3–104, 1978.

82. Performance Standards for Sonic, Infrasonic, and Ultrasonic Radiation Emitting Products: 21 CFR 1050:10 Federal Register 43:7166, 1978.

83. Pilla, A.A., Figueiredo, M., Nasser, P., et al: Non-invasive low intensity pulsed ultrasound: a potent accelerator of bone repair, Proceedings of the 36th Annual Meeting, Orthopaedic Research Society, New Orleans, 1990.

84. Portwood, M.M., Lieberman, S.S., and Taylor, R.G.: Ultrasound treatment of reflex sympathetic dystrophy, Arch. Phys. Med. Rehabil. 68:116, 1987.

85. Quade, A.G., Radzyminski, S.F.: Ultrasound in verruca plantaris, J. Am. Podiatric. Assoc. 56:503, 1966.

86. Reid, D.C., Cummings, G.E.: Factors in selecting the dosage of ultrasound with particular reference to the use of various coupling agents, Physiother. Can. 63:255, 1973.

87. Rimington, S., Draper, D.O., Durrant, E., and Fellingham, G.W.: Temperature changes during therapeutic ultrasound in the precooled human gastrocnemius muscle, J. Ath. Train. 29:325–327, 1994.

88. Rose, S., Draper, D.O., Schulthies, S.S., and Durrant, E.: The stretching window part two: rate of thermal decay in deep muscle following 1 MHz ultrasound, J. Ath. Train. 31:139–143, 1996.

89. Sandler, V., Feingold, P.: The thermal effect of pulsed ultrasound, South African J. Physiother. 37(1):10–12, 1951.

90. Smith, K., Draper, D.O., Schulthies, S.S., and Durrant, E.: The effect of silicate gel hot packs on human muscle temperature. Presented at the 46th Annual Meeting and Clinical Symposium of the National Athletic Trainer's Association; June 15, 1995; Indianapolis, Indiana. Abstract published in J. Ath. Train. 30:S-33, 1995.

91. Snow, C.J., Johnson, K.A.: Effect of therapeutic ultrasound on acute inflammation, Physiother. Can. 40:162, 1988.

92. Starkey, C.: Therapeutic modalities for athletic trainers, Philadelphia, 1993, F.A. Davis.

93. Summer, W., Patrick, M.K.: Ultrasonic therapy, New York, 1964, American Elsevier.

94. ter Haar, C.: Basic physics of therapeutic ultrasound, Physiotherapy 73(3):110–113, 1987.

95. ter Haar, G., Hopewell, J.W.: Ultrasonic heating of mammalian tissue in vivo, Br. J. Cancer 45(suppl V):65–67, 1982.

96. Vaughn, D.T.: Direct method versus underwater method in treatment of plantar warts with ultrasound, Phys. Ther. 53:396, 1973.

97. Vaughen, I.L., Bender, L.F.: Effect of ultrasound on growing bone, Arch. Phys. Med. Rehabil. 40:158, 1959.

98. Ward, A.R.: Electricity fields and waves in therapy, Marrickville, NSW, Australia, 1986, Science Press.

99. Williams, R.: Production and transmission of ultrasound, Physiotherapy 73(3):113–116, 1987.

100. Williams, A.R., McHale, I., and Bowditchm, M.: Effects of MHz ultrasound on electrical pain threshold perception in humans, Ultrasound Med. Biol. 13:249, 1987.

101. Wing, M.: Phonophoresis with hydrocortisone in the treatment of temporomandibular joint dysfunction, Phys. Ther. 62:32–33, 1982.

102. Woolf, N.: Cell, Tissue and disease, ed. 2. London, 1986, Bailliere Tindall.

103. Zarod, A.P., Williams, A.R.: Platelet aggregation in vivo by therapeutic ultrasound, Lancet 1:1266, 1977.

104. Ziskin, M., McDiarmid, T., and Michlovitz, S.: Therapeutic ultrasound, in Michlovitz, S., editor: Thermal agents in rehabilitation, Philadelphia, 1996, F.A. Davis.

Suggested Readings

Abramson, D.I.: Changes in blood flow, oxygen uptake and tissue temperatures produced by therapeutic physical agents. I. Effect of ultrasound, Am. J. Phys. Med. 39:51, 1960.

Aldes, I.H., Grabin, S.: Ultrasound in the treatment of intervertebral disc syndrome, Am. J. Phys. Med. 37:199, 1958.

Allen, K.G.R., Battye, C.K.: Performance of ultrasonic therapy instruments, Physiotherapy 64(6):174–179, 1978.

Antich, T.J.: Physical therapy treatment of knee extensor mechanism disorders: comparison of four treatment modalities, J. Orthop. Sports Phys. Ther. 8:255, 1986.

Aspelin, P., Ekberg, O., Thorsson, O., and Wilhelmsson, M.: Ultrasound examination of soft tissue injury in the lower limb in patients, Am. J. Sports. Med. 20(5):601–603, 1992.

Banties, A., Klomp, R.: Transmission of ultrasound energy through coupling agents, Physiother. Sport, 3:9–13, 1979.

Bare, A., McAnaw, M., and Pritchard, A.: Phonophoretic delivery of

10% hydrocortisone through the epidermis of humans as determined by serum cortisol concentration, Phys. Ther. 76(7): 738–749, 1996.

Bearzy, H.J.: Clinical applications of ultrasonic energy in the treatment of acute and chronic subacromial bursitis, Arch. Phys. Med. Rehabil. 34:228, 1953.

Behrens, B.J., Michlovitz, S.L.: Physical agents: theory and practice for the physical therapist assistant, Philadelphia, 1996, F.A. Davis.

Benson, H.A., McElnay, J.C., and Harland, R.L.: Use of ultrasound to enhance percutaneous absorption of benzydamine, Phys. Ther. 69(2): 113–118, 1989.

Bickford, R.H., Duff, R.S.: Influence of ultrasonic irradiation on temperature and blood flow in human skeletal muscle, Circ. Res. 1:534, 1953.

Billings, C., Draper, D., and Schulthies, S.: Ability of the Omnisound 3000 Delta T to reproduce predictable temperature increases in human muscle, J. Ath. Train. 31(Suppl): S-47, 1996.

Bondolo, W.: Phenylbutazone with ultrasonics in some cases of anhrosynovitis of the knee, Arch. Orthopaed. 73:532–540, 1960.

Borrell, R.M., Parker, R., and Henley, E.J.: Comparison of in vitro temperatures produced by hydrotherapy paraffin wax treatment and fluidotherapy, Phys. Ther. 60:1273–1276, 1984.

Brueton, R.N., Blookes, M., and Heatley, F.W.: The effect of ultrasound on the repair of a rabbit's tibial osteotomy held in rigid external fixation, J. Bone Joint Surg. 69B:494, 1987.

Buchan, J.F.: Heat therapy and ultrasonics, Practitioner, 208: 130–131, 1972.

Buchtala, V.: The present state of ultrasonic therapy, Br. J. Phys. Med. 15:3, 1952.

Bundt, F.B.: Ultrasound therapy in supraspinatus bursitis, Phys. Ther. Rev. 38:826, 1958.

Burns, P.N., Pitcher, E.M.: Calibration of physiotherapy ultrasound generators, Clin. Phys. Physiol. Measure. 5:37 (abstract), 1984.

Byl, N.: The use of ultrasound as an enhancer for transcutaneous drug delivery: phonophoresis, Phys. Ther. 75(6):539–553, 1995.

Callam, M.J., Harper, D.R., Dale, J.J., et al: A controlled trial of weekly ultrasound therapy in chronic leg ulceration, Lancet 2(8552):204, 1987.

Cerino, L.E., Ackerman, E., and Janes, J.M.: Effects of ultrasound on experimental bone tumor, Surg. For. 16:466, 1965.

Cherup, N., Urben, J., and Bender, L.F.: The treatment of plantar warts with ultrasound, Arch. Phys. Med. Rehabil. 44:602, 1963.

Chan, A.K., Siealmann, R.A., and Guy, A.W.: Calculations of therapeutic heat generated by ultrasound in fat-muscle-bone layers, Inst. Electric. Electron. Eng. Trans. Biomed. Eng. BME-2t. 280–284, 1973.

Cline, P.D.: Radiographic follow-up of ultrasound therapy in calcific bursitis, Phys. Ther. 43:16, 1963.

Coakley, W.T.: Biophysical effects of ultrasound at therapeutic intensities, Physiotherapy 94(6):168–169, 1978.

Conger, A.D., Ziskin, M.C., and Wittels, H.: Ultrasonic effects on mammalian multicellular tumor spheroids, Clin. Ultrasound 9:167, 1981.

Conner-Kerr, T., Franklin, M., and Smith, S.: Efficacy of using phonophoresis for the delivery of dexamethasone to human transdermal tissues, JOSPT 23(1):79, 1996.

Costentino, A.B., Cross, D.L., Harrington, R.J., and Sodarberg, G.L.: Ultrasound effects on electroneuromyographic measures in sensory fibres of the median nerve, Phys. Ther. 63(11): 1788–1792, 1983.

Creates, V.: A study of ultrasound treatment to the painful perineum after childbirth, Physiotherapy 73:162, 1987.

Currier, D.F., Greathouse, D., and Swift, T.: Sensory nerve conduction: Effect of ultrasound, Arch. Phys. Med. Rehabil. 59:181, 1978.

DeDeyne, P, Kirsh-Volders, M,: In vitro effects of therapeutic ultrasound on the nucleus of human fibroblasts, Phys. Ther. 75(7): 629–634, 1995.

DiIorio, A., Frommelt, T., and Svendsen, L.: Therapeutic ultrasound effect on regional temperature and blood flow, J. Ath. Train. 31(Suppl):S-14, 1996.

Duarte, L.R.: The stimulation of bone growth by ultrasound, Arch. Orthop. and Trauma Surg. 101:153–159, 1983.

Dyson, M.: The production of blood cell stasis and endothelial damage in the blood vessels of chick embryos treated with ultrasound in a stationary wave field, Ultrasound Med. Biol. 11:133, 1974.

Dyson, M.: The stimulation of tissue regeneration by means of ultrasound, Clin. Sci. 35:273, 1968.

Dyson, M., Pond, J.B.: The effect of pulsed ultrasound on tissue regeneration, Physiotherapy 56(6):134–142, 1970.

Dyson, M., Suckling, J.: Stimulation of tissue repair by ultrasound: a survey of mechanisms involved, Physiotherapy 64:105, 1978.

Dyson, M., ter Haar, G.R.: The response of smooth muscle to ultrasound (abstr). In Proceedings from an International Symposium on Therapeutic Ultrasound, Winnipeg, Manitoba, September 10, 1981.

Dyson, M., Woodward, B., and Pond, J.B.: Flow of red blood cells stopped by ultrasound, Nature 232:572–573, 1971.

Edwards, M.I.: Congenital defects in guinea pigs: prenatal retardation of brain growth of guinea pigs following hyperthermia during gestation, Teratology 2:329, 1969.

Enwemeka, C.S.: The effects of therapeutic ultrasound on tendon healing, Am. J. Phys. Med. Rehabil., 68(6):283–287, 1989.

Falconer, J., Hayes, K.W., and Ghang, R.W.: Therapeutic ultrasound in the treatment of musculoskeletal conditions, Arthritis Care Res. 3(2):85–91, 1990.

Farmer, W.C.: Effect of intensity of ultrasound on conduction of motor axons, Phys. Therapy. 48:1233–1237, 1968.

Faul, E.D., Imig, C.J.: Temperature and blood flow studies after ultrasonic irradiation, Am. J. Phys. Med. 34:370, 1955.

Fieldhouse, C.: Ultrasound for relief of painful episiotomy scars, Physiotherapy 65:217, 1979.

Forrest, G., Rosen, K.: Ultrasound: effectiveness of treatments given under water, Arch. Phys. Med. Rehabil. 70:28, 1989.

Fountain, F.P., Gersten, J.W., and Sengu, O.: Decrease in muscle spasm produced by ultrasound, hot packs and IR, Arch. Phys. Med. Rehabil. 41:293, 1960.

Franklin, M., Smith, S., and Chenier, T.: Effect of phonophoresis with dexamethasone on adrenal function, JOSPT 22(3): 103–107, 1995.

Friedar, S.: A pilot study: the therapeutic effect of ultrasound following partial rupture of achilles tendons in male rats, J. Orthop. Sports Phys. Ther. 10:39, 1988.

Fyfe, M.C.: A study of the effects of different ultrasonic frequencies on experimental oedema, Aust. J. Physiother. 25(5):205–207, 1979.

Fyfe, M.C., Bullock, M.: Acoustic output from therapeutic ultrasound units, Aust. J. Physiother. 32(1):13–16, 1986.

Fyfe, M.C., Chahl, L.A.: The effect of ultrasound on experimental oedema in rats, Ultrasound. Med. Biol. 6:l07, 1980.

Gantz, S.: Increased radicular pain due to therapeutic ultrasound applied to the back, Arch. Phys. Med. Rehabil. 70:493–494, 1989.

Garrett, A.S., Garrett, M.: Letters: ultrasound for herpes zoster pain, J. Roy. College Gen. Practice. Nov, 709, 1982.

Gersten, J.W.: Effect of metallic objects on temperature rises produced in tissues by ultrasound, Am. J. Phys. Med. 37:75, 1958.

Goddard, D.H., Revell, P.A., and Cason, J.: Ultrasound has no anti-inflammatory effect, Ann. Rheum. Dis. 42:582–584, 1983.

Gracewski, S.M., Wagg, R.C., and Schenk, E.A.: High-frequency attenuation measurements using an acoustic microscope, J. Acoustic Soc. Am. 83(6):2405–2409, 1988.

Grant, A., Sleep, J., McIntosh, J., and Ashurst, H.: Ultrasound and pulsed electromagnetic energy treatment for peroneal trauma. A randomized placebo-controlled trial, Br. J. Obstet. Gynecol. 96:434-439, 1989.

Grieder, A., Vinton P., Cinott W., et al: An evaluation of ultrasonic therapy for temperomandibular joint dysfunction, Oral Surg. 31:25, 1971.

Griffin, J.E.: Patients treated with ultrasonic driven cortisone and with ultrasound alone, Phys. Ther. 47:594, 1967.

Griffin, J.E.: Transmissiveness of ultrasound through tap water, glycerin, and mineral oil, Phys. Ther. 60:1010, 1980.

Griffin, J.E., Touchstone, J.C.: Low intensity phonophoresis of cortisol in swine, Phys. Ther. 48(10):1336–1344, 1968.

Griffin, J.E., Touchstone, J.: Ultrasonic movement of cortisol into pig tissue: 1. movement into skeletal muscle, Am. J. Phys. Med. 42:77–85, 1962.

Griffin, J.E., Touchstone, J.C., and Liu, A.: Ultrasonic movement of cortisol into pig tissues; II. peripheral nerve, Am. J. Phys. Med. 4:20, 1965.

Halle, J.S., Scoville, C.R., and Greathouse, D.G.: Ultrasound's effect on the conduction latency of superficial radial nerve in man, Phys. Ther. 61:345, 1981.

Halle, J.S., Franklin, R.J., and Karalfa, B.L.: Comparison of four treatment approaches for lateral epicondylitis of the elbow, J. Orthop. Sports Phys. Ther. 8:62, 1986.

Hamer, J., Kirk, J.A.: Physiotherapy and the frozen shoulder: a comparative trial of ice and ultrasound therapy, N Z Med. 83(3): 191, 1976.

Hansen, T.I., Kristensen, J.H.: Effects of massage: shortwave and ultrasound upon 133Xe disappearance rate from muscle and subcutaneous tissue in the human calf, Scand. J. Rehabil. Medicine. 5:197, 1973.

Harris, S., Draper, D., and Schulthies, S.: The effect of ultrasound on temperature rise in preheated human muscle, J. Ath. Train. 30(Suppl): S-42, 1995.

Hashish, I., Hai, H.K., Harvey, W., et al: Reduction of postoperative pain and swelling by ultrasound treatment, a placebo effect, Pain 33:303–311, 1988.

Hekkenberg, R.T., Oosterbaan, W.A., and van Beekum, W.T.: Evaluation of ultrasound therapy devices, Physiotherapy 72:390, 1986.

Hill, C.R., ter Haar, G.: Ultrasound and non-ionizing radiation protection. In Suess, M.J., editor: WHO Regional Publication, European Series No. 10. World Health Organization, Copenhagen, 1981.

Hogan, R.D., Burke, K.M., and Franklin, T.D.: The effect of ultrasound on microvascular hemodynamics in skeletal muscle: effects during ischemia, Microvasc. Res. 23:370, 1982.

Hone, C-Z., Liu, H.H., and Yu, J.: Ultrasound thermotherapy effect on the recovery of nerve conduction in experimental compression neuropathy, Arch. Phys. Med. Rehabil. 69:410–414, 1988.

Hustler, J.E., Zarod, A.P., and Williams, A.R.: Ultrasonic modification of experimental bruising in the guinea-pig pinna, Ultrasound 16:223–228, 1978.

Imig, C.J., Randall, B.F., and Hines, H.M.: Effect of ultrasonic energy on blood flow, Am. J. Phys. Med. 53:100–102, 1954.

Inaba, M.K., Piorkowski, M.: Ultrasound in treatment of painful shoulder in patients with hemiplegia, Phys. Ther. 52:737, 1972.

Jones. RI: Treatment of acute herpes zoster using ultrasonic therapy, Physiotherapy 70:94, 1984.

Klemp, P., Staberg, B., Korsgard, J., et al: Reduced blood flow in fibromyotic muscles during ultrasound therapy, Scand. J. Rehabil. Med. 15:21–23, 1982.

Kramer, J.F.: Sensory and motor nerve conduction velocities following therapeutic ultrasound, Aust. J. Physiother. 33(4):235–243, 1987.

Kramer, J.F.: Effects of therapeutic ultrasound intensity on subcutaneous tissue temperature and ulnar nerve conduction velocity, Am. J. Phys. Med. 64:9, 1985.

Kramer, J.F: Effect of ultrasound intensity on sensory nerve conduction velocity, Physiother. Can. 37: 5–10, 1985.

Kuitert, J.H., Harr, E.T.: Introduction to clinical application of ultrasound, Phys. Ther. Rev 35:19, 1955.

Kuitert, J.H.: Ultrasonic energy as an adjunct in the management of radiculitis and similar referred pain, Am. J. Phys. Med. 33:61, 1954.

LaBan, M.M.: Collagen tissue: implications of its response to stress in vitro, Arch. Phys. Med. Rehabil. 43:461, 1962.

Lehmann, J.F.: Heating produced by ultrasound in bone and soft tissue, Arch. Phys. Med. Rehabil. 48:397, 1967.

Lehmann, J.F.: Heating of joint structures by ultrasound, Arch. Phys. Med. Rehabil. 49:28, 1968.

Lehmann, J.F.: Therapeutic temperature distribution produced by ultrasound as modified by dosage and volume of tissue exposed, Arch. Phys. Med. Rehabil. 48:662, 1967.

Lehmann, J.F.: Ultrasound effects as demonstrated in live pigs with surgical metallic implants, Arch. Phys. Med. Rehabil. 40:483, 1959.

Lehmann, J.F., Biegler, R.: Changes of potentials and temperature gradients in membranes caused by ultrasound, Arch. Phys. Med. Rehabil. 35:287, 1954.

Lehmann, J.F., Brunner, G.D., and Stow, R.W.: Pain threshold measurements after therapeutic application of ultrasound. microwaves and infrared, Arch. Phys. Med. Rehabil. 39:560, 1958.

Lehmann, J.F., Erickson, D.J., and Martin, G.M.: Comparative study of the efficiency of shortwave, microwave and ultrasonic diathermy in heating the hip joint, Arch. Phys. Med. Rehabil. 40:510, 1959.

Lehmann, J.R., Henrick, J.F.: Biologic reactions to cavitation: a consideration for ultrasonic therapy, Arch. Phys. Med. Rehabil. 34:86, 1953.

Lehmann, J.F., Stonebridge, J.B., de Lateur, B.J., et al: Temperatures in human thighs after hot pack treatment followed by ultrasound, Arch. Phys. Med. Rehabil. 59:472–475, 1978.

Lehmann, J.F., Warren, C.C., and Scham, S.M.: Therapeutic heat and cold, Clin. Orthop. 99:207–245, 1974.

Levenson, J.L., Weissberg, M.P.: Ultrasound abuse: a case report, Arch. Phys. Med. Rehabil. 64: 90–91, 1983.

LIoyd, J.J., Evans, J.A.: A calibration survey of physiotherapy equipment in North Wales, Physiotherapy 74(2):56–61, 1988.

Lota, M.I., Darling, R.C.: Change in permeability of the red blood cell membrane in a homogeneous ultrasonic field, Arch. Phys. Med. Rehabil. 36:282, 1955.

Lyons, M.E., Parker, K.J.: Absorption and attenuation in soft tissues II: experimental results, Inst. Electric. Electron. Eng. Trans. Ultrason. Ferroelect. Freq. Contr. 35:4, 1988.

Madsen, P.W., Gersten, J.W.: Effect of ultrasound on conduction velocity of peripheral nerves, Arch. Phys. Med. Rehabil. 42:645–649, 1963.

Massoth, A., Draper, D., and Kirkendall, D.: A measure of superficial tissue temperature during 1 MHz ultrasound treatments delivered at three different intensity settings, J. Ath. Train. 28(2):166, 1993.

Maxwell, L.: Therapeutic ultrasound and the metastasis of a solid tumor, J. Sport Rehabil. 4(4):273–281, 1995.

Maxwell, L.: Therapeutic ultrasound: its effects on the cellular and molecular mechanisms of inflammation and repair, Physiotherapy 78(6):421–425, 1992.

McDiarmid, T., Burns, P.N., and Lewith, G.T.: Ultrasound and the treatment of pressure sores, Physiotherapy 71:661, 1985.

McLaren, J.: Randomized controlled trial of ultrasound therapy for the damaged perineum (abstr), Clin. Phys. Physiol. Measure 5:40, 1984.

Michlovitz, S.L., Lynch, P.R., and Tuma, R.F.: Therapeutic ultrasound: its effects on vascular permeability (abstr), Fed. Proc. 41:1761, 1982.

Mickey, D., Bernier, J., and Perrin, D.: Ice and ice with nonthermal ultrasound effects on delayed onset muscle soreness, J. Ath. Train. 31(Suppl):S-19, 1996.

Miller, D.L.: A review of the ultrasonic bioeffects of microsonation, gas body activation and related cavitation-like phenomena, Ultrasound Med. Biol. 13(8):443–470, 1987.

Mortimer, A.J., Dyson, M.: The effect of therapeutic ultrasound on calcium uptake in fibroblasts, Ultrasound in Med. Biol. 14:499–508, 1988.

Mummery, C.L.: The effect of ultrasound on fibroblasts in vitro, PhD thesis. London University, 1978.

National Council on Radiation Protection and Measurements (NCRP) Report No 74 (BioloSica) effects of ultrasound, mechanisms and clinical applications, NCRP, Bethesda, Maryland, p. 197, 1983.

Newman, M.K., Kill, M., and Frampton, G.: Effects of ultrasound alone and combined with hydrocortisone injections by needle or hydrospray, Am. J. Phys. Med. 37:206, 1958.

Novak, E.J.: Experimental transmission of lidocaine through intact skin by ultrasound, Arch. Phys. Med. Rehabil. 45:231, 1964.

Oakley, E.M.: Evidence for effectiveness of ultrasound treatment in physical medicine, Br. J. Cancer 45(Suppl V):233–237, 1982.

Olson, S., Bowman, J., and Condrey, K.: Transdermal delivery of hydrocortisone, lidocaine, and menthol in subjects with delayed onset muscle soreness, J. Orthop. Sports Phys. Ther. 19(1):69, 1994.

Paaske, W.P., Hovind, H., and Seyerson, P.: Influence of therapeutic ultrasonic irradiation on blood flow in human cutaneous, subcutaneous, and muscular tissues, Scand. J. Clin. Lab. Invest. 31:389, 1973.

Paul, B.: Use of ultrasound in the treatment of pressure sores in patients with spinal cord injury, Arch. Phys. Med. Rehabil. 41:438, 1960.

Payne, C.: Ultrasound for post-herpetic neuralgia, Physiotherapy 70:96, 1984.

Penderghest, C., Kimura, I., and Sitler, M.: Double blind clinical efficacy study of dexamethasone-lidocaine pulsed phonophoresis on perceived pain associated with symptomatic tendinitis, J. Ath. Train. 31(Suppl): S-47, 1996.

Popspisilova, L., Rottova, A.: Ultrasonic effect on collagen synthesis and deposition in differently localised experimental granulomas, Acta Chirurgica Plastica. 19:148–157, 1977.

Reid, D.C.: Possible contraindications and precautions associated with ultrasound therapy, in Mortimer, A., Lee, N., editors: Proceedings of the International Symposium on Therapeutic Ultrasound, Canadian Physiotherapy Association, Winnipeg, 1981.

Reynolds, N.L.: Reliable ultrasound transmission (letter), Phys. Ther. 72(8):611, 1992.

Roberts, M., Rutherford, J.H., and Harris, D.: The effect of ultrasound on flexor tendon repairs in the rabbit, Hand 14:17, 1982.

Robinson, S., Buono, M.: Effect of continuous-wave ultrasound on blood flow in skeletal muscle, Phys. Ther. 75(2):145–150, 1995.

Roche, C., West, J.: A controlled trial investigating the effects of ultrasound on venous ulcers referred from general practitioners, Physiotherapy 70(12):475–477, 1984.

Rowe, R.J., Gray, I.M.: Ultrasound treatment of plantar warts, Arch. Phys. Med. Rehabil. 46:273, 1965.

Shambereer, R.C., Talbot, T.L., Tipton, H.W., et al: The effect of ultrasonic and thermal treatment of wounds, Plast. Reconstruct. Surg. 68(6):880–870, 1981.

Sicard-Rosenbaum, L., Lord, D., and Danoff, J.: Effects of continuous therapeutic ultrasound on growth and metastasis of subcutaneous murine tumors, Phys. Ther. 75(1):3–12, 1995.

Smith, W., Winn, F., and Farette, R.: Comparative study using four modalities in shinsplint treatments, J. Orthop. Sports Phys. Ther. 8:77, 1986.

Sokoliu, A.: Destructive effect of ultrasound on ocular tissues. In Reid, J.M., Sikov, M.R., editors: Interaction of ultrasound and biological tissues, DHEW Pub (FDA) 73-8008, 1972.

Soren, A.: Evaluation of ultrasound treatment in musculoskeletal disorders, Physiotherapy 61:214–217, 1965.

Soren, A.: Nature and biophysical effects of ultrasound, J. Occup. Med. 7:375, 1965.

Stevenson, J.H.: Functional, mechanical, and biochemical assessment of ultrasound therapy on tendon healing in chicken toe, Plast. Reconstruct. Surg. 77:965, 1986.

Stewart, H.F.: Survey of use and performance of ultrasonic therapy equipment in Pinelles County, Phys. Ther. 54:707, 1974.

Stewart, H.F., Abzug, J.L., and Harris, G.F.: Considerations in ultrasound therapy and equipment performance, Phys. Ther. 80(4):424–428, 1980.

Stoller, D.W., Markholf, K.L., Zager, S.A., and Shoemaker, S.C.: The effects of exercise ice and ultrasonography on torsional laxity of the knee joint, Clin. Orthop. Rel. Res. 174:172–150, 1983.

Stratford, P.W., Cevy, D.R., Gauldie, S., et al: The evaluation of phonophoresis and friction massage as treatments for extensor carpi radialis tendinitis: a randomized controlled trial, Physiother. Can. 41:93, 1989.

Stratton, S.A., Heckmann. R., and Francis, R.S.: Therapeutic ultrasound: its effect on the integrity of a nonpenetrating wound, J. Orthop. Sports Phys. Ther. 5:278, 1984.

Talaat, A.M., El-Dibany, M.M., and El-Garf, A: Physical therapy in the management of myofascial pain dysfunction syndrome, Am. Otol. Rhinol. Laryngol. 95:225, 1986.

Taylor, E., Humphry, R.: Survey of therapeutic agent modality use, Am. J. Occup. Ther. 46(10):924–931, 1991.

ter Haar, G.: Basic physics of therapeutic ultrasound, Physiotherapy 64(4):100–103, 1978.

ter Haar, C., Dyson, M., and Oakley, E.M.: The use of ultrasound by physiotherapists in Britain, 1985, Ultrasound Med. Biol. 13:659, 1987.

ter Haar, G., Wyard, S.J.: Blood cell banding in ultrasonic standing waves: A physical analysis, Ultrasound Med. Biol. 4:111–123, 1978.

van Levieveld, D.W.: Evaluation of ultrasonics and electrical stimulation in the treatment of sprained ankles. A controlled study, Ugesrk-Laeger 141(16):1077–1080, 1979.

Ward, A., Robertson, V.: Comparison of heating of nonliving soft tissue produced by 45 KHz and 1 MHz frequency ultrasound machines, JOSPT 23(4):258–266, 1996.

Warren, C.G., Lehmann, J.F., and Koblanski, N.: Heat and stretch procedures: an evaluation using rat tail tendon, Arch. Phys. Med. Rehabil. 57:122, 1976.

Warren, C.G., Koblanski, I.N., and Sigelmann, R.A.: Ultrasound coupling media: their relative transmissivity, Arch. Phys. Med. Rehabil. 57:218, 1976.

Wells, P.N.: Biomedical ultrasonics, London, 1977, Academic Press.

Wells, P.E., Frampton, V., and Bowsher, D., editors: Pain: management and control in physiotherapy, London, 1988, Heinemann.

Williams, A.R., McHale, I., and Bowditch, M.: Effects of MHz ultrasound on electrical pain threshold perception in humans, Ultrasound Med. Biol. 13:249, 1987.

Williamson, J.B., George, T.K., Simpson, D.C., et al: Ultrasound in the treatment of ankle sprains, Injury 17:76–178, 1986.

Wilson, A.G., Jamieson, S., and Saunders, R.: The physical behaviour of ultrasound, NZ J. Physiotherapy. 12(1):30–31, 1984.

Wood, R.W., Loomis, A.L.: The physical and biological effects of high frequency waves of great intensity, Philosoph. Mag. 4:417, 1927.

Wright, E.T., Haase, K.H.: Keloid and ultrasound, Arch. Phys. Med. Rehabil. 52:280, 1971.

Wyper, D.J., McNiven, D.R., and Donnelly, T.J.: Therapeutic ultrasound and muscle blood flow, Physiotherapy 64:321, 1978.

Zankei, H.T.: Effects of physical agents on motor conduction velocity of the ulnar nerve, Arch. Phys. Med. Rehabil. 47:787–792, 1966.

acoustic impedance Determines the amount of ultrasound energy reflected at tissue interfaces.

acoustic microstreaming The unidirectional movement of fluids along the boundaries of cell membranes resulting from the mechanical pressure wave in an ultrasonic field.

amplitude Describes the magnitude of the vibration in a wave. It is the maximum distance from equilibrium that any particle reaches.

attenuation A decrease in energy intensity as the ultrasound wave is transmitted through various tissues owing to scattering and dispersion.

beam nonuniformity ratio (BNR) Indicates the amount of variability of intensity within the ultrasound beam and is determined by the maximal point intensity of the transducer to the average intensity across the transducer surface.

cavitation The formation of gas-filled bubbles that expand and compress owing to ultrasonically induced pressure changes in tissue fluids.

collimated beam A focused, less divergent beam of ultrasound energy produced by a large diameter transducer.

compressions Regions of high molecular density (i.e., a great amount of ultrasound energy) within the longitudinal wave.

continuous wave ultrasound The sound intensity remains constant throughout the treatment, and the ultrasound energy is being produced 100 percent of the time.

coupling medium A substance used to decrease the acoustical impedance at the air-skin interface and thus facilitates the passage of ultrasound energy.

duty cycle The percentage of time that ultrasound is being generated (pulse duration) over one pulse period, which is also referred to as the mark to space ratio.

effective radiating area The total area of the surface of the transducer that actually produces the sound wave.

hot spots Areas at tissue interfaces that may become overheated.

intensity A measure of the rate at which energy is being delivered per unit area.

longitudinal wave The primary waveform in which ultrasound energy travels in soft tissue, with the molecular displacement along the direction in which the wave travels.

phonophoresis A technique in which ultrasound is used to drive a topical application of a selected medication into the tissues.

piezoelectric effect When an alternating electrical current generated at the same frequency as the crystal resonance is passed through the piezoelectric crystal, the crystal will expand and contract or vibrate at the frequency of the electrical oscillation, thus generating ultrasound at a desired frequency.

power The total amount of ultrasound energy in the beam and is expressed in watts.

pulsed ultrasound The intensity is periodically interrupted with no ultrasound energy being produced during the off period. When using pulsed ultrasound, the average intensity of the output over time is reduced.

rarefactions Regions of lower molecular density (i.e., a small amount of ultrasound energy) within a longitudinal wave.

standing wave As the ultrasound energy is reflected at tissue interfaces with different acoustic impedances, the intensity of the energy is increased as the reflected energy meets new energy being transmitted, forming waves of high energy that can potentially damage surrounding tissues.

stretching window The time period of vigorous heating when tissues will undergo their greatest extensibility and elongation.

transverse wave Occurring only in bone, the molecules are displaced in a direction perpendicular to the direction in which the ultrasound wave is moving.

LAB ACTIVITY

ULTRASOUND

DESCRIPTION:

Therapeutic ultrasound is a physical agent modality utilized in sports medicine for the purpose of elevating tissue temperature, stimulating the repair of musculoskeletal soft tissues, modulating pain, and in the case of phonophoresis, driving medicinal molecules into a local tissue. Ultrasound is a high frequency, inaudible acoustic sound wave that may produce either thermal or nonthermal physiologic effects within the body. When applied to biologic tissues ultrasound may induce significant responses in cells, tissues, and organs. Ultrasound is one of the most widely utilized physical agent modalities in addition to the thermotherapies and electrotherapies.

PHYSIOLOGIC EFFECTS:

Thermal effects
    Elevated tissue temperature
    Increased blood flow
    Increased tissue extensibility
    Increased local metabolism
    Altered nerve conduction velocity
Nonthermal effects
    Cavitation
    Fluid movement
    Increased cellular membrane permeability
    Acoustic microstreaming
    Stimulation of fibroblast activity

THERAPEUTIC EFFECTS:

    Increased collagen tissue extensibility
    Decreased joint stiffness
    Reduction of muscle spasm
    Modulation of pain
    Increased blood flow
    Mild inflammatory response
    Stimulation of tissue regeneration

INDICATIONS:

The primary indication for the use of therapeutic ultrasound by the therapist is in the acute and chronic treatment of soft tissue dysfunction, that is, strains, sprains, contusions with associated symptoms of pain, and muscular spasm. Ultrasound has also been successfully employed to enhance soft tissue and bone healing. Ultrasound can also be employed to percutaneously deliver selected medications to areas of inflammation.

CONTRAINDICATIONS:

- Areas of impaired pain or temperature sensation
- Areas of impaired circulation
- Epiphyseal areas in children
- Not over reproductive organs
- Not over eyes, heart, spinal cord, or cervical/stellate ganglia
- Not over cemented joint prostheses
- Not over malignancies

ULTRASOUND

PROCEDURE	Evaluation		
	1	2	3
1. Check supplies and equipment.			
a. Obtain appropriate ultrasound unit (1 or 3 MHz), towels, and coupling gel.			
2. Question patient.			
a. Verify identity of patient.			
b. Verify the absence of contraindications.			
c. Ask about previous ultrasound treatments and check previous treatment notes.			
3. Position patient.			
a. Place patient in a well-supported, comfortable position.			
b. Expose body part to be treated.			
c. Drape patient to preserve patient's modesty, protect clothing, but allow access to body part.			
4. Inspect body part to be treated.			
a. Check sensation.			
b. Check circulatory status.			
c. Verify that there are no rashes or open wounds.			
d. Assess function of body part (e.g., ROM, strength, irritability).			
5. Apply indicated technique: select continuous or pulsed output and verify output intensity is at 0 before turning unit power on.			
a. Direct Coupling			
i. Apply layer of coupling gel to treatment surface.			
ii. Establish treatment duration dependent on size of area to be treated (i.e., 5 minutes for each 16-square-inch area).			
iii. Maintain contact between soundhead and treatment surface, moving soundhead in circular or linear overlapping strokes at a rate of 2 to 4 inches per second; observe for air bubble formation.			
iv. Adjust treatment intensity: 0.5 to 1.0 W/cm^2 for superficial tissues and 1.0 to 2.0 W/cm^2 for deeper tissues.			
v. Monitor patient response during treatment; if patient reports warmth or ache, reduce intensity by 10 percent and continue treatment.			
b. Bladder Coupling			
i. Fill a balloon or condom with tepid, degassed water.			
ii. Apply layer of coupling gel to bladder.			
iii. Apply layer of coupling gel to treatment surface.			
iv. Place bladder over treatment surface.			
v. Establish treatment duration dependent on size of area to be treated (i.e., 5 min for each 16-square-inch area).			
vi. Maintain contact between soundhead and treatment surface, moving soundhead in circular or linear overlapping strokes at a rate of 2 to 4 inches per second; observe for air bubble formation.			
vii. Adjust treatment intensity: 0.5 to 1.0 W/cm^2 for superficial tissues and 1.0 to 2.0 W/cm^2 for deeper tissues, intensity may need to be increased.			

PROCEDURE	Evaluation		
	1	2	3
viii. Monitor patient response during treatment; if patient reports warmth or ache, reduce intensity by 10 percent and continue treatment.			
c. Underwater Coupling			
i. Fill a plastic or ceramic nonconductive basin with tepid degassed water of sufficient depth to cover treatment surface.			
ii. Immerse the body part into the basin.			
iii. Establish treatment duration dependent on size of area to be treated (i.e., 5 minutes for each 16-square-inch area).			
iv. Maintain soundhead parallel to treatment surface at a distance of 0.5 to 3 cm, moving soundhead in circular or linear overlapping strokes at a rate of 2 to 4 inches per second; observe for air bubble formation on soundhead and wipe away.			
v. Adjust treatment intensity: 0.5 to 1.0 W/cm^2 for superficial tissues and 1.0 to 2.0 W/cm^2 for deeper tissues, intensity may need to be increased.			
vi. Monitor patient response during treatment; if patient reports warmth or ache, reduce intensity by 10 percent and continue treatment.			
d. Phonophoresis			
i. Cleanse treatment surface with alcohol or soap and water.			
ii. Apply medication in glycerol cream, oil, or other vehicle in lieu of coupling gel.			
iii. Establish treatment duration dependent upon size of area to be treated (i.e., 5 minutes for each 16 square inch area).			
iv. Maintain contact between soundhead and treatment surface, moving soundhead in circular or linear overlapping strokes at a rate of 2 to 4 inches per second; observe for air bubble formation.			
v. Adjust treatment intensity: 0.5 to 1.0 W/cm^2 for superficial tissues and 1.0 to 2.0 W/cm^2 for deeper tissues. Intensity may need to be decreased.			
vi. Monitor patient response during treatment; if patient reports warmth or ache, reduce intensity by 10 percent and continue treatment.			
6. Terminate treatment.			
a. Zero out ultrasound unit control before removing soundhead.			
b. Clean soundhead of excess gel or medication in vehicle.			
c. Clean treatment surface of excess gel or medication in vehicle.			
d. Visually inspect the treated area.			
e. Remove draping material and have patient dress.			
7. Assess treatment efficacy.			
a. Ask the patient how the treated area feels.			
b. Record treatment parameters.			
8. Instruct the patient in any indicated exercise.			
9. Return equipment to storage after cleaning.			

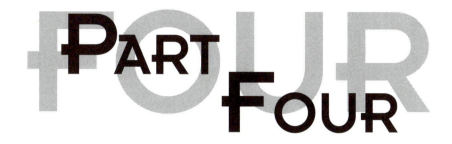

PART FOUR

LIGHT THERAPY

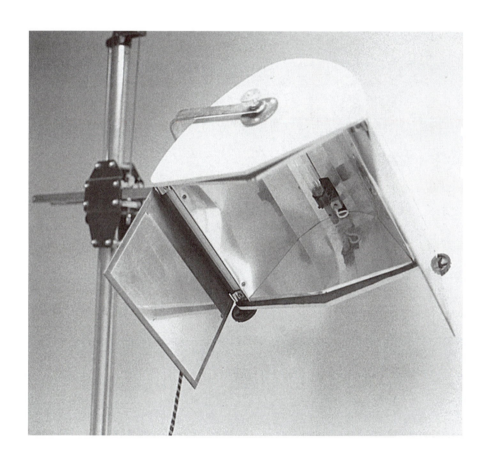

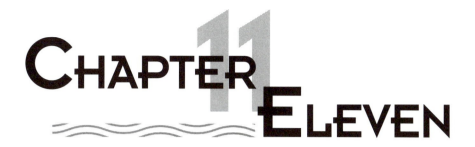

CHAPTER ELEVEN

LOW POWER LASERS

ETHAN SALIBA

SUSAN FOREMAN

OBJECTIVES

Following the completion of this chapter, the student therapist will be able to:

✓ Describe the different types of lasers.
✓ Understand the physical principles used to produce laser light.
✓ Describe the characteristics of the helium neon and gallium arsenide low power lasers.
✓ Describe the therapeutic applications of lasers in wound and soft tissue healing, edema reduction, inflammation, and pain.
✓ Understand the application techniques of low power lasers.
✓ Describe the classifications of lasers.
✓ Describe the safety considerations in the use of lasers.
✓ Describe the precautions and contraindications for low power lasers.

L ASER is an acronym that stands for light amplification of stimulated emissions of radiation. Despite the image presented in science-fiction movies, lasers offer valuable applications in the industrial, military, scientific, and medical environments. Einstein in 1916 was the first to postulate the theorems that conceptualized the development of lasers. The first work with amplified electromagnetic radiation dealt with MASERs (microwave amplification of stimulated emission of radiation). In 1955, Townes and Schawlow showed it was possible to produce stimulated emission of microwaves beyond the optical region of the electromagnetic spectrum. This work with stimulated emission soon extended into the optical region of the electromagnetic spectrum, resulting in the development of devices called optical masers. The first working optical maser was constructed in 1960 by Theodore Maiman when he developed the synthetic ruby laser. Other types of lasers were devised shortly afterward. It was not until 1965 that the term LASER was substituted for optical masers.[27]

Although lasers are relatively new, they have gone through extensive advances and refinements in a very short time. Lasers have been incorporated into numerous

LASER = Light Amplification for the Stimulated Emission of Radiation

laser A device that concentrates high energies into a narrow beam of coherent, monochromatic light; Light Amplification of the Stimulated Emission of Radiation.

everyday applications that range from audio discs and supermarket scanning to communication and medical applications. This chapter provides an overview of lasers, but deals principally with the application of low power lasers as they are used in conservative management of medical conditions.

PHYSICS

Light is a form of electromagnetic energy that has **wavelengths** between 100 and 10,000 nanometers (nm = 10^{-9}) within the electromagnetic spectrum.[27] Visible light ranges from 400 (violet) to 700 nm (red). Beyond the red portion of the visual range is the **infrared** and microwave region, and below the violet end are the ultraviolet, x-ray, gamma, and cosmic ray regions (Fig. 11-1). Light energy is transmitted through space as waves that contain tiny "energy packets" called **photons.** Each photon contains a definite amount of energy, depending on its wavelength (color).

Basics of the atomic theory are used to explain the principles of laser generation. The atom is the smallest particle of an element that retains all the properties of that element. The atom is divisible into fundamental particles called neutrons, protons, and electrons. Neutrons and positively charged protons are contained in the nucleus of the atom. **Electrons,** which are negatively charged, are equal in number to the protons and orbit the nucleus at distinct energy levels.

If an atom gains or loses an electron, it will become a negatively or positively charged ion, respectively. The polarity difference between the positively charged nucleus and negatively charged electrons keeps the electrons orbiting the nucleus at these distinct energy levels. Electrons neither absorb nor radiate energy as long as they are maintained in their distinct orbit. An electron will stay in its lowest energy level **(ground state)** unless it absorbs an adequate amount of energy to move it to one of its higher orbital levels. (Fig. 11-2). If an electron changes orbit, it will either gain or lose a distinct amount (quanta) of energy; it cannot exist between orbits.

If a photon of adequate energy level collides with an electron of an atom, it will cause the electron to change levels. When this occurs, the atom is said to be in an **excited state.** The atom stays in this excited state only momentarily and releases an identical photon (energy level) to the one it absorbed, which returns it to a ground state. This process is called **spontaneous emission** (see Fig. 11-1). Energy levels are particular to the type of atom; therefore, an electron accepts only the precise amount of energy that will move it from one energy level to another. Another means of

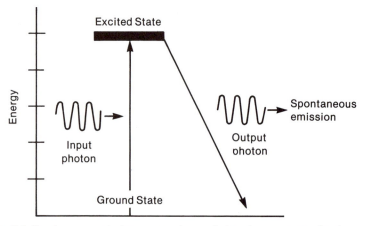

•**Figure 11-1** Spontaneous emission occurs when a photon changes energy level.

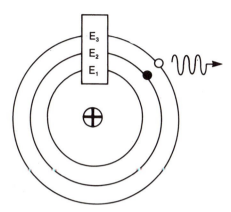

•Figure 11-2 When energy is absorbed by an atom, an orbiting electron can become excited to a higher orbit. As the electron drops back to its original level, energy (photon) is released.

exciting atoms other than with photon collision is with an electrical discharge. The energy is generated by collision of electrons that are accelerated in an electrical field.[17]

STIMULATED EMISSIONS

The concept of **stimulated emission** was postulated by Einstein and is essential to the working principle of lasers. It states that a photon released from an excited atom would stimulate another similarly excited atom to de-excite itself by releasing an identical photon.[27] The triggering photon would continue on its way unchanged, and the subsequent photon released would be identical in frequency, direction, and phase. These two photons would promote the release of additional identical photons as long as other excited atoms were present. A critical factor for this occurrence is having an environment with unlimited excited atoms, which is termed **population inversion.** Population inversion occurs when there are more atoms in an excited state than in a ground state. It is caused by applying an external power source to the lasing medium. The released photons are identical in phase, direction, and **frequency.** To contain them, and to generate more photons, mirrors are placed at both ends of the chamber. One mirror is totally reflective, whereas the other is semipermeable. The photons are reflected within the chamber, which amplifies the light and stimulates the emission of other photons from excited atoms. Eventually, so many photons are stimulated that the chamber cannot contain the energy. When a specific level of energy is attained, photons of a particular wavelength are ejected through the semipermeable mirror. Thus, amplified light through stimulated emissions (LASER) is produced (Fig. 11-3).

The laser light is emitted in an organized manner rather than in a random pattern as from a light bulb. Three properties distinguish the laser from incandescent and fluorescent light sources: **coherence, monochromaticity,** and **collimation.**[27]

Coherence means all photons of light emitted from individual gas molecules are the same wavelength and that the individual light waves are in phase with one another. Normal light, on the other hand, is composed of many wavelengths that superimpose their phases on one another.

Monochromaticity refers to the specificity of light in a single, defined wavelength; if the specificity is in the visible light spectrum, it is only one color. The laser is one of the few light sources that produces a specific wavelength.

stimulated emission When a photon interacts with an atom already in a high energy state and decay of the atomic system occurs, releasing two photons.

coherence Property of identical phase and time relationship. All photons of laser light are the same wavelength.

Three Properties of LASER
- Coherence
- Monochromaticity
- Collimation

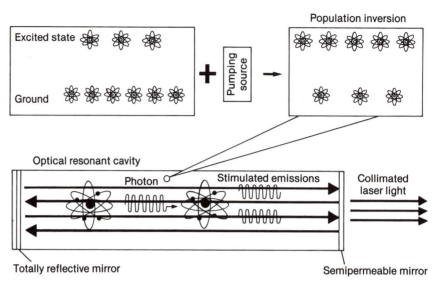

•**Figure 11-3** Pumping is a process of elevating an orbiting electron to a higher level, thus creating population inversion that is essential for laser operation.

divergence The bending of light rays away from each other; the spreading of light.

The laser beam is well collimated, that is, there is minimal divergence of the photons.[1] That means the photons move in a parallel fashion, thus concentrating a beam of light (Fig. 11-4).

TYPES OF LASERS

Lasers are classified according to the nature of the material placed between two reflecting surfaces. There are potentially thousands of different types of lasers, each with specific wavelengths and unique characteristics, depending on the lasing medium utilized. The lasing mediums used to create lasers include the following

Most Commonly Used LASERS
• Helium neon (HeNe)
• Gallium Arsenide (GaAs)

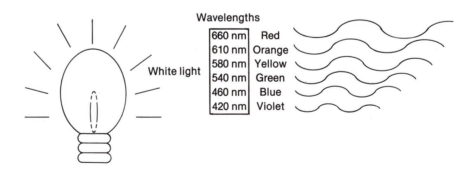

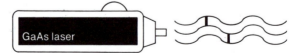

•**Figure 11-4** (*Top*), White light contains electromagnetic energy of all wavelengths (colors) that are superimposed on each other. (*Bottom*), Laser light is monochromatic (single wavelength), coherent (in phase), and collimated (minimal divergence).

categories: crystal and glass (solid-state), gas and excimer, semiconductor, liquid dye, and chemical.

Crystal lasers include the synthetic ruby (aluminum oxide and chromium) and the neodymium, yttrium, aluminum, garnet (Nd:YAG) lasers, among others. Synthetic, rather than natural, materials are used to ensure purity of the medium, which is necessary for the physical characteristics of lasers to occur.[12]

Gas lasers were developed in 1961, shortly after the first ruby laser. The gas lasers developed include the helium neon (HeNe), argon, and carbon dioxide (CO_2) along with numerous others. The HeNe laser is one type of low power device under investigation in the United States for application in physical medicine.

Semiconductor or **diode lasers** were developed in 1962 after the production of gas (HeNe) lasers. The gallium arsenide (GaAs) was the first diode laser developed and is another low power laser under investigation in the United States for application in physical medicine.

Liquid lasers are also known as dye lasers because they use organic dyes as the lasing medium. By varying the mixture of the dyes, the wavelengths of the laser can be varied.

Chemical lasers are usually extremely high powered and frequently used for military purposes.[17]

Lasers can be categorized as either high or low power, depending on the intensity of energy they deliver. High power lasers are also known as "hot" lasers because of the thermal responses they generate. These are used in the medical realms in numerous areas, including surgical cutting and coagulation, ophthalmologic, dermatologic, oncologic, and vascular specialties. The use of low power lasers (also known as "cold" or "soft" lasers) for wound healing and pain management is a relatively new area of application in medicine. These lasers produce a maximal output of less than 1 milliwatt (1 mW = 1/1000 W) in the United States and work by causing photochemical, rather than thermal, effects. No tissue warming occurs. The exact distinction of the power output that delineates a low versus high power laser varies. Low power devices are considered any laser that does not generate an appreciable thermal response. This category can include lasers capable of producing up to 500 W of power (up to a Class IV laser).[5]

Low power lasers, which have been studied and used in Europe for the past 20 to 25 years, have been investigated in the United States for the past decade. The potential applications for low power lasers include treatment of tendon and ligament injury, arthritis, edema reduction, soft tissue injury, ulcer and burn care, scar tissue inhibition, and acutherapy.

EQUIPMENT

Lasers require the following components to be operational.[17]

1. Power supply: Lasers use an electrical power supply that can potentially deliver up to 10,000 V and hundreds of amps.

2. Lasing medium: This is the material that generates the laser light. It can include any type of matter; gas, solid, or liquid.

3. Pumping device: "Pumping" is the term used to describe the process of elevating an orbiting electron to a higher, "excited" energy level (see Fig. 11-3). This creates the population inversion that is essential for laser operation. The pumping device may be high voltage, photoflash lamps, radio-frequency oscillators, or other lasers. The pumping device is very specific to the type of lasing medium being used.

4. Optical resonant cavity: This contains the lasing medium. Once population inversion has occurred, this cavity, which contains the reflecting surfaces, directs the beam propagation.

CASE STUDY 11-1
LOW-POWER LASERS

Background: A 44-year-old man who has had Type I diabetes mellitus for 30 years presents for treatment of a non- or slow-healing lesion on his left foot. He has a mild peripheral sensory neuropathy and developed a blister after going for a long run with new running shoes. The initial injury occurred 3 months ago and there has been no change in the size of the lesion for the past month. The lesion is on the plantar surface of the foot, under the first metatarsal head. It is a full-thickness lesion and is approximately 3 cm in diameter. The patient's medical condition is stable and there are no other complaints.

Impression: Chronic dermal lesion on the left foot.

Treatment Plan: Daily treatment with a helium neon laser was initiated. After cleansing the wound under aseptic conditions, the entire lesion was exposed to the HeNe light at 632.8 nm wavelength. The scanning technique was used to prevent contamination of the wound and equipment. The entire lesion was treated with an energy density of 4.0 J/cm^2.

Response: Photographs were taken on a weekly basis to document the effects of the treatment. After 3 weeks of daily treatment, the frequency was decreased to three sessions per week. After a total of 21 sessions (5 weeks), the lesion was healed. The patient was taught self-care and techniques to prevent further injuries.

The rehabilitation professional employs therapeutic agent modality to create an optimum environment for tissue healing while minimizing the symptoms associated with the trauma or condition.

Discussion Questions
- What tissues were injured or affected?
- What symptoms were present?
- What phase of the injury-healing continuum did the patient present for care in?
- What are the therapeutic agent modality's biophysical effects (direct, indirect, depth, and tissue affinity)?
- What are the therapeutic agent modality's indications and contraindications?
- What are the parameters of the therapeutic agent modality's application, dosage, duration, and frequency in this case study?
- What other therapeutic agent modalities could be used to treat this injury or condition? Why? How?

The helium neon (HeNe) and gallium arsenide (GaAs) lasers are the two principal lasers currently under investigation in the United States for conservative management of medical conditions. The following discussion will concentrate on these two laser types.

HELIUM NEON LASERS

The HeNe gas laser uses a gas mixture of primarily helium with neon in a pressurized tube. This creates a laser in the red portion of the electromagnetic spectrum with a wavelength is 632.8 nm. The power output of the HeNe can vary, but typically runs from 1.0 to 10.0 mW, depending on the gas density used. Larger tubes are necessary for higher-power outputs, and each requires a precise power drive to operate.[5] Laser output can decrease, depending on the care of the equipment, on the number of operating hours, and whether **fiberoptics** are used. For example, rough handling can jar the reflecting surfaces, and a high number of hours in operation or poor fiberoptic quality can diminish the laser output. The HeNe laser in the United States delivers a power output of 1 mW through a fiberoptic tube in a continuous mode. Although the HeNe laser light is well collimated, the utilization of fiberoptics causes a divergence of the beam from 18° to 21°.[5] Fiberoptics can decrease the output delivery 50 percent or more as the light travels from the lasing medium to the tip of the applicator. Fiberoptics are used to make the delivery more convenient because the size of the gas tube would make direct application difficult. HeNe lasers up to 6 mW have been manufactured for clinical use in Canada, which has fewer governmental restrictions than the United States. These higher output lasers, although still considered low power, allow delivery of desired dosages in reduced time.[6]

GALLIUM ARSENIDE LASERS

The gallium arsenide (GaAs) lasers utilize a diode to produce an infrared (invisible) laser at a wavelength of 904 nm. Diode lasers are composed of semiconductor silicone materials that are precisely cut and layered. An electrical source is applied to each side, and lasing action is produced at the junction of the two materials. The cleaved surfaces function as partially reflecting surfaces that will ultimately produce coherent light (Fig. 11-5).[12]

diode laser A solid-state semiconductor used as a lasing medium.

Diode lasers produce a beam that is elliptically shaped so the lasers have a 10° to 35° divergence despite the fact that no fiberoptics are used.[17] The 904 nm laser is delivered in a pulsed mode because of the heat produced at the junction of the diode chips. The GaAs laser manufactured in the United States has a peak power of 2 W but is delivered in a pulsed mode that decreases the average power to 0.4 mW output if delivered at 1000 Hz (see calculations in the Dosage section).

The application of additional layers of materials to other types of diodes allows their operation in a continuous mode at room temperature.[17] The continuous mode results in higher average power outputs from the lasers. Higher output diode lasers are manufactured for clinical applications in Canada and include the following:

780 nm wavelength with a 5 mW output, continuous mode delivery
810 nm wavelength with a 20 mW output, continuous mode delivery
830 nm wavelength with a 30 mW output, continuous mode delivery

These diodes are interchangeable in a single base unit.[6]

The laser units available in the United States have the ability to deliver both HeNe and GaAs lasers. The same device can both measure electrical impedance and deliver electrical point stimulation. The impedance detector allows hypersensitive or acupuncture points to be located. The point stimulator can be combined with laser application when treating pain. The electrical stimulation is believed to provide spontaneous pain relief, whereas the laser provides more latent tissue responses.[7]

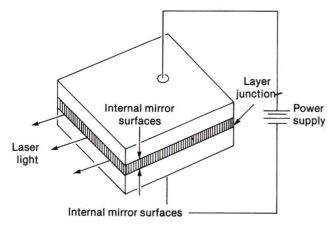

•Figure 11-5 A diode is composed of silicone material that is cleaved and layered. The lasing action occurs at the junction of the layers when an electrical source is applied.

CLINICAL APPLICATIONS FOR LASERS

Since the production of lasers is relatively new, the biologic and physiologic effects of this concentrated light energy are still being explored. The effects of low power lasers are subtle, primarily occurring at a cellular level. Various in vitro and animal studies have attempted to elucidate the interaction of photons with the biologic structures. Although there are few controlled clinical studies in the literature, documented case studies and empirical evidence indicate that lasers are effective in reducing pain and aiding wound healing. The exact mechanisms for action are still uncertain, although proposed physiologic effects include an acceleration in collagen synthesis, a decrease in microorganisms, an increase in vascularization, reduction of pain, and an anti-inflammatory action.[6]

Low power lasers are best recognized for increasing the rate of wound and ulcer healing by enhancing cellular metabolism. Results from animal studies have varied as to the benefits on wound healing, perhaps owing to the fact that the types of lasers, dosages, and protocols used have been inconsistent. In humans, improvement of nonhealing wounds indicates promising possibilities for treatment with lasers.

WOUND HEALING

Early investigations of the effects of low power laser on biologic tissues were limited to in vitro experimentation. Although it was known that high power lasers could damage and vaporize tissues, little was known about the effect of small dosages on the viability and stability of cellular structures. It was found that low dosages ($< 10 \, J/cm^2$) of radiation from low output lasers had a stimulatory action on metabolic processes and cell proliferation compared to incandescent or tungsten light.[2]

Mester conducted numerous in vitro experiments with two lasers in the red portion of the visual spectrum: the ruby laser, wavelength of 694.3 nm, and the HeNe laser, wavelength 632.8 nm. Human tissue cultures showed significant increases in fibroblastic proliferation following stimulation by either laser tested.[18] Fibroblasts are the precursor cells to connective tissue structures such as collagen, epithelial cells, and chondrocytes. When the production of fibroblasts is stimulated, one should expect a subsequent increase in the production of connective tissue. Abergel and associates documented that certain dosages of HeNe and GaAs laser, wavelength 904 nm, caused in vitro human skin fibroblasts to have a threefold increase in procollagen production.[2] This effect was most marked when low-level stimulation (1.94×10^{-7} to $5.84 \times 10^{-6} \, J/cm^2$ of GaAs and dosages of 0.053 to 1.589 J/cm^2 of HeNe) was repeated over 3 to 4 days versus a single exposure. Samples of tissue showed increases in fibroblast and collagenous structures as well as increases in the intracellular material and swollen mitochondria of cells.[18] Furthermore, cells were undamaged in regard to their morphology and structure after exposure to low power laser.[3]

Analysis of the cellular metabolism, with attention to the activity of DNA and RNA, has been made.[2,18,25] Through radioactive markers, it was suggested that laser stimulation enhances the synthesis of nucleic acids and cell division.[8,18] Abergel reported that laser-treated cells had significantly greater amounts of procollagen messenger RNA, further confirming that increased collagen production occurs because of modifications at the transcriptional level.[1]

Low power lasers were used in animal studies to further delineate both the beneficial applications of laser light and its potential harm. In an early study by Mester and associates, mechanical and burn wounds were made on the backs of mice.[19] Similar wounds on the same animals served as the controls, with the experimental wounds subjected to various doses of ruby laser. Although there were no histologic

Indications
Facilitate wound healing
Pain reduction
Increasing the tensile strength of a scar
Decreasing scar tissue
Decreasing inflammation
Bone healing and fracture consolidation

differences among the wounds, the lased wounds healed significantly faster, especially at a dosage of 1 J/cm^2. It was also demonstrated that repeated laser treatments were more effective than a single exposure.

Other researchers investigated the rate of healing and tensile strength of full-thickness wounds when exposed to laser irradiation.[2,13–16,24] There were conflicting reports regarding rates of healing, with some studies showing no change in the rate of wound closure, and others showing significantly faster wound healing.[2,13–16,24] Although the experimental results were conflicting, an explanation for the discrepancy may be an indirect systemic effect of laser energy. Mester showed that it was not necessary to irradiate an entire wound to achieve beneficial results, since stimulation of remote areas had similar results.[18] Kana and associates described an increase in the rate of healing of both the irradiated and nonirradiated wounds on the same animal compared to nonirradiated animals.[14] This systemic effect was most marked with the argon laser. Several studies that investigated the rate of healing on living animal tissue used a second, nontreated control wound on the same animal. The rate of healing may have been confounded by this systemic effect. Whether the systemic effect involves a humoral component, a circulating element, producing immunologic effects has yet to be determined or identified. Bactericidal and lymphocyte stimulation are proposed mechanisms for this phenomenon.

TENSILE STRENGTH

The increased tensile strength of lased wounds was confirmed more often.[2,13,14,16,19,24] Wound contraction, collagen synthesis, and increases in tensile strength are fibroblast-mediated functions and were demonstrated most markedly in the early phase of wound healing. Wounds were tested at various stages of healing to determine their breaking point, and were compared to a control or nonlased wound. Laser-treated wounds had significantly greater tensile strengths, most commonly in the first 10 to 14 days after injury, although they approached the values of the control after that time.[1,16,24] Hypertrophic scars did not result as tissue responses normalized after a 14-day period. HeNe laser of doses ranging from 1.1 to 2.2 J/cm^2 elicited positive results when lased either twice a day or on alternate days. The increased tensile strength corresponds to higher levels of collagen.

IMMUNOLOGIC RESPONSES

These early studies led to the hypothesis that laser exposure could enhance healing of skin and connective tissue lesions, but the mechanism was still unclear. Biochemical analysis and radioactive tracers were used to delineate the immunologic effects of laser light on human tissue cultures. The laser irradiation caused increased phagocytosis by leukocytes with dosages of .05 joules per square centimeter (J/cm^2).[18] This led to the possibility of a bactericidal effect, which was further demonstrated with laser exposures on cell cultures containing *Escherichia coli*, a common intestinal bacteria in humans. The ruby laser had an increased effect both on cell replication and on the destruction of bacteria via the phagocytosis of leukocytes.[18,19] Mester also concluded that there were immunologic effects with the ruby, HeNe, and argon lasers. Specifically, there was a direct stimulatory influence on the T- and B-lymphocyte activity, a phenomenon that is specific to laser output and wavelength. HeNe and Argon lasers gave the best results, with dosages ranging from 0.5 to 1 J/cm^2.[18] Trelles did similar investigations in vitro and in vivo and reported that laser did not have bactericidal effects alone, but when used in conjunction with antibiotics, there were significantly higher bactericidal effects compared to controls.[25]

With the confidence that they would cause little or no harm and that they could serve a therapeutic purpose, low power lasers have been used clinically on human subjects since the 1960s. In Hungary, Mester treated nonhealing ulcers that did not respond to traditional therapy with HeNe and argon lasers with respective wavelengths of 632.8 and 488 nm.[18] The dosages were varied but had a maximum of 4 J/cm². By the time of Mester's publication, 1125 patients had been treated, of which 875 healed, 160 improved, and 85 did not respond. The wounds, which were categorized by etiology, took an average of 12 to 16 weeks to heal. Trelles also showed promising results clinically using the infrared GaAs and HeNe lasers on the healing of ulcers, nonunion fractures, and on herpetic lesions.[25]

Gogia et al., in the United States, treated nonhealing wounds with GaAs lasers pulsed at a frequency of 1000 Hz for 10 sec/cm² with a sweeping technique held about 5 mm from the wound surface.[11] This protocol was used in conjunction with daily or twice daily sterile whirlpool treatments and produced satisfactory results, although statistical information was not reported. Empirical evidence by these authors suggested faster healing and cleaner wounds when subjected to GaAs laser treatment three times per week.

INFLAMMATION

Biopsies of experimental wounds were examined for prostaglandin activity to delineate the effect of laser stimulation on the inflammatory process. A decrease in prostaglandin (PGE_2) is a proposed mechanism in which laser therapy promotes the reduction of edema. During inflammation, prostaglandins cause vasodilation, which contributes to the flow of plasma into the interstitial tissue. By reducing prostaglandins, the driving force behind edema production is reduced.[6] The prostaglandin E and F contents were examined after treatments with HeNe laser at 1 J/cm².[18] In 4 days, both types of prostaglandins accumulated more than the controls. However, at 8 days, the PGE_2 levels decreased, whereas PGF_2 alpha increased. There was also an increased capillarization during this phase. This data indicates that prostaglandin production is affected by laser stimulation, and these changes possibly reflect an accelerated resolution of the acute inflammatory process.[18]

SCAR TISSUE

Macroscopic examination of healed wounds was subjectively described after the laser experiments in most studies. In general, the wounds exposed to laser irradiation had less scar tissue and a better cosmetic appearance. Histologic examination showed greater epithelialization and less exudative material.[15]

Studies that utilized burn wounds showed more regular alignment of collagen and smaller scars. Trelles lased third-degree burns on the backs of hairless mice with GaAs and HeNe lasers and showed significantly faster healing in the lased animals.[25] The best results were obtained with the GaAs laser, because of its greater penetration. Trelles found increased circulation with the production of new blood vessels in the center of the wounds compared to the controls. Edges of the wounds maintained viability and contributed to the epithelialization and closure of the burn. Since there was less contracture associated with irradiated wounds, laser treatment has been suggested for burns and wounds on the hands and neck, where contractures and scarring can severely limit function.

PAIN

Lasers have also been effective in reducing pain and have been shown to affect peripheral nerve activity. Rochkind and others produced crush injuries in rats and treated experimental animals with 10 J/cm^2 of HeNe laser energy transcutaneously along the sciatic nerve projection.[20] The amplitude of electrically stimulated action potentials was measured along the injured nerve and compared with controls up to 1 year later. The amplitude of the action potentials was 43 percent greater after 20 days, which was the duration of laser treatment. By 1 year, all lased nerves demonstrated equal or higher amplitudes than preinjury. The controls followed an expected course of recovery and did not reach normal levels even after 1 year.

The effect of HeNe irradiation on peripheral sensory nerve latency has been investigated on humans by Snyder-Mackler and Bork.[23] This double-blind study showed that exposure of the superficial radial nerve to low dosages of laser resulted in a significantly decreased sensory nerve conduction velocity, which may provide information about the pain-relieving mechanism of lasers. Other explanations for pain relief may be the result of hastened healing, anti-inflammatory action, autonomic nerve influence, and neurohumoral responses (serotonin, norepinephrine) from descending tract inhibition.[6,7]

Chronic pain has been treated with GaAs and HeNe lasers, and positive results have been observed empirically and through clinical research. Walker conducted a double-blind study to document analgesia after exposure to HeNe irradiation in chronic pain patients compared with sham treatments.[28] When the superficial sites of the radial, median, and saphenous nerves as well as painful areas were exposed to laser irradiation, there were significant decreases in pain and less reliance on medication for pain control. These preliminary studies suggest positive results, although pain modulation is difficult to measure objectively.

BONE RESPONSE

Future uses of laser irradiation include the treatment of other connective tissue structures, such as bone and articular cartilage. Schultz et al. studied various intensities of Nd:YAG laser on the healing of partial-thickness articular cartilage lesions in guinea pigs.[21] During the surgical procedure, the lesions were irradiated for 5 sec, with intensities ranging from 25 to 125 J. After 4 weeks, the low-dosage group (25 J) had chondral proliferation, and by 6 weeks the defect had reconstituted to the level of the surface cartilage. Normal basophilia cells were present with staining, indicating normal cellular structures. The higher dosage groups and controls had little or no evidence of restoration of the lesion with cartilage. Bone healing and fracture consolidation have been investigated by Trelles and Mayayo.[26] An adapter was attached to an intramuscular needle so that the laser energy could be directed deeper to the periosteum. Rabbit tibial fractures showed faster consolidation with HeNe treatment of 2.4 J/cm^2 on alternate days. Histologic examination indicated more mature Haversian canals with detached osteocytes in the laser treated bone. There was also a remodeling of the articular line, which is impossible with traditional therapy.[25,26] The use of lasers for the treatment of nonunion fractures has begun in Europe.

CLINICAL CONSIDERATIONS

There have been no ill effects reported from laser treatments for wound healing.[4] More controlled clinical data are needed to determine efficacy and to establish dosimetry that elicits reproducible responses. The impressions of low power lasers are that they have a biostimulative effect on impaired tissues unless higher dosages, in excess of 8 to 10 J/cm^2, are administered.[1] This effect does not influence normal tissue. Beyond these ranges a bioinhibitive effect may occur.

The applications of the low power laser in an athletic training environment are potentially unlimited. Its applications can include wound healing properties on lacerations, abrasions, or infections. Clean procedures should be maintained to prevent cross contamination of the laser tip. Because the depth of penetration of the infrared laser is about 5 cm, other soft tissue injuries can be treated effectively by laser irradiation. Sprains, strains, and contusions have been observed by the authors to have faster healing rates with less pain. Acupuncture and superficial nerve sites also can be lased or combined with electrical stimulation to treat painful conditions.

TECHNIQUES OF APPLICATION

Lasing Techniques
- Gridding
- Scanning

The method of application of laser therapy is relatively simple, but certain principles of dosimetry should be discussed so the clinician can accurately determine the amount of laser energy delivered to the tissues. For general application, only the treatment time and the pulse rate vary. For research purposes, the investigator should measure the exact energy density emitted from the applicator before the treatments. Dosage is the most important variable in laser therapy and may be difficult to determine because of the variables mentioned previously (e.g., hours of operation or condition of the unit).

The laser energy is emitted from a handheld remote applicator. The GaAs laser houses the semiconductor elements in the tip of the applicator, whereas the HeNe lasers contain their componentry inside the unit and deliver the laser light to the target area via a fiberoptic tube. The fiberoptic assembly is fragile and should not be crimped or twisted excessively. The fiberoptics used with the HeNe and the elliptical shape of the GaAs laser create beam **divergence** with both devices. This divergence causes the beam's energy to spread out over a given area so that as the distance from the source increases, the intensity of the beam lessens.

To administer a laser treatment, the tip should be in light contact with the skin and directed perpendicularly to the target tissue while the laser is engaged for the designated time. Commonly, a treatment area is divided into a grid of square centimeters, with each square centimeter stimulated for the specified time. This *gridding technique* is the most frequently utilized method of application and should be used whenever possible. Lines and points should not be drawn on the patient's skin, because this may absorb some of the light energy (Fig. 11-6). If open areas are to be

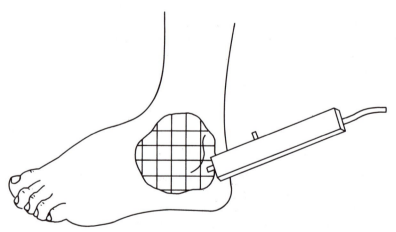

•**Figure 11-6** Grid application of laser. Laser aperture should be perpendicular to the surface. Lase each square centimeter of the injured area for the specified time. The aperture should be in light contact with the skin.

treated, a sterilized clear plastic sheet can be placed over the wound to allow surface contact.

An alternative is a *scanning technique* in which there is no contact between the laser tip and the skin. With this technique, the applicator tip should be held 5 to 10 mm from the wound. Since beam divergence occurs, there is a decrease in the amount of energy as the distance from the target increases. The amount of energy lost becomes difficult to quantify accurately if the distance from the target is variable. Therefore, it is not recommended to treat at distances greater than 1 cm. When using a laser tip of 1 mm with 30° of divergence, the red laser beam of the HeNe should fill an area the size of 1 cm^2 (Fig. 11-7). Although the infrared laser is invisible, the same consideration should be given when using the scanning technique. If the laser tip comes into contact with an open wound, the tip should be cleaned thoroughly with a small amount of bleach or other antiseptic agents to prevent cross-contamination.

The scanning technique should be differentiated from the wanding technique, in which a grid area is bathed with the laser in an oscillating fashion for the designated time. As in the scanning technique, the dosimetry is difficult to calculate if a distance of less than 1 cm cannot be maintained. The wanding technique is not recommended because of irregularities in the dosages.

DOSAGE

PhysioTechnology Ltd. (Topeka, Kansas) is the only manufacturer in the United States that currently produces low power HeNe and GaAs lasers (Fig. 11-8). Table 11-1 describes the contrasting specifications of these lasers. The HeNe laser has a 1.0 mW average power output at the fiber tip and is delivered in the **continuous wave** mode. The GaAs laser has an output of 2 W but has only a 0.4 mW average power when pulsed at its maximum rate of 1000 Hz. The frequency of the GaAs is variable, and the clinician may choose a pulse rate of 1 to 1000 Hz, each with a pulse width of 200 nsec (nsec = 10^{-9}) (Fig. 11-9).

The pulsed modes drastically reduce the amount of energy emitted from the laser. For example, a 2 W laser is pulsed at 100 Hz:

$$\textbf{Average Power} = \textbf{pulse rate} \times \textbf{peak power} \times \textbf{pulse width}$$
$$= 100 \, \text{Hz} \times 2 \, \text{W} \times (2 \times 10^{-7} \, \text{sec})$$
$$= 0.04 \, \text{mW}$$

> **Treatment Tip**
> In treating myofascial trigger points the therapist should use a gridding laser technique with the probe held perpendicular to the skin with light contact. The energy density should be set at 3 J/cm^2. The laser treatment can be combined with electrical stimulation using low frequency (1–5 Hz) high intensity current to produce pain modulation via the release of β-endorphin.

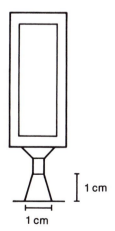

1 cm

1 cm

•**Figure 11-7** Scanning technique. When skin contact cannot be maintained, the remote should be held still in the center of the square centimeter grid at a distance of less than 1 cm. If using the HeNe laser, the red beam should fill a 1-cm^2 grid.

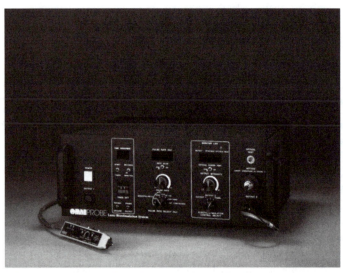

•**Figure 11-8** Low power laser (Physio Technology, Ltd., Topeka, Kansas).

This contrasts the power output of 0.4 mW with the 1000 Hz. Therefore, it can be seen that adjustment of the pulse rate alters the average power, which significantly affects the treatment time if a specified amount of energy is required. In the past it was thought that altering the frequency of the laser would increase its benefits. Recent evidence indicates that the total number of Joules is more important; therefore, higher pulse rates are recommended to decrease the treatment time required for each stimulation point.[6]

The dosage or energy density of laser is reported in the literature as Joules per square centimeter (J/cm^2). One Joule is equal to 1 W/sec. Therefore, dosage is dependent on: (1) the output of the laser in mW; (2) the time of exposure in sec; and (3) the beam surface area of the laser in cm^2.

Dosage should be accurately calculated to standardize treatments and to establish treatment guidelines for specific injuries. The intention is to deliver a specific number of J/cm^2 or mJ/cm^2. After setting the pulse rate, which determines the average power of the laser, only the treatment time per cm^2 needs to be calculated.[6]

$$T_A = (E/P_{av}) \times A$$
$$T_A = \text{treatment time for a given area}$$
$$E = \text{mJ of energy per cm}^2$$
$$P_{av} = \text{Average laser power in mW}$$
$$A = \text{beam area in cm}^2$$

TABLE 11.1 **Parameters of Low-Output Lasers**

	Helium Neon (HeNe)	Gallium Arsenide (GaAs)
Laser type	Gas	Semiconductor
Wavelength	632.8 nm	904 nm
Pulse rate	Continuous wave	1-1000 Hz
Pulse width	Continuous wave	200 nsec
Peak power	3 mW	2 W
Average power	1.0 mW	.04-0.4 mW
Beam area	0.01 cm	0.07 cm
FDA class	Class II laser	Class I laser

Copied with permission from Physio Technology.

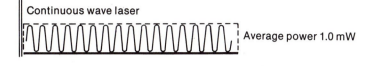

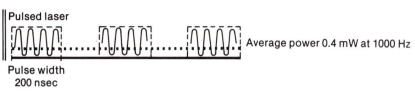

•**Figure 11-9** Continuous wave versus pulsed energies.

For example: To deliver 1 J/cm² with a 0.4 mW average-power GaAs laser with a 0.07 cm² beam area:

$$T_A = (1\,J/cm^2/0.0004\,W) \times 0.07\,cm^2$$
$$= 175\,sec\,or\,2{:}55\,min$$

To deliver 50 mJ/cm² with the same laser, it would only take 8.75 sec of stimulation. Charts are available to assist the clinician in calculating the treatment times for a variety of pulse rates. The GaAs laser can only pulse up to 1000 Hz, resulting in an average energy of 0.4 mW. Therefore, the treatment times may be exceedingly long to deliver the same energy density with a continuous wave laser (Table 11-2).

DEPTH OF PENETRATION

Any energy applied to the body can be absorbed, reflected, transmitted, and refracted. Biologic effects result only from the absorption of energy, and as more energy is absorbed, there is less available for the deeper and adjacent tissues.

Laser light's depth of penetration depends on the type of laser energy delivered. Absorption of HeNe laser energy occurs rapidly in the superficial structures, especially within the first 2 to 5 mm of soft tissue. The response that occurs from absorption is termed the **"direct effect."** The **"indirect effect"** is a lessened response that occurs deeper in the tissues. The normal metabolic processes in the deeper tissues are catalyzed from the energy absorption in the superficial structures to produce the indirect effect. HeNe laser has an indirect effect on tissues up to 8 to 10 mm.[6]

The GaAs, which has a longer wavelength, is directly absorbed in tissues at depths of 1 to 2 cm and has an indirect effect up to 5 cm (Fig. 11-10). Therefore, this laser has better potential for the treatment of deeper soft tissue injuries, such as strains, sprains, and contusions. The radius of the energy field expands as the non-absorbed light is reflected, refracted, and transmitted to adjacent cells as the energy

TABLE 11.2	Treatment Times for Low-Output Lasers							
		Joules per Centimeter Squared (J/cm²)						
Laser Type	Average Power (mW)	0.05	0.1	0.5	1	2	3	4
HeNe (632.8 nm) Continuous wave	1.0	0.5	1.0	5.0	10.0	20.0	30.0	40.0
GaAs (904 nm) Pulsed at 1000 Hz	0.4	8.8	17.7	88.4	176.7	353.4	530.1	706.9

Copied with permission from Physio Technology.

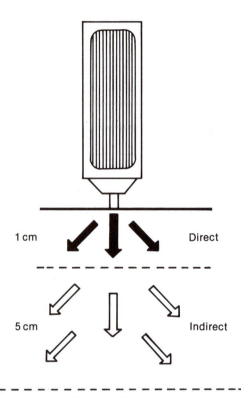

•**Figure 11-10** Depth of penetration with the GaAs laser. Direct penetration is up to 1 cm with the GaAs laser. The stimulation causes an indirect effect up to 5 cm. Penetration is greatest with skin contact.

penetrates. The clinician should stimulate each square centimeter of a "grid," although there will be an overlap of areas receiving indirect exposure.

SUGGESTED TREATMENT PROTOCOLS

Research suggests some laser densities for treating several clinical models. These average from 0.05 to 0.5 J/cm^2 for acute conditions and range from 0.5 to 3 J/cm^2 for more chronic conditions.[6] The responses of the tissues depend on the dosage delivered, although the type of laser used can also influence the effect. The response obtained with different dosages and with different lasers varies considerably among studies, leaving treatment parameters to be determined largely empirically. In the literature, there seems to be little differentiation when comparing the dosages of HeNe and GaAs lasers, although their depths of penetration differ significantly. The laser units produced in the United States have relatively little average power, so the tendency is to administer dosages in millijoules rather than Joules. Three to six treatments may be required before the effectiveness of laser therapy can be determined.

Although higher laser output is recommended to reduce treatment times, overstimulation should be avoided. The Arndt-Schultz principle that states more is not necessarily better is applicable with laser therapy. For this reason, laser should be administered at a maximum of once daily per treatment area. When using large dosages, treatment is recommended on alternate days. If the effects of laser plateau, the frequency of treatments should be reduced or the treatments discontinued for 1 week, at which time the treatment can be reinstated if needed.[25]

PAIN

The use of low power lasers in the treatment of acute and chronic pain can be implemented in various manners. After proper diagnosis of the pain's etiology, the pathology site can be gridded. The entire area of injury should be lased as described previously. Table 11-3 lists some suggested treatment protocols for various clinical conditions. When trigger points are being treated, the probe should be held perpendicular to the skin with light contact. If a specific structure, such as a ligament, is the target tissue, the laser probe should be held in contact with the skin and perpendicular to that structure. When treating a joint, the patient should be positioned so that the joint is open to allow penetration of the energy to the intraarticular areas.

The treatment of acupuncture and trigger points with laser can be augmented with electrical stimulation for pain management. Reference to charts should be made to determine appropriate acupuncture points. The impedance detector in the laser remote enhances the ability to locate these sites. Points should be treated from distal to proximal for best results.

Occasionally patients may experience an increase in pain after a laser treatment. This phenomenon is believed to be the initiation of the body's normal responses to pain that have become dormant.[5] Laser has been found to help resolve the condition by enhancing normal physiologic processes needed to resolve the injury. As stated previously, several treatments should be administered before deeming the modality ineffective in pain management.

Treatment Tip

In treating a new abrasion with a laser, the wound should first be cleaned appropriately and debrided as necessary. A scanning lasing technique with no direct contact should be done around the periphery of the abrasion. It is recommended that a HeNe laser be used at an energy density of 0.5–1 J/cm^2.

WOUND HEALING

Although ulcerations and open wounds are not common in an athletic training environment, contusions, abrasions, and lacerations can be treated with laser to hasten healing time and decrease infection. The wound should be cleaned appropriately and all debris and eschar removed. Heavy exudate that covers the wound will diminish the laser's penetration; therefore, lasing around the periphery of the wound is recommended. The scanning technique should be utilized over open wounds unless a clear plastic sheet is placed over the wound to allow direct contact. Opaque materials can

TABLE 11.3	Suggested Treatment Applications	
Application	**Laser Type**	**Energy Density**
TRIGGER POINT		
Superficial	HeNe	1-3 J/cm^2
Deep	GaAs	1-2 J/cm^2
EDEMA REDUCTION		
Acute	GaAs	0.1-0.2 J/cm^2
Subacute	GaAs	0.2-0.5 J/cm^2
WOUND HEALING (SUPERFICIAL TISSUES)		
Acute	HeNe	0.5-1 J/cm^2
Chronic	HeNe	4 J/cm^2
WOUND HEALING (DEEP TISSUES)		
Acute	GaAs	0.05-0.1 J/cm^2
Chronic	GaAs	0.5-1 J/cm^2
SCAR TISSUE	GaAs	0.5-1 J/cm^2

Copied with permission from Physio Technology.

absorb some of the laser energy and are not recommended. Facial lacerations can be treated with the laser, although care should be taken not to direct the beam into the patient's eyes. Risk of retinal damage from the low power lasers used in the United States is low.

SCAR TISSUE

The laser energy affects only what is metabolically diminished and does not change normal tissue. Hypertrophic scars can be treated with lasers because of the bioinhibitive effects. Bioinhibition requires prolonged treatment times and may be clinically impractical because of the low power output of the lasers used in the United States. Pain and edema associated with pathologic scars have been effectively treated with low power lasers. Thick scars have varied vascularity, which makes laser transmission irregular; therefore, it is often recommended to treat the periphery of the scar rather than directly over it.

EDEMA AND INFLAMMATION

The primary action of laser application for control of edema and inflammation is through the interruption of the formation of intermediate substrates necessary for the production of inflammatory chemical mediators: kinins, histamines, and prostaglandins. Without these chemical mediators, the disruption of the body's homeostatic state is minimized and the extent of pain and edema is diminished. It is also believed that laser energy can optimize cell membrane permeability, which regulates interstitial osmotic hydrostatic pressures. Therefore, during tissue trauma, the flux of fluid into the intercellular spaces would be reduced. Laser treatment is usually applied by gridding over the involved areas or by treating related acupuncture points if the area of involvement is generalized.

SAFETY

Few safety considerations are necessary with the low power laser. However, as the variety of lasers evolved and their uses increased in the United States, it became necessary to develop national guidelines not only for safety but also for therapeutic efficacy. The U.S. Food and Drug Administration's Center for Devices and Radiological Health now regulates the manufacture and sale of lasers in the United States.

Laser equipment commonly is grouped into four FDA classes, with simplified and well-differentiated safety procedures for each.[22]

Class I, or "exempt" lasers, are considered nonhazardous to the body. All invisible lasers with average power outputs of 1 mW or less are Class I devices. These include the GaAs lasers with wavelengths from 820 to 910 nm.[17] The invisible, infrared lasers should contain an indicator light to identify when the laser is engaged.

Class II, or "low-power" lasers are hazardous only if a viewer stares continuously into the source. This class includes visible lasers that emit up to 1 mW average power, such as the HeNe laser.

Class III, or moderate risk lasers, can cause retinal injury within the natural reaction time. The operator and patient are required to wear protective eyewear. However, these lasers cannot cause serious skin injury or produce hazardous diffuse reflections from metals or other surfaces under normal use.[22]

Class IV, or high power lasers, present a high risk of injury and can cause combustion of flammable materials. Other dangers are diffuse reflections that may harm the eyes and cause serious skin injury from direct exposure. These high power lasers seldom are used outside research laboratories and restricted industrial environments.[22]

The low power lasers used in treating sports injuries are categorized as Class I and II laser devices and Class III medical devices. Class III medical devices include new or modified devices not equivalent to any marketed before May 28, 1976.[9] To use a low power laser in the United States on human subjects, a research proposal must be approved by an Institutional Review Board (IRB). The IRB can be established through the manufacturer, a university, or a hospital to obtain an Investigational Device Exemption (IDE). By requiring documentation of the results and side effects of lasers, the FDA regulations serve to generate scientific data to determine safety and efficacy of the device in question.

PRECAUTIONS AND CONTRAINDICATIONS

Lasers deliver nonionizing radiation, therefore, no mutagenic effects on DNA and no damage to the cells or cell membranes have been found.[6] No deleterious effects have been reported after low power laser exposure, including carcinogenic responses, unless applied to already cancerous cells. Tumorous cells may proliferate when stimulated.[10] The following are some suggestions for laser use.

Laser should not be used over cancerous growths.

It is better to underexpose than to overexpose. If clinical results plateau, a reduction in dosage or treatment frequency may facilitate results.

Avoid direct exposure into the eyes because of possible retinal burns. If lasing for extended periods, as with wound healing, safety glasses are recommended to avoid exposure from reflection.

Although no adverse reactions have been documented, the use of laser during the first trimester of pregnancy is not recommended.

A low percentage of patients, especially those with chronic pain, may experience a syncope episode during the laser treatment. Symptoms usually subside within minutes. If symptoms exceed 5 minutes, no further treatments should be given.

Contraindications
Cancerous tumors
Directly over eyes
Pregnancy

CONCLUSION

The use of low power lasers appears to have nothing but positive effects: This in itself should create a state of professional caution in deeming it a panacea modality. Currently, with these power outputs, lasers are recognized as nonsignificant risk devices. However, low power lasers have not been granted recognition by the Food and Drug Administration as being a safe or effective modality. Although many empirical and clinical findings show promising results, more controlled studies are essential to determine the types of lasers and dosages that are required to attain reproducible results.

SUMMARY

1. The first working laser was the ruby laser developed in 1960 and was initially called an optical maser.
2. Visible light wavelengths range from 400 to 700 nanometers. Light is transmitted through space in waves and is comprised of photons emitted at distinct energy levels.
3. An atom is excited when energy is applied and raises an orbiting electron to a higher orbit. When the electron returns to its original orbit, it releases energy in the form of a photon, a process called spontaneous emission.

4. Stimulated emission occurs when the photon is released from an excited atom and promotes the release of an identical photon to be released from a similarly excited atom.

5. For lasers to operate, a medium of excited atoms must be generated. This is termed population inversion and results when an external energy source (pumping device) is applied to the medium.

6. Characteristics of laser light varies from conventional light sources in three manners: laser light is monochromatic (single color or wavelength), coherent (in phase), and collimated (minimal divergence).

7. Laser can be thermal (hot) or nonthermal (low power, soft, or cold). The categories of lasers include solid-state (crystal or glass), gas, semiconductor, dye, or chemical lasers.

8. Helium neon (HeNe; gas) and gallium arsenide (GaAs; semiconductor) lasers are two low power lasers being investigated by the FDA for application in physical medicine. These low power lasers are currently being used in the United States and other countries for wound and soft tissue healing and pain relief.

9. HeNe lasers deliver a characteristic red beam with a wavelength of 632.8 nm. The laser is delivered in a continuous wave and has a direct penetration of 2 to 5 mm and an indirect penetration of 10 to 15 mm.

10. GaAs lasers are invisible and have a wavelength of 904 nm. They are delivered in a pulse mode and have an average power output of 0.4 mW. This laser has a direct penetration of 1 to 2 cm and an indirect penetration to 5 cm.

11. The proposed therapeutic applications of lasers in physical medicine include acceleration of collagen synthesis, decrease in microorganisms, increase in vascularization, and reduction of pain and inflammation.

12. The technique of laser application ideally is done with gentle contact with the skin surface and should be perpendicular to the target surface. Dosage appears to be the critical factor in eliciting the desired response, but exact dosimetry has not been determined. Dosage fluctuates by varying the pulse frequency and the treatment times.

13. The laser is applied by developing an imaginary grid over the target area. The grid is comprised of 1-cm squares and the laser is applied to each square for a predetermined time. Trigger or acupuncture points are also treated for painful conditions.

14. The FDA considers low power lasers as low-risk investigational devices. For use in the United States, they require an IRB approval and informed consent prior to their use.

15. Although no deleterious effects have been reported, certain precautions and contraindications exist. Contraindications include lasing over cancerous tissue, directly into the eyes, and during the first trimester of pregnancy. Occasionally pain may initially increase when laser treatments begin but does not indicate cessation of treatment. A low percentage of patients have experienced a syncope episode during laser treatment, but this is usually self-resolving. If symptoms persist for longer than 5 minutes, future laser treatments are not advised.

16. Future research for determining efficacy and treatment parameters is critically needed to substantiate the application of low power lasers in physical medicine.

REFERENCES

1. Abergel, R.: Biochemical mechanisms of wound and tissue healing with lasers, Second Canadian Low Power Medical Laser Conference, March, 1987.

2. Abergel, R., Lyons, R., and Castel, J.: Biostimulation of wound healing by lasers: Experimental approaches in animal models and in fibroblast cultures, J. Dermatol. Surg. Oncol. 13:127–133, 1987.

3. Bostara, M., Jucca, A., and Olliaro, P.: In vitro fibroblast and

dermis fibroblast activation by laser irradiation at low energy, Dermatologica 168:157–162, 1984.

4. Castel, J.: Laser biophysics, Second Canadian Low Power Medical Laser Conference, Ontario, Canada, March, 1987.

5. Castel, M.: Personal communication, Downsview, Ontario, March, 1989, MEDELCO.

6. Castel, M.: A clinical guide to low power laser therapy, Downsview, Ontario, 1985, PhysioTechnology Ltd.

7. Cheng, R.: Combination laser/electrotherapy in pain management, Second Canadian Low Power Laser Conference, Ontario, Canada, March, 1987.

8. Enwemeka, C.: Laser biostimulation of healing wounds: specific effects and mechanisms of action J. Orthop. Sports Phys. Ther. 9:333–338, 1988.

9. Fact Sheet: Laser biostimulation, Rockville, Maryland, 1984, Center of Devices and Radiological Health, FDA.

10. Farnham, J.: Personal communication, Rockville, Maryland, March, 1989, Center of Devices and Radiological Health, FDA.

11. Gogia, P., Hurt, B., and Zirn, T.: Wound management with whirlpool and infrared cold laser treatment, Phys. Ther. 68:1239–1242, 1988.

12. Hallmark, C., Horn, D.: Lasers: the light fantastic, ed. 2, Blue Ridge Summit, Pennsylvania, 1987, TAB Books.

13. Hunter, J., Leonard, L., and Wilson, R.: Effects of low energy laser on wound healing in a porcine model, Lasers Surg. Med. 3:285–290, 1984.

14. Kana, J., Hutschenreiter, G., and Haina, D.: Effect of low power density laser radiation on healing of open skin wounds in rats, Arch. Surg. 116:293–296, 1981.

15. Longo, L., Evangelista, S., and Tinacci, G.: Effect of diode-laser silver-arsenide-aluminum (Ag-As-Al) 904 nm on healing of experimental wounds, Lasers Surg. Med. 7:444–447, 1987.

16. Lyons, R., Abergel, R., and White, R.: Biostimulation of

17. McComb, G.: The laser cookbook: 88 practical projects, Blue Ridge Summit, Pennsylvania, 1988, TAB Books.

18. Mester, E., Mester, A., and Mester, A.: Biomedical effects of laser application, Laser Surg. Med. 5:31–39, 1985.

19. Mester, E., Spiry, T., and Szende, B.: Effect of laser rays on wound healing, Am. J. Surg. 122:532–535, 1971.

20. Rochkind, S., Nissan, M., and Barr-Nea, L.: Response of peripheral nerve to HeNe laser: experimental studies, Lasers Surg. Med. 7:441–443, 1987.

21. Schultz, R., Krishnamurthy, S., and Thelmo, W.: Effects of varying intensities of laser energy on articular cartilage: a preliminary study, Lasers Surg. Med. 5:577–588, 1985.

22. Sliney, D., Wolkarsht, M.: Safety with lasers and other optical sources: a comprehensive handbook, New York, 1980, Plenum Press.

23. Snyder-Mackler, L., and Bork, C.: Effect of helium neon laser irradiation on peripheral nerve sensory latency, Phys Ther. 68:223–225, 1988.

24. Surinchak, J., Alago, M., and Bellamy, R.: Effects of low-level energy lasers on the healing of full-thickness skin defects, Lasers Surg. Med. 2:267–274, 1983.

25. Trelles, M.: Medical applications of laser biostimulation, Second Canadian Low Power Medical Laser Conference, Ontario, Canada, March, 1987.

26. Trelles, M., and Mayayo, E.: Bone fracture consolidates faster with low power laser, Lasers Surg. Med. 7:36–45, 1987.

27. Van Pelt, W., Stewart, H., and Peterson, R.: Laser fundamentals and experiments, Rockville, Maryland, 1970, U.S. Dept. HEW.

28. Walker, J.: Relief from chronic pain by low power laser irradiation, Neurosci. Lett. 43:339–344, 1983.

wound healing in vivo by a helium neon laser, Ann. Plastic Surg. 18: 47–77, 1987.

Suggested Readings

Abergel, R.: Biostimulation of procollagen production by low energy lasers in human skin fibroblast cultures, J. Invest. Dermatol. 82:395, 1984.

Baxter, G., Bell, A., and Allen, J.: Low level laser therapy: current clinical practice in Northern Ireland, Physiotherapy 77: 171–178, 1991.

Baxter, G.: Therapeutic lasers theory and practice, New York, 1994, Churchill Livingstone.

Beckerman, H., de Bie, R., and Bouter L.: The efficacy of laser therapy for musculoskeletal and skin disorders: a criteria-based meta-analysis of randomized clinical trials, Phys. Ther. 72(7):483–491, 1992.

Bolton, P., Young, S., and Dyson, M.: Macrophage response to laser therapy: a dose response study, Laser Ther. 2:101–106, 1990.

Bolton, P., Young, S., and Dyson, M.: Macrophage responsiveness to laser therapy with varying power and energy densities, Laser Ther. 3:105–112, 1991.

Braverman, B., McCarthy, R., and Ivankovich, A.: Effect on helium neon and infrared laser irradiation on wound healing in rabbits, Lasers Surg. Med. 9:50–58, 1989.

Crous, L., Malherbe, C.: Laser and ultraviolet light irradiation in the treatment of chronic ulcers, Physiotherapy 44:73–77, 1988.

Cummings J.: The effect of low energy (HeNe) laser irradiation on healing dermal wounds in an animal model, Phys. Ther. 65:737, 1985.

Dreyfuss, P., Stratton, S.: The low-energy laser, electro-acuscope, and neuroprobe: treatment options remain controversial, Phys. Sportsmed. 21(8):47–50, 55–57, 1993.

Dyson, M., Young, S.: Effects of laser therapy on wound contraction and cellularity in mice, Laser Surg. Med. 1:125, 1986.

Gogia, P., Marquez, R.: Effects of helium-neon laser on wound healing, Ostomy Wound Manage. 38(6):33, 36, 38–41, 1992.

Hayashi, K., Markel, M., and Thabit, G.: The effect of nonablative laser energy on joint capsular properties: an in vitro mechanical study using a rabbit model, Amer. J. Sports Med. 23(4): 482–487, 1995.

Herbert, K., Bhusate, L., and Scott, D.: Effect of laser light at 820 nm on adenosine nucleotide levels in human lymphocytes, Lasers Life Sci. 3:37–45, 1989.

Karu, T., Tiphlova, S., and Samokhina, M.: Effects of near infrared laser and superluminous diode irradiation on *Escherichia coli* division rate, IEEE J. Quant. Electron. 26:2162–2165, 1990.

Kramer, J., Sandrin, M.: Effect of low-power laser and white light on sensory conduction rate of the superficial radial nerve, Physiother. Can. 45(3):165–170, 1993.

Laakso, L., Richardson, C., and Cramond, T.: Factors affecting low level laser therapy, Aust. J. Physiother. 39(2):95–99, 1993.

Lam T., Abergerl R., and Meeker C.: Biostimulation of human skin fibroblasts: low energy lasers selectively enhance collagen synthesis, Laser Surg. Med. 3:328, 1984.

Lundeberg T., Haker E., and Thomas M.: Effect of laser versus placebo in tennis elbow, Scand. J. Rehabil. Med. 19:135–138, 1987.

Lyons, R., Abergel, R., and White, R.: Biostimulation of wound healing in vivo by a helium neon laser, Ann. Plast. Surg. 18:47–50, 1987.

Malm, M., Lundeberg, T.: Effect of low power gallium arsenide laser on healing of venous ulcers, Scand. J. Reconstruct. Hand Surg. 25:249–251, 1991.

Martin, D.: An investigation into the effects of low level therapy on arterial blood flow in skeletal muscle, Physiotherapy 81(9):562, 1995.

McMeeken, J., Stillman, B.: Perceptions of the clinical efficacy of laser therapy, Aust. J. Physiother. 39(2):101–106, 1993.

Mester, E., Jaszsagi-Nagy, E.: The effects of laser radiation on wound healing and collagen synthesis, Studia Biophysica 35(3):227, 1973.

Nussbaum, E., Biemann, I., and Mustard, B.: Comparison of ultrasound/ultraviolet-C and laser for treatment of pressure ulcers in patients with spinal cord injury, Phys. Ther. 74(9):812–823, 1994.

Palmgren, N., Dahlin, J., and Beck, H.: Low level laser therapy of infected abdominal wounds after surgery, Lasers Surg. Med. 3(Suppl):11, 1991.

Rockhind, S., Russo, M., and Nissan, M.: Systemic effect of low power laser on the peripheral and central nervous system, cutaneous wounds, and burns, Lasers Surg. Med. 9:174–182, 1989.

Saperia, D., Glassberg, E., and Lyons, R.: Stimulation of collagen synthesis in human fibroblast cultures, Laser Life Sci. 1:61–77, 1986.

Vasseljen, O.: Low-level laser versus traditional physiotherapy in the treatment of tennis elbow, Physiotherapy 78(5):329–334, 1992.

Waylonis, G., Wilke, S., and O'Toole, D.: Chronic myofascial pain: management by low-output helium-neon laser therapy, Arch. Phys. Med. Rehabil. 69(12):1017–1020, 1988.

Young, S.: Macrophage responsivity to light therapy, Lasers Surg. Med. 9:497–505, 1989.

Young, S., Dyson, M., and Bolton, P.: Effect of light on calcium uptake by macrophages. Presented at the Fourth International Biotherapy Association Seminar on Laser Biostimulation, Guy's Hospital, London, 1991.

GLOSSARY

coherence Property of identical phase and time relationship. All photons of laser light are the same wavelength.

collimate To make parallel.

continuous wave An uninterrupted opposed to pulsed beam of laser light.

diode laser A solid-state semiconductor used as a lasing medium.

direct effect The tissue response that occurs from energy absorption.

divergence The bending of light rays away from each other; the spreading of light.

electron Fundamental particle of matter possessing a negative electrical charge and small mass.

excited state State of an atom that occurs when outside energy causes the atom to contain more energy than normal.

fiberoptic A solid glass or plastic tube that conducts light along its length.

frequency The number of cycles or pulses per second.

ground state The normal, unexcited state of an atom.

indirect effect A decreased response that occurs in deeper tissues.

infrared A portion of the electromagnetic spectrum between the visible and microwave regions. Wavelengths range from 780 to 100,000 nm.

laser A device that concentrates high energies into a narrow beam of coherent, monochromatic light (Light Amplification by the Stimulated Emission of Radiation).

monochromaticity The condition that occurs when a light source produces a single color or wavelength.

photon The basic unit of light; a packet or quanta of light energy.

population inversion A condition where more atoms exist in a high energy, excited state than those atoms that are in a normal ground state. This is required for lasing to occur.

spontaneous emission This occurs when an atom in a high energy state emits a photon and drops to a more stable ground state.

stimulated emission This occurs when a photon interacts with an atom already in a high energy state and decay of the atomic system occurs, releasing two photons.

wavelength The distance from peak to the same point on the next peak of an electromagnetic or acoustic wave.

LAB ACTIVITY

LOW-POWER LASER

DESCRIPTION:

Low-power lasers produce a coherent, monochromatic, collimated light beam. They are used in the United States principally for pain modulation and wound healing. The two principal wavelengths used are 632.8 nm, produced by the helium neon (HeNe) laser, and 94 nm, produced by the gallium arsenide (GaAs) laser. Low-power (cold) lasers are distinguished from high-power (hot) lasers by the lack of thermal effects by the low-power lasers.

The mechanism of action of low-power laser energy is not clear. Whether the absorbed photons stimulating protein synthesis, thus promoting tissue healing, have a bactericidal effect on the wound or increase angiogenesis has not been established. The potential mechanisms for pain modulation are even less clear.

Although it has been suggested that laser energy may have indirect effects on tissue up to 5 cm deep, there is no convincing evidence of penetration this deep. How light energy absorbed by the superficial cells is conducted to underlying cells when the energy is nonionizing and nonthermal has not been explained.

It must be made crystal clear that the use of low power lasers for these purposes has not been approved by the U.S. Food and Drug Administration, the regulating body for medical devices. Individuals using low power lasers for these purposes must have an Investigational Device Exemption and should obtain informed consent from each patient before using the laser.

The physiologic and therapeutic effects of low power laser stimulation are not well established. Therefore, the indications, which are derived from the physiologic effects, are somewhat speculative.

PHYSIOLOGIC EFFECTS:

Increased collagen synthesis by fibroblasts
Decreased nerve conduction velocity

THERAPEUTIC EFFECTS:

Increased rate of wound closure
Increased tensile strength of wounds
Decreased perception of pain

INDICATIONS:

Low-power laser stimulation may be helpful to optimize the rate of wound closure, modulate musculoskeletal pain, and remodel established scar tissue.

CONTRAINDICATIONS:

There are no established contraindications to low-power laser application, but the light should not be directed at the eyes.

LOW POWER LASER			
PROCEDURE	Evaluation		
	1	2	3
1. Check supplies.			
a. Obtain towels or sheets for draping.			
b. Check laser equipment for charged battery, broken or frayed cables, and so on.			

PROCEDURE	Evaluation		
	1	2	3
2. Question patient.			
a. Verify identity of patient (if not already verified).			
b. Verify the absence of contraindications.			
c. Ask about previous exposure to laser therapy; check treatment notes.			
3. Position patient.			
a. Place patient in a well-supported, comfortable position.			
b. Expose body part to be treated.			
c. Drape patient to preserve patient's modesty, protect clothing, but allow access to body part.			
4. Inspect body part to be treated.			
a. Check light touch perception.			
b. Assess function of body part (e.g., ROM, irritability).			
5. Apply laser stimulation.			
a. Determine the area to be treated and visualize a grid overlying the treatment area. The grid should be divided into 1-cm squares.			
b. If the gridding technique is to be used, place the tip of the probe in light contact with the skin and administer the light to each square centimeter of area for the appropriate time to obtain the desired dosage.			
c. If the scanning technique is to be used, hold the tip of the probe within 1 cm of the skin and make sure the aperture of the probe is positioned such that the laser beam will be perpendicular to the skin. Administer the light to each square centimeter of area for the appropriate time to obtain the desired dosage.			
d. Insure that the laser energy will not be directed at the patient's eyes.			
e. If the patient reports anything unusual, such as discomfort at the treatment site, nausea, and so on, discontinue treatment.			
f. Continue to monitor the patient during the duration of the treatment.			
6. Complete treatment.			
a. When the treatment time is over, discontinue application of the laser energy.			
b. Remove material used for draping, assist the patient in dressing as needed.			
c. Have the patient perform appropriate therapeutic exercise as indicated.			
d. Clean the treatment area and equipment according to normal protocol.			
7. Assess treatment efficacy.			
a. Ask the patient how the treated area feels.			
b. Visually inspect the treated area for any adverse reactions.			
c. Perform functional tests as indicated.			

CHAPTER 12 TWELVE

ULTRAVIOLET THERAPY

J. MARC DAVIS

OBJECTIVES

Following completion of this chapter, the student therapist will be able to:

- ✓ Describe the position of ultraviolet radiation (UVR) in the electromagnetic spectrum and the relationship of UVR to other forms of electromagnetic energy.
- ✓ Understand how UVR raises energy levels within irradiated objects.
- ✓ Understand the effect of UVR on individual cells and human tissue and explain the tanning process.
- ✓ Describe the effect of long-term exposure to UVR and the effect of UVR on the eyes.
- ✓ Explain the physical setup and procedures for operating a UVR device, including safety precautions, the skin test, the inverse square law, and the cosine law.
- ✓ Understand various clinical uses of UVR.

Ultraviolet radiation (UVR) is one of the oldest medical modalities. The physicians of ancient Egypt and Greece attributed many healing powers to sunlight, and in fact life itself would not be possible without the interaction of solar UVR and plant photosynthesis. Before this century the sun was the only satisfactory source of UVR, but now a wide selection of UVR generators is available.

This chapter serves to familiarize the student therapist with the properties of UVR, explain how UVR affects human tissue, and explore different UVR treatment apparatus and techniques. Subsequently, the therapist should be able to understand why UVR therapy can be effective in treating certain maladies, and therefore be able to correctly choose UVR therapy when it is the appropriate treatment for a given problem.

ULTRAVIOLET RADIATION

Ultraviolet radiation is the portion of the electromagnetic spectrum that ranges from 2000 to 4000 Å and is bordered below 2000 Å by x-ray and above 4000 Å by visible light (see Fig. 1-2). The UVR portion of the electromagnetic spectrum is further divided into three sections: UV-A, UV-B, and UV-C. Shortwave UV (UV-C, also called extreme UV, and far UV) ranges from 2000 to 2900 Å and is bactericidal.[28,34] UV-B (called middle UV and the sunburn spectrum) ranges from 2900 to 3200 Å and is associated with sunburn and age-related skin changes.[27-33] UV-A (near UV) ranges from 3200 to 4000 Å. Until recently little or no physiologic effect was attributed to UV-A, but recent research and clinical use of UV-A are showing possible benefits and hazards for UV-A exposure. The UVR apparatus most likely to be encountered in a clinical setting would generate UVR in the UV-B or UV-C range or in both ranges.[13]

The beneficial effects of UVR as a treatment modality are mediated by its limited absorption. Ultraviolet radiation is absorbed within the first 1 to 2 mm of human skin and most of the physiologic effects are superficial.[8] Therefore, the most effective use of UVR therapy is in the treatment of various skin disorders such as acne and psoriasis.[5,12,16]

EFFECT ON CELLS

Ultraviolet radiation is a form of energy. As such, when it contacts any surface, skin included, it must be either reflected or absorbed and transmitted. If UVR strikes the skin at a 90-degree angle, 90 to 95 percent of the energy will be absorbed. Most will be absorbed within the epidermis of the skin (80–90%), whereas the rest will reach the dermis.[8] As the UVR is absorbed within the tissue it causes the energy level of exposed atoms to increase. These atoms will quickly return to their normal energy state; however, the presence of excess energy causes chemical excitation within the cells of the exposed tissue. This chemical excitation is the cause of the various effects of UVR on living cells and tissue. Even a single exposure to UVR will cause chemical excitation within exposed cells, which leads to physiologic changes within these cells.

These physiologic changes are the result of a photochemical event that is the end product of the UVR-induced chemical excitation. This photochemical event results in an alteration of cell biochemistry and cellular metabolism. The synthesis of **DNA** and **RNA** is affected, leading to alterations in protein and enzyme production. As a consequence, cell protein structure can be altered, and this alteration of cellular protein and DNA may leave the cell inactive or dead.[28-33]

Fortunately, defenses have evolved that protect microorganisms and cells that are exposed to a constant barrage of UVR from the sun. The damaged cells may be restored by enzymatic action or by simple deterioration of the damaged portion; the damaged segment may be replaced by normal material, or it may be bypassed when the cell reproduces.[28] DNA synthesis within cells of the human epidermis is suppressed for 24 to 48 hours following exposure to UVR in the range of 2500 to 2700 Å and is then followed by a period of increased DNA synthesis.[28,33]

keratin The fibrous protein that forms the chemical basis of the epidermis.

EFFECT ON NORMAL HUMAN TISSUE

SHORT-TERM EFFECT ON SKIN

Normal human skin consists of two layers, the superficial epidermis and the underlying dermis (Fig. 12-1). The epidermis is avascular and composed mostly of well-organized layers of **keratinocytes.** These produce **keratin,** the fibrous protective protein of the skin. The keratinocytes are produced from cells of the basal layer of the epidermis and then move upward through the epidermis. The dermis is divided into two layers, the papillary layer that contains a rich blood supply, and the reticular

keratinocytes A cell that produces keratin.

CROSS SECTION OF SKIN

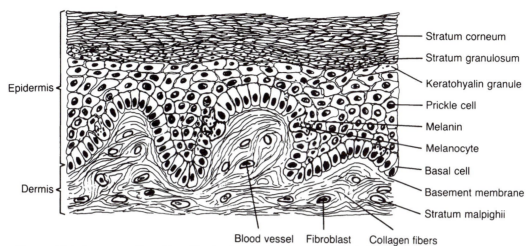

•**Figure 12-1** A cross section of the skin showing the dermis and epidermis layers.

layer that is composed of heavy connective tissue and contains fibroblasts, histiocytes, and most cells.

When human skin is exposed to UVR, the individual cells react as previously described. However, the skin is a protective organ, covering the entire human exterior, and it will respond in a generalized manner over the entire area that is irradiated. This generalized response culminates in the development of an acute inflammatory reaction. The end results of an active inflammation within the skin are **erythema** (the reddening of the skin associated with sunburn), **pigmentation** (tanning), and increased epidermal thickness.[8,17,28,33]

Inflammation is the response of any human tissue, skin included, to an irritating or injurious substance or event. In the case of UVR exposure, the irritating substances are the end products of the previously described photochemical event and may include damaged DNA, RNA, and cell proteins. The inflammatory process removes these injurious and irritating substances from the skin. Since the appearance of these irritating substances does not occur immediately following UVR exposure, the inflammatory response is delayed. Normally it begins several hours after irradiation and peaks 8 to 24 hours following exposure.[28]

This inflammatory response is characterized by local vasodilation and increased capillary permeability. Theoretically this is caused by (1) the absorption of UVR by keratinocytes, leading to the release of substances that diffuse to the papillary dermis and cause vasodilation; or (2) the absorption of UVR by mast cells in the dermis that in turn release histamine, resulting in vasodilation.[8,17,28] Erythema is caused by this vasodilation and the subsequent increase of blood within the dermis. The increased capillary permeability permits certain proteins to move from the capillaries into the dermis. This results in a change in osmotic pressure; consequently, water is drawn into the area and edema occurs. Leukocytes, lymphocytes, and monocytes pass into the dermis and to a small degree into the epidermis. These cells phagocytize (consume or engulf) dead cells and other debris. At 24 hours the inflammatory process is completed, and at 30 hours the rebuilding begins. The reparative process is characterized by increased activity of the keratinocytes and results in a thickening of the epidermis **(hyperplasia)**.[28] This is protective; areas covered with a thick epidermis, such as the soles of the feet, do not sunburn.

The acute effects of UVR exposure can be exacerbated if certain chemicals or medications are present on the skin or in the body. **Photosensitization** is a process in which a person becomes overly sensitive to UVR as a result of the excitation of a chemical by UVR exposure.[8] Any person taking a photosensitizing medication is

pigmentation Tanning of the skin from sun exposure.

hyperplasia An increase in the size of a tissue; in the skin, an increased thickness of the epidermis.

CASE STUDY 12-1
ULTRAVIOLET THERAPY

Background: A 25-year-old man developed a psoriatic plaque over the region of the posterior aspect of his left elbow. After an unsuccessful regimen of oral medications and topical ointments, his dermatologist referred him for a regimen of ultraviolet therapy. The lesion measured 3 × 5 centimeters extending over the olecranon region. The patient was otherwise in a normal state of health and exhibited full active ROM and strength of the left upper extremity.

Impression: Active psoriasis.

Treatment Plan: After establishing the patient's MED (minimal erythemal dosage) as 30 sec during an initial treatment session; a progressive program of exposure was begun to the posterior left elbow. Exposure began at 1 MED and increased by 1/2 MED each treatment session conducted on alternate days. When the patient reached 6 MED exposure, treatment was suspended pending physician reassessment.

Response: There was an increase in erythema noted around the margins of the lesion subsequent to initial UV exposure. Subsequent sessions did not produce any notable change from this initial response. A gradual reduction in plaque size was noted over the course of exposures, having decreased by 30 percent at the time treatment was suspended.

The rehabilitation professional employs therapeutic agent modalities to create an optimum environment for tissue healing while minimizing the symptoms associated with the trauma or condition.

Discussion Questions

- What tissues were injured or affected?
- What symptoms were present?
- What phase of the injury healing continuum did the patient present for care in?
- What are the therapeutic agent modality's biophysical effects (direct, indirect, depth, and tissue affinity)?
- What are the therapeutic agent modality's indications and contraindications?
- What are the parameters of the therapeutic agent modality's application, dosage, duration, and frequency in this case study?
- What other therapeutic agent modalities could be utilized to treat this injury or condition? Why? How?

very susceptible to the effects of UVR and should be treated accordingly. It should be noted that such an adverse reaction can occur even after limited exposure to natural sunlight. A list of common photosensitizing agents follows:

Antibacterial and microbial agents
> Tetracyclines: a group of broad-spectrum antibiotics
> Sulfonamides: a group of synthetic antimicrobial drugs
> Griseofulvin (Fulvicin, Grifulvin, Grisactin): an antibiotic with an additional antifungal action

Thiazide diuretics: A group of drugs that act on the kidney to increase sodium and water in the urine
> Chlorothiazide (Diuril)
> Hydrochlorothiazide (Hydrodiuril, Oretic, Esidrix)
> Methychlorothiazide (Enduron)

Other medications
> Phenothiazines (Thorazine): widely used tranquilizers
> Psoralens: a group of dermal pigmenting agents
> Sulfonylureas (Dymelor, Diabinese)
> Diphenhydramine (Benadryl): an antihistamine

Miscellaneous
    Sunscreens
    Tar
    Oral contraceptives
    Certain cosmetics[8,27,28]

TANNING

Tanning is the increase of pigmentation within the skin and is a protective mechanism activated by UVR exposure. An increase of **melanin,** the pigment responsible for darkening, within the skin causes the tan (see Fig. 12-1). The melanin functions as a biologic filter of UVR by scattering the radiation, absorbing the UVR, and dissipating the absorbed energy as heat.[33] The process of tanning is divided into two phases: immediate and delayed tanning.

Immediate tanning appears most often in darkly pigmented individuals and occurs immediately following UVR exposure. Immediate tanning represents the darkening of melanosomes already present in the skin. It begins to fade 1 hour after exposure and is hardly noticeable 3 to 8 hours later.[28,33] Delayed tanning is the result of the formation of new pigment (melanin) through the process of melanogenesis. The process is initiated by production of erythema (sunburn) within the skin. Melanogenesis occurs within the melanocytes of the basal layer of the epidermis (see Fig. 12-1), and the end products of this process are melanosomes, new pigment granules. These melanosomes are transferred from the melanocytes via nerve cells to nearby keratinocytes. As the keratinocytes gradually move outward to the skin's surface, the new pigment also migrates to the periphery. Delayed tanning usually becomes apparent 72 hours after UVR exposure.

Human skin color is a baseline that is influenced by various environmental factors (exposure to solar radiation, occupation, leisure activities) and the genetically determined level of melanin within the skin.[8,34] Individuals of all races have the same number of melanocytes per unit area, but darker individuals are able to produce greater amounts of melanin.[7]

Artificial Tanning Devices

In the past decade, artificial tanning devices have become popular in the spa and health club industry. These tanning salons, beds, and booths usually consist of an array of long tubes positioned in a frame that allows for exposure of the entire body.[23] The manufacturers claim that these devices produce only UVR in the UV-A spectrum and therefore are safe. However, the production of this type of UV-A generator is largely unregulated, and the effects of long-term exposure to UV-A are unknown. There is no standard of training required for the owners of these machines, and their knowledge of the tanning process and the dangers of UVR might be nonexistent. Caution should be exercised before allowing anyone to be overexposed to UVR, either from sunlight or from an artificial source.

LONG-TERM EFFECT ON SKIN

The most serious effects of long-term UVR exposure are premature aging of the skin and skin cancer.[20,30,31] Lightly pigmented individuals are more susceptible to these maladies. Premature aging of the skin is characterized by dryness, cracking, and a decrease in the elasticity of the skin, and it results from a change in the epidermis called solar elastosis. An alteration in the skin's elastic fibers causes solar elastosis and has been tentatively linked to UVR-induced DNA damage.[28]

Skin cancer is the most common malignant tumor found in humans and has been epidemiologically and clinically associated with solar UVR.[1,28,30,34] Damage to

erythema A redness of the skin caused by capillary dilation.

melanin A group of dark brown or black pigments that occur naturally in the eye, skin, hair, and other animal tissues.

Phases of Tanning
- Immediate
- Delayed

DNA is suspected as the cause of skin cancer, but the exact cause is yet unknown. The major types of skin cancer are basal cell carcinoma, which rarely metastasizes (spreads to other areas); squamous cell carcinoma, which metastasizes in 5 percent of all cases; and malignant melanoma, which metastasizes in a majority of cases.[28,30] Fortunately, the rate of cure exceeds 95 percent with early detection and treatment.

Sunscreens*

sun protection factor (SPF) A sunscreen's effectiveness in absorbing sunburn-inducing radiation.

Sunscreens applied to the skin can help prevent many of the damaging effects of UVR. A sunscreen's effectiveness in absorbing the sunburn-inducing radiation is expressed as the **sun protection factor (SPF)**. An SPF of 6 indicates that you can be exposed to UVR six times longer than without a sunscreen before you will receive a minimal erythemal dose. Higher numbers provide greater protection. However, individuals who have a family or personal history of skin cancer may experience significant damage to skin even when wearing an SPF 15 sunscreen. Therefore, these individuals should wear an SPF 30 sunscreen.

Sunscreen should be worn regularly by anyone who spends time outside. This is particularly true for individuals with fair complexions, light hair, blue eyes, or those whose skin burns easily. People with dark complexions should also wear sunscreens to prevent such damage. Sunscreens should also be worn by anyone with a personal or family history of skin cancer.

It has been clearly shown that sun exposure causes premature aging of the skin (wrinkling, freckling, prominent blood vessels, coarsening of skin texture), induces the formation of precancerous growths, and increases the risks of developing basal and squamous cell skin cancers. Blistering sunburns in one's youth also increase the risk of developing melanoma, a potentially fatal skin cancer. Since 60 to 80 percent of our lifetime sun exposure is often obtained before the age of 20, everyone over 6 months of age should use sunscreens. Sunscreens specifically labeled for children are no different than adult products. Adult sunscreens are not too strong for children's skin. It is estimated that the incidence of skin cancer would be reduced at least 70 percent if sunscreens were regularly used in childhood. Daily sunscreen use not only decreases or prevents photo damage but promotes repair of sun-damaged skin.

Cancers of Skin
- Basal cell carcinoma
- Squamous cell carcinoma
- Malignant melanoma

Sunscreens are needed most during March to November, but should preferably be used year round. They are needed most between 10 AM and 4 PM and should be applied 15 to 30 minutes before sun exposure.

Approximately 80 to 90 percent of the basal and squamous cell skin cancers occur on the face, neck, ears, and back of the hands. Although clothing and hats will provide some protection from the sun, they are not a substitute for sunscreens. (A typical white cotton T-shirt provides an SPF of only 5.) Reflected sunlight from water, sand, and snow may effectively increase sun exposure and the risk of burning.

EFFECT ON EYES

For centuries it has been known that sunlight can have an adverse effect on vision. Snow blindness, the result of solar UVR being reflected from the snow to the unprotected eyes of winter outdoor enthusiasts, was first described in 375 BC.[33] Ultraviolet radiation exposure of the eyes causes an acute inflammation called **photokeratitis**. It is a delayed reaction occurring from 6 to 24 hours after exposure, but occasionally develops within 30 minutes. Conjunctivitis (inflammation of the mucous membrane that lines the inside of the eyelid) develops, accompanied by erythema of adjacent facial skin, and the injured person reports the sensation of a foreign body on the eye. Photophobia, increased tear production, and spasm of the ocular muscles may

photokeratitis An inflammation of the eyes caused by exposure to UVR.

(*Used with permission from Chapel Hill Dermatology, P.A., Chapel Hill, North Carolina.)

occur.[28,34] The acute reaction lasts from 6 to 24 hours, and all symptoms will generally clear by 48 hours with few residual effects. The eye, unlike the skin, does not develop a tolerance to UVR. The development of cataracts has been attributed to UVR, especially in wavelengths of greater than 2900 Å.[32,34]

SYSTEMIC EFFECTS

The only systemic effect that can be objectively attributed to UVR is the photosynthesis of vitamin D following irradiation of the skin by UVR in the UV-D range.[19,32] The process is activated when the skin is irradiated by UVR at approximately 300 Å wavelength. This activates a complicated biochemical pathway that travels from the skin to the liver and kidneys and results in vitamin D being delivered to bones, intestines, various organs, and muscles. Vitamin D is responsible for regulating calcium and phosphorus, and after UVR exposure the absorption of these elements increases within the intestines and results in increased amounts of calcium and phosphorus within the blood. Consequently, UVR can be used as a treatment for disorders of calcium and phosphorus metabolism, such as rickets and tetany. Presently, the treatment of choice for such problems is dietary supplementation; however, if this is not effective, UVR is an acceptable alternative.

> Systemic effect is photosynthesis of vitamin D.

Although no other systemic effects can be objectively attributed to UVR exposure, there are several psychologic benefits and problems that may result from exposure. Many people relish the immediate sensation of warmth and relaxation that results from resting in the sun on a nice summer day; a general sense of well-being and good health surrounds the individual. Ideally, this happy experience is not overindulged, resulting in a painful sunburn. Moderation is the key to preventing damage to the skin; this includes gradually increasing exposure to the sun and prudent use of sunscreens.

Europeans, especially those living in northern latitudes, are probably the world's most active sunbathers. During the spring and summer months, they will congregate in sunny areas and feed on the sunlight that is so unavailable during their dark winters. The use of artificial UVR for tanning purposes is great in these areas, certainly for the sense of well-being that follows brief UVR exposure and also for questionable medical reasons. The use of artificial UVR to preserve the summer's tan is also on the increase in the United States and can be witnessed in the rapidly increasing number of tanning salons and spas. The apparatus most likely to be employed in one of these establishments will produce UVR in the UV-A wavelength, and the management of the salon will be quick to point out that this is a safe alternative to natural sunlight. An individual can certainly achieve tanning from these devices, although not as effectively as from UV-B exposure, but the research is still cloudy on the safety of long-term exposure to UV-A.

Needless to say, the psychologic effect from the extreme skin damage from long-term exposure to UVR can be devastating. The peaches-and-cream complexion of a 20-year-old beauty queen can turn to withered leather at 40 if caution is not used out of doors and in the tanning salon. A diagnosis of skin cancer will surely throw a person's psychologic health into a downward spiral.

APPARATUS

Since the beginning of this century many types of UVR generators have been developed, including the carbon arc lamp, fluorescent lamp, xenon compact arc lamp, and mercury arc lamps. Of these, the mercury arc lamps are the most common, and they have been found to be safe, effective, and easy to operate.

UVR Generators
- Carbon arc lamp
- Xenon compact arc lamp
- Fluorescent ultraviolet lamp (blacklight)
- Mercury arc lamp

Mercury arc lamp most commonly used.

The **carbon arc lamp** is composed of two carbon electrodes that consist of carbon and certain inorganic salts and metals. Initially the two electrodes are in contact when the current is applied and then are moved slightly apart, causing the current to arc across this small gap. As the salts and metals within the electrodes become heated, UVR is emitted, the majority between 3500 and 4000 Å. The electrode gradually burns, and so the lamp will deteriorate and the electrodes must be replaced. This burning is noisy and causes an unpleasant odor, and the device requires a high electrical input.

The **xenon compact arc lamp** is composed of xenon gas enclosed in a vessel in which it is compressed to 20 times atmospheric pressure. An electric arc is passed through the gas, causing increased temperature. When the gas is heated to 6000°C (10,832°F), the atoms become incandescent and emit infrared, visible, and ultraviolet light waves. Most of the UVR is in the range of 3200 to 4000 Å. Caution must be exercised when using a device with gas under such high pressure, because rupture of the containing vessel could endanger the patient and operator.

The **mercury arc lamps** are divided into two categories, low-pressure and high-pressure mercury arcs. Both consist of mercury (a heavy metal in a liquid state) contained in a quartz envelope. When an electric arc is passed through the envelope, the mercury becomes vaporized and at 8000°C (14,432°F) the atoms become incandescent and emit ultraviolet, infrared, and visible light. In the low-pressure lamp, also called the cold quartz lamp, the temperature of the mercury electrons is greater than the mercury vapor, and the temperature of the quartz envelope is about 60°C—hot, but not dangerous. The UVR spectrum produced by low pressure lamps is limited to 1849 and 2537 Å. The 1849 Å wavelength is blocked by the quartz envelope, or it would combine with oxygen and produce ozone; 95 percent of the UVR produced by these lamps is the 2537 Å wavelength, which is highly germicidal. The low pressure mercury arc lamp does not require a warm up or cool down period, and it is used mainly where the bactericidal effect of UVR is desired.

A high pressure mercury arc occurs when the mercury vapor temperature equals the mercury electron temperature and the pressure within the envelope reaches 1 atmosphere or more.[31] The quartz envelopes of these lamps become quite hot and may be cooled by a water jacket or circulating air; subsequently these are called hot quartz lamps. The UVR spectrum produced peaks at 2537, 2800, 2967, 3025, 3130, and 3660 Å.[8,17,32,33] The 2537 Å wavelength is absorbed by the increased density of the mercury vapor and does not pass from the lamp. Most of the UVR produced falls within the UV-B range. These lamps require a warm up period before reaching peak efficiency and a cool down period after the current is stopped before the lamp can be restarted. The high pressure mercury arc lamps are mainly used to produce erythema and the accompanying photochemical reactions.

The **fluorescent ultraviolet lamp**, or "blacklight," is actually a low pressure mercury lamp. It consists of a tube of UV-transmitting glass that is coated with phosphors. The phosphors are fluorescing substances that absorb the UVR and then reemit it at a longer wavelength. Most of the UVR emitted ranges from 3000 to 4000 Å, within the high UV-B and entire UV-A range.[32] These lamps are low-powered and generally used in multiples. These lamps are used where exposure of several people simultaneously is desired.

The **mercury arc lamps** are the most likely kind of UVR lamp to be used in a clinical setting, and generally the lamps will be either a standing model or a hand-held model. The standing model consists of a mercury arc lamp surrounded by a reflector. The opening below the lamp and reflector can be closed by the use of shutters. The lamp, reflector, and shutters are supported by a column, and the height of the column is adjustable. At the base of the column is a housing that contains the electrical controls contained within the configuration of the unit (Fig. 12-2). The

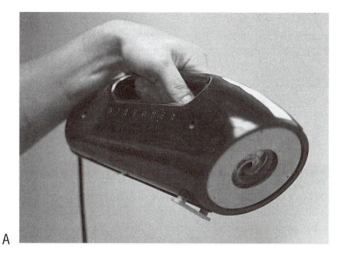

A

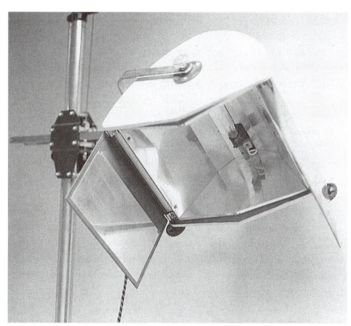

B

•**Figure 12-2** A. A handheld cold quartz ultraviolet lamp. B. A standing hot quartz ultraviolet lamp. Note the open shutters.

handheld unit is used for very local treatments and produces the bactericidal spectral bond of 2536 Å. It is very effective for treating local skin infections and, with the addition of a special lens, is used for diagnostic purposes.

TECHNIQUE OF APPLICATION

Before operation of any UVR generator, therapists must thoroughly familiarize themselves with the equipment; the operation manual must be understood and available if needed. Faulty operation of the equipment can endanger both the patient and the operator.[21] The lamp and reflector must be kept clean by wiping with gauze and methyl alcohol or by following the manufacturer's instructions. The quality of UVR is greatly diminished by dirty lamps and reflectors. The entire device must be completely inspected prior to use to ensure safe operation.

The effectiveness of the apparatus must be determined before UVR therapy can begin. The lamps in these devices deteriorate over time and accumulation of dirt and other residues on the lamp and reflector can also alter the effect of the UVR. Two lamps of the same model may have two differing effects, depending on the age of the lamp and its condition. The effectiveness of the lamp is assessed by determining the skin sensitivity to UVR of the patient to be treated. This sensitivity is measured by the **minimal erythemal dose.** The minimal erythemal dose is the exposure time needed to produce a faint erythema of the skin 24 hours after exposure.[8,30] Prior to testing, the patient should be questioned regarding photosensitizing drugs, and the area of skin to be tested should be cleaned. The area of the test should have pigmentation similar to the area to be treated. The forearm is a common choice for the test site.

For the skin test, the patient should be positioned comfortably, and eye protection must be provided to the patient and the operator. The goggles must fit snugly, since UVR can be reflected behind the lens of ordinary sunglasses. The patient may be instructed to close his or her eyes as an added precaution. The patient is draped except for the test site; a good quality bed sheet or bath towel provides an adequate barrier to UVR. A piece of typing paper with five cutouts 1-inch square and 1 inch apart is placed over the test site (Fig. 12-3). If necessary the lamp is warmed up with the protective shutters closed. The lamp is positioned over the patient with care being taken to adjust the height of the lamp from the patient to the same level as for treatment. With the lamp in position, the shutters are opened and the cutouts covered at 15-sec intervals so that the five portions of the skin will be exposed for 15, 30, 45, 60, and 75 sec. The patient returns in 24 hours, and a visual inspection determines the minimal erythemal dose. This information is used as the basis for determining treatment time.[4]

Areas tested that reveal no erythema 24 hours after testing have received a suberythemal dose, whereas those demonstrating erythema at 24 hours have received the minimal erythemal dose. At 48 hours if erythema is still present, a first-degree erythemal dose has been given, and a second-degree erythemal dose has been given if erythema persists from 48 to 72 hours. If the erythema lasts past 72 hours after testing, then a third-degree erythemal dose has been given. The third-degree erythemal dose is pathologic and causes destruction of the skin. Second- and

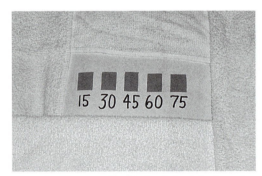

•**Figure 12-3** The ultraviolet skin test. The patient's back is draped and has been sequentially exposed to ultraviolet radiation for 15, 30, 45, 60, and 75 seconds.

third-degree doses are seldom used except in the case of stubborn skin infections, and when they are used, the skin surrounding the area of treatment should be well protected from exposure. First- and second-degree doses can be estimated; first-degree erythemal doses approximately correspond to two and a half times the minimal erythemal dose, and second-degree doses correspond to five times the minimal erythemal dose.[8,22]

Since human skin adapts to UVR exposure, the minimal erythemal dose will gradually increase with repeated treatments. Therefore, it is necessary to gradually increase exposure time in order to achieve the same reaction. Once the treatment time has been determined, it is increased 5 sec per treatment with the height of the lamp remaining constant. Conversely, treatment time should be reduced 5 sec for each day missed, or it should be set back to the original minimal erythemal dose.

In order to give consistent treatments, the operator needs to be aware of the two laws of physics that apply directly to UVR treatments, the inverse square law and the cosine law. The inverse square law states that the strength of radiation of light from a point source varies inversely with the square of the distance from the source.[6,8,32] If the lamp is set closer to the patient than during the skin test, a stronger dose is given; if it is set further away, a weaker dose is given. The distance of the lamp from the patient must be kept constant if the intensity of the treatments is to be equal. The height of the lamp is generally standardized at each clinic, usually ranging from 24 to 40 inches.[7] My preference is to set the height of the lamp at 30 inches.

The cosine law states that for maximum absorption of radiant energy, the source must be perpendicular to the absorbing surface (the patient being the absorbing surface).[8,32] A deviation of 10 degrees causes no major alteration in the amount of energy absorbed. Therefore, care should be taken in positioning the lamp and patient during testing and treatment.

Once the minimal erythemal dose has been established, treatment can commence. As with the skin test, the treatment area should be warm and provide maximum privacy since the patient may be partially or fully disrobed. Goggles, stopwatch, measuring tape, and draping must be readily available. The patient should be carefully draped so that areas not to receive UVR exposure are protected. Besides the eyes, the nipples and genitalia should be protected. It should be taken into account that UVR can be reflected from white linen and shiny equipment surfaces. If needed, the UVR apparatus should be warmed up with the protective shutter in place. The patient and operator are ready to begin treatment when the patient is comfortable, properly draped, and has his or her eyes protected. The lamp is positioned at proper height and angle, and the operator has his or her goggles in place and stopwatch ready. Treatment commences when the operator simultaneously opens the shutters and activates the stopwatch. At the end of the predetermined treatment time, the shutters are closed, the lamp is extinguished, and the patient is allowed to remove the goggles and dress. Accurate records noting the height of the lamp, time of exposure, and condition of the area treated must be kept. Also, the same lamp should be used for subsequent treatments, since lamp deterioration causes differing intensities from UVR sources of even the same manufacturer's model.

Consistency is crucial if safe and effective UVR treatments are to be given.[21] The setup of the patient and equipment should not vary without adequate reason. Usually the only variable is the length of treatment (exposure) and that is determined by and based on the skin test, the treatment prescription, the lesion to be treated, and the progression of treatment. If the length of treatment is in doubt, it is always best to yield to brevity rather than to endanger a patient.

minimal erythemal dose The amount of time of exposure to UVR necessary to cause a faint erythema 24 hours after exposure.

CLINICAL USE

Ultraviolet radiation therapy is used to obtain one or more of the following effects: increased vitamin D production, stimulation of the skin, sterilization, tanning, hyperplasia, and exfoliation (peeling).[32] The use of UVR is indicated for treatment of infectious and noninfectious skin diseases and for the excitation of calcium metabolism.[8] The development of antibiotics and other medications has greatly reduced the clinical use of UVR, since these drugs are very effective and simple to employ in the treatment of disease. Today the most common use of UVR is in the treatment of dermatologic conditions such as psoriasis and acne and hard to cure infectious skin conditions such as pressure sores.[14,15,26] The protocol for treating certain maladies with UVR follows.

PSORIASIS

The Goekerman technique developed in 1925 is still widely used.[35] This consists of applying a crude tar ointment (2–5%) over the patches of psoriasis the night prior to treatment. The next morning the tar is removed, except for a thin film, and the area is irradiated with a UV-B source at minimal erythemal dosage.[3,8] The exposure time is gradually increased, and the treatment is usually carried out for several weeks. In the past decade, a UV-A source and the photosensitizing drug psoralen have been used to treat psoriasis.[12] This technique is called PUVA therapy.

PUVA Therapy

This is a treatment for psoriasis that consists of ingestion of oral methoxsalen, a psoralen, and exposure of the affected site to a UV-A light source. The methoxsalen increases the patient's sensitivity to UVR, and in the presence of UV-A it binds with DNA and inhibits DNA synthesis.[9] Unfortunately, several studies point to an increased risk of developing skin cancer following PUVA therapy, and problems with the safety of the UV-A sources have been uncovered.[2,9,10,29] Still, in selected cases PUVA therapy is considered by the American Academy of Dermatology to be safe, but its use should be limited to physicians with training in photochemotherapy.[2]

DISTURBANCES OF CALCIUM AND PHOSPHORUS ABSORPTION

Conditions such as osteomalacia (rickets) and tetany can be treated with irradiation by a UV-B source. These disturbances of absorption are caused by a vitamin D deficiency. As previously discussed, vitamin D is produced following irradiation of the skin. Whole body irradiation is indicated if diet and oral supplementation of calcium and phosphorus do not produce improvement.[19,32]

PRESSURE SORES

Unlike most infectious skin disorders, pressure sores do not respond readily to antibiotic therapy. Irradiation of the lesion by low pressure mercury or cold quartz lamp, which produces UVR of the bactericidal 2537 Å wavelength, can be an effective means of treating this problem. Handheld lamps are most useful, since they can be used to produce a very localized reaction. Exposure time should be sufficient to produce a second- or third-degree erythemal dose response.[8,11,32] Care must be taken to protect the surrounding skin.

STERILIZATION

Bacteria are destroyed when exposed to UVR in the range of 2500 to 2700 Å. This technique has been used to sterilize the air in operating rooms and to sterilize water. The technique is quite safe if human exposure to the UVR source is kept to a minimum.

DIAGNOSIS

A UVR source fitted with a special filter, a Wood's filter, can be used to aid in the diagnosis of certain skin disorders. The filter blocks all the UVR except that in the range of 3600 to 3700 Å. This wavelength is most effective in causing exposed areas to fluoresce. The test is performed in a darkened room, and since all animal tissues fluoresce, the exposure to the filtered UVR will cause the exposed tissue to appear to be a specific color.[32] However, if an infection is present, the color of the area will correspond to the **fluorescence** of the infecting organism rather than the expected normal color. This abnormal coloration can be evaluated, and a tentative diagnosis made.

INDICATIONS

Acne: General body irradiation may help, minimal erythemal dose applied three times per week

Aseptic wounds: Suberythemal dose applied every 3 days[3,8,20,25,30]

Folliculitis: Suberythemal dose applied every 3 days until clear

Pityriasis rosea: General body irradiation, minimal erythemal dose applied three times per week[18]

Tinea capitum: Local first-degree erythemal reaction, repeated when initial response clears

Septic wounds: Local second-degree erythemal response, repeated every 3 days

Sinusitis: General body irradiation

Psoriasis	Sterilization
Pressure sores	Tanning
Osteomalacia	Hyperplasia
Diagnosis of skin disorders	Exfoliation
Increased vitamin D production	

CONTRAINDICATIONS

Porphyrias	Pellagra
Lupus erythematosus	Sarcoidosis
Xeroderma pigmentosum	Acute psoriasis
Acute eczema	Herpes simplex
Renal and hepatic insufficiencies	Diabetes
Hyperthyroidism	Generalized dermatitis
Advanced arteriosclerosis	

Active and progressive pulmonary tuberculosis[3,8,20,24,25,32]

The use of UVR therapy in physical therapy has been limited in recent years. Many indications for its use, such as acne, skin infections, and fungal infections, are adequately treated with medication. This does not mean that UVR should be excluded from the clinic; it most certainly has beneficial effects that could be used by therapists. However, considering the small number of potential patients and the limited budgetary resources most clinics have available, UVR equipment will remain a low-priority item.

SUMMARY

1. Ultraviolet radiation is that portion of the electromagnetic spectrum that ranges from 2000 to 4000 Å.
2. Exposure to UVR causes a photochemical reaction within living cells and can cause alterations of DNA and cell proteins.
3. The irradiation of human skin causes an acute inflammation that is characterized by an erythema, increased pigmentation, and hyperplasia.
4. The effects of long-term exposure to UVR are premature aging of the skin and skin cancer.
5. The eye is extremely sensitive to UVR and will develop photokeratitis following exposure.
6. Many types of equipment are manufactured that produce UVR, but the majority used clinically are of the low- and high pressure mercury lamp variety.

REFERENCES

1. Bergner, T., Przybilla, B.: Malignant melanoma in association with phototherapy, Dermatology 184(1):59–61, 1992.
2. Bickford, E.: Risks associated with the use of UV-A irradiators, Photochem. Photobiol. 30(2):199–202, 1979.
3. Burdick Corp.: Burdick syllabus, ed. 7, Milton, Wisconsin, 1969.
4. Downer, A.: Physical therapy procedures, ed. 3, Springfield, Illinois, 1981, Charles C Thomas.
5. Gilmour, J., Vestey, J., and Norval, M.: The effect of UV therapy on immune function in patients with psoriasis, Br. J. Dermatol. 129(1):28–38, 1993.
6. Goats, G.: Appropriate use of the inverse square law, Physiotherapy 74(1):8, 1988.
7. Goldman, L.: Introduction to modern phototherapy, Springfield, Illinois, 1978, Charles C Thomas.
8. Griffin, J., Karsalis, T.: Physical agents for physical therapists, ed. 2, Springfield, Illinois, 1982, Charles C Thomas.
9. Hall, L.: Current status of oral PUVA therapy for psoriasis, J. Am. Acad. Dermatol. 1(2):106–107, 1979.
10. Harbor, L.: PUVA therapy status, J. Am. Acad. Dermatol. 1(2):150, 1979.
11. High, A., High, J.: Treatment of infected skin wounds using ultra-violet radiation: an in-vitro study, Physiotherapy 69(10):359–360, 1983.
12. Hudson-Peacock, M., Diffey, B., and Farr, P.: Photoprotective action of emollients in ultraviolet therapy of psoriasis, Br. J. Dermatol. 130(3):361–365, 1994.
13. Kitchen, S., Partridge, C.: A review of ultraviolet radiation therapy, Physiotherapy 77(6):423–432, 1991.
14. Kloth, L.: Physical modalities in wound management: UVC, therapeutic heating and electrical stimulation, Ostomy Wound Manage. 41(5):18–20, 22–24, 26–27, 1995.
15. Kowalzick, L., Kleinheinz, A., and Weichenthal, M.: Low dose versus medium dose UV-A1 treatment in severe atopic eczema, Acta Dermato-Venereologica 75(1):43–45, 1995.
16. Kottke, F.: Krusen's handbook of physical medicine and rehabilitation, ed. 3, Philadelphia, 1983, W.B. Saunders.
17. Kovacs, R.: Light therapy, Springfield, Illinois, 1950, Charles C Thomas.
18. Leenutaphong, V., Jiamton, S.: UVB phototherapy for pityriasis rosea: a bilateral comparison study, J. Amer. Acad. Dermatol. 33(6):996–999, 1995.
19. Lemke, E.: The influence of UV irradiation on vitamin D metabolism in children with chronic renal diseases, Int. Urol. Nephrol. 25(6):595–601, 1993.
20. Lewis, G.: Practical dermatology, Philadelphia, 1967, W.B. Saunders.
21. Low, J., Bazin, S., and Docker, M.: Guidelines for the safe use of ultraviolet therapy equipment, Physiotherapy 80(2):89–90, 1994.
22. Low, J.: Quantifying the erythema due to UVR, Physiotherapy 72(1):60–64, 1986.
23. Lowe, N.: Home ultraviolet phototherapy, Semin. Dermatol. 11(4):284–286, 1992.
24. Mayer,. E.: Clinical application of sunlight and artificial radiation, Baltimore, 1926, Williams & Wilkins.
25. Mayer, E.: The curative value of light, New York, 1932, D. Appleton.

26. Owoeye, I., Adeyemi-Doro, H.: The therapeutic effect of ultra-violet irradiation on traumatic open wounds: an experimental investigation, J. Nigeria Soc. Physiol. 13(1):33–44, 1995.

27. Parish, P.: The doctors and patients handbook of medicines and drugs, New York, 1980, Alfred A. Knopf.

28. Parrish, J.: UV-A biological effects of ultraviolet radiation, New York, 1979, Plenum.

29. Pittekow, M.: Skin cancer in patients with psoriasis treated with coal tar, Arch. Dermatol. 117:465–468, 1981.

30. Rook, A.: Textbook of dermatology, Oxford, 1979, Blackwell Scientific.

31. Stewart, W.: Dermatology: diagnosis and treatment of cutaneous disorders, St. Louis, 1978, C.V. Mosby.

32. Stillwell, G.: Therapeutic electricity and ultraviolet radiation, Baltimore, 1983, Williams & Wilkins.

33. Urbach, F.: The biologic effects of ultraviolet radiation, London, 1969, Pergamon.

34. U.S. Dept. of HEW, Public Health Service: Occupational exposure to ultraviolet radiation, Washington, D.C., 1972, National Institute for Occupational Safety and Health, HSM73-1 1009.

35. Williams, R.: PUVA therapy vs. Goeckerman therapy in the treatment of psoriasis: a pilot study, Physiother. Can. 37(6): 361–366, 1985.

SUGGESTED READINGS

Bryant, B.: Treatment of psoriasis, Am. J. Hosp. Pharm. 37: 814–820, 1980.

Cerio, R., Low, J.: Successful treatment by general ultra-violet radiation of pruritus due to biliary cirrhosis, Physiotherapy. 73(12):689, 1987.

Challner, A., Corless, D., and Davis, A: Personnel monitoring exposure to UV radiation, Clin. Exp. Dermatol. 1:175–179, 1976.

Challner, A., Duffey, B.: Problems associated with ultraviolet dosimetry in the photochemotherapy of psoriasis, Br. J. Dermatol. 97:643–648, 1977.

Collins, P., Ferguson, J.: Narrow-band UVB (TL-01) phototherapy: an effective preventative treatment for the photodermatoses, Br. J. Dermatol. 132(6):956–963, 1995.

Corless, D., Gupta, S.: Response of plasma 25 hydroxyvitamin D to ultraviolet irradiation in long stay geriatric patients, Lancet 223:649–651, 1978.

Dietzel, F.: Effects of non-ionizing electromagnetic radiation on the development and intrauterine implantation of the rat, In Tyler, A.E., editor: Biological effects of nonionizing radiation, Ann. NY Acad. Sci. 247:367, 1975.

Diffey, B.: Ultraviolet radiation and skin cancer: are physiotherapists at risk? Physiotherapy 75(10):615–616, 1989.

Dootson, G., Norris, P., and Gibson, C.: The practice of ultraviolet phototherapy in the United Kingdom, Br. J. Dermatol. 131(6):873–877, 1994.

Everett, M., Olson, R., and Sayer, R.: Ultraviolet erythema, Arch. Dermatol. 92:713, 1975.

Fischer, T.: Comparative treatment of psoriasis with UV-light trioxsalen plus UV-light and coal tar plus UV-light, Acta Dermatol. Venereol. 57:345–350, 1977.

Fitzpatrick, T., Pathak, A., Magnus,. I.: Abnormal reactions of man to light, Ann. Rev. Med. 14:195, 1963.

Giese, A., editor: Photophysiology, vol. V, New York, 1970, Academic Press.

Giese, A., editor: Photophysiology, vol. IV, New York, 1968, Academic Press.

Giese, A., editor: Photophysiology, vol. VI, New York, 1971, Academic Press.

Giese, A., editor: Photophysiology, vol. VII, New York, 1972, Academic Press.

Gordon, M., editor: Pigment cell biology, New York, 1959, Academic Press.

Green, C., Diffey, B., and Hawk, J.: Ultraviolet radiation in the treatment of skin disease, Phys. Med. Biol. 37(1):1–20, 1992.

Grynbaum, B.: Prevention of ultraviolet induced erythema, Arch. Phys. Med. Rehabil. 31:587–592, 1950.

Hardie, R., Hunter, J.: Psoriasis, Br. J. Hosp. Med. 20:13–23, 1978.

Holick, M., Clark, M.: The photogenesis and metabolism of vitamin D, Fed. Proc. 37: 12:2567–2574, 1978.

Hollaender, A., editor: Radiation biology, vol. II, New York, 1955, McGraw-Hill.

Holti, G.: Measurements of the vascular responses in skin at various time intervals after damage with histamine and ultraviolet radiation, Clin. Sci. 14:143–155, 1955.

Jarratt, M., Knox, J.: Photodynamic action: theory and applications. Prog. Dermatol. 8:1, 1974.

Jekler, J., Bergbrant, I., and Faergemann, J.: The in vivo effect of UVB radiation on skin bacteria in patients with atopic dermatitis, Acta Dermato-Venereol. 72(1):33–36, 1992.

Jekler, J.: Phototherapy of atopic dermatitis with ultraviolet radiation, Acta Dermato-Venereol. 72(1):1–37, 1992.

Kelner, A.: Photoreactivation of ultraviolet irradiated *Escherichia coli*, with special reference to the dose reduction principle and to ultraviolet induced mutation, J. Bacteriol. 58:11–22, 1949.

Lebwohl, M., Martinez, J.: Effects of topical preparations on the erythemogenicity of UVB: implications for psoriasis phototherapy, J. Amer. Acad. Dermatol. 32(3):469–471, 1995.

Licht, S., editor: Therapeutic electricity and ultraviolet radiation, ed. 2, New Haven, 1967, Elizabeth Licht.

Lynch, W.: Clinical results of photochemotherapy, Cutis 20: 477–480, 1977.

MacKinnon, J., Cleek, P.: The penetration of ultraviolet light through transparent dressings: a case report, Phys. Ther. 64(2):204, 1984.

Macleod, M., Blacklock, N.: UVL induced changes in calcium absorption and excretion and in serum vitamin D₃ levels measured in black skinned and caucasian males, J. R. Nav. Med. Serv. 65:75–78,1979.

Marisco, A.: Ultraviolet light and tar in the Goeckermann treatment of psoriasis, Arch. Dermatol. 112:1249–1250, 1976.

Montagna, W., Labitz, W., editors: The epidermis, New York, 1964, Academic Press.

Morison, W.: Controlled study of PUVA and adjunctive therapy in the management of psoriasis, Br. J. Dermatol. 98:125–132, 1978.

Moseley, H., Thomas, R., and Young, M.: UVB lamps: a burning issue, Br. J. Dermatol. 128(6):704–706, 1993.

Nussbaum, E., Biemann, I., and Mustard, B.: Comparison of ultrasound/ultraviolet-C and laser for treatment of pressure ulcers in patients with spinal cord injury, Phys. Ther. 74(9):812–825, 1994.

Ohayashi, T., Yoshimoto, S., and Yasamura, M.: Effect of wavelength on the photochemical reaction of ergocalciferol (vitamin D₂) irradiated by monochromatic ultraviolet light, J. Nutr. Sci. Vitaminol. 23:281–290, 1977 (in English).

Parrish, J.: Photochemotherapy of psoriasis with oral methoxsalen and longwave ultraviolet light, N. Engl. J. Med. 291:1207–1222, 1974.

Pathak, M., Harber, J., and Seiji, M.: editors: Sunlight and man, Tokyo, 1974, University of Tokyo Press.

Peak, M.: Inactivation of transforming DNA by ultraviolet light: II. Protection by histadine, Mutat. Res. 20:137–141, 1973.

Roenig, H.: Comparison of phototherapy systems for photochemotherapy, Cutis 20:485–489, 1977.

Rogers, S.: Effect of PUVA on serum 25-OH vitamin D in psoriatics, Br. Med. J. 833:34, 1979.

Rolston, K., Gold, M., and Elson M.: Ultraviolet: a treatment of pruritus secondary to hyperbilirubinemia, Dermatol. Nurs. 2(1):31–32, 1990.

Salem, L.: Theory of photochemical reactions, Science 191:822, 1976.

Sams, W., Winkleman, R.: The effect of ultraviolet light on isolated cutaneous blood vessels, J. Invest. Dermatol. 53:79–83, 1969.

Sauer, G., editor: Manual of skin diseases, ed. 3, Philadelphia, 1973, J.B. Lippincott.

Segal, S.: PUVA: a caution, Pediatrics 62:253, 1978.

Sjovall, P., Christensen, O.: Treatment of chronic hand eczema with UV-B Handylux in the clinic and at home, Contact Dermatolitis 31(1):5–8, 1994.

Smith, K., Skelton, H., and Yeager, J.: Ultraviolet radiation therapy and HIV disease, J. Amer. Acad. Dermatol. 33(5 Pt 1):841–842, 1995.

Sulzberger, W., Wolf, J., and Witten, V.: Dermatology: diagnosis and treatment, ed. 2, Chicago, 1961, Year Book.

Task Force Committee on Photobiology of the National Program for Dermatology, Harber, L.C., Chairman, Arch. Dermatol. 109:833–839, 1974.

Taylor, R.: Clinical study of ultraviolet in various skin conditions, Phys. Ther. 52:279–282, 1972.

Telles, J., Coakley, C., and Kluger, A.: Bureau of Radiological Health. Food and Drug Administration: Possible hazards from high intensity discharge mercury vapor and metal halide lamps, Nov., 1977.

Thomsen, D.: Phototherapy: treatment with light, Science News 105:404, 1974.

Urbach, F., editor: Biological effects of ultraviolet radiation, New York, 1969, Pergamon; UV radiation, Clin. Exp. Dermatol. 1:175–179, 1976.

Van Der Leun, J.: Theory of ultraviolet erythema, Photochem. Photobiol. 4:453–458, 1965.

Van Pelt, W., Payne, W., and Peterson, R.: A review of selected bioeffects thresholds for various spectral ranges of light, DH EW Publ. no. (FDA) 74-8010.

Weber, G.: Combined 8-methoxypsoralen and black light therapy of psoriasis: technique and results, Br. J. Dermatol. 90:317–323, 1974.

Wurtman, R.: The effects of light on the human body, Sci. Am. 233:69, 1975.

Young, P.: Turning on light turns off disease, National Observer, May 29, 1976.

Glossary

DNA Deoxyribonucleic acid; the substance found in the chromosomes of the cell nucleus that carries the genetic code of the cell.

erythema A redness of the skin caused by capillary dilation.

fluorescence The capacity of certain substances to radiate when illuminated by a source of a given wavelength; a light of a different wavelength (color) than that of the irradiating source when illuminated by a given wavelength.

hyperplasia An increase in the size of a tissue; in the skin, an increased thickness of the epidermis.

keratin The fibrous protein that forms the chemical basis of the epidermis.

keratinocytes A cell that produces keratin.

melanin A group of dark brown or black pigments that occur naturally in the eye, skin, hair, and other animal tissues.

minimal erythemal dose The amount of time of exposure to UVR necessary to cause a faint erythema 24 hours after exposure.

photokeratitis An inflammation of the eyes caused by exposure to UVR.

photosensitization A process in which a person becomes overly sensitive to UVR.

RNA Ribonucleic acid; an acid found in the cell cytoplasm and nucleolus. It is intimately involved in protein synthesis.

sun protection factor (SPF) A sunscreen's effectiveness in absorbing sunburn-inducing radiation.

LAB ACTIVITY

ULTRAVIOLET

DESCRIPTION:

Electromagnetic energy in the ultraviolet (UV) wavelength range has several medically accepted uses; however, it is rare for a sports therapist to treat a patient with ultraviolet. In the past, UV was considered a heating physical agent because of the sensation of warmth that it produced. However, the warmth is extremely superficial, and UV is not considered a heating physical agent.

Ultraviolet energy is absorbed by the epidermis and, to a limited extent, the dermis. The primary effect is to produce an increase in the synthesis of vitamins D_2 and D_3, and an increase in melanin content of the epidermis as a protective response.

There is also evidence that UV energy stimulates cells of the reticuloendothelial system in the dermis of the skin. This may enhance the immune response to bacterial infection, thus helping the body overcome the infection.

Prior to initiating a course of treatment with UV, the individual patient's sensitivity to UV must be determined. Because the total energy delivered to the patient is a function of the duration of exposure, the distance from the source to the patient, and the angle of intercept of the UV light with the skin, two of these three variables must remain constant. The easiest one to vary is the time of exposure; therefore, distance and angle should remain constant from the time of determination of appropriate dosage throughout the duration of the treatment. The appropriate beginning dose of UV is the time, distance, and angle that produces a minimal erythemal dose (MED). One MED is the time of exposure that produces an erythemal reaction within 8 hours of exposure and that disappears within 24 hours of exposure. This can be determined by exposing an area of skin that is not normally exposed to sunlight (e.g., the anterior surface of the forearm, lower abdomen) to UV for specific durations. The best way to do this is to cover the area with paper or cloth that has six small (approx 1 cm diameter) holes cut in it; five of the holes are covered, while the skin exposed by the sixth hole is exposed to the UV for 30 sec. After 30 sec, the adjacent hole is uncovered for 30 sec, then another hole is uncovered every 15 sec. This results in exposures of 120, 105, 90, 75, 60, and 30 sec. The areas exposed should be marked so that the patient can report which area turns red within 8 hours and resolves within 24 hours.

PHYSIOLOGIC EFFECTS:

Vitamin D synthesis enhanced
Melanin deposition enhanced
Bactericidal

THERAPEUTIC EFFECTS:

Skeletal deposition of calcium enhanced
Desquamation of epithelium enhanced
Infectious organisms may be destroyed

INDICATIONS:

The principal indications for UV radiation are dermatologic conditions such as psoriasis and acne. Dietary approaches are generally used to correct Vitamin D deficiencies.

CONTRAINDICATIONS:

- Hypersensitivity to UV radiation

ULTRAVIOLET			
PROCEDURE	Evaluation		
	1	2	3
1. Check supplies.			
a. Obtain sheet or towels for draping, stopwatch, UV protection goggles for patient and therapist.			
b. Check lamp for frayed power cords, integrity of lamp and shields, and so on.			
c. Verify that the intensity control is at zero.			
2. Question patient.			
a. Verify identity of patient (if not already verified).			
b. Verify the absence of contraindications.			
c. Ask about previous ultraviolet treatments, check treatment notes.			
3. Position patient.			
a. Place patient in a well-supported, comfortable position.			
b. Expose body part to be treated; have patient remove all jewelry from the area.			
c. Drape patient to preserve patient's modesty and protect clothing, but allow access to body part. Insure that only the area you want to expose to UV is exposed; draping is crucial.			
4. Inspect body part to be treated.			
a. Check for precancerous skin lesions (e.g., keratoses).			
b. If treating for acne, attempt to quantify the number of lesions; if treating a wound, measure the size of the wound.			
5. Determine minimal erythemal dose (MED) of ultraviolet light on initial treatment day.			
a. Cut six 1-cm^2 holes of different shapes in a piece of cloth (e.g., stockinette) or stiff paper (e.g., file folder).			
b. Cover an area of the body away from the treatment area that has not been exposed to ultraviolet in the past few weeks (e.g., the abdomen or anterior forearm) with the paper or cloth.			
c. Position lamp such that the bulb is parallel to the body part being treated (such that the energy will strike the body at a 90° angle) and is about 75 cm away from the patient.			
d. Inform the patient that he or she should feel only a mild warmth; if it is hot, he or she should inform you. Start the lamp.			
e. Expose the first window for 30 sec, then uncover the second window for an additional 30 sec; continue exposing remaining windows every 15 sec. If six windows are used, the first window will have been exposed for 120 sec, the last for only 15 sec.			
f. The MED is the duration of exposure that produces redness within 8 hours and disappears within 24 hours. Inform the patient to inspect the test area over the next 24-hour period and report the results on the next visit.			
6. Apply ultraviolet light.			

PROCEDURE	Evaluation		
	1	2	3
a. Position lamp such that the bulb is parallel to the body part being treated (such that the energy will strike the body at a 90° angle) and is about 75 cm away from the patient.			
b. Inform the patient that he or she should feel only a mild warmth; if it is hot, he or she should inform you. Start the lamp.			
c. Expose the treatment area for the appropriate time (i.e., one MED for the first treatment, with an increase of 35% per treatment; if 1 day's treatment is missed, exposure should be the same as the last treatment).			
7. Complete the treatment.			
a. When the treatment time is over, move the lamp away from the patient and turn the output control to zero; dry the area with a towel.			
b. Remove material used for draping, assist the patient in dressing as needed.			
c. Clean the treatment area and equipment according to normal protocol.			
8. Assess treatment efficacy.			
a. Ask the patient how the treated area feels.			
b. Visually inspect the treated area for any adverse reactions.			
c. Perform functional tests as indicated.			

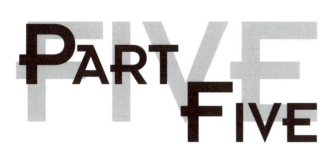

PART FIVE

MECHANICAL MODALITIES

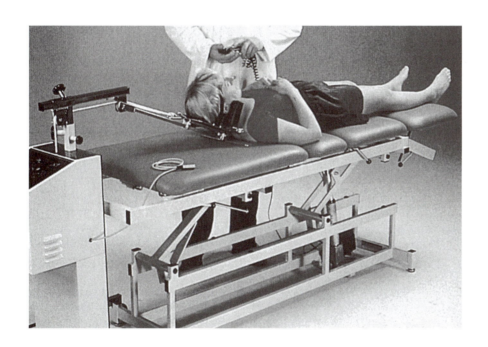

CHAPTER 13 THIRTEEN

SPINAL TRACTION

DANIEL N. HOOKER

OBJECTIVES

Following completion of this chapter, the student therapist will be able to:

✓ Discuss the effect and therapeutic value of traction on bone, muscle, ligaments, joint structures, nerve, blood vessels, and intervertebral disk.
✓ Describe the parameters of traction.
✓ Discuss the effect that changing a parameter might have on treatment results.
✓ Outline the setup procedure for mechanical, positional, and manual traction to both the lumbar and cervical spine.

Traction has been used since ancient times in the treatment of painful spinal conditions, but the literature on traction and its clinical effectiveness is limited.[6,8,12,22,27,33,39] Most of the clinical studies go into great depth about the pathology being treated and give only a cursory description of the traction setup, making duplication of the traction method difficult. Traction can be defined as a drawing tension applied to a body segment.[4]

EFFECTS ON SPINAL MOVEMENT

Traction encourages movement of the spine both overall and between each individual spinal segment.[2] Changes in overall spinal length and the amount of separation or space between each vertebra have been shown in studies of both the lumbar and the cervical spine (Fig. 13-1).[1,6,21,26,27,32,33]

The amount of movement varies according to the position of the spine, the amount of force, and the length of time the force is applied. Separations of 1 to 2 mm per intervertebral space have been reported. This change is very transient and the spine quickly returns to the previous intervertebral space relationships when traction is released and the erect posture is assumed.[10,17,21,27] Decreases in pain, paresthesia, or tingling while traction is applied may be caused by the physical separation of the vertebral segments and the resultant decrease in pressure on sensitive

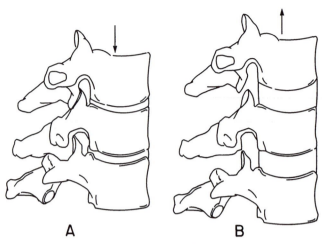

•**Figure 13-1** A. Spine in normal resting position. B. Spine under traction load with overall increase in length and overall increased separation between vertebrae.

structures. If these changes occur while the patient is being treated with traction, the prognosis for the patient is good and traction should be continued as part of the treatment plan.[2,5,26] Any lasting therapeutic changes must be assumed to occur from adjustments or adaptations of the structures around the vertebrae in response to the traction.

EFFECTS ON BONE

Wolff's law Bone remodels itself and provides increased strength along the lines of the mechanical forces placed on it.

Bone changes, according to **Wolff's law,** usually occur in response to compressive or distractive loads. Traction places a distractive load on each of the vertebrae affected by the traction load. Although bone tissue adapts relatively quickly, bony changes do not occur fast enough to cause the symptom changes that occur with traction application. An intermittent traction with a rhythmic on and off load cycle not only provides distraction load but also promotes movement. The major effect of traction on the bone may come from the increase in spinal movement that reverses any immobilization-related bone weakness by increasing or maintaining bone density.

EFFECTS ON LIGAMENTS

viscoelastic properties The property of a material to show sensitivity to rate of loading.

The ligamentous structures of the spinal column is stretched by traction. Structural changes of the ligaments occur relatively slowly in response to mechanical stresses because ligaments have **viscoelastic properties** that allow them to resist shear forces and return to their original form following the removal of a deforming load.[2,5,25]

With rapid loading, the ligaments become stiffer or resistant to changes in length and are able to absorb a high load or force before failure occurs. With this type of loading, overstress could produce a significant injury.[5] The Wild West and the cervical traction of horse thieves gives us a notable example of this type of loading. The sudden drop of body weight as the horse rides out and leaves the thief suspended by a rope around his neck places a rapid load on the ligaments and bones of the cervical spine. This overstress produces no adaptive change as it overwhelms the ligamentous and bony structures, causing a fracture dislocation of the upper cervical spine with spinal cord compression, resulting in the death of the thief.

Slow loading rates allow the ligament to lengthen as it absorbs the force of the load. Overstress can still produce injury but it is not be as severe as in the high loading rates. The amount of **ligament deformation** accompanying a low rate of loading is higher than in rapid loading situations. Loading should be applied slowly and comfortably.[5] The ligament deformation allows the spinal vertebrae to move apart.

In ligaments shortened or contracted by an injury or a long-term postural problem, traction is important in restoring normal length. The traction force provides the stress that encourages the ligament to make adaptive changes in length and strength. The traction force in this instance would have to be heavy enough to stimulate adaptive changes but not heavy enough to overwhelm the ligament. In acute severely sprained ligaments, a traction force may overwhelm the ligament and have a negative effect on the healing process. Traction treatment should be a part of an overall treatment program that includes strengthening and flexibility exercises.[2]

When they are stretched, the ligaments put pressure on or move other structures within the ligamentous structure (**proprioceptive nerves**) and external to the ligament structure (**disk material, synovial fringes,** vascular structures, nerve roots). This pressure or movement can have a tremendous impact on painful problems if pressure on a sensitive structure (nerve, vascular) is reduced. Activation of the proprioceptive system also relieves pain by providing a gating effect similar to a transcutaneous electrical nerve stimulation treatment.[2,8]

proprioceptive nervous system System of nerves that provide information on joint movement, pressure, and muscle tension.

EFFECTS ON THE DISK

The mechanical tension created by the traction has an excellent effect on **disk protrusions** and disk-related pain. Normally, the disk helps to dissipate compressive forces while the spine is in an erect posture (Fig. 13-2A).

In the normal disk, internal pressure increases but the nucleus pulposus (fluid-like center of the fibrocartilaginous vertebral disk) does not move with changes in the weight-bearing forces as the spine moves from flexion to extension.[27] When an injury occurs to the disk structures and the disk loses its normal fullness, the vertebrae can move closer together. The annular fibers bulge just as an underinflated car tire bulges when compared with a normally inflated one (Fig. 13-2B).[27]

If the disk is damaged and movement occurs in a weight-bearing position, the disk nucleus will shift according to fluid-dynamic principles. Pressure on one side squeezes the nucleus in the opposite direction (Fig. 13-2C). If tears develop in the annular fibers, the nucleus will tend to take the path of least resistance and move in this direction (Fig. 13-2D).

Traction that increases the separation of the vertebral bodies decreases the central pressure in the disk space and encourages the **disk nucleus** to return to a central position. The mechanical tension of the **annulus fibrosus** and ligaments surrounding the disk also tends to force the nuclear material and cartilage fragments toward the center.[2,8,12,17,22,25,27]

Movement of these materials relieves pain and symptoms if they are compressing nervous or vascular structures. Decreasing the compressive forces also allows for better fluid interchange within the disk and spinal canal.[2,8] The reduction in **disk herniation** is unstable and the herniation tends to return when compressive forces return (Fig. 13-2D, E).[21,22]

The positive effect of traction in this instance may be destroyed by allowing the patient to sit after treatment. Minimizing compressive forces after treatment may be

disk protrusion The abnormal projection of the disk nucleus through some or all of the annular rings.

Annulus fibrosus The interlacing cross fibers of fibroelastic tissue that are attached to adjacent vertebral bodies that contain the nucleus pulposus.

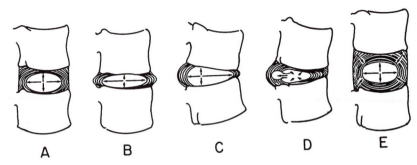

•**Figure 13-2** Fluid dynamics of the intervertebral disk. A. Normal disk in noncompressed position; internal pressure, indicated by arrows, is exerted relatively equally in all directions. The internal annular fibers contain the nuclear materials. B. Sitting or standing with compression of an injured disk causes the nucleus to become flatter. Pressure in this instance still remains relatively equal in all directions. C. In an injured disk, movement in the weight-bearing position causes a horizontal shift in the nuclear material. If this was forward bending, the bulge to the left would take place at the posterior annular fibers, whereas the anterior annular fibers would be slackened and narrow. D. Weakness of the annular wall would allow the nuclear material to create a herniation and possibly put pressure on sensitive structures in the area. E. When placed under traction, the intervertebral space expands, lowering the disk pressure. The taut annulus creates a centripetally directed force. Both these factors encourage the nuclear material to move and decrease the herniation and its effects.

equally as important to the treatment's success as the traction.[2] The sitting posture increases the disk pressure, causing the nucleus to follow the path of least resistance and a return of the disk herniation.

EFFECTS ON ARTICULAR FACET JOINTS

facet joints Articular joints of the spine.

The articular joints of the spine (**facet joints**) can be affected by traction, primarily through increased separation of the joint surfaces. **Meniscoid structures,** synovial fringes, or osteochondral fragments (calcified bone chips) impinged between joint surfaces are released and a dramatic reduction in symptoms is noticed when joint surfaces are separated. Increased joint separation decompresses the articular cartilage, allowing the synovial fluid exchange to nourish the cartilage. The separation may also decrease the rate of degenerative changes from osteoarthritis. Increased proprioceptive discharge from the facet joint structures provides some decrease in pain perception.[2,5,10,22]

meniscoid structures A cartilage tip found on the synovial fringes of some facet joints.

EFFECTS ON THE MUSCULAR SYSTEM

Ligaments may be progressively stretched with traction.

The vertebral muscles can be effectively stretched by traction provided that the positions of the spine during traction are selected to optimize the stretch of particular muscle groups. The initial stretch should come from body positioning, and the addition of traction then provides some additional stretch. **Electromyographic recordings** of the spinal erector muscles during traction showed some decrease in EMG activity in most patients, indicating a muscular relaxation.[11,24] This effect can be enhanced by palpating the erector muscles and focusing the patient's attention on relaxing them. The muscular stretch lengthens tight muscle structures, or creates relaxation of contraction, allowing better muscular blood flow, and also activates

CASE STUDY 13-1
SPINAL TRACTION

Background: A 49-year-old man developed lower cervical pain 4 days ago following a pick-up game of basketball; although the patient runs on a regular basis, playing basketball is not part of his normal exercise regimen. He has been referred for symptomatic treatment of his mechanical neck pain; there are no neural deficits, and no signs of a disk lesion. The patient is experiencing pain in the midline of the lower cervical area, and across the upper trapezius area bilaterally. His active range of motion is normal, but is painful at the end of range in all planes, and overpressure increases the symptoms. Extension (back bending) is the most painful motion.

Impression: Soft-tissue injury of the lower cervical spine.

Treatment Plan: To assist in pain relief, a 3-day-per-week course of intermittent mechanical cervical traction was initiated. The patient was positioned supine on the traction table, and the traction unit was adjusted to produce approximately 20 degrees of cervical flexion during traction. For the initial session, 20 pounds of traction was applied, with four progressive steps up, and four regressive steps down. Each traction cycle consisted of 15 seconds of tension, followed by 20 seconds of rest. Total treatment time was 20 minutes. The target traction force was increased by 10 percent each session, to a maximum of 40 pounds. In addition to the traction, active exercise was prescribed.

Response: The patient reported a transient increase in symptoms following the first two sessions, then a gradual resolution of the symptoms. There was a marked reduction in symptoms immediately following the third session; the relief persisted for approximately 2 hours. Cervical traction was discontinued after a total of six sessions, and the patient was instructed in a home exercise program. Two weeks later, the patient was asymptomatic.

The rehabilitation professional employs therapeutic agent modality to create an optimum environment for tissue healing while minimizing the symptoms associated with the trauma or condition.

Discussion Questions

- What tissues were injured or affected?
- What symptoms were present?
- What phase of the injury-healing continuum did the patient present for care in?
- What are the therapeutic agent modality's biophysical effects (direct, indirect, depth, and tissue affinity)?
- What are the therapeutic agent modality's indications and contraindications?
- What are the parameters of the therapeutic agent modality's application, dosage, duration, and frequency in this case study?
- What other therapeutic agent modalities could be used to treat this injury or condition? Why? How?

---

muscle proprioceptors, providing even more of a gating influence on the pain. All these properties lead to a decrease in muscular irritation.[2,10,11,13,20,23]

EFFECTS ON THE NERVES

The nerve is the structure at which traction's effects are most often directed. Pressure on nerves or roots from bulging disk material, irritated facet joints, bony spurs, or narrowed foramen size causes the neurologic malfunctioning often associated with spinal pain. Tingling is usually the first clinical sign indicating that there is pressure on a nerve structure. If the pressure is not relieved or if damage of the nerve as a result of trauma or anoxia has resulted in an inflammation, the tingling may not respond to traction.[10,12,26,27,32,34]

Unrelieved pressure on a nerve causes slowing and eventual loss of impulse conduction. The signs of motor weakness, numbness, and loss of reflex become progres-

nerve root impingement Abnormal encroachment of some body tissue into the space occupied by the nerve root.

sively more apparent and are indicative of nerve degeneration. Pain, tenderness, and muscular spasm are also associated with continued pressure on the nerve.

Anything that decreases the pressure on the nerve increases the blood's circulation to the nerve, decreasing edema and allowing the nerve to return to normal functioning. Some degenerative changes are reversible, depending on the amount of degeneration and the amount of fibrosis that occur during the repair process.[2,10,32,34]

EFFECTS ON THE ENTIRE BODY PART

The previous discussion outlined the effect of traction on the major systems involved in spine-related pain and dysfunction. The complexity and interrelationships among these systems make determining specific causes of pain and dysfunction very difficult. Traction is not specific to one system but has an effect on each system, and collectively the effect can be very satisfactory. Traction can affect the pathologic process in any of the systems, and then all the structures involved can begin to normalize. Traction should not stand alone as a treatment but should be considered as part of an overall treatment plan, and each component of any spine-related dysfunction should be treated with other appropriate modalities.[1,2,5,8,20,26,27,28,32]

CLINICAL APPLICATION

The discussion of specific traction setups is organized according to lumbar and cervical traction. Each of these areas will contain discussions of postural, manual, and machine-assisted traction. The traction setups mentioned in this chapter should be used as starting points in a treatment plan. The parameters of time, position, and traction force should be adapted to the patient, rather than forcing the patient to adapt to a predetermined traction setup.

The treatment plan should include the clinical criteria for judging the success and continued use of traction. Positive changes should occur within 5 to 8 treatment days if traction is going to be successful; for example, if a patient has a positive straight leg raise sign (i.e., pain in the back with a passive straight leg raise). This is a measurable clinical criterion that can be used to judge the treatment's success. If the straight leg raise test is positive at 20 degrees of hip flexion before and after traction, and after successive treatments the straight leg raise test is positive at increasing degrees of hip flexion, then the treatment can be considered successful.

LUMBAR TRACTION

Traction is most often used to treat nerve root impingement.

Spinal nerve root impingement, from a variety of causes ranging from disk herniation or prolapse to spondylolisthesis, is the leading diagnosis for which traction is prescribed. Traction has also been used to treat joint hypomobility, arthritic conditions of the facet joints, mechanically produced muscle spasm, and joint pain.[2,11,12,26,27,34,36,39]

Lumbar Positional Traction

Normal spinal mechanics allow movements to occur that narrow or enlarge the intervertebral foramina. If the patient is placed in the backlying position with hips and knees flexed, the lumbar spine bends forward and the spinous processes sepa-

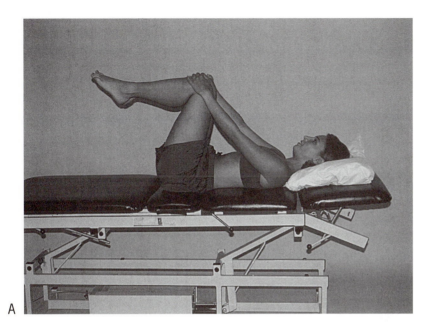

A

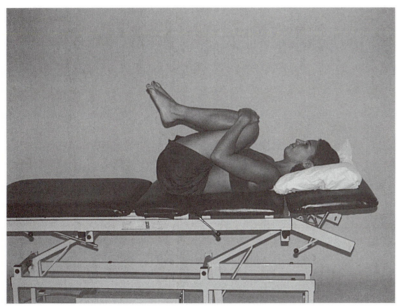

B

•**Figure 13-3** A. Positional traction; B. Knees to chest posture can be used to increase the size of the lumbar intervertebral foramen bilaterally.

rate. This movement increases the size of the **intervertebral foramen** bilaterally (Fig. 13-3). The flexed postures used to treat low-back pain are examples of this positional traction.

The greatest **unilateral foramen opening** occurs by positioning the patient sidelying with a pillow or blanket roll between the iliac crest and the lower border of the rib cage. The side on which increased foramen opening is desired should be superior. The roll should be close to the level of the spine where the traction separation is desired. The spine side bends around the roll (Fig. 13-4). The patient's hips

unilateral foramen opening Enlargement of the foramen on one side of a vertebral segment.

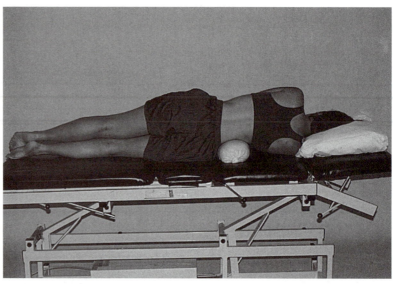

•**Figure 13-4** Positional traction; patient positioned sidelying with a blanket roll between iliac crest and rib cage. This increases the intervertebral foramen size of the left side of the lumbar spine.

and knees are then flexed until the lumbar spine is in a forward-bent position (Fig. 13-5, A). This accentuates the opening of a foramen. Maximal opening can be achieved by adding trunk rotation toward the side of the superior shoulder (Fig. 13-5B).[27,32–34]

Positional traction is normally used when the patient is on a very restricted activity program because of low-back pain. The positions are used on a trial and error basis to determine maximum comfort and to attempt to relieve pressure on nerve roots.

The results of the patient evaluation should be used to determine whether the painful side should be up or down when using the sidelying positional traction technique. Protective scoliosis is the most obvious sign that will help determine patient position. If the patient leans away from the painful side, the painful side should be up (Fig. 13-6A). If the patient leans toward the painful side, the painful side should be down (Fig. 13-6B).

The location of the pressure from the disk herniation was previously believed to cause these signs. Further research suggests that hand dominance may be more of a factor than herniation location in producing this scoliosis. However, the patient may be more compliant with the treatment regime if simple mechanical explanations such as pushing the herniation back into place are used.[29]

Patients with these symptoms may also be good candidates for unilateral traction.[2,5,26,27,31,32] Facet irritation is capable of causing similar scoliotic curves; in most instances the scoliosis is convex toward the painful side.

Inversion Traction

Inversion traction, another positional traction, is used for prevention and treatment of back problems. Specialized equipment or simply hanging upside down from a chinning bar places a person in the inverted position. The spinal column is lengthened because of the stretch provided by the weight of the trunk. The force of the trunk in this position is usually calculated to be approximately 40 percent of body weight (Fig. 13-7).[14]

When the person is comfortable and able to relax, the length of the spinal column increases. These length changes coincides with decreases in spinal muscle activity.[1,2,6,7,16,18,19,24]

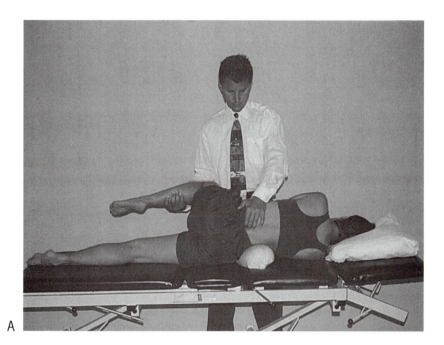

A

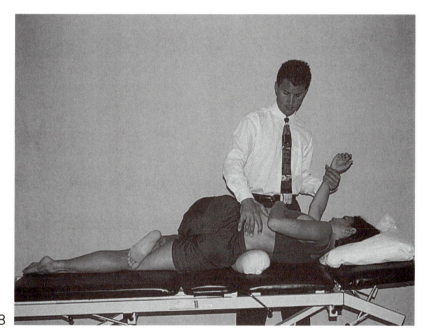

B

•**Figure 13-5** Positional traction; maximum opening of the intervertebral foramen of the left side of the patient's lumbar spine is achieved by flexing the upper hip and knee and rotating the patient's shoulders so he is looking over the left shoulder (left rotation).

No research-supported protocols exist for this method of traction, although a slow progression of time in the inverted position seems to be best. One study suggests the electromyographic activity decreases after 70 seconds in the inverted position. If the patient is comfortable completely inverted, 70 seconds may be used as a minimum treatment time. The inverted position may be repeated two or three times at a treatment session, with a 2- to 3-minute rest between bouts. Longer treatment times also may enhance results. Maximum treatment times range from 10 to 30 minutes. Setup procedures are equipment-dependent and the manufacturer's proto-

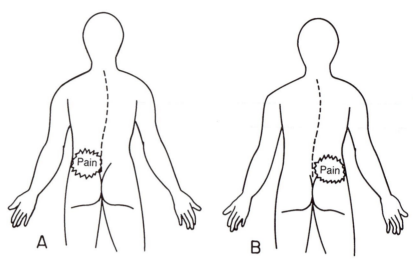

•**Figure 13-6** A. Patient leaning away from the painful side. The patient's left side should be placed up while sidelying over a blanket roll to open up the upper foramen or the nerve roots away from the lateral herniation or both. B. Patient leaning toward the painful side. The patient's left side should be placed up while sidelying over a blanket roll to pull the nerve roots away from a medial herniation.

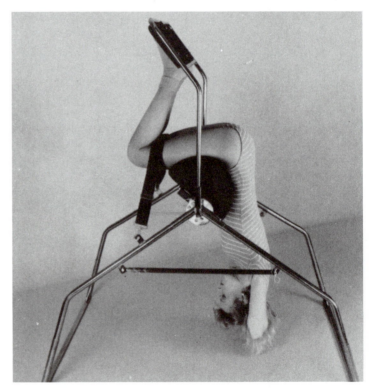

•**Figure 13-7** Inversion traction apparatus.
(courtesy Lossing Orthopaedic, Minneapolis, Minnesota 55404).

cols should be followed and modified as necessary to meet the needs of the patient.[1,2,3,9,24]

Blood pressure should be monitored while the patient is in the inverted position. If a rise of 20 mm of mercury above the resting diastolic pressure is found, the therapist should stop the treatment for that session.[2,3,24]

Contraindications include hypertensive (140/90) individuals and anyone with heart disease or glaucoma. Patients with sinus problems, diabetes, thyroid conditions, asthma, migraine headaches, detached retinas, or hiatal hernias should consult their physicians before treatment is initiated.

Recent surgery or musculoskeletal problems to the lower limb may require modification of the inversion apparatus. In addition, meals or snacks should not be eaten during the hour before treatment to keep the patient comfortable.

One method of testing the patient's tolerance to the inverted position is to have the patient assume the hand-knee position and put his or her head on the floor, holding that position for 60 seconds. Any vertigo, dizziness, or nausea may indicate that this patient is a poor candidate for inversion and that the treatment progression should be very slow (Fig. 13-8).[1–3,6,7,9,16,18,19,24]

Manual Lumbar Traction

Manual lumbar traction is used for lumbar spine problems to test the patient's tolerance to traction, to arrive at the most comfortable treatment setup, to make the traction as specific to one vertebral level as possible, and to provide the specificity needed for a traction mobilization of the spine. If the patient's back pain is diminished by having the therapist flex the patient's hips and knees to 90 degrees each and apply enough pressure under the calves to lift the buttocks off the table, then the patient is a good candidate for spine 90-90 degree traction. The disadvantage is that maintaining the large forces necessary for separation of the lumbar vertebrae for a period of time is difficult and energy-consuming for the therapist.[2,31,32]

Having a split table will eliminate most of the friction between the patient's body segments and the treatment table and is essential for effective delivery of manual lumbar traction (Fig. 13-9).[2,5,21,32,34] The therapist's effort does not cause separation of the vertebral segments unless the frictional forces are overcome first.

Level Specific Manual Traction

To make the traction specific to a vertebral level, the patient is positioned sidelying on the split table. For traction specific to L3-4, L4-5, and L5-S1 levels, the patient's lumbar spine is flexed, using the patient's upper leg as a lever. The therapist palpates

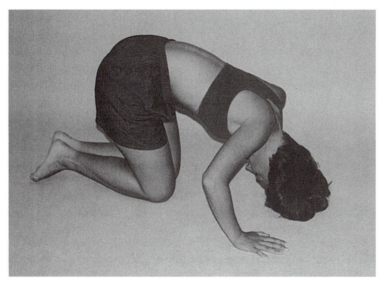

•**Figure 13-8** Inversion tolerance test position. Any vertigo, dizziness, or nausea may indicate that this patient is a poor candidate for inversion treatment.

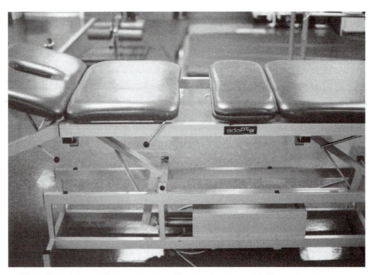

•**Figure 13-9** Split table with movable section to decrease frictional forces.

the interspinous area between two spinous processes. The upper spinous process is the one at which maximum effect is desired. When the lumbar spine flexes and the therapist feels the motion of the lower spinous process with the palpating hand, the foot is placed against the opposite leg so that further flexion is not allowed (see Fig. 13-5A). The patient's trunk is rotated by the therapist until motion of the upper spinous process is felt by the therapist. Trunk rotation should be passively produced by the therapist, positioning the patient's upper arm with hand on the rib cage, and pulling on the patient's lower arm, creating trunk rotation toward the upper arm. In this case it is rotation to the left (see Fig. 13-5B).

If lumbar levels T12, L1, L1-2, and L2-3 are to be given specific traction, the patient is again positioned sidelying. These levels require positioning in reverse order from the lower levels. First the trunk is rotated, then the lumbar spine is flexed.[2,5]

In both instances the rotation and flexion tighten and lock joint structures in which these motions have taken place, leaving the desired segment with more movement available than the upper or lower levels. When traction is applied, greater movement of the desired level occurs, whereas movement at other levels is minimized because of the joint locking created by the preliminary positioning.

The split table is then released and the therapist palpates the spinous processes of the selected intervertebral level, places his or her chest against the anterior superior iliac spine of the patient's upper hip, and leans toward the patient's feet. Enough force is used to cause a palpable separation of the spinous processes (Fig. 13-10). Intermittent movement is most easily accomplished, whereas sustained traction becomes physically more difficult.[2,5]

Unilateral Leg Pull Manual Traction

Unilateral leg pull traction has been used in the treatment of hip joint problems or difficult lateral shift corrections. A thoracic countertraction harness is used to secure the patient to the table. The therapist grabs the patient's ankle and brings the patient's hip into 30-degree flexion, 30-degree abduction, and full external rotation. A steady pull is applied until a noticeable distraction is felt (Fig. 13-11).[5]

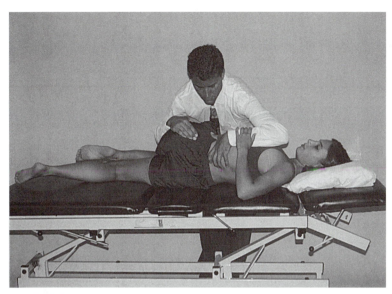

•**Figure 13-10** Manual lumbar traction with maximum effect at a specific level. The therapist has positioned the patient for maximum effect and is palpating the interspinous area between the two spinous processes where maximum traction effect is desired. The therapist then places his or her chest against the anterior superior iliac spine and the patient's upper hip. The split table is released and the therapist leans toward the patient's feet, using enough force to cause a palpable separation of the spinous processes at the desired level.

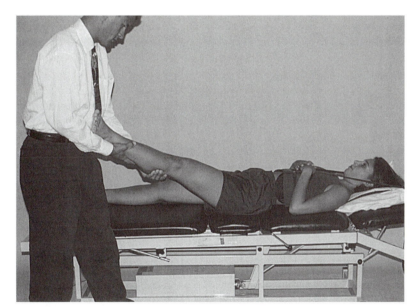

•**Figure 13-11** Unilateral leg pull traction. With the patient secured to the table with a thoracic countertraction harness, the therapist brings the patient's hip into 30-degree flexion, 30-degree abduction, and maximum external rotation. A steady pull is then applied.

In suspected sacroiliac joint problems, a similar setup can be used. A banana strap is placed through the groin on the side to be stretched. This strap will secure the patient in position. The therapist grabs the patient's ankle, brings his or her hip into 30-degree flexion and 15-degree abduction, and then applies a sustained or intermittent pull to create a mobilizing effect on the sacroiliac joint (Fig. 13-12).[5]

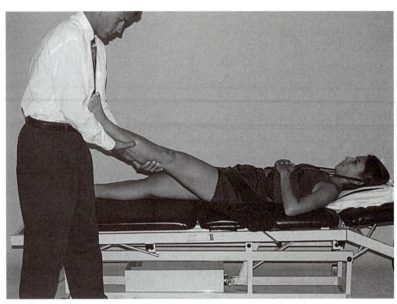

•**Figure 13-12** Unilateral leg pull traction for sacroiliac joint problems. A strap is placed through the groin and secured to the table. The therapist brings the patient's hip into 30-degree flexion and 15-degree abduction, and then applies a traction force to the leg.

As a preliminary to mechanical traction, manual traction is helpful in determining what degree of lumbar flexion, extension, or sidebending is most comfortable and will also give an indication of the treatment's success. The most comfortable position is usually the best therapeutic position.[5,31,33]

Patient comfort may have a bigger impact on the traction's results than the angle of pull, the force used, the mode, or the duration of the treatment. The inability of the patient to relax in any traction setup affects the traction's ability to cause a separation of the vertebrae. The lack of vertebral separation minimizes some of the traction's therapeutic benefits.[5,31,33]

Mechanical Lumbar Traction

Traction will return disk nucleus to a central position.

When using mechanical traction, the therapist will have to select and adjust the following parameters of the traction equipment and patient position.

1. Body position: prone, supine, hip position, bilateral, or unilateral direction of pull
2. Force used
3. Intermittent traction: traction time and rest time
4. Sustained traction
5. Duration of treatment
6. Progressive steps
7. Regressive steps

Traction can relieve pressure on a nerve root.

The research on mechanical lumbar traction gives us a strong protocol for using traction to decrease disk protrusion and nerve root symptoms. The protocols for use in other pathologies are not supported by research, but clinical empiricism and inference from some of the research give a good working protocol. The therapist will need to match the traction treatment to the patient's symptoms and make adjustments based on the clinical results.[5,12,25,31]

Patient Setup and Equipment

A split table or other mechanism to eliminate friction between body segments and the table surface is a prerequisite to effective lumbar traction. Otherwise, most of the force applied would be spent overcoming the coefficient of friction (see Fig. 13-9).[1,2,5,15,21,32,34]

A nonslip traction harness is needed to transfer the traction force comfortably to the patient and to stabilize the trunk while the lumbar spine is placed under traction. A harness lined with a vinyl material is best because it adheres to the patient's skin and does not slip like the cotton-lined harness. Clothing between the harness and the skin will also promote slipping. The vinyl-sided harness does not have to be as constricting as the cotton-backed harness to prevent slippage, thus increasing the patient's comfort (Fig. 13-13).[5,32,34]

The harness can be applied when the patient is standing next to the traction table prior to treatment. The pelvic harness is applied so the contact pads and upper belt are at or just above the level of the iliac crest (Fig. 13-14).

Shirts should never be tucked under the pelvic harness because some of the tractive force would be dissipated pulling on the shirt material. The contact pads should be adjusted so that the harness loops provide a posteriorly directed pull, encouraging lumbar flexion (Fig. 13-15). The harness firmly adheres to the patient's hips.[5,32,34]

The rib belt is then applied in a similar manner with the rib pads positioned over the lower rib cage in a comfortable manner. The rib belt is then snugged up and the patient is positioned on the table (Fig. 13-16).[5,32,34]

The standing application of the traction harness is easier and more effective if the patient is to be placed in prone position for treatment (Fig. 13-17).[5,33,34] The traction harness can also be applied by laying it out on the traction table and having the patient lie down on top of it. The pads are then adjusted and the belts snugged with the patient lying down.

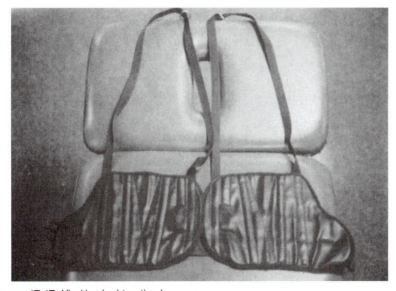

•**Figure 13-13** Vinyl-backed traction harness.

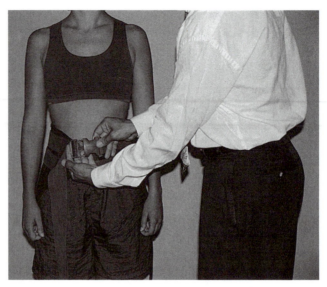

•**Figure 13-14** Pelvic harness for mechanical lumbar traction. The contact pads are applied so that the upper belt is at or just above the level of the iliac crest.

Body Position

Body position has been reported to have a substantial impact on traction results, but this has been empirically derived rather than research supported. The therapist needs a satisfactory understanding of the mechanics of the lumbar spine to make decisions about position that will best affect a patient's symptoms.[2,5,22,27,32,34]

Generally, the neutral spinal position allows for the largest intervertebral foramen opening, and it is usually the position of choice whether the patient is prone or supine. Extension beyond neutral lumbar spine causes the bony elements of the

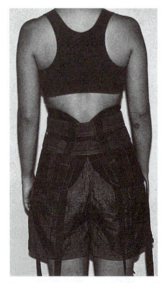

•**Figure 13-15** The traction straps from the pelvic harness should bracket the patient's buttocks if a lumbar flexion pull is desired. If a straight pull is desired, the pelvic harness should be adjusted so that the straps bracket the patient's lateral hip area.

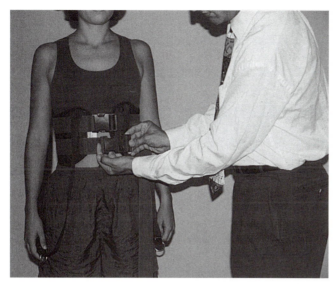

•**Figure 13-16** Thoracic countertraction harness. Rib pads are positioned over the lower rib cage.

foramen to create a narrower opening. Lumbar spinal flexion beyond neutral causes the ligamentum flavum and other soft tissues to constrict the foramen's opening (Fig. 13-18).[31,33]

Saunders recommends the prone position with a normal to slightly flattened lumbar lordosis (an abnormal anterior curve) as the position of choice in disk pro-

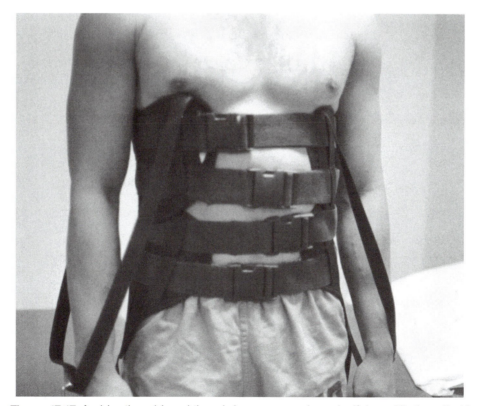

•**Figure 13-17** Applying the pelvic and thoracic harnesses may be easier if done while the patient is standing.

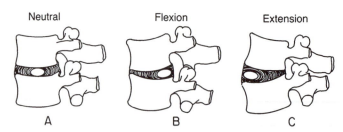

•**Figure 13-18** A. Neutral lumbar spine position allows for the largest intervertebral foramen opening before traction is applied. B. Flexion puts pressure on the disk nucleus to move posterior, although it may tend to increase the posterior opening. Other soft tissue may also close the foramen opening. C. Extension beyond neutral tends to close the foramen down as the bony arches come closer together.

trusions.[32,34] The amount of lordosis may be controlled by using pillows under the abdomen. The prone position also allows the easy application of other modalities to the pain area and an easier assessment of the amount of spinous process separation (Fig. 13-19).[5,32,34]

In traction applied to a patient in the supine position, hip position was found to affect vertebral separation. As hip flexion increased from 0 to 90 degrees, traction produced a greater posterior intervertebral space separation (Fig. 13-20).[30]

Unilateral pelvic traction also has been recommended when a stronger force is desired on one side of the spine. Patients with protective scoliosis, unilateral joint dysfunction, or unilateral lumbar muscle spasm with scoliosis may do quite well with this approach. Only one side of the pelvic harness is hooked to the traction device to accomplish this technique (Fig. 13-21).[32]

In patients with protective scoliosis, when the patient leans away from the painful side, the traction should be applied on the painful side. When the patient leans toward the painful side, the traction should be applied on the nonpainful side (see Fig. 13-6).

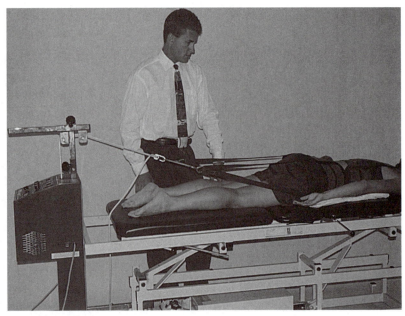

•**Figure 13-19** Mechanical lumbar traction; patient in the prone position with a pillow under the abdomen to help control lumbar spine extension.

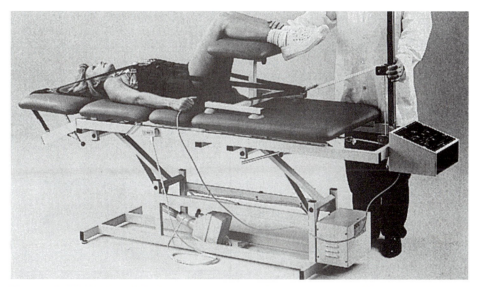

•**Figure 13-20** Mechanical lumbar traction; patient in the supine position with hips flexed to approximately 90 degrees.

In patients with scoliosis caused by muscle spasm, the traction force should be applied from the side with the muscle spasm (Fig . 13-22). In unilateral facet joint dysfunction, the traction should be applied from the side of most complaint.[33]

Overall, patient positioning for traction should be varied according to a patient's needs and comfort. Experimentation with positioning is encouraged so that the traction's effect on the patient will be maximized. Patient comfort is far more important than relative position in making patient position decisions. If the patient cannot relax, the traction will not be successful in causing vertebral separation.[5,32,34]

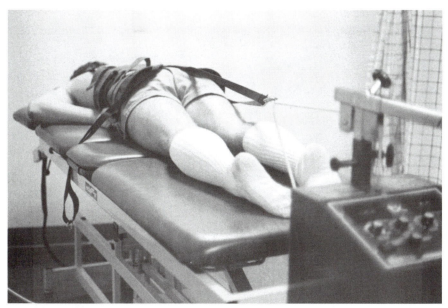

•**Figure 13-21** Mechanical lumbar traction with a unilateral pull; only one of the pelvic straps is hooked to the traction device.

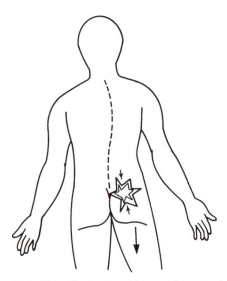

•**Figure 13-22** In a patient with scoliosis caused by muscle spasm (right), the unilateral traction force should be applied using only the right pelvic strap.

Traction Force

Several researchers have indicated that no lumbar vertebral separation will occur with traction forces less than one-quarter of the patient's body weight. The traction force necessary to cause effective vertebral separation will range between 65 and 200 pounds.[1,2,21,22,32,34] This force does not have to be used on the first treatment, and progressive steps both during and between treatments are often necessary to comfortably reach these therapeutic loads. A force equal to half the patient's body weight is a good guideline to use in selecting a force high enough to cause vertebral separation. These high-weight levels pose no danger, as cadaver research indicates a force of 440 pounds or greater is necessary to cause damage to the lumbar spine components (Fig. 13-23).[21,22]

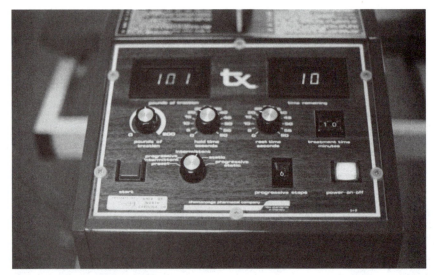

•**Figure 13-23** Traction device set for traction with 100 pounds of static traction for 10 minutes with six progressive steps.

Caution must be used when using traction of the lumbar spine, because there is a tendency for the nucleus pulposus gel to imbibe fluid from the vertebral body, thus increasing pressure within the disk. This happens in a very short period of time. When pressure is released and weight is applied to the disk, this excess fluid increases pressure on the annulus and exacerbates the patient's symptoms. Therefore, it is recommended that during an initial treatment with lumbar traction a maximum of 30 pounds be used to determine whether traction will have a negative effect on the symptoms.[10]

The research has been aimed at forces necessary to cause vertebral separation. Traction certainly has effects that are not associated with vertebral separation, and if these effects are desired, less force may be necessary to get them.

Intermittent versus Sustained Traction

Good results have been reported with both intermittent and sustained traction. In most cases of lumbar disk problems, sustained traction seems to be the treatment of choice. Partial reduction in disk protrusions was observed in 4 minutes of sustained traction.[21,22,26,32,34] Good results also were reported using intermittent traction in the treatment of ruptured intervertebral disk.[11]

Separation of the posterior intervertebral space was noted with a 10-second-hold intermittent traction.[30] Posterior intervertebral separations using 100 pounds of force were similar when intermittent and sustained traction modes were compared.[22] The electromyographic activity of the sacrospinalis musculature showed similar patterns when sustained and intermittent traction were compared.[11]

Traction can stretch paraspinal muscles.

Sustained traction is favored in treating intervertebral disk herniation because sustained traction allows more time with the disk uncompressed to cause the disk nuclear material to move centripetally and reduce the disk herniation's pressure on nerve structures. When used for this purpose, sustained traction may be superior to intermittent traction.[5,32,34]

In deciding on sustained versus intermittent traction, the therapist should follow the guidelines for treating diagnosed disk herniations with sustained traction, whereas most other traction-appropriate diagnoses may be treated with intermittent traction. Intermittent traction, in any case, is usually more comfortable when using higher forces, and increased comfort is one of the primary considerations because there is no conclusive evidence supporting the choice of one method over the other.[1,2,5,12,22,30,32,34]

The timing of the traction and rest phases of intermittent traction has not been researched. Short traction phases (less than 10 seconds) cause only minimal interspace separation but will activate joint and muscle receptors and create facet joint movements.[5,8] Longer traction phases (more than 10 seconds) tend to stretch the ligamentous and muscular tissues long enough to overcome their resistance to movement and create a longer-lasting mechanical separation. When using high traction forces, the comfort of the patient may dictate the adjustment of the traction time. Also, a longer total treatment time is tolerated with intermittent traction.[5,8,10,22,32]

Rest phase times should be relatively short but should also be comfort-oriented. The rest time should be adjusted to allow the patient to recover and feel relaxed before the next traction cycle. The therapist should monitor the traction patient frequently to adjust traction and rest time adjustments to maintain the patient in a relaxed comfortable state.

Duration of Treatment

The total treatment times of sustained traction and intermittent traction are only partially research-based. With sustained traction, Mathews found reduction in disk protrusion after 4 minutes with further reduction at 20 minutes.[21] Complete reduction in protrusions was seen at 38 minutes. Other researchers found no difference in separation of the cervical spine when times of 7, 30, and 60 seconds were compared.[8,21,22]

When dealing with suspected disk protrusions, the total treatment time should be relatively short. As the disk space widens, the pressure inside the disk decreases and the disk nucleus moves centripetally. The projected time for pressure within a disk to equalize is 8 to 10 minutes. At this point the nuclear material is no longer moving centripetally. With longer time in this position, osmotic forces equalizes the pressure within the disk with that of the surrounding tissue. When the pressure equalization occurs, the traction effect on the protrusion is lost. The intradisk pressure may increase when the traction is released if the traction stays on too long. This increased pressure results in increased symptoms. This situation has not been reported when treatment times are kept at 10 minutes or less.[32,34] If this reaction does occur, shorter treatment times or long-hold intermittent traction (60 seconds' traction, 10 to 20 seconds' rest) may be necessary to control the symptoms.

Some sources advocate traction times of up to 30 minutes.[5,21,22] The contradiction in philosophy may be because of pathology or the individual anatomy of each patient. However, an adverse reaction to traction (i.e., a dramatic increase in symptoms when the traction is released) is something the therapist should try to avoid.

Total treatment time for sustained traction when treating disk-related symptoms should start at less than 10 minutes. If the treatment is successful in reducing symptoms, the time should be left at 10 minutes or less. If the treatment is partially successful or unsuccessful in relieving symptoms, the therapist may increase the time gradually over several treatments to 30 minutes.

Progressive and Regressive Steps

Some traction equipment is built with progressive and regressive modes. The machine progressively increases the traction force in a preselected number of steps. A gradual increase in pressure lets the patients accommodate slowly to the traction and helps him or her to stay relaxed. A gradual progression of force also allows the therapist to release the split table after the slack in the system has been taken up by several progressions (Fig. 13-24).[2,5,28]

Regressive steps do just the opposite and allow the patient to come down gradually from the high loads. Again, patient comfort is the primary consideration because no research supports any protocol (Fig. 13-25).[2,5,28]

Some equipment has the capability to be programmed for progressive and regressive steps and also to have minimum traction forces, allowing a sustained force with intermittent peaks (Fig. 13-26).[2,5,28] To achieve such traction setups with a machine that is not programmable, manual operation and timing are necessary.

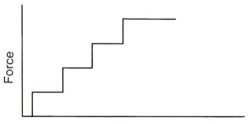

•**Figure 13-24** Progressive steps for lumbar traction of X pounds. Four steps are used: the first is X pounds, the second $\frac{2}{4}$ X, and so on. Each lasts for an equal time.

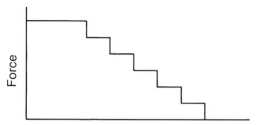

•**Figure 13-25** Regressive steps for lumbar traction of X pounds. Six equal regressive steps are used: the first drops the traction force from X to $\frac{5}{6}$ X, the second to $\frac{4}{6}$ X, and so on. Each lasts for an equal time.

Throughout the discussion on lumbar traction, patient comfort comes up again and again in regard to the parameters of the treatment setup. One of the primary keys to successful traction treatment is the relaxation of the patient. The use of appropriate modalities before and during the traction treatment adds to the total effectiveness of the treatment plan. Bracing or appropriate exercise after traction may also enhance the results and prolong the benefits gained. Better technology and more research will help refine the traction art and provide better results from this type of treatment.

CERVICAL TRACTION

The objectives for using traction in the cervical region do not vary much from the objectives for using traction in the lumbar region. Reasonable objectives for cervical traction include stretch of the muscles and joint structures of the vertebral column, enlargement of the intervertebral spaces and foramina, centripetally directed forces on the disk and soft tissue around the disk, mobilization of vertebral joints, increases and changes in joint proprioception, relief of compressive effects of normal posture, and improvement in arterial venous and lymphatic flow.[5,10,22,31,36-38] In the clinical setting, diagnoses and symptoms requiring traction are found infrequently.[26] These diagnoses are usually found in older populations. The literature provides a relatively clear protocol to use in trying to achieve vertebral separation using a mechanical traction apparatus.

The patient should be supine or long-sitting with the neck flexed between 20 and 30 degrees (Fig. 13-27). A sitting posture can be used; however, this is clinically more cumbersome and is not supported by the research as an optimal position of cervical traction.[35]

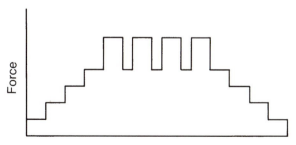

•**Figure 13-26** Progressive and regressive steps with a minimum sustained traction force.

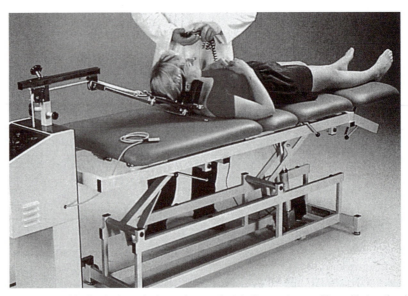

•**Figure 13-27** Mechanical cervical traction; patient in the supine position with traction harness placed so that maximum pull is exerted on the occiput and the patient is in a position of approximately 20 to 30 degrees of neck flexion.

A traction force above 20 pounds, applied intermittently for a minimum of 7 seconds' traction time and with adequate rest time for recovery is recommended. This traction should be continued over 20 to 25 minutes. Higher forces up to 50 pounds may produce increased separation, but the other parameters should remain the same. The average separation at the posterior vertebral area is 1 to 1.5 mm per space while the anterior vertebral area separates approximately 0.4 mm per space. Greater separations are expected in the younger than in the older population. Within 20 to 25 minutes from the time traction is stopped and normal sitting or standing postures are resumed, the vertebral separation returns to its previous heights. The upper cervical segments do not separate as easily as lower cervical segments.[8,10,22] This traction force can be applied either manually or mechanically.

Mechanical Traction Protocol

The traction harness must be arranged comfortably so that the majority of pull is placed on the occiput rather than the chin (see Fig. 13-27). Some cervical traction harnesses do not have a chin-piece. These harnesses may have an advantage, provided that the traction force is effectively transferred to the structures of the cervical spine.[8,10]

For diagnoses or symptoms that require stretching the posterior neck and ligamentous structures, the following parameters should be used (Fig. 13-28).

1. The neck-trunk angle should be positioned at less than 30 degrees. Various rotations and sidebendings also can be used.
2. Force should be 20 pounds or more applied intermittently with a 20-second traction time.
3. Treatment duration should be 10 minutes or longer.
4. The addition of pain reducing and heating modalities will add to the benefits gained by the traction.[1,2,5,10,22]

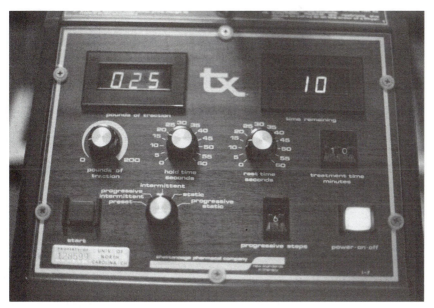

•Figure 13-28 Control panel of traction machine with parameters adjusted for intermittent cervical traction.

Manual Cervical Traction

In most cases involving sprains and strains, simple manual traction used to produce a rhythmic longitudinal movement is very successful in helping decrease pain, muscle spasm, stiffness, and inflammation and also in reducing joint compressive forces. Manual traction is infinitely more adaptable than mechanical traction, and changes in the direction, force, duration of the traction, and patient position can be made instantaneously as the therapist senses relaxation or resistance.[1,2,5,8,22]

The patient's head and neck are supported by the therapist. The hand should cradle the neck and provide adequate grip for the effective transfer of the traction force to the mastoid processes. One hand should be placed under the patient's neck with the thenar eminence (base of the thumb) in contact with one mastoid process and the fingers cradling the neck reaching across toward the other mastoid process (Fig. 13-29A).[2]

The therapist then provides a gentle (< 20 lbs) pull in a cephalic direction. Intervertebral separation is not desired because of the damage to the ligaments or capsule. A head halter or similar harness may be used to deliver the force also (Fig. 13-29B).

The force should be intermittent, with the traction time between 3 and 10 seconds. The rest time may be very brief, but the tractive force should be released almost completely. The total treatment time should be between 3 and 10 minutes.[1,2,5,8]

When pain limits or affects movement, a bout of traction should be followed by a reassessment of the painful motion to determine increases or decreases in pain or motion. Successive bouts of traction can be used as long as the symptoms are improving. When the symptoms stabilize or are worse on the reassessment, the traction should be discontinued.[5]

A variety of patient head and neck positions can be used in cervical traction. Different head and neck positions place some vertebral structures under more tension than others. Satisfactory knowledge of cervical kinesiology and biomechanics

Treatment Tip
Manual traction is considerably more adaptable than mechanical traction, and changes in the direction, force, duration of the traction, and patient position can be made instantaneously as the therapist senses relaxation or resistance on the part of the patient.

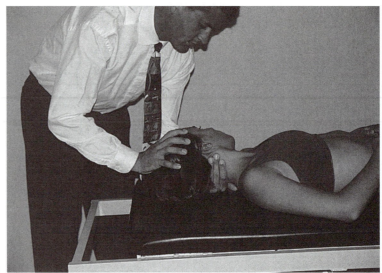

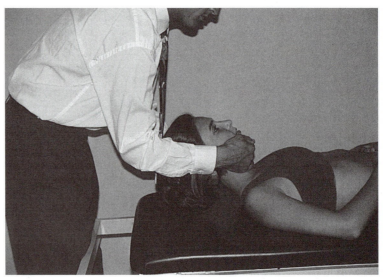

•**Figure 13-29** A. Manual cervical traction; B. patient in the supine position with the therapists's fingertips and thenar eminence contacting the mastoid process of the patient's skull.

and skill in joint mobilization are required before the therapist should experiment with extensive position changes (Fig. 13-30).[2,5,8]

Protection of the neck with a soft collar is often desirable at the completion of the traction treatment, to prevent extremes of motion, minimize compressive forces, and encourage muscle relaxation in cases of strain or sprain. Instructions for sleeping positions and regular support postures are also important in caring for patients with cervical problems.[2,5]

Wall-Mounted Traction

A mechanical traction device can be very costly and is beyond the budgetary limitations of many institutions. Thus, knowledge of techniques of manual traction are necessary. A third option is a wall-mounted traction device that can provide cervical traction. These units are relatively inexpensive and can be effective if used appropri-

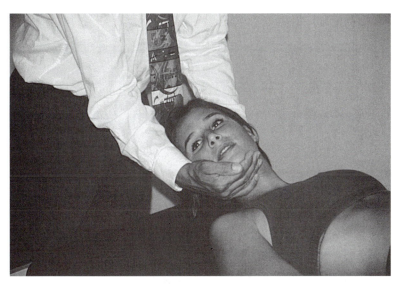

•**Figure 13-30** Manual cervical traction. The patient is positioned with neck in flexion and with some neck rotation to the right. Laterally flexed positions also may be used.

ately. Weight application can be accomplished using weight plates, sand bags, or water bags. The patient should be placed in a comfortable position (sitting, prone) with 10 to 20 pounds of traction applied for 20 to 25 minutes. Static traction is most easily employed, although intermittent traction may also be used, if desired, by simply lifting the weight and releasing tension periodically (Fig. 13-31).

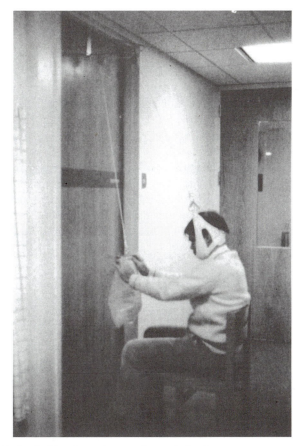

•**Figure 13-31** Cervical traction using a wall-mounted unit.

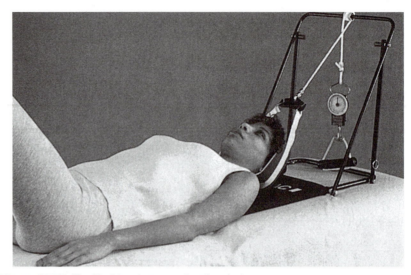

•Figure 13-32 The Necktrac home-use traction device.
(courtesy Lossing Orthopedic, Minneapolis, Minnesota 55418).

The Necktrac is another example of a fairly inexpensive home-use traction device (Fig. 13-32).

Indications and Contraindications for Spinal Traction

Indications
    Impingement on a nerve root
    Disk herniation
    Spondylolisthesis
    Narrowing within the intervertebral fora-
    men
    Osteophyte formation
    Degenerative joint diseases
    Subacute pain
    Joint hypomobility
    Discogenic pain
    Muscle spasm or guarding
    Muscle strain
    Spinal ligament or connective tissues
    contractures
    Improvement in arterial, venous, and lym-
    phatic flow

Contraindications
    Acute sprains or strains
    Acute inflammation
    Fractures
    Vertebral joint instability
    Any condition in which movement exacer-
    bates the existing problem
    Tumors
    Bone diseases
    Osteoporosis
    Infections in bones or joints
    Vascular conditions
    Pregnancy
    Cardiac or pulmonary problems

INDICATIONS AND CONTRAINDICATIONS

As discussed throughout this chapter, there are a number of conditions for which spinal traction may be useful, including cases where there is impingement on a nerve root resulting from disk herniation, spondylolisthesis, narrowing within the intervertebral foramen, or osteophyte formation; degenerative joint diseases, subacute pain; joint hypomobility; discogenic pain; and muscle spasm.

Traction, except as a light mobilization, is contraindicated in acute sprains or strains (first 3–5 days), acute inflammation, or in any conditions in which movement is either undesirable or exacerbates the existing problem. In cases of vertebral joint instability, traction may perpetuate the instability or cause further strain. Certainly, the serious problems associated with tumors, bone diseases, osteoporosis, and infections in bones or joints are also contraindications. Patients who can potentially experience problems relating to the fitting of a harness, such as those with vascular conditions, pregnant females, or those with cardiac or pulmonary problems, should also avoid traction.

SUMMARY

1. Traction has been used to treat a variety of cervical and lumbar spine problems. The effect of traction on each system involved in the complex anatomic make-up of the spine needs to be considered when selecting traction as a part of a therapeutic treatment plan.

2. The traction protocol should be set up to manage a particular problem rather than applied in the same manner regardless of the patient or pathology. Trac-

tion is a flexible modality with an infinite number of variations available. This flexibility allows the therapist to adjust protocols to match the patient's symptoms and diagnosis.

3. Traction is capable of producing a separation of vertebral bodies; a centripetal force on the soft tissues surrounding the vertebrae; a mobilization of vertebral joints; a change in proprioceptive discharge of the spinal complex; a stretch of connective tissue; a stretch of muscle tissue; an improvement in arterial, venous, and lymphatic flow; and a lessening of the compressive effects of posture. Any of these effects can change the symptoms of the patient under treatment and help to normalize the patient's lumbar or cervical spine.

REFERENCES

1. Bridger, R.: Effect of lumbar traction on stature, Spine 15:522–524, 1990.

2. Burkhardt, S.: Course notes, cervical and lumbar traction seminar, Morgantown, West Virginia, 1983.

3. Cooperman, J., Scheid, D.: Guidelines for the use of inversion, Clin. Manage. 4(1):6, 1984.

4. Dorland's illustrated medical dictionary, ed. 24, Philadelphia, 1965, W.B. Saunders.

5. Erhard, R.: Course notes, cervical and lumbar traction seminar, Morgantown, West Virginia, 1983.

6. Gianakopoulos, G.: Inversion devices: their role in producing lumbar distraction, Arch. Phys. Med. Rehabil. 68:100–102, 1985.

7. Goldman, R.: The effects of oscillating inversion on systemic blood pressure pulse, intraocular pressure and central retinal arterial pressure, Phys. Sports Med. 13(3):93–96, 1985.

8. Grieve, G.: Neck traction, Physiotherapy 6:260–265, 1982.

9. Gudenhoven, R.: Gravitational lumbar traction, Arch. Phys. Med. Rehabil. 59:510–512, 1978.

10. Harris, P.: Cervical traction: review of the literature and treatment guidelines, Phys. Ther. 57:910–914, 1977.

11. Hood, C.: Comparison of EMG activity in normal lumbar sacrospinalis musculature during continuous and intermittent pelvic traction, JOSPT 2:137–141, 1981.

12. Hood, L., Chrisman, D.: Intermittent pelvic traction in the treatment of the ruptured intervertebral disk, Phys. Ther. 48:21–30, 1968.

13. Jett, D.: Effect of intermittent, supine cervical traction on the myoelectric activity of the upper trapezius muscle in subjects with neck pain, Phys. Ther. 65:1173–1176, 1985.

14. Klatz, R.: Effects of gravity inversion on hypertensive subjects, Phys. Sports Med. 13(3):85–89, 1985.

15. KeKosz, U.: Cervical and lumbopelvic traction, Post Grad. Med. 80(8):187–94, 1986.

16. Kent, B.: Anatomy of the trunk, Part I, Phys. Ther. 54:722–744, 1974.

17. Kent, B.: Anatomy of the trunk, Part II, Phys. Ther. 54:850–859, 1974.

18. LaBan, M.: Intermittent traction: a progenitor of lumbar radicular pain, Arch. Phys. Med. Rehabil. 73:295–296, 1992.

19. LeMarr, J.: Cardiorespiratory responses to inversion, Phys. Sports Med. 11(11):51–57, 1983.

20. Letchuman, R., Deusinger, R.: Comparison of sacrospinalis myoelectric activity and pain levels in patients undergoing static and intermittent lumbar traction, Spine 18:1261–1365, 1993.

21. Mathews, J.: Dynamic discography: a study of lumbar traction, Ann. Phys. Med. 9:275–279, 1968.

22. Mathews, J.: The effects of spinal traction, Physiotherapy 58:64–66, 1972.

23. Murphy, M.: Effects of cervical traction on muscle activity, JOSPT 13:220–225, 1991.

24. Nosse, L.: Inverted spinal traction, Arch. Phys. Med. Rehabil. 59:367–370, 1978.

25. O'Donoghue, D.: Treatment of injuries to patients, ed. 3, Philadelphia, 1978, W.B. Saunders.

26. Onel, D.: Computed tomographic investigation of the effects of traction on lumbar disc herniations, Spine 14:82–90, 1989.

27. Paris, S.: Course notes, Basic course in spinal mobilization, Atlanta, Georgia, 1977.

28. Petulla, L.: Clinical observations with respect to progressive/regressive traction, JOSPT 7:261–263, 1986.

29. Porter, R., Miller, C.: Back pain and trunk list, Spine 11:596–600, 1986.

30. Reilly, J.: Pelvic femoral position on vertebral separation produced by lumbar traction, Phys. Ther. 59:282–286, 1979.

31. Roaf, R.: A study of the mechanics of spinal injuries, J. Bone Joint Surg. 42B:810–819, 1960.

32. Saunders, D.: Lumbar traction, JOSPT 1:36–45, 1979.

33. Saunders, D.: Unilateral lumbar traction, Phys. Ther. 61:221–225, 1981.

34. Saunders, D.: Use of spinal traction in the treatment of neck and back conditions, Clin. Orthop. 179:31–38, 1983.

35. Stoddard, A: Traction for cervical nerve root irritation, Physiotherapy 40:48–49, 1954.

36. Sood, N.: Prone cervical traction, Clin. Manage. Phys. Ther. 7(6):37, 1987.

37. Varma, S.: The role of traction in cervical spondylosis, Physiotherapy 59:248–249, 1973.

38. Walker, G.: Goodley polyaxial cervical traction: a new approach to a traditional treatment, Phys. Ther. 66:1255–12259, 1986.

39. Weinert, A., Rizzo, T.: Non-operative management of multi-level lumbar disk herniations in an adolescent patient, Mayo Clin. Proc. 67:137–141, 1992.

Suggested Readings

Alice, M., Wong, M., and Chaupeng, I.: The traction angle and cervical intervertebral separation, Spine 17(2):136, 1992.

Beurskens, A., de Vet, H., and Koke, A.: Efficacy of traction for non-specific low back pain: a randomised clinical trial, Lancet 346(8990):1596–1600, 1995.

Beurskens, A., van der Heijden, G., and de Vet, H.: The efficacy of traction for lumbar back pain: design of a randomized clinical trial, J. Man. Physiol. Ther. 18(3):141–147, 1995.

Creighton, D.: Positional distraction, a radiological confirmation, J. Manual Man. Ther. 1(3):83–86, 1993.

Gilworth, G.: Cervical traction with active rotation: Physiotherapy 77(11):782–784, 1991.

Hariman, D.: The efficacy of cervical extension-compression traction combined with diversified manipulation and drop table adjustments in the rehabilitation of cervical lordosis: a pilot study, J. Man. Physiol. Ther. 18(5):323–325, 1995.

Harrison, D., Jackson, B., and Troyanovich, S.: The efficacy of cervical extension-compression traction combined with diversified manipulation and drop table adjustments in the rehabilitation of cervical lordosis: a pilot study, J. Man. Physiol. Ther. 1995.

Letchuman, R., Deusinger, R.: Comparison of sacrospinalis myoelectric activity and pain levels in patients undergoing static and intermittent lumbar traction, Spine 18(10):1361–1365, 1993.

Ljunggren, A., Walker, L., and Weber, H.: Manual traction vs. isometric exercise in patients with herniated intervertebral lumbar disks, Physiother. Theory Pract. 8:207, 1992.

Nanno, M.: Effects of intermittent cervical traction on muscle pain. Flowmetric and electromyographic studies of the cervical paraspinal muscles, J. Nippon Med. School 61(2):137–147, 1994.

Pal, B., Magnion, P., and Hossian, M.: A controlled trial of continuous lumbar traction in the treatment of back pain and sciatica, Br. J. Rheumatol. 25:181, 1989.

Pellecchia, G.: Lumbar traction: a review of the literature, [review] JOSPT 20(5):262–267, 1994.

Pio, A., Rendina, M., and Benazzo, F.: The statics of cervical traction, J. Spinal Disord. 7(4):337–342, 1994.

Terahata, N., Ishihara, H., and Ohshima, H.: Effects of axial traction stress on solute transport and proteoglycan synthesis in the porcine intervertebral disc in vitro, Eur. Spine J. 3(6):325–330, 1994.

Tesio, L., Merlo, A.: Autotraction versus passive traction: an open controlled study in lumbar disc herniation, Arch. Phys. Med. Rehabil. 74(8):871–876, 1993.

Trudel, G.: Autotraction, Arch. Phys. Med. Rehabil. 75(2):234–235, 1994.

van der Heijden, G., Beurskens, A., and Koes, B.: The efficacy of traction for back and neck pain: a systematic, blinded review of randomized clinical trial methods, Phys. Ther. 75(2):93–104, 1995.

Wong, A., Leong, C., and Chen, C.: The traction angle and cervical intervertebral separation, Spine 17(2):136–138, 1992.

Glossary

annulus fibrosus The interlacing cross-fibers of fibroelastic tissue that are attached to adjacent vertebral bodies that contain the nucleus pulposus.

anoxia Reduction of oxygen in body tissues below physiologic levels.

disk herniation The protrusion of the nucleus pulposus through a defect in the annulus fibrosus.

disk material Cartilaginous material from vertebral body surfaces, disk nucleus, or annulus fibrosus.

disk nucleus The protein polysaccharide gel that is contained between the cartilaginous endplates of the vertebrae and the annulus fibrosus.

disk protrusion The abnormal projection of the disk nucleus through some or all of the annular rings.

facet joints Articular joints of the spine.

fibrosis The formation of fibrous tissue in the injury repair process.

ligament deformation Lengthening distortion of ligament caused by traction loading.

meniscoid structures A cartilage tip found on the synovial fringes of some facet joints.

nerve root impingement Abnormal encroachment of some body tissue into the space occupied by the nerve root.

proprioceptive nervous system System of nerves that provides information on joint movement, pressure, and muscle tension.

spondylolisthesis Forward displacement of one vertebra over another.

synovial fringes Folds of synovial tissue that move in and out of the joint space.

traction Drawing tension applied to a body segment.

unilateral foramen opening Enlargement of the foramen on one side of a vertebral segment.

viscoelastic properties The property of a material to show sensitivity to rate of loading.

Wolff's law Bone remodels itself and provides increased strength along the lines of the mechanical forces placed on it.

LAB ACTIVITY

MECHANICAL TRACTION

DESCRIPTION:

Mechanical traction has been used since ancient times in the treatment of painful spinal conditions. Simply, traction is applying tension to a body segment though a rope attached to various straps, halters, or devices. The therapeutic effect of traction is a function of the position of the spine, amount of traction force, and length of time the force is applied. Mechanical traction results in longitudinal separation of cervical or lumbar spinal segments with associated ligament, discal, neural, and muscular structures.

THERAPEUTIC EFFECTS:

Separation of spinal segments
Elongation of muscle, ligament, and capsular tissue
Reduced intradiscal pressure

INDICATIONS:

Mechanical traction is indicated to reduce the signs and symptoms of spinal compression. Appropriately applied mechanical traction can stretch facet joint capsules, increase the dimension of the intervertebral foramen thus increasing space for nerve roots, and alter intradiscal pressure. Paraspinal muscle tissues can also be elongated contributing to a reduction in the pain-spasm cycle, which frequently accompanies spinal dysfunction.

CONTRAINDICATIONS:

- Spinal infection or malignancy
- Rheumatoid arthritis
- Osteoporosis
- Spinal hypermobility
- Acute stage injury
- Cardiac or respiratory insufficiency
- Pregnancy

MECHANICAL TRACTION			
PROCEDURE	Evaluation		
	1	2	3
1. Check supplies and equipment.			
a. Assemble towels, halters, harnesses, and belts.			
2. Question patient.			
a. Verify identity of patient.			
b. Verify the absence of contraindications.			
c. Ask about previous traction treatments and review treatment record.			
3. Apply and adjust appropriate halters, harnesses and belts for indicated traction treatment.			
a. Cervical: Apply head halter beneath the occiput and mandible, attach to spreader bar.			

PROCEDURE	Evaluation		
	1	2	3
b. Lumbar: Attach pelvic harness snugly about the waist, beginning just above the iliac crests, thoracic rib belt snugly about the lower rib cage.			
c. Attach traction apparatus to unit: Take up and adjust for slack in the line.			
4. Position patient for indicated traction treatment.			
a. Cervical: supine lying with neck flexed 20 to 30 degrees.			
b. Lumbar: supine hooklying with hips flexed and legs supported by pillows or stools.			
c. Lumbar: prone lying in neutral.			
d. Insure proper body alignment and pull off traction apparatus.			
4. Apply indicated traction poundage.			
a. Cervical: Adjust traction poundage beginning with 20# or as tolerated by the patient, (range 20–50 pounds).			
b. Lumbar: Adjust traction poundage beginning with 65# or as tolerated by the patient (range 65–200 pounds).			
5. Adjust traction duty cycle and treatment duration.			
a. Sustained: less than 10 minutes.			
b. Intermittent: 3 to to 10 seconds, on/off for 20 to 30 minutes			
6. Complete the treatment.			
a. Zero out equipment, turn power off.			
b. Slacken traction line.			
c. Remove the traction harness, halter, or belt.			
d. Have patient sit up slowly.			
e. Assess treatment efficacy.			
f. Record treatment parameters.			
7. Instruct the patient in any indicated exercise.			
8. Return equipment to storage after cleaning.			

CHAPTER 14 FOURTEEN

INTERMITTENT COMPRESSION DEVICES

DANIEL N. HOOKER

OBJECTIVES

Following completion of this chapter the student therapist will be able to:

- ✓ Discuss the effects of external compression on the accumulation and the reabsorption of edema following an athletic injury.
- ✓ Outline the setup procedure for intermittent external compression.
- ✓ Describe the effects that changing a parameter might have on edema reduction.
- ✓ Know when intermittent compression devices may best be used.

Edema accumulation following trauma is one of the clinical signs at which considerable attention is directed in first aid and therapeutic rehabilitation programs. **Edema** is defined as the presence of abnormal amounts of fluid in the extracellular tissue spaces of the body. Intermittent compression is one of the clinical modalities used to help reduce the accumulation of edema.

There are two distinct kinds of tissue swelling that are usually associated with injury. **Joint swelling,** marked by the presence of blood and joint fluid accumulated within the joint capsule, is one kind. This type of swelling occurs immediately following injury to a joint. Joint swelling is usually contained by the joint capsule and has the appearance and feel of a water balloon. If pressure is placed on the swelling, the fluid moves but it immediately returns when the pressure is released.

Lymphedema is the other variety of swelling encountered in athletic injuries. This type of swelling in the subcutaneous tissues results from an excessive accumulation of **lymph** and usually occurs over several hours following the injury. Intermittent compression can be used with both varieties, but it is usually more successful with **pitting edema.** The lymphatic system is the primary body system that deals with these injury induced changes.

THE LYMPHATIC SYSTEM

PURPOSES OF THE LYMPHATIC SYSTEM

The lymphatic system has four major purposes.

1. The fluid in the interstitial spaces is continuously circulating. As plasma and plasma proteins escape from the small blood vessels, they are picked up by the lymphatic system and returned to the blood circulation.

2. The lymphatic system acts as a safety valve for fluid overload and helps keep edema from forming. As the interstitial fluid increases, the interstitial fluid pressure increases, which causes an increase in the local lymph flow. The local lymphatic system can be overwhelmed by sudden local increases in the interstitial fluid and pitting edema will be the result.[33]

3. The homeostasis of the extracellular environment is maintained by the lymphatic system. The lymphatic system removes excess protein molecules and waste from the interstitial fluid. The large protein molecules and fluids that can not reenter the circulatory vessels gain entry back into the blood circulation through the terminal lymphatics.

4. The lymphatic system also cleanses the interstitial fluid and provides a blockade to the spread of infection or malignant cells in the lymph nodes. The lymph nodes' ability is not clearly understood and is highly variable.[16]

STRUCTURE OF THE LYMPHATIC SYSTEM

The lymphatic system is a closed vascular system of **endothelial cell-lined** tubes that parallel the arterial and nervous system. The lymphatic capillaries are made of single layered endothelial cells with **fibrils** radiating from the junctions of the endothelial cells (Fig. 14-1). These fibrils support the lymphatic capillaries and anchor them to the surrounding connective tissue. The capillary is surrounded by the interstitial fluid and tissues. These lymphatic capillaries are called the terminal lymphatics and they provide the entry way into the lymphatic system for the excess interstitial fluid and plasma proteins.

These lymphatic capillaries join together in a network of lymphatic vessels that eventually lead to larger collecting vessels in the extremities. The collecting vessels connect with the thoracic duct or the right lymphatic duct, which join the venous system in the left and right cervical area. As the lymph flows centrally up the system, the lymph moves through one or more lymph nodes. These nodes remove the foreign substances and are the primary area of lymphocyte activity.[16]

endothelial cell Cells that line the cavities of vessels.

lymph A transparent slightly yellow liquid found in the lymphatic vessels.

fibrils Connective tissue fibers supporting the lymphatic capillaries.

Capillary

Lymph vessel

Plasma

Plasma protein

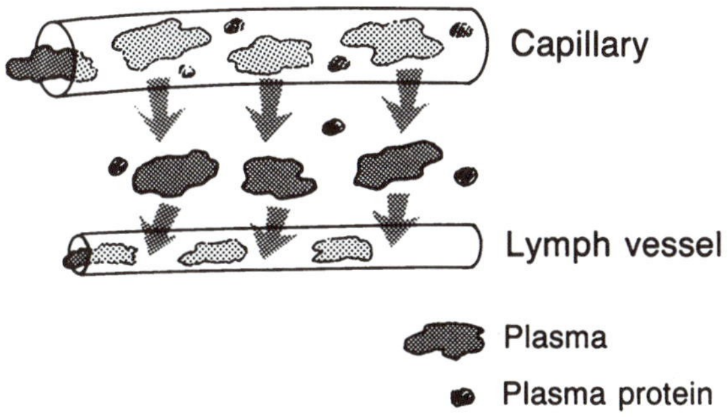

•**Figure 14-1** Plasma proteins outside the capillaries attract fluid to the intercellular space, leading to an abnormal "wet state" in the intercellular spaces. Plasma is absorbed back into the lymphatic spaces and away from the injured area.

PERIPHERAL LYMPHATIC STRUCTURE AND FUNCTION

Deep and superficial lymphatic collecting systems are found in the extremities. The terminal lymphatics in the skin and subcutaneous tissue drain into the superficial branches. Lymph channels in the fascial and bony layers drain into the deep branches.

In the superficial branches, the dermis is packed with two types of lymphatic channels. The channels closer to the surface have no valves, whereas those lying under the dermis and in the subcutaneous tissue do have valves. The valves are located approximately 1 centimeter apart and are similar in construction to the valves in veins. These structures prevent the back flow of lymph when pressure is applied. As with the blood vessels, the lymph system is concentrated on the medial side of the limbs.[16]

As the lymphatic system changes from the entry channels to the collecting channels, the lymphatic vessel changes to look similar to venous tissue. These vessels have smooth muscle and appear to have innervation from the sympathetic nervous system.

As the fluid or tissues move in the interstitial spaces, they push or pull on the fibrils supporting the terminal lymphatics (Fig. 14-2). This activity forces the endothelial cells to gap apart at their junctions, creating an opening in the terminal lymphatics for the entry of interstitial fluid, cellular waste, large protein molecules, plasma proteins, extracellular particles, and cells into the lymphatic channels. These junctions are constantly being pushed and pulled open and are then allowed to close, depending on the local activity. Once the interstitial fluid and proteins enter these channels, they become lymph. Terminal lymphatics in inflamed areas are dilated and an increased number of gaps in the capillary are present (see Fig. 14-2).[11,16, 20,41,42]

If no tissue activity or interstitial volume increase takes place, these endothelial junctions remain closed. The interstitial fluid, however, can still enter the terminal lymphatics by moving across the endothelial cell, or by being transported across in a vesicle or cell organelle. This permeability is similar to the small blood vessels or capillaries (see Fig. 14-1).

Muscle activity, active and passive movements, elevated positions, respiration, and blood vessel pulsation, all aid in the movement of lymph by compressing the lymphatic vessels and allowing gravity to pull the lymph down the channels. The valves help by maintaining a unidirectional flow of lymph in response to pressure. The collecting lymph channels all have smooth muscle in their walls. These muscles can provide contractible activity that promotes lymph flow. These muscles

Movement of Lymph Occurs because of
- Muscle activity
- Active and passive motion
- Elevation
- Respiration
- Contraction of vessels

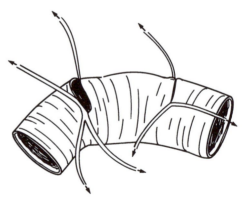

•**Figure 14-2** Lymphatic capillary with pore open to allow movement of plasma protein out of the intercellular space. As the intercellular fluid accumulates, the fibrils radiating from the seams in the lymphatic capillary pull the seam open to create a pore large enough for plasma proteins to enter.

have a natural firing frequency that simulates a rhythmic pumping action. There are also studies that indicate increased lymph flow during heating of animal limbs.[1–7,9,10,12,13,19,36,37,39–44]

INJURY EDEMA

Following a closed injury, changes in and around the site of the injury occur that have an impact on the accumulation of extracellular fluid and proteins in the local interstitial spaces. The direct effects of the injury include cell death, bleeding, the release of chemical mediators to initiate and guide the healing process, and changes in local tissue electric currents. The first stage of the healing process is inflammation, which is characterized by local redness, heat, swelling, and pain. In addition, loss of function frequently occurs.

These changes are brought about by changes in the local circulation. Local edema is formed by the plasma, plasma proteins, and cell debris from the damaged cells all moving into the interstitial spaces. This sudden volume change is compounded by the intact local circulatory responses to the chemical mediators of the inflammatory process. The hormones released by the injured cells stimulate the small arterioles, capillaries, and venules to vasodilate, enlarging the size of the vascular pool. This causes the local blood flow to slow down and the pressure within the blood vessels to increase. The endothelial cells in the blood vessel walls then separate or become more loosely bound to their neighboring cell. The permeability of the vessel increases, allowing more plasma, plasma proteins, and leucocytes to escape into the local area. The increase in the plasma proteins in the interstitial spaces causes the osmotic pressure to push more plasma into the area, forming an inflammatory exudate. This exudate forms too quickly for the lymphatic system to maintain the local equilibrium and pitting edema is formed (Fig. 14-3). This small increase in the plasma protein in the intercellular spaces causes an increase in the intercellular fluid volume by several hundred percent.[1,2,3,7,15,21,42,43]

This fluid in the form of a gel is trapped by both collagen fibers and proteoglycan molecules. The gel prevents the free flow of fluid, as seen in the joint fluid example. Clinically, this state is recognized as pitting edema. After finger pressure on the swollen part is released, a slight pit is left at the finger's previous location. Fluid is squeezed out of the intercellular space and time is needed for the fluid to move slowly back into that space (Fig. 14-3).

As the intercellular fluid becomes greater, the lymph begins to flow. If the edema causes an overdistention of the lymph capillaries, the entry pores become

edema The presence of abnormal amounts of fluid in the extracellular tissue spaces of the body.

pitting edema A type of swelling that leaves a pitlike depression when the skin is compressed.

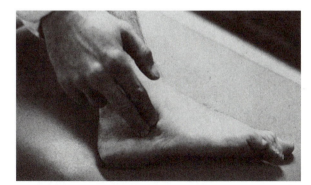

•Figure 14-3 Ankle with pitting edema. Finger pressure squeezes fluid out of the intercellular space; an indentation is left when the pressure is removed.

CASE STUDY 14-1
INTERMITTENT COMPRESSION

Background: A 48-year-old male developed pain and edema in his right foot and ankle subsequent to stepping in a hole in his yard while mowing his lawn. He was treated at his local hospital's emergency room. He failed to comply with their instructions to elevate and ice the injured extremity and reported to his family physician 48 hours later with a moderately swollen and ecchymotic right ankle. The patient reported the obvious swelling, localized tenderness over the lateral aspect of the ankle, and difficulty with weight-bearing during ambulation. Physical examination revealed point tenderness at the ATF (anterior talofibular ligament), 2+ effusion—figure 8 girth increased by 3/4 inch versus uninvolved side, and reduced ROM of dorsiflexion to 0 degrees/plantarflexion to 35 degrees. The ankle was stable to anterior drawer and talar tilt tests.

Impression: Subacute grade I inversion sprain right ankle.

Treatment Plan: In addition to reinstruction in home care principles; a course of intermittent compression was initiated to the right foot/ankle to mobilize the residual effusion/edema. The right lower extremity was elevated, pre-treatment circumferential measurements taken, and stockingnette placed over the extremity. Treatment consisted of 60 mmHg pressure applied intermittently for 30 seconds on/10 seconds off cycles for 30 minutes duration. Post-treatment circumferential measures were taken and the patient was encouraged to attempt active and active-assisted ankle pumping exercise. Patient was fitted with a compression stocking and thermoplastic ankle stirrup for ambulation weight-bearing as tolerated.

Response: Post initial treatment, patient's circumferential measures were reduced by 1/4 inch. Dorsiflexion range of motion increased by 5 degrees. Over the course of five treatment sessions, effusion was resolved and active range of motion approached normal limits. Strengthening exercises were implemented and the patient continued to ambulate with the aid of the ankle stirrup. At the time of discharge the patient was essentially symptom free, independent in performing his strengthening regimen and had returned to his yard work.

The rehabilitation professional employs therapeutic agent modalities to create an optimum environment for tissue healing while minimizing the symptoms associated with the trauma or condition.

Discussion Questions

- What tissues were injured or affected?
- What symptoms were present?
- What phase of the injury-healing continuum did the patient present for care in?
- What are the therapeutic agent modality's biophysical effects (direct, indirect, depth, and tissue affinity)?
- What are the therapeutic agent modality's indications and contraindications?
- What are the parameters of the therapeutic agent modality's application, dosage, duration, and frequency in this case study?
- What other therapeutic agent modalities could be utilized to treat this injury or condition? Why? How?

ineffective and lymphedema results. Constriction of lymph capillaries or larger lymphatic vessels from increased pressure also discourage lymph flow and cause intercellular fluid to increase.[1,2,3,7,15,21,42,43]

Using computerized tomography cross sectional images, Airaksinen et al. reported a 23 percent increase in the subcutaneous tissue, thickened skin, and muscular atrophy in patients following lower leg fracture and casting. They reported an 8 percent edema decrease in the subcutaneous compartment after intermittent compression. The mean area of the subfascial compartment remained the same but the density of the muscle tissue increased after treatment. This study indicates that injury edema follows the path of least resistance and that tissues that have the least natural pressure exerted on them demonstrate the greatest accumulation of extra fluid. The skin and subcutaneous tissue appear to be the major site for pitting edema; the deep muscle and connective tissue have enough pressure to inhibit major accumulations in the deeper tissues.[3]

Clinical measurement of edema is reasonably accurate and correlates extremely well with both CT scan and volumetric measures. The standard clinical circumferential measurement of limb and joint are adequate to determine the treatment effects.[3,5]

Edema compounds the extent of an injury by causing the secondary hypoxic cellular death in the tissues surrounding the injured area. The edema increases the distance nutrients and oxygen must travel to nourish the remaining cells. This in turn adds to the injury debris in the damaged area and causes further edema to accumulate, thus perpetuating the cycle.[9]

Other ill effects of edema include the physical separation of torn tissue ends, pain, and restricted joint range of motion. Recovery times become more prolonged. If the edema persists, further problems with extremity function can occur, including infection, muscle atrophy, joint contractures, interstitial fibrosis, and reflex sympathetic dystrophy.[7,11,13]

TREATMENT

Good first aid can minimize edema (Fig. 14-4). The use of ice, compression, electricity, elevation, and early gentle motion retards the accumulation of fluid and keeps the lymphatic system operating at an optimum level. Any treatment that encourages the lymph flow will decrease plasma protein content in the intercellular spaces and therefore decrease edema. The standard methods of treatment in most clinical settings include elevation, compression, and muscular contraction.

The force of gravity can be used to augment normal lymph flow. The swollen part can be elevated so that gravity does not resist the flow of lymph but encourages its movement. Elevation of the injured swollen part above heart level is all that is necessary. The higher the elevation, the greater the effect on the lymph flow.[31,34]

In an uninjured population, placing the legs in an elevated position significantly decreased ankle volume after 20 minutes, although the dependent position signifi-

Edema Is Best Treated with
- Elevation
- Compression
- Weight bearing exercise
- Cryotherapy

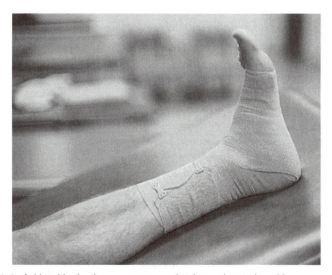

•**Figure 14-4** Ankle with elastic wrap compression in an elevated position.

cantly increased ankle volumes. These findings could be expected to be the same in injured subjects, but the dependent position may markedly increase volume, whereas the elevated position may decrease volumes less well because of the injury to the tissue. In studies using postacute ankle sprain edema, elevation alone provided a significant posttreatment reduction in ankle volume.[5,24,31,34]

Rhythmic internal compression provided by muscle contraction also squeezes the lymph through the lymph vessels, improving its flow back to the vascular system. This muscle contraction can be accomplished through isometric or active exercise or through electrically induced muscle contraction. Several authors also advocate the use of non-contractable electric current for edema control and reduction. (See Chapter 5 for a discussion of electrical therapy for edema control.) When elevation is combined with muscle contraction, lymph flow benefits.[4,6,12]

External pressure also can be used to increase lymph flow. Massage, elastic compression, and intermittent pressure devices are the most often used external pressure devices. This external compression not only moves the lymph along but also may spread the intercellular edema over a larger area, enabling more lymph capillaries to become involved in removing the plasma proteins and water. External pressure from horseshoe, pads, and elastic wraps are also helpful in minimizing the accumulation or reaccumulation of edema in the injured area.[9,41,42,43]

Gardner has proposed that weight bearing activities activate a powerful venous pump.[15] The pump consists of the venae comitantes of the lateral plantar artery. It is emptied immediately on weight bearing and flattening of the plantar arch. Because this emptying occurs so rapidly, they believe that this process is mediated by the release of an **endothelial-derived relaxing factor** (EDRF) and is not related to muscular activity of the limb. The EDRF is liberated by sudden pressure changes and it diffuses locally. Its major action is to relax the smooth muscle and stimulate blood flow rates in the veins.[18]

This phenomenon may explain the rapid decrease in edema that occurs when patients switch from a non-weight-bearing gait to a weight bearing gait. Using this venous pump on lower leg edema is a reason to include early weight bearing in a variety of injury treatment protocols.

Using an intermittent compression device to decrease postacute injury edema has recently been shown to have a good effect. The addition of cryotherapy to the intermittent compression has shown the best results in the reduction of postacute injury edema.[1,2,3,5,19,20,24,29,35,36,44]

CLINICAL PARAMETERS

There are three parameters available for adjustment when using most intermittent pressure devices: (1) inflation pressure; (2) on-off time sequence; and (3) total treatment time (Fig. 14-5). There are also intermittent pressure devices with multiple compartments that inflate distal to proximal with gradual reduced pressure in each compartment. These devices try to mimic the massage strokes used in edema removal.[19,20,24,39] Reduction in post acute injury edema does not require this graded sequential action, nor is post injury edema reduction significantly enhanced by these devices.[24,39] All intermittent compression devices seem to have similar influences on edema.

Little research has been done comparing adjustments of these parameters with volumetric results. Empiricism and clinical trials have been used to design the established protocols. Pressure settings have been loosely correlated with blood pressure and patient comfort to arrive at the therapeutic pressure. A pressure approximating the patient's diastolic blood pressure has been used in most treatment protocols. The

---

Treatment Tip

When using intermittent compression following an acute ankle sprain, the compression boot should be applied with the inflation pressure set at about 60 mm, the on/off time at 30 sec on 30 sec off, and a total treatment time of 20 minutes initially. The on/off times and total treatment time can be increased over the next several days as tolerated.

Treatment Parameters
- Inflation pressure
- On/off times
- Total treatment time

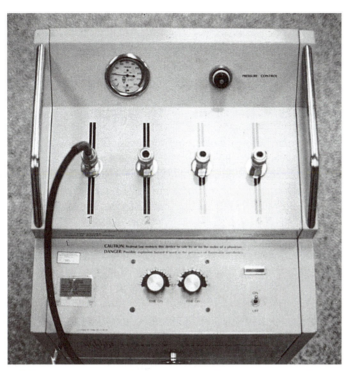

•**Figure 14-5** Pressure gauge and pressure control knob on an intermittent compression unit.

arterial capillary pressures are approximately 30 mmHg, and any pressure that exceeds this should encourage reabsorption of the edema and movement of the lymph. Maximum pressure should correspond to the systolic blood pressure. Higher pressure would shut off arterial blood flow and create a potentially uncomfortable tissue response as a result of low blood flow.[1,2,3,11,13,21,22]

More may not necessarily be better. Enough pressure is needed to squeeze the lymphatic vessels and force the lymph to move. This should be accomplished with relatively low pressures, for example, 30 to 40 mmHg. The other mechanism in operation is the force of the hydrostatic pressure and pressure in the range of 40 to 50 mmHg should suffice to raise the interstitial fluid pressure higher than the blood vessel pressures.[13,21,22]

On and off time sequences are even more variable, with some protocols calling for a sequence of 30 seconds on, 30 seconds off; 1 minute on, 2 minutes off; whereas others reverse this to 2 minutes on, 1 minute off. Others use a 4 minutes on to 1 minute off ratio. If lymphatic massage is the primary vehicle used in this therapy, shorter on-off time sequences may have an advantage. The hydrostatic pressure vehicles require the longer on times. These time periods are not research-based, and the therapist is left to his or her own empirical judgment as to the optimum time sequence for each patient. Patient comfort should be the primary deciding factor here. Total treatment times have some basis in research, but again this is convenience or empirically based in many instances. Most of the protocols for primary lymphedema call for 3- to 4-hour treatments. This time frame has been effective for many patients.[1,2,3,5,12,13,19,20,22,24,29,31,32,35,36,39,44]

Researchers have shown a marked increase in lymph flow on initiation of massage; this flow decreases over a 10-minute period and stops when the massage is discontinued.[28,34] Clinical studies show significant gains in limb volume reduction after 30 minutes of compression.[1,2,3,5,12,24,29,35,36,44] In most situations, a 10- to

Treatment Tip
Joint swelling is usually contained in the joint capsule and feels very much like a water balloon. The fluid is easily moved around by simply applying pressure on one side of the joint. Lymphedema occurs in the subcutaneous tissues has more of a gel-like feeling to it and leaves an indentation after finger pressure is removed.

30-minute treatment seems adequate unless the edema is overwhelming in volume or is resistant to treatment. More treatment times per day may also be an advantage in controlling and reducing edema from various musculoskeletal injuries.

PATIENT SETUP AND INSTRUCTIONS

Patient setup using an intermittent compression device is relatively simple. The patient should have the appropriate-sized compression appliance fitted on the extremity in an elevated position (Fig. 14-6). The compression sleeves come as either half-leg, full-leg, full-arm, or half-arm. The deflated compression sleeve is connected to the compression unit via a rubber hose and connecting valve.

Once the machine has been turned on, three parameters may be adjusted; on/off time, inflation pressure, and treatment time. The on time should be adjusted between 30 to 120 seconds (Fig. 14-7). The off time is left at 0 until the sleeve is inflated and the treatment pressure is reached and then may be adjusted between 0 and 120 seconds. When the unit cycles off, the patient should be instructed to move the extremity. A 30-seconds-on, 30-seconds-off setting seems to be both effective and comfortable for the patient. Some compression devices slowly reach the target pressure, whereas others respond more rapidly. It is important that the on and off times take the machine characteristics into account.

When using electrical stimulation in combination with compression, always adjust the current intensity with the sleeve fully pressurized, as this may affect electrode contact and current density (Fig. 14-8).

The treatment should last between 20 and 30 minutes. Patients do not seem to comfortably tolerate treatments lasting longer than 30 minutes. On completion of the treatment, the extremity should be measured to see if the desired results have been achieved. The part should be wrapped with elastic compression wraps to help maintain the reduction. If the edema is not reduced, another treatment may be needed after a short recovery time. If not contraindicated, weight bearing should be encouraged to stimulate the venous pump.

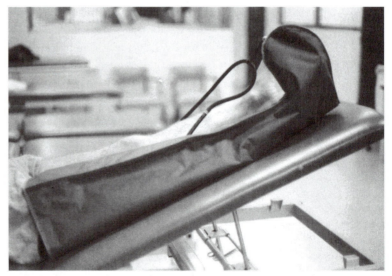

•**Figure 14-6** Uninflated compression appliance applied to a patient's leg in an elevated position.

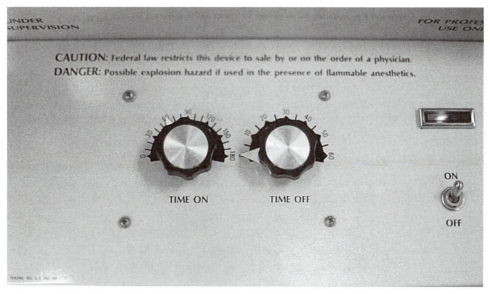

•**Figure 14-7** Time setting control knobs for on and off cycles of an intermittent compression unit. This illustrates the setting at the beginning of the treatment when the appliance is uninflated. The off time knob is increased when the proper inflation pressure is reached.

COLD AND COMPRESSION COMBINATION

Some manufacturers have coupled intermittent pressure with a coolant (either water or Freon). These devices have the advantage of cooling the injured part as well as compressing it. The Jobst Cryotemp is a controlled cold-compression unit that has a temperature adjustment ranging between 10 and 25°C. Cooling is accomplished by circulating cold water through the sleeve.

The combination of cold and compression has been shown to be clinically effective in treating some edema conditions.[5,12,21,24,25,29,35,36] A study comparing a technique using an intermittent compression unit, cold, and elevation with one using an elastic wrap, cold, and elevation showed that the use of the cold-compression device was more effective in edema reduction.[5]

Treatment Tip
Using electrical stimulating currents to induce muscle pumping contractions should facilitate removal of edema. Also it is well documented that using cold in conjunction with compression is clinically effective in treating cases of lymphedema.

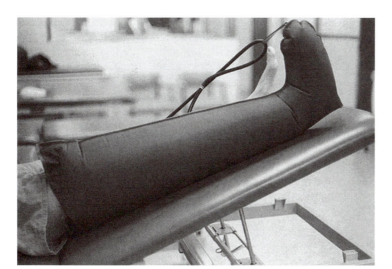

•**Figure 14-8** Inflated pressure sleeve.

LINEAR COMPRESSION PUMPS

Intermittent compression pumps have incorporated sequentially inflated multiple compartment designs for some time.[16,17,29] Recently, these designs have also included a programmable gradient design, such as the Wright Linear Pump (Fig. 14-9). This was designed to incorporate the massage effect of a distal to proximal pressure with a gradual decrease in the pressure gradient.[20]

The highest pressure is in the distal sleeve and, according to the manufacturer's recommendation, is determined by the mean value of systolic to diastolic pressure at the outset of a specifically determined 48-hour protocol whose purpose is to determine the effectiveness of the device in individual cases.[20] The middle cell is set 20 mm lower than the distal cell, and the proximal cell pressure is reduced an additional 20 mm.

The length of each pressure cycle is 120 seconds. The distal cell is pressurized initially and continues pressurization for 90 seconds. Twenty seconds later the middle cell is inflated, and after another 20 seconds the proximal cell inflates. A final 30-second period allows pressure in all three cells to return to 0, after which the cycle repeats itself.

Only a few studies have shown the efficacy of using decreasing pressure in a distal to proximal direction relative to previously existing compression sleeves.[15,16] In a study comparing linear compression and cold and compression, Lemly found both effective in reducing edema but no significant difference between the devices.[24]

Intermittent compression may also be used in conjunction with a low-frequency pulsed or surging electrical stimulating current setup to produce muscle pumping

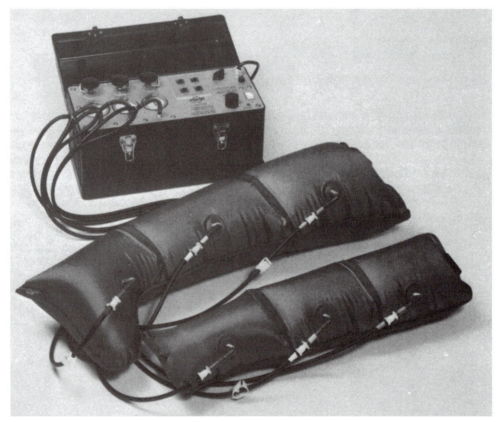

•**Figure 14-9** The Wright Linear Pump is a programmable gradient sequential pressure system.

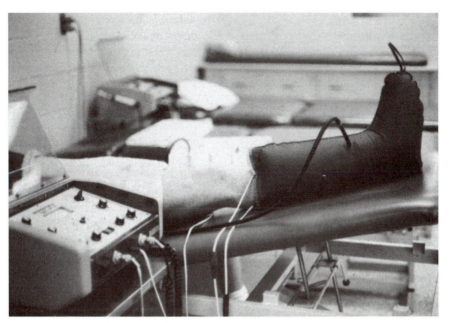

•**Figure 14-10** Intermittent compression used in combination with electrical stimulating currents to reduce edema.

contractions. The combination of these two modalities should facilitate resorption of injury byproducts by the lymphatic system (Fig. 14-10).[12]

INDICATIONS AND CONTRAINDICATIONS FOR USE

Intermittent compression has been recommended for treating lymphedema; traumatic edema that occurs following injury to soft tissue; chronic edema that occurs in patients with certain types of neurological diseases owing to an inability to move a limb; stasis ulcers that develop with the presence of fluid in the interstitial spaces for long periods of time; swelling that occurs with limb amputation; patients on dialysis owing to renal insufficiency that tend to develop edema in the extremities and hypothesion; patients with arterial insufficiency, such as in cases of intermittent claudications to increase venous return; edema and contractures in the hand that result from stroke or surgery; and to stimulate proteoglycan synthesis in human cartilage.[17,23,27,30,32,38] It has also been used postoperatively to reduce the possibility of developing a deep vein thrombosis resulting from inactivity and coagulation; and to facilitate wound healing following surgery by reducing swelling.[8,26,28]

The therapist should avoid using intermittent compression in patients with known deep vein thrombosis, local superficial infection, congestive heart failure, acute pulmonary edema, and displaced fractures.[14]

Indications and Contraindications for Intermittent Compression

Indications
   Lymphedema
   Traumatic edema
   Chronic edema
   Stasis ulcers
   Intermittent claudications
   Facilitate wound healing following surgery

Contraindications
   Deep vein thrombosis
   Local superficial infection
   Congestive heart failure
   Acute pulmonary edema
   Displaced fractures

SUMMARY

1. Edema following injury or surgery can be managed effectively using a compression pump program.
2. This treatment, along with external elastic supports, elevation, weight bearing, and exercise will help reverse edema and prevent its reaccumulation.

3. Treatment parameters are better understood from clinic empiricism than from research studies. Although trying to use the physiologic principles of edema accumulation and reduction to create minimum and maximum values, specific manipulations of on-off times, pressure, and total treatment time should use patient comfort as the primary guide.

REFERENCES

1. Airaksinen, O.: Changes in post-traumatic ankle joint mobility, pain and edema following intermittent pneumatic compression therapy, Arch. Phys. Med. Rehabil. 70:341–344, 1989.

2. Airaksinen, O.: Treatment of post-traumatic edema in lower legs using intermittent pneumatic compression, Scand. J. Rehabil. Med. 20:25–28, 1988.

3. Airaksinen, O.: Intermittent pneumatic compression therapy in post-traumatic lower limb edema: computed tomography and clinical measurements, Arch. Phys. Med. Rehabil. 72:667–670, 1991.

4. Angus, J., Prentice, W., and Hooker, D.: A comparison of two intermittent external compression devices and their effect on post acute ankle edema, J. Ath. Train. 29(2):179, 1994.

5. Brewer, K., Prentice, W., and Hooker, D.: The effects of intermittent compression and cold on reducing edema in post-acute ankle sprains, Unpublished master's thesis, University of North Carolina, Chapel Hill, North Carolina, 1990.

6. Brown, S.: Ankle edema and galvanic muscle stimulation, Phys. Sports Med. 9:137, 1981.

7. Carriere, B.: Edema—its development and treatment using lymph drainage massage, Clin. Manage. Phys. Ther. 8(5):19–21, 1988.

8. Clark, W.: Pneumatic compression of the calf and post operative deep vein thrombosis, Lancet 2:5, 1974.

9. Duffley, H., Knight, K.: Ankle compression variability using elastic wrap, elastic wrap with a horseshoe, edema II boot and air stirrup brace, Ath. Train. 24:320–323, 1989.

10. Elkins, E., Herrick, J., and Grindley, J.: Effect of various procedures on the flow of lymph, Arch. Phys. Med. Rehabil. 34:31–39, 1953.

11. Evans, P.: The healing process at the cellular level: a review, Physiotherapy 66:256–259, 1980.

12. Flicker, M.: An Analysis of cold intermittent compression with simultaneous treatment of electrical stimulation in the reduction of post acute ankle lymphaedema, Unpublished master's thesis, University of North Carolina, Chapel Hill, North Carolina, May, 1993.

13. Foldi, E., Foldi, M., and Weissleder, H.: Conservative treatment of lymphoedema of the limbs, Angiology 36:171–180, 1985.

14. Fond, D., Hecox, B.: Intermittent pneumatic compression, In Hecox, B., Mehreteab, T., and Weisberg, J., editors: Physical agents; a comprehensive text for physical therapists, Norwalk, Connecticut, 1994, Appleton & Lange.

15. Gardner, A.: Reduction of post-traumatic swelling and compartment pressure by impulse compression of the foot, JBJS 72-B:810–815, 1990.

16. Gnepp, D.: Lymphatics 263–298 in Staub, N., Taylor, A., editors: Edema, New York, 1984, Raven.

17. Henry, J., Windos, T.: Compensation of arterial insufficiency by augmenting the circulation with intermittent compression of the limbs, Am. Heart J. 70(1):77–88, 1965.

18. Hurley, J.: Inflammation 463–488. In Staub, N., Taylor, A., editors: Edema, New York, 1984, Raven.

19. Kim-Sing, C., Basco, V.: Postmastectomy lymphedema treated with the Wright Linear Pump, Can. J. Surg. 30(5):368–370, 1987.

20. Klein, M., Alexander, M., and Wright, J.: Treatment of lower extremity lymphedema with the Wright Linear Pump: a statistical analysis of a clinical trial, Arch. Phys. Med. Rehabil. 69:202–206, 1988.

21. Kobl, P., Denegar, C.: Traumatic edema and the lymphatic system, Ath. Train. 18:339–341, 1983.

22. Kruse, R., Kruse, A., Britton, R.: Physical therapy for the patient with peripheral edema: procedures for management, Phys. Ther. Rev. 80:29–33, 1960.

23. Lafeber, F.: Intermittent hydrostatic compressive force stimulates exclusively the proteoglycan synthesis of osteoarthritic human cartilage. Br. J. Rheumatol. 31(7):437–442, 1992.

24. Lemley, T., Prentice, W., and Hooker, D.: A comparison of two intermittent compression devices on pitting ankle edema, J. Ath. Train. 28(2):156–157, 1993.

25. Liu, N., Olszewski, W.: The influence of local hyperthermia on lymphedema and lymphedematous skin of the human leg, Lymphology 26:28–37, 1993.

26. Matzdorff, A.: Green, D.: Deep vein thrombosis and pulmonary embolism: prevention, diagnosis, and treatment, Geriatrics 47(8):48–52, 55–57, 62–63, 1992.

27. McCulloch, J.: Intermittent compression for the treatment of a chronic stasis ulceration: a case report, Phys. Ther. 61:1452–1453, 1981.

28. Pflug, J.: Intermittent compression: a new principle in the treatment of wounds, Lancet 2(3):15, 1974.

29. Quillen, W., Rouiller, L.: Initial management of acute ankle sprains with rapid pulsed pneumatic compression and cold, JOSPT 4:39–43, 1982.

30. Redford, J.: Experiences in the use of a pneumatic stump shrinker, Int. Clin. Inform. Bull. Prosth. Orthot. 12:1, 1973.

31. Rucinski, T., Hooker, D., and Prentice, W.: The effects of

intermittent compression on edema in post-acute ankle sprains, JOSPT 14(2):65–69, August 1991.

32. Sanderson, R., Fletcher, W.: Conservative management of primary lymphedema, Northwest Med. 64:584–588, 1965.

33. Seki, K.: Lymph flow in human leg, Lymphology 12:2–3, 1979.

34. Sims, D.: Effects of positioning on ankle edema, JOSPT 8:30–33, 1986.

35. Sloan, J., Giddings, P., and Hain, R.: Effects of cold and compression on edema, Phys. Sports Med. 16(8):116–120, 1988.

36. Starkey, J.: Treatment of ankle sprains by simultaneous use of intermittent compression and ice packs, Am. J. Sports Med. 4:142–144, 1976.

37. Stillwell, G.: Further studies on the treatment of lymphedema, Arch. Phys. Med. Rehabil. 38:435–441, 1957.

38. van Veen, S., Hagen, J., and van Ginkel, F.: Intermittent compression stimulates cartilage mineralization, Bone 17(5):461–465, 1995.

39. Wakim, K.: Influence of centripetal rhythmic compression on localized edema of an extremity, Arch. Phys. Med. Rehabil. 36:98–103, 1955.

40. Wilkerson, J.: Contrast baths and pressure treatment for ankle sprains, Phys. Sports Med. 7:143, 1979.

41. Wilkerson, J.: Treatment of ankle sprains with external compression and early mobilization, Phys. Sports Med. 13(6): 83–90, 1985.

42. Wilkerson, J.: External compression for controlling traumatic edema, Phys. Sports Med. 13(6):97–106, 1985.

43. Wilkerson, J.: Treatment of the inversion ankle sprain through synchronous application of focal compression and cold, Ath. Train. 26:220–237, 1991.

44. Winsor, T., Selle, W.: The effect of venous compression on the circulation of the extremities, Arch. Phys. Med. Rehabil. 34:559–565, 1953.

Suggested Readings

Christen, Y., Reymond, M.: Hemodynamic effects of intermittent pneumatic compression of the lower limbs during laparoscopic cholecystectomy, Amer. J. Surg. 170(4):395–398, 1995.

DePrete, A., Cogliano, T., and Agostinucci, J.: The effect of circumferential pressure on upper motoneuron reflex excitability in healthy subjects, Phys. Ther. 74(5)(Suppl): S70, 1994.

Hamzeh, M., Lonsdale, R., and Pratt, D.: A new device producing ambulatory intermittent pneumatic compression suitable for the treatment of lower limb edema: a preliminary report, J. Med. Eng. Technol. 17(3):110–113, 1993.

Hofman D.: Intermittent compression treatment for venous leg ulcers, J. Wound Care 4(4):163–165, 1995.

Jacobs, M.: Leg volume changes with EPIC and posturing in dependent pregnancy edema: external pneumatic intermittent compression, Nurs. Res. 35(2):86–89, 1986.

Lachmann, E., Rook, J., and Tunkel, R.: Complications associated with intermittent pneumatic compression, Arch. Phys. Med. Rehabil. 73(5):482–485, 1992.

Majkowski, R., Atkins, R.: Treatment of fixed flexion deformities of the knee in rheumatoid arthritis using the Flowtron intermittent compression stocking, Br. J. Rheumatol. 31(1):41–43, 1992.

McCulloch, J.: Physical modalities in wound management: ultrasound, vasopneumatic devices and hydrotherapy, Ostomy Wound Manage. 41(5):30–32, 34, 36–7, 1995.

Murphy, K.: The combination of ice and intermittent compression system in the treatment of soft tissue injuries, Physiotherapy 74(1):41, 1988.

Smith, P.: The use of intermittent compression in treatment of fixed flexion deformities of the knee, Physiotherapy 75(8):494, 1989.

Yates, P., Cornwell, J., and Scott, G.: Treatment of haemophilic flexion deformities using the Flowtron intermittent compression system, Br. J. Haematol. 82(2):384–387, 1992.

Glossary

edema The presence of abnormal amounts of fluid in the extracellular tissue spaces of the body.

endothelial cell Cells that line the cavities of vessels.

endothelial-derived relaxing factor Relaxes smooth muscle and stimulates blood flow rates in veins.

fibrils Connective tissue fibers supporting the lymphatic capillaries.

joint swelling Accumulation of blood and joint fluid within the joint capsule.

lymph A transparent slightly yellow liquid found in the lymphatic vessels.

lymphedema Swelling of subcutaneous tissues as a result of accumulation of excessive lymph fluid.

pitting edema A type of swelling that leaves a pitlike depression when the skin is compressed.

LAB ACTIVITY

INTERMITTENT COMPRESSION

DESCRIPTION:

Intermittent compression pumps are mechanical units that inflate double-layered fabric sleeves shaped to fit the extremities in order to apply external pressure to facilitate the body's reabsorption of edema resulting from injury or trauma. Units allow the regulation of inflation pressure, on/off time sequence, and total treatment time.

Physiological Effects:

Movement of interstitial fluid to venous and lymphatic drainage sites
Temporary decrease in peripheral blood flow

Therapeutic Effects:

Reduction of soft tissue edema
Decreased pain
Increased range of motion

Indications:

The therapist will most frequently employ intermittent compression pumps in the treatment of soft tissue edema that accompanies musculoskeletal trauma. It may also be utilized in cases of venous insufficiency and lymphedema.

Contraindications:

- Infections
- Arterial insufficiency
- Possibility of blood clots
- Cardiac or kidney dysfunction
- Obstructed lymphatic channels

INTERMITTENT COMPRESSION			
PROCEDURE	Evaluation		
	1	2	3
1. Check supplies.			
a. Obtain compression pump, pneumatic sleeve, and cotton stockingnette.			
2. Question patient.			
a. Verify identity of patient.			
b. Verify the absence of contraindications.			
c. Take the patient's blood pressure.			
d. Ask about previous treatments and review treatment notes.			
3. Position patient.			
a. Place patient in a well-supported, comfortable position.			
b. Elevate the extremity to be treated.			

PROCEDURE	Evaluation		
	1	2	3
4. Inspect the patient's skin and extremity sensation.			
a. Perform circumferential measures of part to be treated.			
b. Cover extremity with stockingette, insure there are no wrinkles.			
5. Apply compression sleeve over the stockingnette covered extremity.			
6. Explain the procedure to the patient.			
7. Begin the indicated procedure.			
a. Attach sleeve to compression pump via tubing.			
b. Turn pump "on" and inflate to: <60 mm for the lower extremity <50 mm for the upper extremity **Warning: Do not exceed diastolic bp.**			
c. Adjust the compression pump to cycle in a 3:1 ratio of on and off time.			
d. Set duration of treatment from 30 minutes to 1 hour.			
e. Encourage the patient to wiggle his or her fingers or toes during the off cycle.			
f. Remove the sleeve at least once during the course of treatment to inspect skin and allow joint motion.			
8. Complete the treatment.			
a. Remove the sleeve and stockingnette.			
b. Inspect the skin and check peripheral circulation.			
c. Perform circumferential measures.			
d. Record results of treatment.			
e. Assess treatment efficacy.			
9. Wrap extremity to retain edema reduction and perform any indicated exercise.			
10. Return equipment to storage after cleaning.			

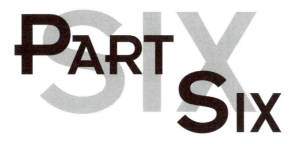

PART SIX

MANUAL MODALITIES

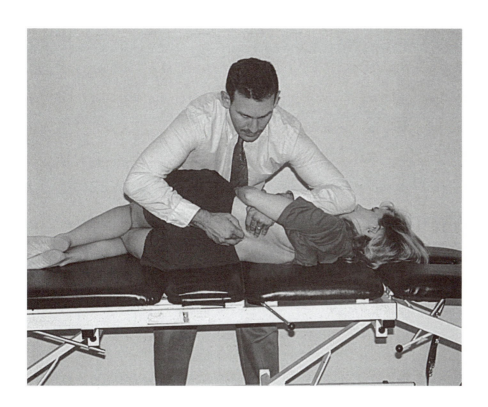

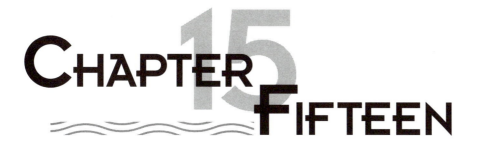

CHAPTER FIFTEEN

THERAPEUTIC MASSAGE

WILLIAM E. PRENTICE

CLAIRBETH LEHN

OBJECTIVES

Following completion of this chapter, the student therapist will be able to:

- ✓ Discuss the physiologic effects of massage differentiating between reflexive and mechanical effects.
- ✓ Be aware of specific treatment guidelines and considerations when administering massage.
- ✓ Discuss the various strokes involved with classic Hoffa massage.
- ✓ Describe connective tissue massage.
- ✓ Discuss how acupressure massage is most effectively used and identify the relationship between acupuncture and trigger points.
- ✓ Explain how myofascial release can be used to restore normal functional movement patterns.
- ✓ Discuss special massage techniques, including Rolfing and Tragering.

THE VALUE OF MANUAL THERAPY TECHNIQUES

Manual therapy techniques, including massage, joint mobilization, and traction, as well as proprioceptive neuromuscular facilitation techniques, are being used more frequently in rehabilitation by the therapist. In recent years, therapists have tended to get caught up in some of the technological advances that have been made available in rehabilitation equipment. These "high tech" devices to a great extent have taken the place of what many consider to be the greatest tool available in the rehabilitation repertoire, our hands. It seems, however, that the pendulum is beginning to swing back in the other direction, and more therapists are incorporating manual therapy techniques into their rehabilitation regimens. Thus, the in-depth discussions of massage in this chapter, joint mobilization and traction techniques in Chapter 16, and PNF techniques in Chapter 17 are essential.

THE EVOLUTION OF MASSAGE AS A TREATMENT MODALITY

The earliest available medical records seem to indicate that massage played an important role in the treatment of sick and injured people.[20] A natural reaction when a part of the body hurts is to rub the injured area with a hand.

In early writings pertaining to medical treatments little difference is shown between massage, as we know it, and general exercise of the body. In fact, although there are very detailed descriptions of techniques, one has a great deal of difficulty in making a determination as to exactly what is meant because the terminology is unfamiliar. Language changes with time.

In Europe during the Middle Ages the influence of the Church of Rome and its religious teachings discouraged the use of massage as a healing practice. This brought the art to somewhat of a halt until enlightened individuals strove to bring medical knowledge into the forefront and scholars in the medical fields started to again delve into how and why the body functions as it does.

The word massage is derived from two sources. One is the Arabic verb *mass*, to touch, and the other is the Greek word *massein*, to knead. However, history shows that this was not an art exclusive to the Greeks and Arabs. The general knowledge of massage was also known and practiced by the Egyptians, Romans, Japanese, Persians, and Chinese.

In Sweden in the early part of the nineteenth century, Peter H. Ling (1776 to 1839), the acknowledged founder of curative gymnastics, used massage as a branch of gymnastics. He appears to be the founder of modern-day massage techniques with some incorporation of French massage techniques into his system.[9]

Massage techniques have changed dramatically in the past 50 years. They are based on the research and teachings of Albert Hoffa (1859–1907), James B. Mennell (1880–1957), and Gertrude Beard (1887–1971). Medical practitioners of the twentieth century have added a scientific basis to massage along with additional techniques and terms. In modern-day preventative and rehabilitative therapy, massage is a widely used therapeutic modality that seems to be gaining renewed interest.[25]

massage The act of rubbing, kneading, or stroking the superficial parts of the body with the hand or with an instrument.

PHYSIOLOGIC EFFECTS OF MASSAGE

Physiologic Effects of Massage
- Reflexive
- Mechanical

Massage is a mechanical stimulation of the tissues by means of rhythmically applied pressure and stretching.[46] Over the years many claims have been made relative to the therapeutic benefits of massage in the athletic population, although few are based on well-controlled and designed studies.[4] Patients have used massage to increase flexibility and coordination as well as increase pain threshold; decrease neuromuscular excitability in the muscle being massaged; stimulate circulation, thus improving energy transport to the muscle; facilitate healing and restore joint mobility; and remove lactic acid, thus alleviating muscle cramps.[22,26,27,35,41] Conclusive evidence of the efficacy of massage as an ergogenic aid in the athletic population is lacking.[19]

How these effects may be accomplished is determined by the specific approaches used with massage techniques and how they are applied. Generally, the effects of massage may be either reflexive or mechanical.[8] The effect of massage on the nervous system differs greatly according to the method employed, pressure exerted, and duration of applications. Through the reflex mechanism, sedation is induced. Slow, gentle, rhythmical, and superficial effleurage may relieve tension and soothe, rendering the muscles more relaxed. This indicates an effect on sensory and motor nerves locally and some central nervous system response. The mechanical approach seeks to make mechanical or histological changes in myofascial structures through direct force applied superficially.[8]

REFLEXIVE EFFECTS

The first approach in massage therapy involves a reflexive mechanism. The reflexive approach attempts to exert effects through the skin and superficial connective tissues. Mobilization of soft tissue stimulates sensory receptors in the skin and superficial fascia.[8] If hands are passed lightly over the skin, a series of responses occur as a result of the sensory stimulus of cutaneous receptors. This reflex mechanism is believed to be an autonomic nervous system phenomenon.[3] The reflex stimulus can occur alone (i.e., unaccompanied by the mechanical mechanism). Mennell calls this the "reflex effect."[34] In itself, it is not an effect but the cause of an effect (i.e., causes sedation, relieves tension, increases blood flow).

Reflexive Effects
- Pain
- Circulation
- Metabolism

Effects on Pain

The effect of massage on pain is probably regulated by both the gate control theory and through the release of endogenous opiates (see Chapter 3). In gate control, cutaneous stimulation of large diameter afferent nerve fibers effectively blocks transmission of pain information carried in small diameter nerve fibers. Stimulation of painful areas in the skin or myofascia can facilitate the release of β-endorphins and enkephalin, which essentially effect the transmission of pain associated information in descending spinal tracts.

Effects on Circulation

The effect of massage on the circulation of the blood, according to Pemberton, takes place through a reflex influence on blood vessels from a sympathetic division in the nervous system.[36] He believes that vessels in the muscular system are emptied during massage, not only by being squeezed but also by this reflex action. Very light massage (effleurage) produces an almost instantaneous reaction through transient dilation of lymphatics and small capillaries. Heavier pressure brings about a more lasting dilation. If capillary dilation occurs, blood volume and blood flow increase, producing an increase in temperature in the area being massaged.[14]

Massage increases lymphatic flow.[16] In the lymphatic system, movement of fluid depends on forces outside of the system. Such factors as gravity, muscle contraction, movement, and massage can affect the flow of lymph. Increased lymphatic flow assists in the removal of edema.[7] When administering massage to an edematous part, elevation also helps to increase lymph flow.

Effects on Metabolism

Massage does not alter general metabolism appreciably.[36] There is no change in acid-base equilibrium of blood. Massage does not appear to have any significant effects on the cardiovascular system.[5] Massage metabolically augments a chemical balance. The increased circulation means increased dispersion of waste products and an increase of fresh blood and oxygen. The mechanical movements assist in the removal and hastens the resynthesis of lactic acid.

MECHANICAL EFFECTS

The second approach to massage is mechanical in nature. Techniques that stretch a muscle, elongate fascia, or mobilize soft tissue adhesions or restrictions are all

CASE STUDY 15-1
MASSAGE

Background: A 30-year-old stockbroker complains of chronic cervical myalgia ("My neck hurts."). There was no prior history of trauma and his family physician reported that his x-rays were within normal limits without evidence of degenerative changes or loss of disk space height. The patient reports no radiation of pain into the shoulders or upper extremities, but did complain of restriction in rotating his head to the left. The patient stated that he spends many hours each day at work cradling a telephone with his right side.

Impression: "Occupational Neck:" Right Upper Trapezius and Sternocleidomastoid Muscle Spasm

Treatment Plan: The patient was placed in a forward seated position with the head and neck supported by pillows on the treatment plinth. The arms were likewise supported by a pillow in the lap. A small amount of prewarmed massage lotion was applied to the right upper quarter region and a Hoffa massage commenced with light effleurage stroking begun to the SCM and upper trapezius muscles. The light effleurage stroking was followed by several minutes of deep effleurage strokes, which identified several "trigger point" areas in each muscle. Petrissage was directed at each 'trigger point' area for approximately 30 seconds, then the massage concluded with several more minutes of deep, then superficial effleurage strokes. At the completion of the massage, excess lotion was removed, then the patient was instructed in cervical and upper quarter active range of motion exercise. The patient was encouraged to perform his home range of motion exercises each AM and PM.

Response: The patient reported immediate relief of his symptoms following the initial session of massage. He reported the ability to fully turn and bend his head and neck. The patient returned for two additional sessions of massage treatment and was educated as to postural habits that triggered his condition. He continued his range of motion exercises twice a day, added isometric strengthening exercises to his daily regimen and monitored his postural habits at work. His employer subsequently added once weekly visits by a massage therapist as an employee benefit.

The rehabilitation professional employs therapeutic agent modalities to create an optimum environment for tissue healing while minimizing the symptoms associated with the trauma or condition.

Discussion Questions

- What tissues were injured or affected?
- What symptoms were present?
- What phase of the injury-healing continuum did the patient present for care in?
- What are the therapeutic agent modality's biophysical effects (direct, indirect, depth, and tissue affinity)?
- What are the therapeutic agent modality's indications and contraindications?
- What are the parameters of the therapeutic agent modality's application, dosage, duration, and frequency in this case study?
- What other therapeutic agent modalities could be utilized to treat this injury or condition? Why? How?

mechanical techniques. The mechanical effects are always accompanied by some reflex effects. As the mechanical stimulus becomes more effective, the reflex stimulus becomes less effective. Mechanical techniques should be performed after reflexive techniques. This is not to imply that mechanical techniques are more aggressive forms of massage. However, mechanical techniques are most often directed at deeper tissues, such as adhesions or restrictions in muscle, tendons, and fascia.

Effects on Muscle

The basic goal of massage on muscle tissue is to "maintain the muscle in the best possible state of nutrition, flexibility, and vitality so that after recovery from trauma or disease the muscle can function at its maximum."[46] Muscle massage is done either for mechanical stretching of the intramuscular connective tissue or to relieve pain and discomfort associated with myofascial trigger points. Massage has been shown to increase blood flow to skeletal muscle, and thus to increase venous return.[13,47] It has also been shown to retard muscle atrophy following injury.[40] Massage has also been shown to increase the range of motion in hamstring muscles owing to the combined decrease in neuromuscular excitability and stretching of muscle and scar tissue.[11] Massage does not increase strength or bulk of muscle, nor does it increase muscle tone.

Effect on Skin

Effects of massage on the skin include an increase in skin temperature, possibly as a result of direct mechanical effects, and indirect vasomotor action. It has also been found that increased sweating and decreased skin resistance to galvanic current result from massage.

If skin becomes adherent to underlying tissues and scar tissue is formed, friction massage usually can be used to mechanically loosen the adhesions and soften the scar. Massage toughens yet softens the skin. It acts directly on the surface of the skin to remove dead cells that result from prolonged casting of 6 to 8 weeks.

The effect of massage on scar tissue is that it stretches and breaks down the fibrous tissue. It can break down adhesions between skin and subcutaneous tissue and stretch contracted or adhered tissue.

PSYCHOLOGIC EFFECTS OF MASSAGE

The psychologic effects of massage can be as beneficial to some patients as the physiologic effects. The "hands on" effect helps patients feel as if someone is helping them. A general sedative effect can be most beneficial for the patient. Massage has been shown to lower psycho-emotional and somatic arousal such as tension and anxiety.[28] The therapist's approach should inspire a feeling of confidence in the patient, and the patient should respond with a feeling of well being—a feeling of being helped.

MASSAGE TREATMENT CONSIDERATIONS AND GUIDELINES

The therapist must have the basic essential knowledge of anatomy and of the particular area being treated. The physiology of the area to be treated and the total function of the patient must be considered. There should be an understanding of the existing pathology so that the process by which repair occurs is known. The therapist needs a thorough knowledge of massage principles and skillful techniques, as well as manual dexterity, coordination, and concentration in the use of massage techniques. The therapist also needs to exhibit such traits as patience, a sense of caring for the patient's welfare, and courteousness both in speech and manner.

Perhaps the most important tools in massage therapy are the hands of the clinician. They must be clean, warm, dry, and soft. The nails must be short and smooth. Washing of the hands before and after treatment must take place for sanitary reasons. If the therapist's hands are cold, they should be placed in warm water for a short period. Rubbing them together briskly helps to warm them too.

Positioning is also important for the clinician. Correct positioning will allow relaxation, prevent fatigue, and permit free movement of arms, hands, and the body.

Indications and Contraindications for Therapeutic Sports Massage

Indications
  Increase coordination
  Decrease pain
  Decrease neuromuscular excitibility
  Stimulate circulation
  Facilitate healing
  Restore joint mobility
  Remove lactic acid
  Alleviate muscle cramps
  Increase blood flow
  Increase venous return
  Retard muscle atrophy
  Increase range of motion
  Edema
  Myofascial trigger points
  Stretching scar tissue
  Adhesions
  Muscle spasm
  Myositis
  Bursitis
  Fibrositis
  Tendinitis
  Revascularization
  Raynaud's disease
  Intermittent claudication
  Dysmenorrhea
  Headaches
  Migraines

Contraindications
  Arteriosclerosis
  Thrombosis
  Embolism
  Severe varicose veins
  Acute phlebitis
  Cellulitis
  Synovitis
  Abscesses
  Skin infections
  Cancers
  Acute inflammatory conditions

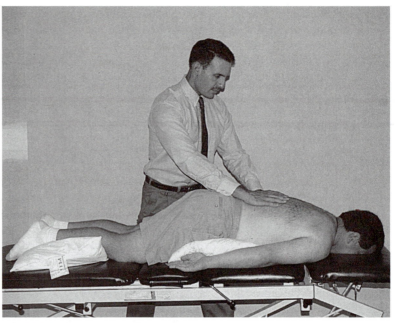

•**Figure 15-1** Position of therapist for stroking.

Good posture will also help prevent fatigue and backache. The weight should rest evenly on both feet with the body in good postural alignment. When massaging a large area, the weight should shift from one foot to the other. You must be able to fit your hands to the contour of the area being treated. A good position is required to allow the correct application of pressure and rhythmic strokes during the procedure (Fig. 15-1).

The following points are important to consider when administering massage.

1. Pressure regulation should be determined by the type and amount of tissue present. It must also be governed by the patient's condition and which tissues are to be affected. The pressure must be delivered from the body, through the soft parts of the hands, and it is adjusted to contours of the patient's body parts.

2. Rhythm must be steady and even. The time for each stroke and time between successive strokes should be equal.

3. Duration depends on the pathology, size of the area being treated, speed of motion, age, size, and condition of the patient. One also should observe the response of the patient to determine duration of the procedure. Massage of the back or the neck area might take 15 to 30 minutes. Massage of a large joint (such as a hip or shoulder) may require less than 10 minutes.

4. If swelling is present in an extremity, treatment should begin with the proximal part. The purpose of this is to help facilitate the lymphatic flow proximally. The subsequent effects of distal massage in removing fluid or edema will be more efficient since the proximal resistance to lymphatic flow will be reduced. This technique has been referred to as the "uncorking effect."

5. Massage should never be painful, except possibly for friction massage, nor should it be given with such force that it causes ecchymosis (discoloration of the skin resulting from contusion).

6. In general, the direction of forces should be applied in the direction of the muscle fibers (Fig. 15-2).

7. During a session, one should begin and end with effleurage. The maneuvers should increase progressively to the greatest energy possible and end by decreasing energy maneuvers.

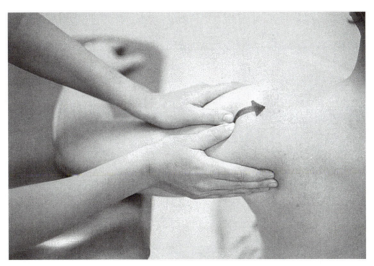

•**Figure 15-2** In the application of massage, forces should be applied in the direction of muscle fibers.

8. The therapist must consider the position in which massage can best be given and be sure the patient is warm and in a comfortable, relaxed position.

9. The body part may be elevated if this is necessary and possible (Fig. 15-3).

10. The therapist should be in a position in which the whole body, as well as hands and arms, can be relaxed and the procedure accomplished without strain (see Fig. 15-1).

11. Sufficient lubricant should be used so that the therapist's hands will move smoothly along the skin surface (except in friction). The use of too much lubricant should be guarded against.

12. Massage should begin with superficial stroking; this stroke is used to spread the lubricant over the part being treated.

13. Each stroke should start at the joint or just below the joint (unless massage over joints is contraindicated) and finish above the joint so that strokes will overlap.

14. The pressure should be in line with venous flow followed by a return stroke without pressure. The pressure should be in the centripetal direction (Fig. 15-4).

15. Care should be used over body areas. Hands should be relaxed and pressure adjusted to fit the contour of the area being treated.

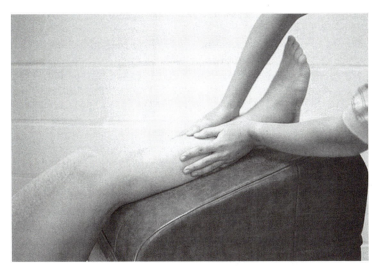

•**Figure 15-3** The part being massaged should be elevated.

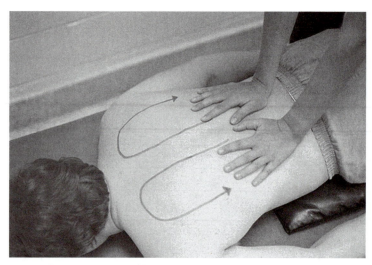

•**Figure 15-4** Massage pressure should be in line of venous flow followed by a return stroke without pressure.

16. Bony prominences and painful joints should be avoided if possible.
17. All strokes should be rhythmic. The pressure strokes should end with a swing off, in a small half circle, in order that the rhythm will not be broken by an abrupt reversal.

EQUIPMENT

Table

A firm table, easily accessible from both sides, is most desirable. The height of the table should be reasonably comfortable for the therapist; leaning over or reaching up to perform the required movements should not be necessary. An adjustable table is almost a must in this situation. To facilitate cleaning and disinfecting, a washable plastic surface is much preferred. There should be a storage area close by for linens and lubricant. If the table is not padded, a mattress or foam pad should be used for the comfort of the patient.

Linens and Pillows

The patient should be draped with a sheet, so only that part to be massaged is uncovered (Fig. 15-5). Towels should be handy for removing the lubricant. A cotton sheet between the plastic surface of the table and the patient is required to absorb perspiration and for patient comfort. The surface of the plastic material is generally too cool for comfort. Pillows should be available to support the patient.

Lubricant

Some type of lubricant should be used in almost all massage movements to overcome friction and avoid irritations by ensuring smooth contact of hands and skin. If the patient's skin is too oily, it may be desirable to wash the skin first.

The lubricant should be of a type that is absorbed slightly by the skin but does not make it so slippery that the clinician finds it difficult to perform the required strokes. A light oil is recommended for lubrication. One that works well is a combination of one part beeswax to three parts coconut oil. These ingredients should be melted together and allowed to cool (Fig. 15-6). It is best to use oil in situations in which (1) the clinician's or patient's skin is too dry; (2) a cast has recently been

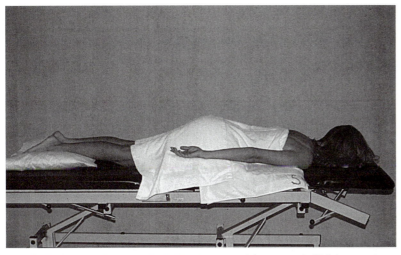

•**Figure 15-5** Draping of prone patient. Towels are used for removal of lubricants, sheets are used for draping, and pillows are placed under hips and ankles for patient comfort.

removed; (3) scar tissue is present; or (4) there is excess hair. Some types of oil that may be used are olive oil, mineral oil, cocoa butter, or hydrolanolin. The "warm creams" or analgesic creams are skin irritants and if used in conjunction with massage may cause a burn, depending on the skin type of the patient. These are also thought to cause blood to come to the surface of the skin, moving away from the muscles, which is exactly the opposite of what we are trying to accomplish through the massage techniques.

Alcohol may be used to remove the lubricant after massage. It is suggested that alcohol be placed in the clinician's hands before application to avoid the dramatic temperature drop that occurs when alcohol is applied directly to the patient.

Sometimes unscented powder should be used if the clinician's hands tend to perspire, or it may be used to prevent skin irritation.

Lubricant is not desired, nor should it be used, when applying friction movements, since a firm contact between the skin and hands of clinician must take place.

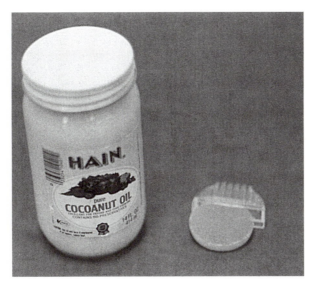

•**Figure 15-6** Example of lubricant to be used, beeswax and coconut oil.

PREPARATION OF THE PATIENT

The position of the patient is probably the most important aspect of ensuring a beneficial relaxation of the muscles from massage. The patient should be in a relaxed, comfortable position. Lying down, when possible, is most beneficial to the patient, and this also permits gravity to assist in the venous flow of the blood.

The part involved in the treatment must be adequately supported. It may be elevated, depending on the pathology. When the patient is being treated in the prone position, for massage of the neck, shoulders, back, buttocks, or back of the legs, a pillow or a roll should be placed under the abdomen. Another pillow should be placed under the ankles so that the knees are slightly flexed (see Fig. 15-5). If the patient is in the supine position, small pillows should be placed under the head and under the knees (Fig. 15-7).

Sometimes the prone position will be too painful for a patient to assume for massaging a shoulder, upper back, or neck. A position that may be more comfortable is sitting in a chair, facing the table while leaning forward and supported by pillows on the table. Forearms and hands are on the table for additional support (Fig. 15-8). The therapist can administer the massage while standing behind the patient (Fig. 15-8).

The body areas not being treated should be covered to prevent the patient from being chilled (see Fig. 15-5). Clothing should be removed from the part being treated. Towels should cover any clothes near the area being treated to protect them from the lubricant (see Fig. 15-5).

SPECIFIC MASSAGE TECHNIQUES

HOFFA MASSAGE

Albert Hoffa's text, published in 1900, provides the basis for the various massage techniques that have developed over the years.[21] Hoffa massage is essentially the classical massage technique that uses a variety of superficial strokes, including **effleurage, petrissage, tapotment,** and **vibration.** Although some clinicians consider this technique to be mechanical, the strokes may be lighter and more superficial, thus making them more reflexive in nature. This technique opens the door for more mechanical techniques that are directed toward underlying tissues.

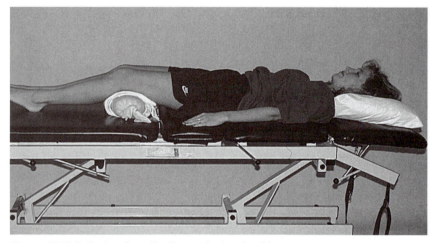

•**Figure 15-7** Patient supine with pillow under head and knees.

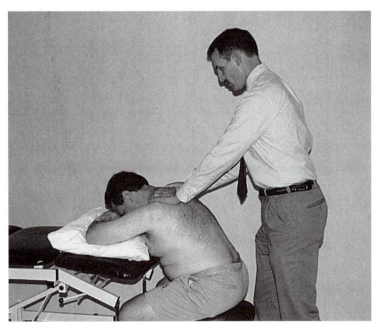

•**Figure 15-8** Patient resting in a chair facing table and leaning forward is supported by pillows on the table with forearms and hands on the table for support. Therapist stands behind the patient.

Effleurage

This massage maneuver glides over the skin lightly without attempting to move the deep muscle masses. The main physiologic effect occurs when stroking is begun at the peripheral areas and moves toward the heart. The return flow of the venous and lymphatic systems is probably helped by this process. Circulation to the skin surface also is increased by stroking; the success is traced to the increased rate of metabolic exchange in the peripheral areas.

The primary purpose of effleurage is to accustom the patient to the physical contact of the clinician. Initially effleurage serves to evenly distribute the lubricant. It also allows sensitive fingers to search for areas of muscle spasm or soreness and to locate trigger points and pressure points that can help in determining the type of procedures to be used during the massage.

At the start of the massage, the stroke should be performed with a light pressure, coming from the flat of the hand with fingers slightly bent and thumbs spread (Fig. 15-9). Once the unidirectional flow is established, going either centripetally or centrifugally, it should be continued throughout the treatment. Movement of the stroke should be toward the heart, and contact should be maintained with the patient at all times to enhance relaxation (Fig. 15-10).

Deep stroking massage is also a form of effleurage, except it is given with more pressure to produce a mechanical effect, as well as a reflexing effect (Fig. 15-11).

Every massage begins and ends with effleurage. Stroking should also be used between other techniques. Stroking relaxes, decreases the defensive tension against harder massage techniques, and has a generally mentally soothing effect.

effleurage To stroke; any stroke that glides over the skin without attempting to move the deep muscle masses.

Petrissage

Petrissage consists of kneading manipulations that press and roll the muscles under the fingers or hands. There is no gliding over the skin except between progressions

petrissage Massage technique that is a kneading manipulation.

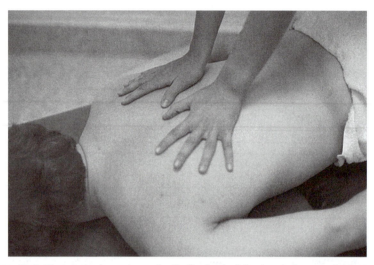

•**Figure 15-9** The stroke is performed with the heel of the hand, fingers slightly bent and thumbs spread.

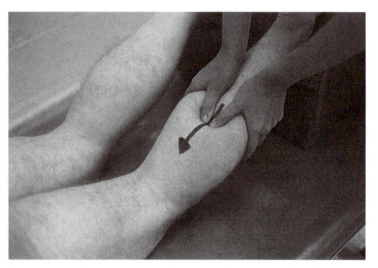

•**Figure 15-10** The kneading stroke is directed toward the heart, and contact should be maintained with the patient.

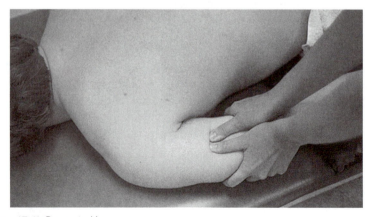

•**Figure 15-11** Deep stroking massage.

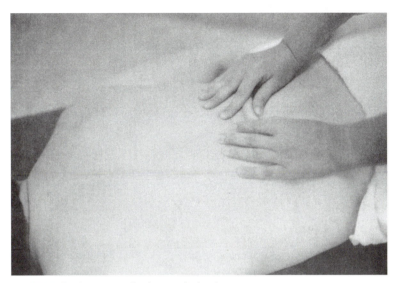

•**Figure 15-12** Petrissage application on the back.

from one area to another. The muscles are gently squeezed, lifted, and relaxed. The hands may remain stationary or may travel slowly along the length of the muscle or limb. The purpose of petrissage is to increase venous and lymphatic return and to press metabolic waste products out of affected areas through intensive, vigorous action. This form of massage can also break up adhesions between the skin and underlying tissue, loosen adherent fibrous tissue, and increase elasticity of the skin.

Petrissage can be described as a kneading technique. It is the repeated grasping, application of pressure, releasing in a lifting or rolling motion, then moving an adjacent area (Fig. 15-12). Smaller muscles may be kneaded with one hand (Fig. 15-13). Larger muscles, such as the hamstrings or muscle groups, will require the use of both hands (Fig. 15-14). When kneading, the hands should move from the distal to the proximal point of the muscle insertion grasping parallel to or at right angles to the muscle fibers (see Fig. 15-10).

Treatment Tip
In treating a tight muscle the therapist may choose to use a petrissage stroke that involves a deep kneading technique. Petrissage is often used to break up adhesions in the underlying muscle and also to assist the lymphatic system in removing waste from the area.

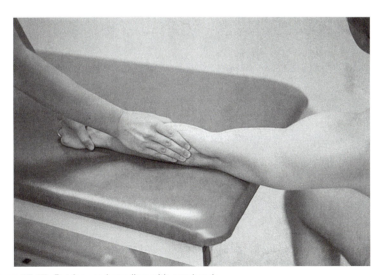

•**Figure 15-13** Petrissage kneading with one hand.

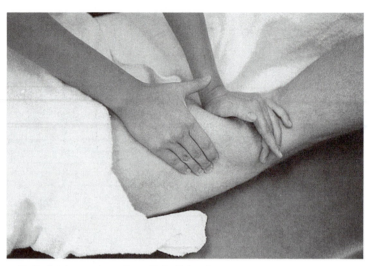

•**Figure 15-14** Petrissage kneading with both hands.

Tapotment or Percussion

tapotement A percussion massage; any series of brisk blows following each other in a rapid alternating fashion: hacking, cupping, slapping, beating, tapping, and pinching.

Percussion movements are a series of brisk blows, administered with relaxed hands and following each other in rapid alternating movements. This technique has a penetrating effect that is used to stimulate subcutaneous structures. Percussion is often used to increase circulation or to get a more active flow of blood. Peripheral nerve endings are stimulated so that they convey impulses more strongly with the use of percussion techniques.

Types of percussion techniques are hacking-alternate striking of patient with the ulnar border of the hand (Fig. 15-15); slapping-alternate slapping with fingers (Fig. 15-16); beating-half-closed fist using the hypothenar eminence of the hand (Fig. 15-17); tapping with the tips of the fingers (Fig. 15-18); and clapping or cupping using fingers, thumb, and palm together to form a concave surface (Fig. 15-19). Clapping or cupping is used primarily in postural drainage.

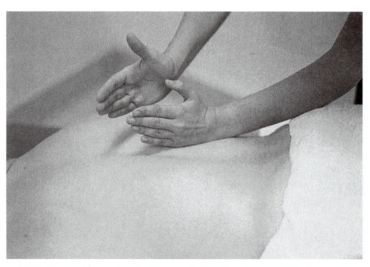

•**Figure 15-15** Percussion stroke of striking with the ulnar border of the hand.

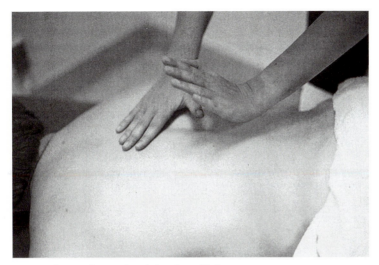

•**Figure 15-16** Percussion stroke of slapping with fingers.

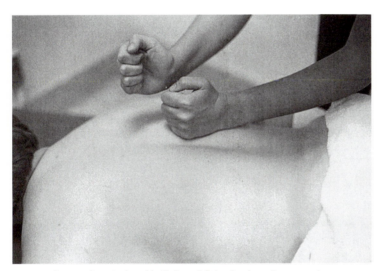

•**Figure 15-17** Percussion stroke of half-closed fist using hypothenar eminence.

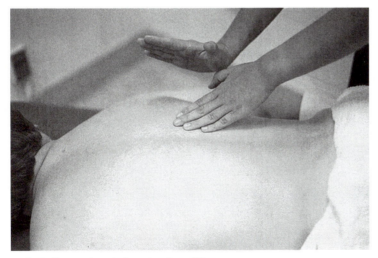

•**Figure 15-18** Percussion stroke using tips of fingers.

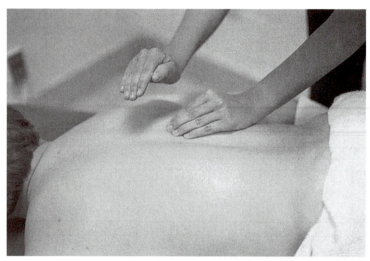

•**Figure 15-19** Percussion stroke of cupping using fingers, thumb, and palm together.

Vibration

Vibration technique is a fine tremulous movement, made by the hand or fingers placed firmly against a part; this causes the part to vibrate. The hands should remain in contact with the patient and a rhythmical trembling movement will come from the whole forearm, through the elbow (Fig. 15-20).

Routine

The following is an example of a massage progression or routine.

1. Superficial stroking
2. Deep stroking
3. Kneading
4. Optional friction or tapotement
5. Deep stroking
6. Superficial stroking

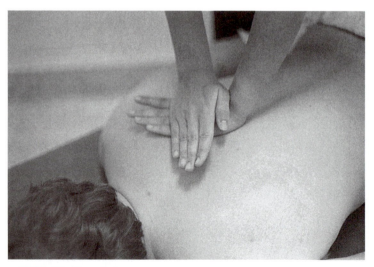

•**Figure 15-20** Vibration stroke.

The various individual classic massage techniques alone, however, do not make for a good massage. A proper program, intensity, tempo, and rhythm, as well as the proper starting, climax, and closing of the massage, are all important too. The form of the massage depends on the individual requirements of the patient.

Indications and Contraindications for Massage

The areas of treatment that we most often see patients for are muscle, tendon, and joint conditions. Adhesions, muscle spasm, myositis, bursitis, fibrositis, tendinitis or tenosynovitis, and postural strain of the back all generally fall into this category.

Areas of concern that indicate that you should not treat a patient with massage include arteriosclerosis, thrombosis or embolism, severe varicose veins, acute phlebitis, cellulitis, synovitis, abscesses, skin injections, and cancers. Acute inflammatory conditions of the skin, soft tissues, or joints are also contraindications.

FRICTION MASSAGE

James Cyriax and Gillean Russell have used a technique called deep **friction massage** to affect musculoskeletal structures of ligament, tendon, and muscle to provide therapeutic movement over a small area.[12] The purposes for friction movements are to loosen adherent fibrous tissue (scar), aid in the absorption of local edema or effusions, and reduce local muscular spasm. Inflammation around joints is softened and more readily broken down so that the formation of adhesions is prevented. Another purpose is to provide deep pressure over trigger points to produce reflex effects. This technique is performed by the tips of the fingers, the thumb, or the heel of the hand, according to the area to be covered, making small circular movements (Fig. 15-21). The superficial tissues are moved over the underlying structures by keeping the hand or fingers in firm contact with the skin (Fig. 15-22).

Transverse friction massage is a technique for treating chronic tendon inflammations.[12] Inflammation is an important part of the healing process. It must occur before the healing process can advance to the fibroblastic stage. In chronic inflammations, however, the inflammatory process "gets stuck" and never really accomplishes what it is supposed to. The purpose of transverse friction massage is to try and increase the inflammation to a point where the inflammatory process is com-

> **friction massage** A technique performed by small circular movements that penetrate into the depth of a muscle, not by moving the finger on the skin, but by moving the tissues under the skin.

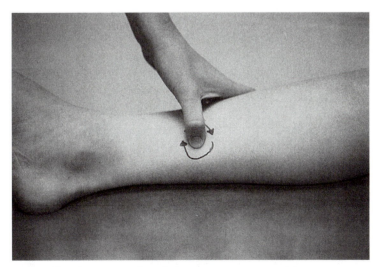

•**Figure 15-21** Thumb movement in a circle on an acupressure point.

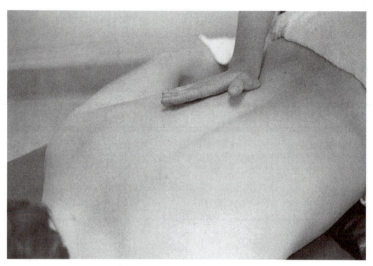

•**Figure 15-22** Superficial friction applied to the back by using the heel of the hand.

plete and the injury can progress to the later stages of the healing process. This technique is used most often in chronic overuse problems such as lateral or medial humeral epicondylitis, "jumper's knee," and rotator cuff tendinitis.

The technique involves placing the tendon on a slight stretch. Massage is done using the thumb or index finger to exert intense pressure in a direction perpendicular to the direction of the fibers being massaged (Fig. 15-23). The massage should last for 7 to 10 minutes and should be done every other day. Since transverse friction massage is a painful technique, it may help to apply ice to the treatment area prior to massage for analgesic purposes.

CONNECTIVE TISSUE MASSAGE

Connective tissue massage (Bindegewebsmassage) was developed by Elizabeth Dicke, a German physical therapist who suffered from decreased circulation in her right lower extremity for which amputation was advised. In trying to relieve her lower back pain, she massaged the area with pulling strokes. She found that with the

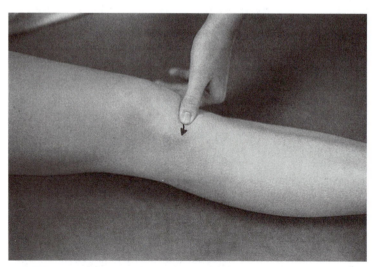

•**Figure 15-23** Transverse tendon friction massage on the patellar tendon.

continued stroking there was a relaxation of the muscular tension and a prickling warmth in the area. She continued the technique on herself, and after 3 months, she had no low back pain and she had restored circulation to her right leg.

Connective tissue massage is a stroking technique carried out in the layers of connective tissue on the body surface. This stimulates the nerve endings of the autonomic nervous system. Afferent impulses travel to the spinal cord and the brain, and this causes a change in reaction susceptibility.[34]

Connective tissue is an organ of metabolism; therefore, abnormal tension in one part of the tissue is reflected in other parts. All pathologic changes involve an inflammatory reaction in the affected part. One of the changes caused by inflammatory reaction is accumulation of fluid in the affected area. The area where these changes can most readily be detected is on the body surface. These changes are often seen as flattened areas or depressed bands that may be surrounded by elevated areas. The flat areas are the areas of main response and the connective tissue is tight, resisting pulling in any direction with movement.

The technique of connective tissue massage is not used as much in the United States as it is in European countries, especially Germany. As more results are seen, especially in the treatment of diseases associated with the pathology of circulation, this technique should become more widely accepted and used in this country.

General Principles of Connective Tissue Massage

Position of the Patient

The patient is usually in the sitting position for a connective tissue massage. Occasionally a patient may be treated in a sidelying or prone position when he or she cannot be treated in a sitting position.

Position of the Therapist

The therapist should be in a position, seated or standing, that provides good body mechanics, is comfortable, and avoids fatigue.

Application Technique

The basic stroke of pulling is performed with the tips, or pads, of the middle and ring fingers of either hand. Fingernails must be very short. The stroking technique is characterized by a tangential pull on the skin and subcutaneous tissues away from the fascia with the fingers. This technique should cause a sharp pain in the tissue. The stroke is a pull, not a push of the tissue. No lubricant is used. All treatments are started by the basic strokes from the coccyx to the first lumbar vertebra. Treatments last about 15 to 25 minutes. After 15 treatments, which are carried out two to three times per week, there should be a rest period of at least 4 weeks.

Other Considerations

Before any logical plan for treatment can be made, it is important to determine where any alterations in the optimum function of connective tissue have taken place, where the changes started, and, if possible, the cause of the alteration.

Evaluation is a most important part of an effective connective tissue massage program. The technique of stroking with two fingers of one hand along each side of the vertebral column will give much information about the sensory changes that are caused by alterations in the tension of surface tissues.

Indications and Contraindications

There are numerous arterial and venous disorders that may respond to connective tissue massage. Specific disabilities include: (1) scars on the skin; (2) fractures and arthritis in the bones and joints; (3) lower back pain, and torticollis in the muscles; (4) varicose symptoms, thrombophlebitis (subacute), hemorrhoids, and edema in the blood and lymph; (5) Raynaud's disease, intermittent claudication, frostbite, and trophic changes in the circulatory system. Connective tissue massage can also be used for myocardial dysfunctions, respiratory disturbances, intestinal disorders, ulcers, hepatitis, infections of the ovaries and uterus (subacute), amenorrhea, dysmenorrhea, genital infantilism, multiple sclerosis, Parkinson's disease, headaches, migraines, and allergies. Connective tissue massage is recommended to help in the process of revascularization following orthopedic complications such as fractures, dislocations, and sprains.

Contraindications to connective tissue massage include tuberculosis, tumors, and mental illnesses that result from psychologic dependence.

Connective tissue massage must be learned and performed initially under the direct supervision of someone who has been taught these highly specialized techniques. More detailed information about connective tissue massage can be found listed in the references.[15,29,42]

ACUPRESSURE AND TRIGGER POINT MASSAGE

acupressure The technique of using finger pressure over acupuncture points to decrease pain.

Acupressure is a type of massage based on the ancient Chinese art of acupuncture. Acupuncture, along with herbal medicine, composes traditional Chinese medicine. Only recently has the amount of research, publication, and interest in acupuncture in Western medical literature increased dramatically.

The Chinese make no distinction between arteries, veins, or nerves when explaining the functions of the body.[30] They concentrate instead on an elaborate system of forces whose interplay is thought to regulate all bodily functions. The traditional, philosophical Chinese explanation has little correlation with the more scientifically oriented Western concepts of medicine, which rely heavily on anatomic and physiologic principles. Consequently, utilization of acupuncture as a therapeutic technique in Western medical practice has encountered considerable skepticism.

The Chinese believe that an essential life force known as Qi (pronounced che) exists in everyone and controls all aspects of life. Qi is governed by the interplay of two opposing forces, the yang (positive) forces and the yin (negative) forces. Disease and pain result from some imbalance between the two.[31] The yin and yang flow through passageways or lines within the body called jing by the Chinese and known as meridians in the west. The twelve meridians within the body are named according to the part of the body with which they are associated. The meridians on one side of the body are duplicated by those on the other; however, two additional meridians exist that cannot be paired.[32]

1. Lung (L)
2. Large intestine (LI)
3. Stomach (ST)
4. Spleen (SP)
5. Heart (H)
6. Small intestine (SI)
7. Urinary bladder (UB)
8. Kidney (K)
9. Pericardium (P)
10. Triple warmet (TW)
11. Gall bladder (GB)
12. Liver (LIV)
13. Governing vessel (GV) (not paired)
14. Conception vessel (CV) (not paired)

Along these meridians lie the acupuncture points that are associated with each particular meridian. These points are named according to the meridian on which they lie. Whenever there is pain or illness, certain points on the surface of the body become tender.[32] When pain is eliminated or the disease is cured, these tender points seem to disappear.[1] According to acupuncture theory, stimulation of specific points through needling can dramatically reduce pain in areas of the body known to be associated with a particular point. Thousands of acupuncture points have been identified by the Chinese. In the Nei Ching, a classical text on Chinese medicine, 365 points that lie on the meridians have been enumerated.[23] Additional acupuncture points have been identified on the auricle as well as the hand.

There is some evidence for the actual physical existence of these points.[45] The electrical resistance of the skin at certain points corresponding to the acupuncture points is lower than that of the surrounding skin, especially when a disease state is present. Examining acupuncture points by sectioning indicated increased nerve endings at these points. Russian investigators have reportedly discovered differences in skin temperature at these points. Despite this evidence, there is no definite physical attribute of all acupuncture points nor is there a thoroughly demonstrated mode of action for the technique. Whatever the explanation, it appears that the locations and effects of stimulating specific acupuncture points for the relief of pain were determined empirically.[33]

In Western medicine, the counterpart of the acupuncture point is the **trigger point.** Trigger points may be found in skeletal muscle and tendons, in myofascia, in ligaments and capsules surrounding joints, in periosteum, and in the skin. Trigger points may activated and become painful because of some trauma to the muscle occurring either from direct trauma or from overuse that result in some inflammatory response.[44] Like acupuncture points, pain is usually referred to areas that follow as specific pattern associated with a particular point. Stimulation of these points has also been demonstrated to result in the relief of pain.[17]

Acupuncture and trigger points are not necessarily one and the same. However, a study by Melzack, Fox, and Stillwell attempted to develop a correlation coefficient between acupuncture and trigger points on the basis of two criteria: spatial distribution and associated pain patterns.[33] They found a remarkably high correlation coefficient of 0.84, which suggested that acupuncture and trigger points used for pain relief, although discovered independently, labeled by totally different methods, and derived from such historically different concepts of medicine, represent a similar phenomenon and may be explained by the same underlying neural mechanisms.[33]

Physiologic explanations of the effectiveness of acupressure massage may likely be attributed to some interaction of the various mechanisms of pain modulation discussed in Chapter 3.[1] There is considerable evidence that intense, low-frequency stimulation of these points triggers the release of β-endorphin.[37,39,42]

Acupressure Massage Techniques

By using acupuncture charts (Fig. 15-24) or trigger point charts specific points are selected, which are described in the literature as having some relationship to the area of pain.[44] The charts provide the therapist with a general idea of where these points are located. Two techniques may be used to specifically locate acupressure and trigger points. Since it is known that electrical impedance is reduced at these points, an ohmmeter may be used to locate the points. Perhaps the easiest technique is simply to palpate the area until either a small fibrous nodule or a strip of tense muscle tissue that is tender to the touch is felt.[6,9,10]

Once the point is located, massage is begun using the index or middle fingers, the thumb, or perhaps the elbow. Small friction-like circular motions are used on the point. The amount of pressure applied to these acupressure points should be determined by patient tolerance; however, it must be intense and will likely be painful to

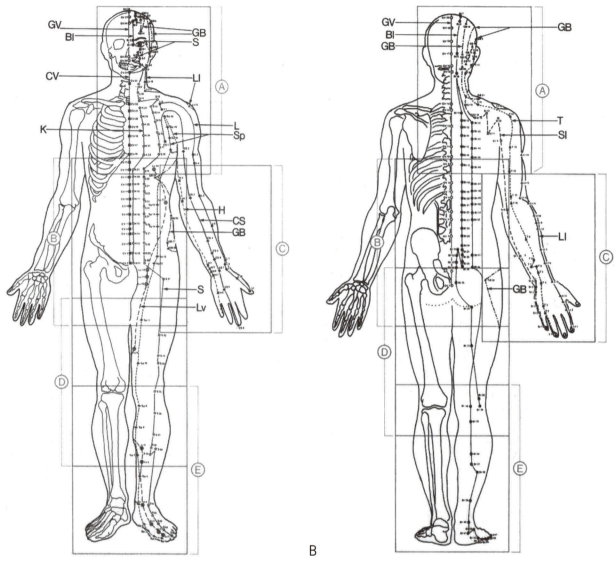

•Figure 15-24 Acupuncture point charts should be used to locate specific points.

the patient. Generally, the more pressure the patient can tolerate, the more effective the treatment.

Effective treatment times range from 1 to 5 minutes at a single point per treatment. It may be necessary to massage several points during the treatment to obtain the greatest effects. If this is the case, it is best to work distal points first and to move proximally.

During the massage, the patient will report a dulling or numbing effect and will frequently indicate that the pain diminishes or subsides totally during the massage. The lingering effects of acupressure massage vary tremendously from patient to patient. The effects may last for only a few minutes in some but may persist in others for several hours.

MYOFASCIAL RELEASE

Myofascial release is a term that refers to a group of techniques used for the purpose of relieving soft tissue from the abnormal grip of tight fascia.[24] It is essentially a form of stretching that has been reported to have significant impact in treating a

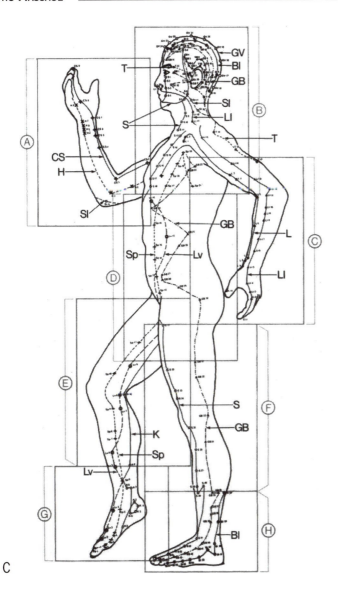

C

variety of conditions. Some specialized training is necessary for the therapist to understand specific techniques of myofascial release, in addition to an in-depth understanding of the fascial system.[2]

Fascia is a type of connective tissue that surrounds muscles, tendons, nerves, bones, and organs. It is essentially continuous from head to toe and is interconnected in various sheaths or planes. Fascia is composed primarily of collagen along with some elastic fibers. During movement the fascia must stretch and move freely. If there is damage to the fascia owing to injury, disease, or inflammation, it will not only affect local adjacent structures but may also affect areas far removed from the site of the injury. Thus it may be necessary to release tightness in both the area of injury as well as in distant areas.[24] It will tend to soften and release in response to gentle pressure over a relatively long period of time.[24]

Myofascial release has also been referred to as soft tissue mobilization, although technically all forms of massage involve mobilization of soft tissue. Soft tissue mobilization should not be confused with joint mobilization, although it must be emphasized that the two are closely related. Joint mobilization is used to restore normal joint arthrokinematics, and specific rules exist regarding direction of movement and

myofascial release A group of techniques used for the purpose of relieving soft tissue from the abnormal grip of tight fascia.

joint position based on the shape of the articulating surfaces. Myofascial restrictions are considerably more unpredictable and may occur in many different planes and directions. Myofascial treatment is based on localizing the restriction and moving into the direction of the restriction regardless of whether that follows the arthrokinematics of a nearby joint.[8] Thus, myofascial manipulation is considerably more subjective and relies heavily on the experience of the clinician.

Myofascial manipulation focuses on large treatment areas, whereas joint mobilization focuses on a specific joint. Releasing myofascial restrictions over a large treatment area can have significant impact on joint mobility.[18] Once a myofascial restriction is located, the massage should be directly through the restriction. The progression of the technique is from superficial to deep. Once more superficial restrictions are released, the deep restrictions can be located and released without causing any damage to superficial tissues. Joint mobilization should follow myofascial release and will likely be more effective once soft tissue restrictions are eliminated.

As the extensibility is improved in the myofascia, elongation and stretching of the musculotendinous unit should be incorporated. In addition, strengthening exercises are recommended to enhance neuromuscular reeducation, which helps promote new, more efficient movement patterns. As freedom of movement improves, postural reeduction may help to ensure the maintenance of the less restricted movement patterns.

Generally, acute cases tend to resolve in just a few treatments. The longer a condition has been present, the longer it will take to resolve. Occasionally dramatic results will occur immediately after treatment. It is usually recommended that treatment should be performed at least three times per week.[11]

Treatment Considerations

Protecting the Hands

The hands are the primary treatment modality in all forms of massage. Certainly, in myofascial release they are constantly subjected to stress and strain and consideration must be given to protection of the therapist hands. It is essential to avoid constant hyperextension or hyperflexion of any joints, which may lead to hypermobility. If it is necessary to work in deeper tissues where more force is necessary, then the fist or elbow may be substituted for the thumb and fingers.[8]

Use of Lubricant

It is necessary to use a small amount of lubricant, particularly if large areas are to be treated using long stroking movements. Enough lubricant should be used to allow for traction while reducing painful friction without allowing slipping of the hands on the skin.[8]

Positioning of the Patient

As with the other forms of massage, it is critical to appropriately position the patient such that the effects of the treatment may be maximized. Pillows or towel rolls may be a great aid in establishing and effective treatment position even before the hands contact the patient (Fig. 15-25). The therapist should make certain that good body mechanics and positioning are considered to protect the therapist as well as the patient.

ROLFING

Rolfing, also referred to as structural integration, is a system devised by Ida Rolf that is used to correct inefficient structure or to "integrate structure." The goal of this

---

Treatment Tip
To treat a myofascial trigger point a therapist could try several different techniques that have proven to be effective including circular pressure massage, a spray and stretch technique, or a combination of ultrasound and electrical stimulation.

Hands are the most important tool in massage.

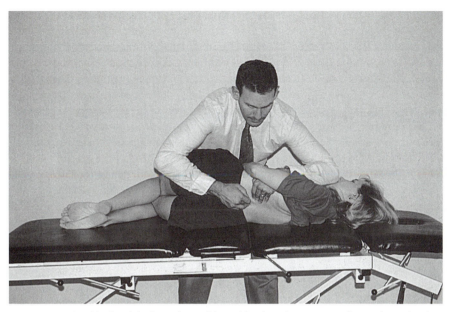

•Figure 15-25 Myofascial release is a mild combination of pressure and stretch used to free soft tissue restrictions.

technique is to balance to body within a gravitational field through a technique involving manual soft tissue manipulation.[8] The basic principle of treatment is that if balanced movement is essential at a particular joint yet nearby tissue is restrained, both the tissue and the joint will relocate to a position that accomplishes a more appropriate equilibrium.[38]

Rolfing is a standardized approach that is administered without regard to symptoms or specific pathologies. The technique involves 10 hour-long sessions, each of which emphasizes some aspect of posture with the massage directed toward the myofascia. The ten sessions include the following.

1. Respiration
2. Balance under the body (legs and feet)
3. Sagittal plane balance: lateral line from front to back
4. Balance left to right: base of body to midline
5. Pelvic balance: rectus abdominis and psoas
6. Weight transfer from head to feet: sacrum
7. Relationship of head to rest of body: occiput and atlas
8. **and 9.** Upper half of the body to lower half of the body relationship
10. Balance throughout the system

Once these ten treatments are completed advanced sessions may be performed in addition to periodic "tune-up" sessions.

A major aspect of this treatment approach is to integrate the structural with the psychological. An emotional state may be seen as the projection of structural imbalances. The easiest and most efficient method for changing the physical body is through direct intervention in the body. Changing the structural imbalances can alter the psychological component.[38]

Rolfing A system devised to correct inefficient structure by balancing the body within a gravitational field through a technique involving manual soft tissue manipulation.

TRAGER

Developed by Milton Trager, **Tragering** combines mechanical soft tissue mobilization and neurophysiological reeducation.[43] Unlike Rolfing, Trager has no standard-

Trager A technique that attempts to establish neuromuscular control so that more normal movement patterns can be routinely performed.

ized protocols or procedures. The Trager system uses gentle, passive, rocking oscillations of a body part. This is essentially a mobilization technique emphasizing traction and rotation as a relaxation technique to encourage the patient to relinquish control. This relaxation technique is followed by a series of active movements designed to alter the patient's neurophysiological control of movement, thus providing a basis for maintaining these changes. This technique does not attempt to make mechanical changes in the soft tissues but rather to establish neuromuscular control, so that more normal movement patterns can be routinely performed. Essentially it uses the nervous system to make changes rather than making mechanical changes in the tissues themselves.

SUMMARY

1. Massage, as we know it today, is an improved and more scientific version of the various procedures that go back thousands of years to the Greeks, Egyptians, and others.

2. Massage is the mechanical stimulation of tissue by means of rhythmically applied pressure and stretching. It allows the therapist, as a health care provider, to assist a patient to overcome pain and to relax through the application of the therapeutic massage techniques.

3. Massage has effects on the circulation, the lymphatic system, the nervous system, the muscles, myofascia, the skin, scar tissue, psychologic responses, relaxation feelings, and pain.

4. Hoffa massage is the classic form of massage and uses strokes that include effleurage, petrissage, percussion, or tapotement, and vibration.

5. Friction massage is used to increase the inflammatory response, particularly in cases of chronic tendinitis or tenosynovitis.

6. Massage of acupuncture and trigger points is used to reduce pain and irritation in anatomical areas known to be associated with specific points.

7. Connective tissue massage is a reflex zone massage. It is a relatively new form of treatment in this country and has its best effects on circulatory pathologies.

8. Myofascial release is a massage technique used for the purpose of relieving soft tissue from the abnormal grip of tight fascia.

9. Rolfing is a system devised to correct inefficient structure by balancing the body within a gravitational field through a technique involving manual soft tissue manipulation.

10. Trager attempts to establish neuromuscular control so that more normal movement patterns can be routinely performed.

REFERENCES

1. Baldry, P.E.: Acupuncture, trigger points and musculoskeletal pain, London, 1993, Churchill Livingstone.

2. Barnes, J.: Five years of myofascial release, Phys. Ther. Forum 6(37):12–14, 1987.

3. Barr, J., Taslitz, N.: Influence of back massage on autonomic functions, Phys. Ther. 50:1679–1691, 1970.

4. Birukov, A.: Training massage during contemporary sports loads, Soviet Sports Rev. 22:42–44, 1987.

5. Boone, T., Cooper, R., and Thompson, W.: A physiologic evaluation of the sports massage, Ath. Train. 26(1):51–54, 1991.

6. Brickey, R., Yao, J.: Acupuncture and transcutaneous electrical stimulation techniques, Course Manual in Acutherapy Post Graduate Seminars, Raleigh, North Carolina, 1978.

7. Cafarelli, E.: Vibratory massage and short-term recovery from muscular fatigue, Int. J. Sports Med. 11:474, 1990.

8. Cantu, R., Grodin, A.: Myofascial manipulation: theory and clinical applications, Gaithersburg, Maryland, 1992, Aspen.

9. Castel, J.: Pain management with acupuncture and transcutaneous electrical nerve stimulation techniques and photo stimulation (Laser), course manual, 1982.

10. Cheng, R., Pomerantz, B.: Electroacupuncture analgesia could be mediated by at least two pain relieving mechanisms: endorphin and non-endorphin systems, Life Sci. 25:1957–1962, 1979.

11. Crosman, L., Chateauvert, S., and Weisberg, J.: The effects of massage to the hamstring muscle group on range of motion, J. Orthop. Sport Phys. Ther. 6:168, 1984.

12. Cyriax, J., Russell, G.: Textbook of orthopedic medicine, vol. II., ed. 10, Baltimore, 1980, Williams & Wilkins.

13. Dubrovsky V.: Changes in muscle and venous blood flow after massage, Soviet Sports Rev. 18:134–135, 1983.

14. Ebel, A., Wisham, L.: Effect of massage on muscle temperature and radiosodium clearance, Arch. Phys. Med. 33:399–405, 1952.

15. Ebner, M.: Connective tissue manipulations, Malibar, Florida, 1985, R.E. Krieger.

16. Elkins, E.: Effects of various procedures on flow of lymph, Arch. Phys. Med. 34:31–39, 1953.

17. Fox, E., Melzack, R.: Transcutaneous electrical stimulation and acupuncture: comparison of treatment for low back pain, Pain 2:357–373, 1976.

18. Gordon, P.: Myofascial reorganization, Brookline, Massachusetts, 1988, The Gordon Group.

19. Harmer, P.: The effect of preperformance massage on stide frequency in sprinters, Ath. Train. 26(1):55–59, 1991.

20. Head, H.: Die Sensibilitatsstssstorungen der Haut bei viszeral Erkran Kungen, Berlin, 1898.

21. Hoffa, A.: Technik der massage, ed 14. Stuttgart, 1900, Ferdinand Enke.

22. Hungerford, M., Bornstein, R.: Sports massage, Sports Medm Guide 4:4–6, 1985.

23. Hwang Ti Nei Ching (translation), Berkeley, 1973, University of California Press.

24. Juett, T.: Myofascial release—an introduction for the patient, Phys. Ther. Forum 7(41):7–8, 1988.

25. King, R.: Performance massage, Champaign, Illinois, 1993, Human Kinetics.

26. Kopysov, V.: Use of vibrational massage in regulating the precompetition condition of weight lifters, Soviet Sports Rev. 14:82–84, 1979.

27. Kuprian, W.: Massage. In Kuprian, W., editor: Physical therapy for sports, Philadelphia, 1981, W.B. Saunders.

28. Longworth, J.: Psychophysiological effects of slow stroke back massage in normotensive females, Adv. Nurs. Sci. 10:44–61, 1982.

29. Licht, S.: Massage, manipulation and traction, New Haven, Connecticut, 1960, Elizabeth Licht.

30. Man, P., Chen, C.: Acupuncture aesthesia—a new theory and clinical study, Curr. Ther. Res. 14:390–394, 1972.

31. Manaka, Y.: On certain electrical phenomena for the interpretation of Chi in Chinese literature, Am. J. Chin. Med. 3:71–74, 1975.

32. Mann, F.: Acupuncture: the ancient Chinese art of healing and how it works scientifically, New York, 1973, Random House.

33. Melzack, R., Stillwell, D., and Fox, E.: Trigger points and acupuncture points for pain: correlations and implications, Pain 3:3–23, 1977.

34. Mennell, J.: Physical treatment, ed. 5, Philadelphia, 1968, Blakiston.

35. Morelli, M., Seaborne, P.T., and Sullivan, S.J.: Changes in H-reflex amplitude during massage of triceps surae in healthy subjects, J. Orthop. Sports Phys. Ther. 12(2):55–59, 1990.

36. Pemberton, R.: The physiologic influence of massage. In Mock, H.E., Pemberton, R., and Coulter, J.S., editors: Principles and practices of physical therapy, vol. I, Hagerstown, Maryland, 1939, W.F. Prior.

37. Prentice, W.: The use of electroacutherapy in the treatment of inversion ankle sprains, J. Nat. Athl. Train. Assoc. 17(1):15–21, 1982.

38. Rolf, I.: Rolfing: the integration of human structures, Rochester, Vermont, 1977, Healing Arts Press.

39. Sjolund, B., Eriksson, M.: Electroacupuncture and endogenous morphines, Lancet 2:1085, 1976.

40. Suskind, M., Hajek, N., and Hinds, H.: Effects of massage on denervated muscle, Arch. Phys. Med. 27:133–135, 1946.

41. Sullivan, S.: Effects of massage on alpha motorneuron excitability, Phys. Ther. 71:555, 1991.

42. Tappan, F.: Healing massage techniques: holistic, classic, and emerging methods, East Norwalk, Connecticut, 1988, Appleton & Lange.

43. Trager, M.: Trager psychophysical integration and mentastics, Trager J. 5:10, 1982

44. Travell J., Simons, D.: Myofascial pain and dysfunction: the trigger point manual, Baltimore, 1983, Williams & Wilkins.

45. Wei, L.: Scientific advances in Chinese medicine, Am. J. Chin. Med. 7:53–75, 1979.

46. Wood, E., Becker, P.: Beard's massage, Philadelphia, 1981, W.B. Saunders.

47. Wyper, D., McNiven, D.: Effects of some physiotherapeutic agents on skeletal muscle blood flow, Phys. Ther. 62:83–85, 1976.

SUGGESTED READINGS

Barnes, M., Personius, W., and Gronlund, R.: An efficacy study on the effect on myofascial release treatment technique on obtaining pelvic symmetry, Phys. Ther. 19(1):56, 1994.

Bean, B., Henderson, H., and Martinsen, M.: Massage: how to do it and what it can do for you, Scholastic Coach 52(5):10–11, 1982.

Beard, G., Wood, E.: Massage: principles and techniques, Philadelphia, 1964, W.B. Saunders.

Beard, G.: A history of massage technique, Phys. Ther. Rev. 32:613–624, 1952.

Beck, M.: Theory and practice of therapeutic massage, Albany, New York, 1994, Malidy.

Breakey, B.: An overlooked therapy you can use ad lib, RN 45:7, 1982.

Chamberlain, G.: Cyriax's friction massage: a review, J. Orthop. Sports Phys. Ther. 4(1):16–22, 1982.

Cyriax, J.: Textbook of orthopedic medicine, vol. I, ed. 8, New York, 1982, Macmillan.

Day, J., Mason, P., and Chesrow, S.: Effect of massage on serom level of β-endorphin and β-lipotrophin in healthy adults, Phys. Ther. 67:926–930, 1987.

Ebner, M.: Connective tissue massage, Physiotherapy 64:208–210, 1978.

Ehrett, S.: Craniosacral therapy and myofascial release in entry-level physical therapy curricula, Phys. Ther. 68(4):534–540, 1988.

Ernst, E., Matra, A., Magyarosy, I.: Massages cause changes in blood fluidity, Physiotherapy 73:43–45, 1987.

Fritz, S.: Fundamentals of therapeutic massage, St. Louis, 1995, Mosby.

Goats, G.: Massage: the scientific basis of an ancient art: Part 1. The techniques, Br. J. Sports Med. 28(3):149–152, 1994.

Goldberg, J., Seaborne, D., and Sullivan, S.: The effect of therapeutic massage on H-reflex amplitude in persons with a spinal cord injury, Phys. Ther. 74(8):728–737, 1994.

Hall, D.: A practical guide to the art of massage, Runner's World, 14(10):58–59, 1979.

Hammer, W.: The use of transverse friction massage in the management of chronic bursitis of the hip or shoulder, J. Man. Physiol. Ther. 16(2):107–111, 1993.

Hanten, W., Chandler, S.: Effects of myofascial release leg pull and sagittal plane isometric contract-relax techniques on passive straight-leg raise angle, JOSPT 20(3):138–144, 1994.

Hollis, M.: Massage for therapists, Oxford, England, 1987, Blackwell Scientific.

Hovind, H., Neilson, S.: Effect of massage on blood flow in skeletal muscle, Scand. J. Rehabil. Med. 6:74–77, 1974.

Kewley, M.: What you should know about massage, Int. Swim. September:29–30, 1982.

Kirshbaum, M.: Using massage in the relief of lymphoedema, Prof. Nurse 11(4):230–232, 1996.

Malkin, K.: Use of massage in clinical practice, Br. J. Nurs. 3(6):292–294, 1994.

Manheim, C., Lavett, D.: The myofascial release manual, Thorofare, New Jersey, 1989, Slack.

Martin, D.: Massage, Jogger 10(5):8–15, 1978.

McConnell, A.: Practical massage, Nurs. Times. 91(36):S2–14, 1995.

McKeechie, A.A.: Anxiety states; a preliminary report on the value of connective tissue massage, J. Psychosomat. Res. 27(2):125–129, 1983.

Meagher, J., Boughton, P.: Sportsmassage, New York, 1980, Doubleday & Co.

Morelli, M., Seaborne, D., and Sullivan, S.: H-reflex modulation during manual muscle massage of human triceps surae, Arch. Phys. Med. Rehabil. 72(11):915–999, 1991.

Morelli, M., Seaborne, P.T., and Sullivan, S.J.: H-reflex modulation during massage of triceps surae in healthy subjects, Arch. Phys. Med. Rehabil. 72:915, 1991.

Newman, T., Martin, D., and Wilson, L.: Massage effects on muscular endurance, J. Ath. Train. 31(Suppl):S-18, 1996.

Pellecchia, G., Hamel, H., and Behnke, P.: Treatment of infrapatellar tendinitis: a combination of modalities and transverse friction massage versus iontophoresis, J. Sport Rehabil. 3(2):135–145, 1994.

Phaigh, R., Perry, P.: Athletic massage, New York, 1984, Simon & Schuster.

Pope, M., Phillips, R., and Haugh, L.: A prospective randomized three-week trial of spinal manipulation, transcutaneous muscle stimulation, massage and corset in the treatment of subacute low back pain, Spine 19(22):2571–2577, 1994.

Rogoff, J.: Manipulation, traction and massage, ed. 2, Baltimore, 1980, Williams & Wilkins.

Ryan, J.: The neglected art of massage. Phys. Sports Med. 18(12):25, 1980.

Smith, L., Keating, M., and Holbert, D.: The effects of athletic massage on delayed onset muscle soreness, creatine kinase, and neutrophil count: a preliminary report, JOSPT 19(2):93–99, 1994.

Stamford, B.: Massage for patients, Phys. Sports Med. 13(10):178, 1985.

Steward, B., Woodman, R., and Hurlburt, D.: Fabricating a splint for deep friction massage, JOSPT 21(3):172–175, 1995.

Sucher, B.: Myofascial manipulative release of carpal tunnel syndrome: documentation with magnetic resonance imaging, J. Amer. Osteopath. Assn. 93(12):1273–1278, 1993.

Sucher, B.: Myofascial release of carpal tunnel syndrome, J. Amer. Osteopath. Assn. 93(1):92–94, 100–101, 1993.

Tappan, F.: Healing massage techniques: a study of eastern and western methods, Reston, Virginia, 1978, Reston Publishing.

Tiidus, P., Shoemaker, J.: Effleurage massage, muscle blood flow and long-term post-exercise strength recovery, Int. J. Sports Med. 16(7):478–483, 1995.

Trevelyan, J.: Massage, Nurs. Times 89(19):45–47, 1993.

van Schie, T.: Connective tissue massage for reflex sympathetic dystrophy: a case study, NZ J. Physiother. 21(2):26, 1993.

Wakim, K.G., Martin, G.M., and Terrier, J.C.: The effects of massage in normal and paralyzed extremities, Arch. Phys. Med. 30:135–144, 1949.

Weber, M., Servedio, F., and Woodall, W.: The effects of three modalities on delayed onset muscle soreness, JOSPT 20(5):236–242, 1994.

Wiktorrson-Moeller, M., Oberg, B., and Ekstrand, J.: Effects of warming up, massage and stretching on range of motion and muscle strength in the lower extremity, Am. J. Sports Med. 11:249–251, 1983.

Yates, J.: Physiological effects of therapeutic massage and their application to treatment, British Columbia, 1989, Massage Therapists Association.

acupressure The technique of using finger pressure over acupuncture points to decrease pain.

Bindegewebsmassage Reflex zone massage; uses a pulling stroke across connective tissue to effect change.

effleurage To stroke; any stroke that glides over the skin without attempting to move the deep muscle masses. The hand is molded to the part, stroking with more or less constant pressure, usually upward. Any degree of pressure may be applied, varying from the lightest possible touch to very deep pressure.

friction massage A technique that affects fibrositic adhesions in tendon, muscle, or ligament. It is performed by small circular movements that penetrate into the depth of a muscle, not by moving the finger on the skin, but by moving the tissues under the skin.

massage The act of rubbing, kneading, or stroking the superficial parts of the body with the hand or with an instrument for the purpose of modifying nutrition, restoring power of movement, or breaking up adhesions.

myofascial release A group of techniques used for the purpose of relieving soft tissue from the abnormal grip of tight fascia.

petrissage Massage technique that is a kneading manipulation. Consists of repeatedly grasping and releasing the tissue with one or both hands or parts thereof, in a lifting, rolling, or pressing movement. The outside characteristic of this movement as contrasted to stroking movements is that the pressure is applied intermittently.

Rolfing A system devised to correct inefficient structure by balancing the body within a gravitational field through a technique involving manual soft tissue manipulation.

tapotement A percussion massage; any series of brisk blows following each other in a rapid alternating fashion: hacking, cupping, slapping, beating, tapping, and pinchment. It is used when stimulation is the objective.

Trager A technique that attempts to establish neuromuscular control so that more normal movement patterns can be routinely performed.

vibration A shaking massage technique; a fine tremulous movement made by the hand or fingers placed firmly against a part that will cause the part to vibrate. Often used for a soothing effect; may be stimulating when more energy is applied.

LAB ACTIVITY

MASSAGE

DESCRIPTION:

Massage is most likely the oldest form of mechanical therapy for injury. Even very small children know that rubbing an injured area tends to diminish the pain. As with essentially all physical agents, the massage itself does not produce healing, but the therapeutic effects can assist during the healing process.

There are many types of massage, each with proponents and detractors. The different types of massage have different proposed physiological and therapeutic effects, although there is a great deal of overlap. In essence, all forms of massage involve the application of mechanical force to various tissues of the body, usually with the therapist's hands. Massage may exert an influence on the injured or dysfunctional tissue via either via a direct mechanical action or neurological reflexes.

PHYSIOLOGICAL EFFECTS:

Increase in large diameter afferent neural input
Increase in venous outflow
Increase in lymph outflow

THERAPEUTIC EFFECTS:

Decreased pain
Decreased soft tissue swelling and congestion
Remodeling of collagen

INDICATIONS:

The indications for massage vary depending on the type of massage used. In general, pain, swelling, and connective tissue contracture are the indications for massage.

CONTRAINDICATIONS:

There are probably no absolute contraindications to massage. Obviously, precautions should be used in the case of fractures, open wounds, and severe pain. The amount of pressure applied can be regulated based on the irritability of the tissue and the desired effect.

MASSAGE			
PROCEDURE	Evaluation		
	1	2	3
1. Check supplies.			
a. Obtain sheet or towels for draping.			
b. Obtain lubricant as indicated.			
2. Question patient.			
a. Verify identity of patient (if not already verified).			
b. Verify the absence of contraindications.			
c. Ask about previous massage treatments, check treatment notes.			

PROCEDURE	Evaluation		
	1	2	3
3. Position patient.			
a. Place patient in a well-supported, comfortable position. Positioning is particularly crucial for massage.			
b. Expose body part to be treated.			
c. Drape patient to preserve patient's modesty, protect clothing, but allow access to body part.			
4. Inspect body part to be treated.			
a. Check light touch perception.			
b. Check circulatory status (pulses, capillary refill).			
c. Verify that there are no open wounds or rashes.			
d. Assess function of body part (e.g., ROM, irritability).			
5a. Apply Hoffa massage			
a. After applying lubricant, effleurage is applied with a stroking motion from distal to proximal with light to moderate pressure; the deeper tissue is not moved. The initial strokes serve to distribute the lubricant over the treatment area.			
b. Petrissage is a kneading type motion, where the muscles are lifted and rolled.			
c. Tapotment is a series of percussion movements with the tips of the fingers, the ulnar border of the hands, the heel of the hands, or cupped hands.			
d. Vibration is a rapid oscillation or tremor of the hands when they are in firm contact with the skin.			
5b. Apply transverse friction massage.			
a. No lubricant is used.			
b. The tendon or ligament is placed on a slight stretch.			
c. Using deep pressure, such that the skin and thumb or finger, move together over the deeper tissue, apply a back-and-forth motion perpendicular to the fibers of the tendon or ligament.			
d. The duration of the massage should be up to 10 minutes, or as tolerated by the patient.			
5c. Apply connective tissue massage (Bindegewebsmassage).			
a. No lubricant is used.			
b. Using the tips of the third and fourth digits, the skin and subcutaneous tissues are pulled away from the fascia.			
c. The massage extends from the coccyx to the upper lumbar area, and each pulling stroke should produce a transient, sharp pain.			
d. Duration of treatment should be 15 to 25 minutes or as tolerated by the patient.			
5d. Acupressure/Trigger Point Massage.			
a. No lubricant is used.			
b. Technique is similar to transverse friction massage, but is applied to a trigger or acupuncture point (found using a chart, or by palpation). Trigger points usually are nodular-like lumps in a muscle, and often feel gritty.			

PROCEDURE	Evaluation		
	1	2	3
c. Using the tip of any digit, or even the olecranon process, the skin is moved on the trigger point; no motion should take place between the therapist and the patient's skin. The motion is circular, and is confined to the point.			
d. Pressure will be painful, and as hard as the patient can tolerate. The pressure may produce pain radiating to distant areas.			
e. Duration of the massage is between 1 and 5 minutes per point.			
6. Complete treatment.			
a. On completion of the massage, remove any lubricant with a towel.			
b. Remove material used for draping, assist the patient in dressing as needed.			
c. Have the patient perform appropriate therapeutic exercise indicated.			
d. Clean the treatment area and equipment according to normal protocol.			
7. Assess treatment efficacy.			
a. Ask the patient how the treated area feels.			
b. Visually inspect the treated area for any adverse reactions.			
c. Perform functional tests as indicated.			

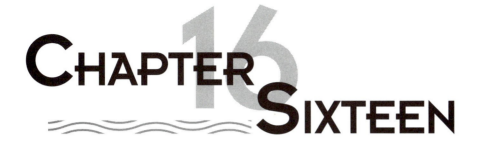

CHAPTER SIXTEEN

JOINT MOBILIZATION AND TRACTION

WILLIAM E. PRENTICE

OBJECTIVES

After completion of this chapter, the student therapist should be able to:

- ✓ Differentiate between physiological movements and accessory motions.
- ✓ Discuss joint arthrokinematics.
- ✓ Discuss how specific joint positions can enhance the effectiveness of the treatment technique.
- ✓ Discuss the basic techniques of joint mobilization.
- ✓ Identify Maitland's five oscillation grades.
- ✓ Discuss indications and contraindications for mobilization.
- ✓ Discuss the use of various traction grades in treating pain and joint hypomobility.
- ✓ Explain why traction and mobilization techniques should be used simultaneously.
- ✓ Demonstrate specific techniques of mobilization and traction for various joints.

Following injury to a joint, there will almost always be some associated loss of motion. That loss of movement may be attributed to a number of pathological factors, including contracture of inert connective tissue (e.g., ligaments and joint capsule); resistance of the contractile tissue or musculotendinous unit (e.g., muscle, tendon, and fascia) to stretch; or some combination of the two.[5,6] If left untreated the joint will become hypomobile and eventually begin to show signs of degeneration.[20]

Joint mobilization and *traction* are manual therapy techniques that are slow, passive movements of articulating surfaces.[7] They are used to regain normal active joint range of motion, restore normal passive motions that occur about a joint, reposition or realign a joint, regain a normal distribution of forces and stresses about a joint, or reduce pain, all of which will collectively improve joint function.[17] Joint mobilization and traction are two extremely effective and widely utilized techniques in injury rehabilitation.

THE RELATIONSHIP BETWEEN PHYSIOLOGICAL AND ACCESSORY MOTIONS

Osteokinematic movements = physiologic movement
Arthrokinematic motions = accessory motions

For the therapist supervising a rehabilitation program, some understanding of the biomechanics of joint movement is essential. There are basically two types of movement that govern motion about a joint. Perhaps the better known of the two types of movement are the physiological movements that result from either concentric or eccentric active muscle contractions that move a bone or joint. This type of motion is referred to as osteokinematic motion. A bone can move about an axis of rotation or a joint into flexion, extension, abduction, and rotation. The second type of motion is accessory motion. Accessory motions refer to the manner in which one articulating joint surface moves relative to another. Physiological movement is voluntary, whereas accessory movements normally accompany physiological movement.[2] The two occur simultaneously. Although accessory movements cannot occur independently, they may be produced by some external force. Normal accessory component motions must occur for full-range physiological movement to take place. If any of the accessory component motions are restricted, normal physiological cardinal plane movements will not occur.[14,15] A muscle cannot be fully rehabilitated if the joint is not free to move and vice versa.[20]

Physiologic Movements
• Flexion/extension
• Abduction/adduction
• Rotation

Traditionally in rehabilitation programs we have tended to concentrate more on passive physiological movements without paying much attention to accessory motions. The question is always being asked, "How much flexion or extension is this patient lacking?" Rarely will anyone ask "How much is rolling or gliding restricted?"

It is critical for the therapist to closely evaluate the injured joint to determine whether motion is limited by physiological movement constraints involving musculotendinous units or by limitation in accessory motion involving the joint capsule and ligaments. If physiological movement is restricted, the patient should engage in stretching activities designed to improve flexibility. Stretching exercises should be used whenever there is resistance of the contractile or musculotendinous elements to stretch. Stretching techniques are most effective at the end of physiological range of movement; they are limited to one direction, and they require some element of discomfort if additional range of motion is to be achieved. Stretching techniques make use of long lever arms to apply stretch to a given muscle.[9]

If accessory motion is limited by some restriction of the joint capsule or ligaments, the therapist should incorporate mobilization techniques into the treatment program. Mobilization techniques should be used whenever there are tight inert or noncontractile articular structures; they can be used effectively at any point in the range of motion, and they can be used in any direction in which movement is restricted. Mobilization techniques use a short lever arm to stretch ligaments and joint capsules, placing less stress on these structures, and consequently are somewhat safer to use than stretching techniques.[3]

JOINT ARTHROKINEMATICS

Accessory Motions
• Spinning
• Rolling
• Gliding

Accessory motions are also referred to as joint arthrokinematics, which include spin, roll, and glide (Fig. 16-1).[1,10,12]

Spin occurs around some stationary longitudinal mechanical axis and may be in either a clockwise or counterclockwise direction. An example of spinning is motion of the radial head at the humeroradial joint as occurs in forearm pronation/supination (see Fig. 16-1A).

Rolling occurs when a series of points on one articulating surface comes in contact with a series of points on another articulating surface. An analogy would be to

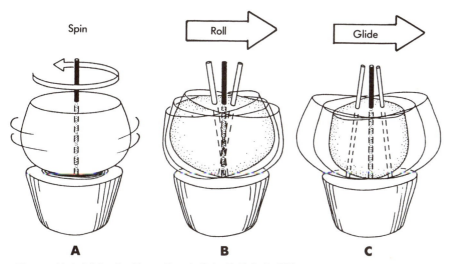

•**Figure 16-1** Joint arthrokinematics. A. Spin. B. Roll. C. Glide.

picture a rocker of a rocking chair rolling on the flat surface of the floor. An anatomical example would be the rounded femoral condyles rolling over a stationary flat tibial plateau (see Fig. 16-1B).

Gliding occurs when a specific point on one articulating surface comes in contact with a series of points on another surface. Returning to the rocking chair analogy, the rocker slides across the flat surface of the floor without any rocking at all. Gliding is sometimes referred to as translation. Anatomically, gliding or translation occurs during an anterior drawer test at the knee when the flat tibial plateau slides anteriorly relative to the fixed rounded femoral condyles (see Fig. 16-1C).

Pure gliding can occur only if the two articulating surfaces are congruent where either both are flat or both are curved. Since virtually all articulating joint surfaces are incongruent, meaning that one is usually flat while the other is more curved, it is more likely that gliding will occur simultaneously with a rolling motion. Rolling does not occur alone because this would result in compression or perhaps dislocation of the joint.

Although rolling and gliding usually occur together, they are not necessarily in similar proportion, nor are they always in the same direction. If the articulating surfaces are more congruent, more gliding will occur, whereas if they are less congruent, more rolling will occur.

Rolling will always occur in the same direction as the movement. For example, in the knee joint when the foot is fixed on the ground, the femur will always roll in an anterior direction when moving into knee extension and conversely will roll posteriorly when moving into flexion (Fig. 16-2).

The direction of the gliding component of motion is determined by the shape of the articulating surface that is moving. If you consider the shape of two articulating surfaces, one joint surface can be determined to be convex in shape, whereas the other may be considered to be concave in shape. In the knee, the femoral condyles are considered the convex joint surface, whereas the tibial plateau are the concave joint surface. In the glenohumeral joint, the humeral head is the convex surface, whereas the glenoid fossa is the concave surface.

This relationship between the shape of articulating joint surfaces and the direction of gliding is defined by the **Convex-Concave Rule**. If the concave joint surface is moving on a stationary convex surface, gliding will occur in the same direction as the rolling motion. Conversely, if the convex surface is moving on a stationary concave surface, gliding will occur in an opposite direction to rolling. Hypomobile joints

spin Occurs around some stationary longitudinal mechanical axis and may be in either a clockwise or counterclockwise direction.

rolling Occurs when a series of points on one articulating surface comes in contact with a series of points on another articulating surface.

gliding Occurs when a specific point on one articulating surface comes in contact with a series of points on another surface.

convex-concave rule Defines the relationship between the shape of articulating joint surfaces and the direction of gliding.

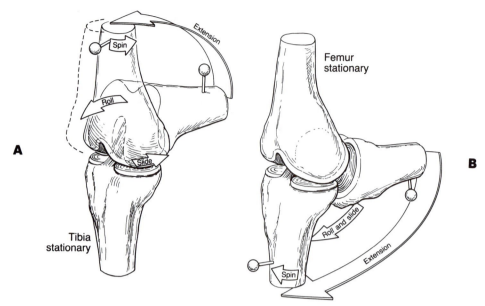

•**Figure 16-2** Convex-concave rule. A, Convex moving on concave. B, Concave moving on convex.

are treated by using a gliding technique. Thus it is critical to know the appropriate direction to use for gliding.

JOINT POSITIONS

loose-packed position The articulating joint surfaces are maximally separated.

Each joint in the body has a position in which the joint capsule and the ligaments are most relaxed, allowing for a maximum amount of **joint play**.[10,11] This position is called the resting position. It is essential to know specifically where the resting position is since testing for joint play during an evaluation, and treatment of the hypomobile joint using either mobilization or traction are both usually performed in this position. Table 16-1 summarizes the appropriate resting positions for many of the major joints.

Placing the joint capsule in the resting position allows the joint to assume a loose-packed position in which the articulating joint surfaces are maximally separated. A close-packed position is one in which there is maximal contact of the articulating surfaces of bones with the capsule and ligaments tight or tense. In a loose-packed position the joint will exhibit the greatest amount of joint play, whereas the close-packed position allows for no joint play. Thus the loose-packed position is most appropriate for mobilization and traction (Fig. 16-3).

close-packed position There is maximal contact of the articulating surfaces of bones with the capsule and ligaments tight or tense.

Both mobilization and traction techniques use a translational movement of one joint surface relative to the other. This translation may be in one of two directions; it may be either perpendicular or parallel to the treatment plane. The treatment plane falls perpendicular to, or at a right angle to, a line running from the axis of rotation in the convex surface to the center of the concave articular surface (Fig. 16-4).[10,11] Thus the treatment plane lies within the concave surface. If the convex segment moves, the treatment plane remains fixed. However, the treatment plane will move along with the concave segment. Mobilization techniques use glides that translate one articulating surface along a line parallel with the treatment plane. Traction techniques translate one of the articulating surfaces in a perpendicular direction to the treatment plane. Both techniques use a **loose-packed joint position**.[10]

TABLE 16-1
Shape, Resting Position, and Treatment Planes of Various Joints

Joint	Convex Surface	Concave Surface	Resting Position	Treatment Plane
Sternoclavicular	Clavicle*	Sternum*	Anatomical position	In sternum
Acromioclavicular	Clavicle	Acromion	Anatomical position, in horizontal plane at 60 degrees to sagittal plane	In acromion
Glenohumeral	Humerus	Glenoid	Shoulder abducted 55 degrees, horizontally adducted 30 degrees, rotated so forearm is in horizontal plane	In glenoid fossa in scapular plane
Humeroradial	Humerus	Radius	Elbow extended, forearm supinated	In radial head perpendicular to long axis of radius
Humeroulnar	Humerus	Ulna	Elbow flexed 70 degrees, forearm supinated 10 degrees	In olecranon fossa, 45 degrees to long axis of ulna
Radioulnar (Proximal)	Radius	Ulna	Elbow flexed 70 degrees, forearm supinated 35 degrees	In radial notch of ulna, parallel to long axis of ulna
Radioulnar (Distal)	Ulna	Radius	Supinated 10 degrees	In radius, parallel to long axis of radius
Radiocarpal	Proximal carpal bones	Radius	Line through radius and third metacarpal	In radius, perpendicular to long axis of radius
Metacarpophalangeal	Metacarpal	Proximal phalanx	Slight flexion	In proximal phalanx
Interphalangeal	Proximal phalanx	Distal phalanx	Slight flexion	In proximal phalanx
Hip	Femur	Acetabulum	Hip flexed 30 degrees, abducted 30 degrees, slight external rotation	In acetabulum
Tibiofemoral	Femur	Tibia	Flexed 25 degrees	On surface of tibial plateau
Patellofemoral	Patella	Femur	Knee in full extension	Along femoral groove
Talocrural	Talus	Mortise	Plantarflexed 10 degrees	In the mortise in anterior/posterior direction
Subtalar	Calcaneus	Talus	Subtalar neutral between inversion/eversion	In talus, parallel to foot surface
Intertarsal	Proximal articulating surface	Distal articulating surface	Foot relaxed	In distal segment
Metatarsophalangeal	Tarsal bone	Proximal phalanx	Slight extension	In proximal phalanx
Interphalangeal	Proximal phalanx	Distal phalanx	Slight flexion	In distal phalanx

*In the sternoclavicular joint the clavicle surface is convex in a superior/inferior direction and concave in an anterior/posterior direction.

JOINT MOBILIZATION TECHNIQUES

The techniques of joint mobilization are used to improve joint mobility or to decrease joint pain by restoring accessory movements to the joint and thus allow full, nonrestricted, pain-free range of motion.[16,23]

Mobilization techniques may be used to attain a variety of either mechanical or neurophysiological treatment goals: reducing pain; decreasing muscle guarding; stretching or lengthening tissue surrounding a joint, in particular capsular and ligamentous tissue; reflexogenic effects that either inhibit or facilitate muscle tone or stretch reflex; and proprioceptive effects to improve postural and kinesthetic awareness.[1,8,15,18,20]

Mobilization should be done in loose-packed position.

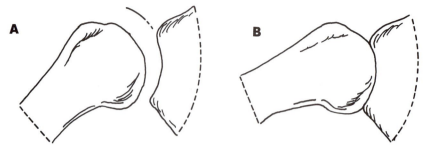

•**Figure 16-3** Joint capsule resting position. A. Loose-packed position. B. Close-packed position.

physiological movements Result from an active muscle contraction that moves an extremity through traditional cardinal planes.

accessory motions Refer to the manner in which one articulating joint surface moves relative to another.

Movement throughout a range of motion can be quantified with various measurement techniques. **Physiological movement** is measured with a goniometer and composes the major portion of the range. Accessory motion is thought of in millimeters, although precise measurement is difficult.

Accessory movements may be hypomobile, normal, or hypermobile.[4] Each joint has a range of motion continuum with an anatomical limit (AL) to motion that is determined by both bony arrangement and surrounding soft tissue (Fig. 16-5). In a hypomobile joint, motion stops at some point referred to as a pathological point of limitation (PL), short of the anatomical limit caused by pain, spasm, or tissue resistance. A hypermobile joint moves beyond its anatomical limit because of laxity of the surrounding structures. A hypomobile joint should respond well to techniques of mobilization and traction. A hypermobile joint should be treated with strengthening exercises, stability exercises, and, if indicated, taping, splinting, or bracing.[19,20]

In a hypomobile joint, as mobilization techniques are used into the range of motion restriction some deformation of soft tissue capsular or ligamentous structures occurs. If a tissue is stretched only into its elastic range, no permanent structural changes will occur. However, if that tissue is stretched into its plastic range permanent structural changes will occur. Thus, mobilization and traction can be used

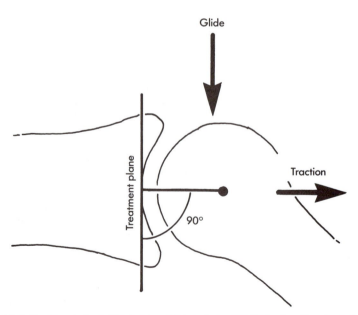

•**Figure 16-4** Treatment plane. The treatment plane is perpendicular to a line drawn from the axis of rotation to the center of the articulating surface of the concave segment.

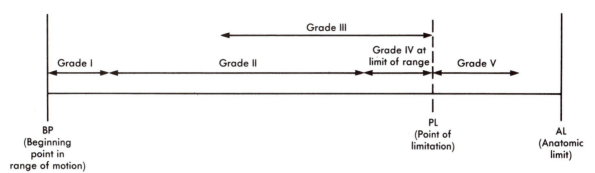

•**Figure 16-5** Maitland's five grades of motion. PL (point of limitation); AL (anatomical limit).

stretch tissue and break adhesions. If used inappropriately they can also damage tissue and cause sprains of the joint.[20]

Treatment techniques designed to improve accessory movement are generally slow, small-amplitude movements; the amplitude being the distance that the joint is moved passively within its total range. Mobilization techniques use these small-amplitude oscillating motions that glide or slide one of the articulating joint surfaces in an appropriate direction within a specific part of the range.

Maitland has described various grades of oscillation for joint mobilization. The amplitude of each oscillation grade falls within the range of motion continuum between some beginning point (BP) and the AL.[14,15] Figure 16-5 shows the various grades of oscillation that are used in a joint with some limitation of motion. As the severity of the movement restriction increases, the PL will move to the left, away from the AL. However, the relationships that exist among the five grades in terms of their positions within the range of motion remain the same. The five mobilization grades are defined as follows.

Grades I and II used for pain.

1. Grade I: A small-amplitude movement at the beginning of the range of movement. Used when pain and spasm limit movement early in the range of motion.[25]
2. Grade II: A large-amplitude movement within the midrange of movement. Used when spasm limits movement sooner with a quick oscillation than with a slow one or when slowly increasing pain restricts movement halfway into the range.

Grades III and IV used for stiffness.

3. Grade III: A large-amplitude movement up to the PL in the range of movement. Used when pain and resistance from spasm, inert tissue tension, or tissue compression limit movement near the end of the range.
4. Grade IV: A small-amplitude movement at the very end of the range of movement. Used when resistance limits movement in the absence of pain and spasm.
5. Grade V: A small-amplitude, quick thrust delivered at the end of the range of movement, usually accompanied by a popping sound, which is called a manipulation. Used when minimal resistance limits the end of the range. Manipulation is most effectively accomplished by the velocity rather than the force of the thrust.[21] Most authorities agree that manipulation should be used only by individuals trained specifically in these techniques, because a great deal of skill and judgment are necessary for safe and effective treatment.[22]

Joint mobilization uses these oscillating gliding motions of one articulating joint surface in whatever direction is appropriate for the existing restriction. The appropriate direction for these oscillating glides is determined by the Convex-Concave Rule described previously. When the concave surface is stationary and the convex surface is mobilized, a glide of the convex segment should be in the direction opposite to the restriction of joint movement (Fig. 16-6A).[10,11,24] If the convex articular surface is stationary and the concave surface is mobilized, gliding of the concave segment should be in the same direction as the restriction of joint move-

Joint manipulation should not be done by anyone who has not had specific training in this technique.

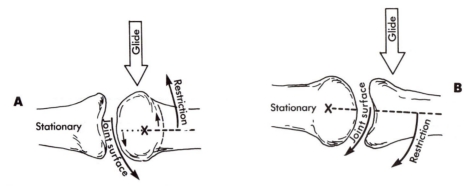

•**Figure 16-6** Gliding motions. A. Glides of the convex segment should be in the direction opposite to the restriction. B. Glides of the concave segment should be in the direction of the restriction.

Indications and Contraindications for Using Joint Mobilization and Traction

Indications
  Hypomobility
  Stiffness
  Joint contractures
  Joint pain
  ROM limitation

Contraindications
  Inflammatory arthritis
  Malignancy
  Bone disease
  Neurological involvement
  Bone fracture
  Congenital bone deformities
  Vascular disorders of the vertebral artery

ment (Fig. 16-6B). For example, the glenohumeral joint is considered a convex joint with the convex humeral head moving on the concave glenoid. If shoulder abduction is restricted, the humerus should be glided in an inferior direction relative to the glenoid to alleviate the motion restriction. When mobilizing the knee joint, the concave tibia should be glided anteriorly in cases where knee extension is restricted. If mobilization in the appropriate direction exacerbates complaints of pain or stiffness, the therapist should apply the technique in the opposite direction until the patient can tolerate the appropriate direction.[24]

Typical mobilization of a joint may involve a series of three to six sets of oscillations lasting between 20 and 60 seconds each, with one to three oscillations per second.[14,15]

INDICATIONS FOR MOBILIZATION

In Maitland's system, grades I and II are used primarily for treatment of pain, and grades III and IV are used for treating stiffness. Pain must be treated first and stiffness second.[15] Painful conditions should be treated on a daily basis. The purpose of the small-amplitude oscillations is to stimulate mechanoreceptors within the joint that can limit the transmission of pain perception at the spinal cord or brain stem levels.

Joints that are stiff or hypomobile and have restricted movement should be treated three to four times per week on alternating days with active motion exercise. The therapist must continuously reevaluate the joint to determine appropriate progression from one oscillation grade to another.

Indications for specific mobilization grades are relatively straightforward. If the patient complains of pain before the therapist can apply any resistance to movement, it is too early, and all mobilization techniques should be avoided. If pain is elicited when resistance to motion is applied, mobilization using grades I and II is appropriate. If resistance can be applied before pain is elicited, mobilization can be progressed to grades III and IV. Mobilization should be done with both the patient and the therapist positioned in a comfortable and relaxed manner. The therapist should mobilize one joint at a time. The joint should be stabilized as near one articulating surface as possible, while moving the other segment with a firm, confident grasp.

CONTRAINDICATIONS FOR MOBILIZATION

Techniques of mobilization and manipulation should not be used haphazardly. These techniques should generally not be used in cases of inflammatory arthritis,

CASE STUDY 16-1
JOINT MOBILIZATION

Background: An 18-year-old high school multi-sport athlete underwent a capsulabral repair of his right shoulder following a traumatic dislocation during a wrestling meet. Postoperative rehabilitation proceeded uneventfully. At 8 weeks shoulder range of motion was within normal limits with the exception of abduction, which was limited to 165 degrees and external rotation, which was limited to 75 degrees. Strength was assessed as 4/5 on the manual muscle test and functional upper extremity exercises were well tolerated.

Impression: Postoperative glenohumeral capsular restriction at extremes of range of motion.

Treatment Plan: A short course of mobilization was initiated for the right glenohumeral joint focused on increasing abduction and external rotation. Grade III/IV oscillations were applied to the anterior and inferior capsule for three 20-second bouts of mobilization per treatment session. Mobilization was applied on an every other day basis for 10 days. The patient continued dynamic strengthening exercises with emphasis on end range stability.

Response: At the conclusion of 2 weeks of treatment, the patient demonstrated full active and passive range of motion of the right shoulder and continued with strengthening activities for the shoulder girdle.

The rehabilitation professional employs therapeutic agent modalities to create an optimum environment for tissue healing while minimizing the symptoms associated with the trauma or condition.

Discussion Questions
- What tissues were injured or affected?
- What symptoms were present?
- What phase of the injury healing continuum did the patient present for care in?
- What are the therapeutic agent modality's biophysical effects (direct, indirect, depth, and tissue affinity)?
- What are the therapeutic agent modality's indications and contraindications?
- What are the parameters of the therapeutic agent modality's application, dosage, duration, and frequency in this case study?
- What other therapeutic agent modalities could be utilized to treat this injury or condition? Why? How?

malignancy, bone disease, neurological involvement, bone fracture, congenital bone deformities, and vascular disorders of the vertebral artery. Again, manipulation should be performed only by those therapists specifically trained in the procedure because some special knowledge and judgment are required for effective treatment.[24]

JOINT TRACTION TECHNIQUES

Traction refers to a technique involving pulling on one articulating segment to produce some separation of the two joint surfaces. Although mobilization glides are done parallel to the treatment plane, traction is performed perpendicular to the treatment plane (Fig. 16-7). Like mobilization techniques, traction may be used to either decrease pain or to reduce joint hypomobility.[26]

Kaltenborn has proposed a system using traction combined with mobilization as a means of reducing pain or mobilizing hypomobile joints.[9] As discussed earlier, all joints have a certain amount of joint play or looseness. Kaltenborn referred to this looseness as slack. Some degree of slack is necessary for normal joint motion. Kaltenborn's three traction grades are defined as follows (Fig. 16-8).

Traction and mobilization should be done in conjunction with one another.

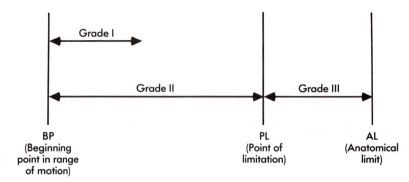

•**Figure 16-7** Traction versus glides. Traction should be perpendicular to the treatment plane, while glides are parallel to the treatment plane.

If movement is limited by tight muscles, stretching.

1. Grade I traction (loosen): Traction that neutralizes pressure in the joint without actual separation of the joint surfaces. The purpose is to produce pain relief by reducing the compressive forces of articular surfaces during mobilization and is used with all mobilization grades.
2. Grade II traction (tighten, or "take up the slack"): Traction that effectively separates the articulating surfaces and takes up the slack or eliminates play in the joint capsule. Grade II is used in initial treatment to determine joint sensitivity.
3. Grade III traction (stretch): Traction that involves actual stretching of the soft tissue surrounding the joint to increase mobility in a hypomobile joint.

If movement is limited by tight ligaments and joint capsule, traction and mobilization.

Grade I traction should be used in the initial treatment to reduce the chance of a painful reaction. It is recommended that 10-second intermittent Grades I and II traction be used, distracting the joint surfaces up to a Grade III traction and then releasing distraction until the joint returns to its resting position.

Kaltenborn emphasizes that Grade III traction should be used in conjunction with mobilization glides to treat joint hypomobility (Fig. 16-9).[10] Grade III traction stretches the joint capsule and increases the space between the articulating surfaces, placing the joint in a loose-packed position. Applying grade III and grade IV oscillations within the patient's pain limitations should maximally improve joint mobility (see Fig. 16-8).

MOBILIZATION AND TRACTION TECHNIQUES

Mobilization perpendicular to treatment plane.

Figures 16-10 through 16-73 provide descriptions and illustrations of various mobilization and traction techniques. These figures should be used to determine appropriate hand positioning, stabilization (S), and the correct direction for gliding (G), traction (T), and rotation (R). The information presented in this chapter should be used as a reference base for appropriately incorporating joint mobilization and traction techniques into the rehabilitation program.

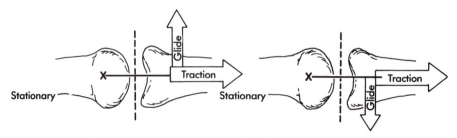

•**Figure 16-8** Kaltenborn's grades of traction. PL, point of limitation; AL, anatomical limit.

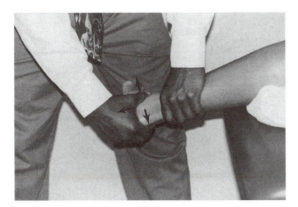

•**Figure 16-9** Traction and mobilization. Traction and mobilization should be used together.

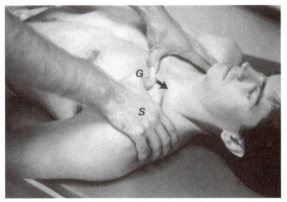

•**Figure 16-10** Posterior and superior clavicular glides. When posterior or superior clavicular glides are done at the sternoclavicular joint, use the thumbs to glide the clavicle. Posterior glides are used to increase clavicular retraction, and superior glides increase clavicular retraction and clavicular depression.

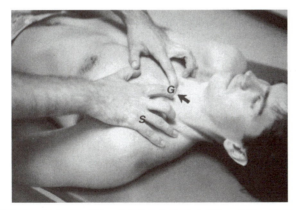

•**Figure 16-11** Inferior clavicular glides. Inferior clavicular glides at the sternoclavicular joint use the index fingers to mobilize the clavicle, which increases clavicular elevation.

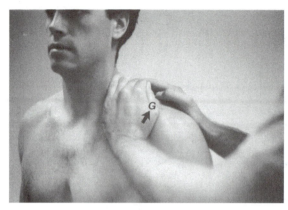

•**Figure 16-12** Posterior clavicular glides. Posterior clavicular glides done at the acromio-clavicular (AC) joint apply posterior pressure on the clavicle while stabilizing the scapula with the opposite hand. They increase mobility of the AC joint.

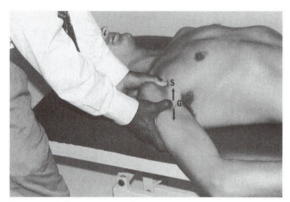

•**Figure 16-13** Anterior/posterior glenohumeral glides. Anterior/posterior glenohumeral glides are done with one hand stabilizing the scapula, and the other gliding the humeral head. They initiate motion in the painful shoulder.

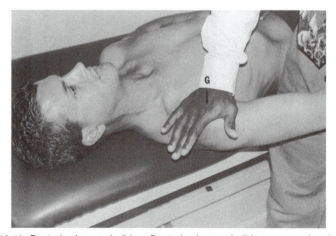

•**Figure 16-14** Posterior humeral glides. Posterior humeral glides use one hand to stabilize the humerus at the elbow and the other to glide the humeral head. They increase flexion and medial rotation.

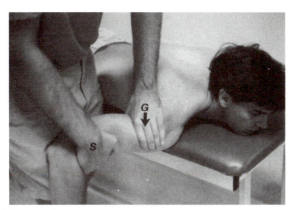

•**Figure 16-15** Anterior humeral glides. In anterior humeral glides the patient is prone. One hand stabilizes the humerus at the elbow, and the other glides the humeral head. They increase extension and lateral rotation.

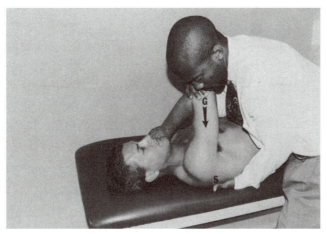

•**Figure 16-16** Posterior humeral glides. Posterior humeral glides may also be done with the shoulder at 90 degrees. With the patient in supine position, one hand stabilizes the scapula underneath while the patient's elbow is secured at the sports therapist's shoulder. Glides are directed downward through the humerus. They increase horizontal adduction.

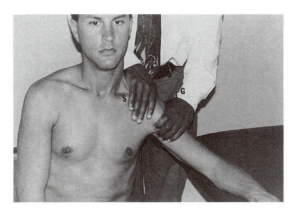

•**Figure 16-17** Inferior humeral glides. For inferior humeral glides the patient is in the sitting position with the elbow resting on the treatment table. One hand stabilizes the scapula, and the other glides the humeral head inferiorly. These glides increase shoulder abduction.

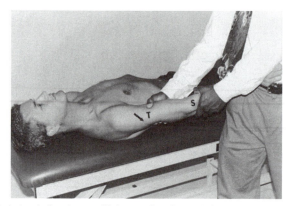

•**Figure 16-18** Lateral glenohumeral joint traction. Lateral glenohumeral joint traction is used for initial testing of joint mobility and for decreasing pain. One hand stabilizes the elbow while the other applies lateral traction at the upper humerus.

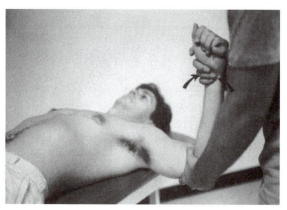

•**Figure 16-19** Medial and lateral rotation oscillations. Medial and lateral rotation oscillations with the shoulder abducted at 90 degrees can increase medial and lateral rotation in a progressive manner according to patient tolerance.

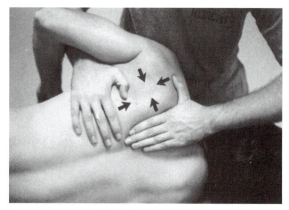

•**Figure 16-20** General scapular glides. General scapular glides may be done in all directions, applying pressure at either the medial, inferior, lateral, or superior border of the scapula. Scapular glides increase general scapulothoracic mobility.

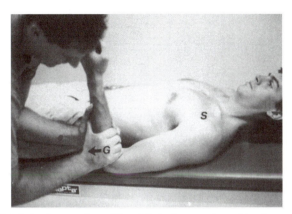

•**Figure 16-21** Inferior humeroulnar glides. Inferior humeroulnar glides increase elbow flexion and extension. They are performed using the body weight to stabilize proximally with the hand grasping the ulna and gliding inferiorly.

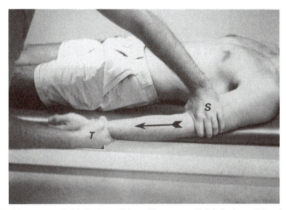

•**Figure 16-22** Humeroradial inferior glides. Humeroradial inferior glides increase the joint space and improve flexion and extension. One hand stabilizes the humerus above the elbow; the other grasps the distal forearm and glides the radius inferiorly.

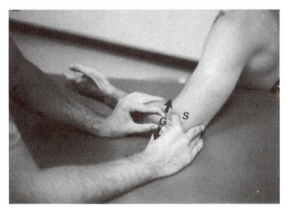

•**Figure 16-23** Proximal anterior/posterior radial glides. Proximal anterior/posterior radial glides use the thumbs and index fingers to glide the radial head. Anterior glides increase flexion, whereas posterior glides increase extension.

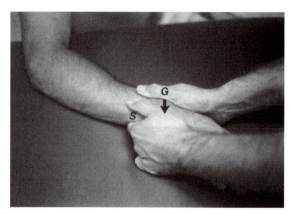

•**Figure 16-24** Distal anterior/posterior radial glides. Distal anterior/posterior radial glides are done with one hand stabilizing the ulna and the other gliding the radius. These glides increase pronation.

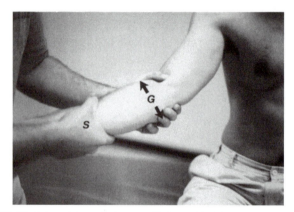

•**Figure 16-25** Medial and lateral ulnar oscillations. Medial and lateral ulnar oscillations increase flexion and extension. Valgus and varus forces are used with a short lever arm.

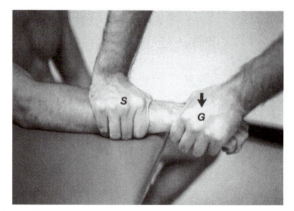

•**Figure 16-26** Radiocarpal joint anterior glides. Radiocarpal joint anterior glides increase wrist extension.

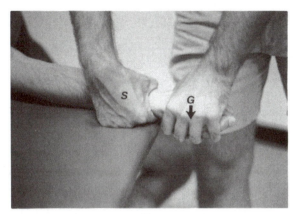

•**Figure 16-27** Radiocarpal joint posterior glides. Radiocarpal joint posterior glides increase wrist flexion.

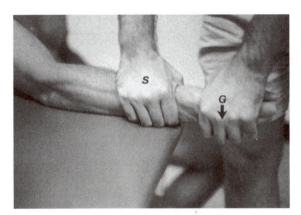

•**Figure 16-28** Radiocarpal joint ulnar glides. Radiocarpal joint ulnar glides increase radial deviation.

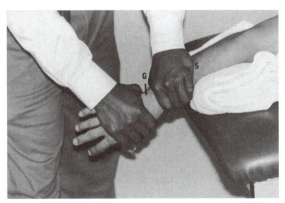

•**Figure 16-29** Radiocarpal joint radial glides. Radiocarpal joint radial glides increase ulnar deviation.

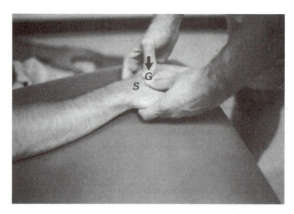

•**Figure 16-30** Carpometacarpal joint anterior/posterior glides. Carpometacarpal joint anterior/posterior glides increase mobility of the hand.

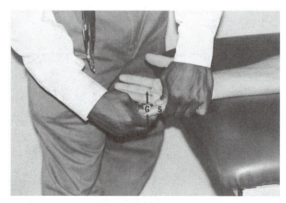

•**Figure 16-31** Metacarpophalangeal joint anterior/posterior glides. In metacarpophalangeal joint anterior or posterior glides, the proximal segment, in this case the metacarpal, is stabilized and the distal segment is mobilized. Anterior glides increase flexion of the MP joint. Posterior glides increase extension.

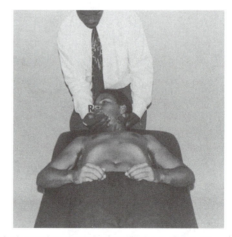

•**Figure 16-32** Cervical vertebrae rotation oscillations. Cervical vertebrae rotation oscillations are done with one hand supporting the weight of the head and the other rotating the head in the direction of the restriction. These oscillations treat pain or stiffness when there is some resistance in the same direction as the rotation.

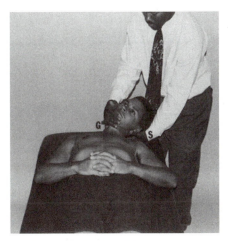

•**Figure 16-33** Cervical vertebrae sidebending. Cervical vertebrae sidebending may be used to treat pain or stiffness with resistance when sidebending the neck.

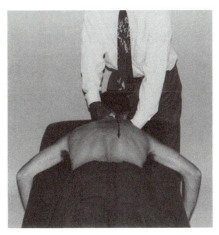

•**Figure 16-34** Unilateral cervical facet anterior/posterior glides. Unilateral cervical facet anterior/posterior glides are done using pressure from the thumbs over individual facets. They increase rotation or flexion of the neck toward the side where the technique is used.

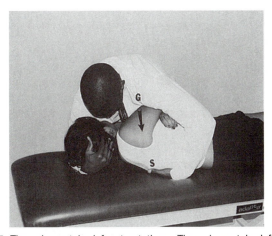

•**Figure 16-35** Thoracic vertebral facet rotations. Thoracic vertebral facet rotations are accomplished with one hand underneath the patient providing stabilization and the weight of the body pressing downward through the rib cage to rotate an individual thoracic vertebra. Rotation of the thoracic vertebrae is minimal, and most of the movement with this mobilization involves the rib facet joint.

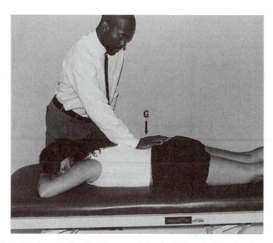

•**Figure 16-36** Anterior/posterior lumbar vertebral glides. In the lumbar region, anterior/posterior lumbar vertebral glides may be accomplished at individual segments using pressure on the spinous process through the pisiform in the hand. These decrease pain or increase mobility of individual lumbar vertebrae.

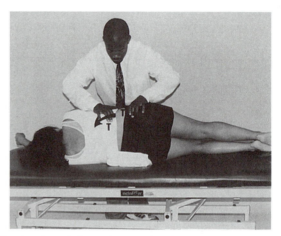

•**Figure 16-37** Lumbar lateral distraction. Lumbar lateral distraction increases the space between transverse process and increases the opening of the intervertebral foramen. This position is achieved by lying over a support, flexing the patient's upper knee to a point where there is gapping in the appropriate spinal segment, then rotating the upper trunk to place the segment in a close-packed position. Then finger and forearm pressure are used to separate individual spaces. This pressure is used for reducing pain in the lumbar vertebrae associated with some compression of a spinal nerve.

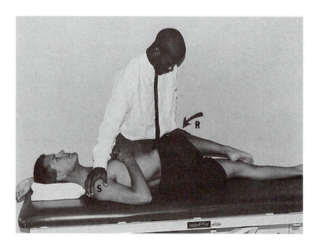

•**Figure 16-38** Lumbar vertebral rotations. Lumbar vertebral rotations decrease pain and increase mobility in lumbar vertebrae. These rotations should be done in a sidelying position.

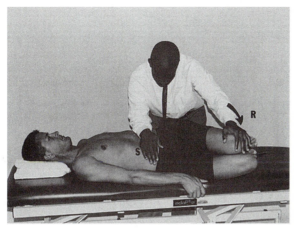

•**Figure 16-39** Lateral lumbar rotations. Lateral lumbar rotations may be done with the patient in supine position. In this position, one hand must stabilize the upper trunk, while the other produces rotation.

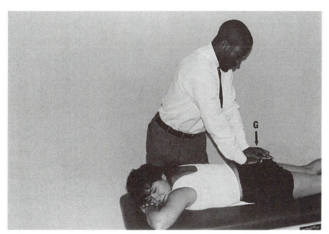

•**Figure 16-40** Anterior sacral glides. Anterior sacral glides decrease pain and reduce muscle guarding around the sacroiliac joint.

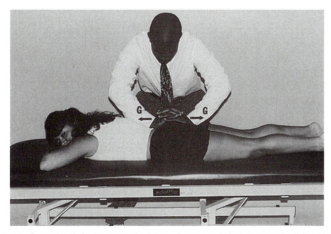

•**Figure 16-41** Superior/inferior sacral glides. Superior/inferior sacral glides decrease pain and reduce muscle guarding around the sacroiliac joint.

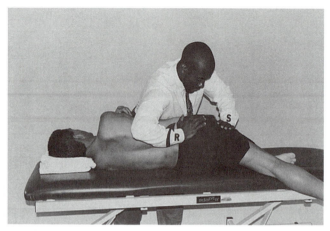

•**Figure 16-42** Anterior innominate rotation. An anterior innominate rotation in a sidelying position is accomplished by extending the leg on the affected side then stabilizing with one hand on the front of the thigh while the other applies pressure anteriorly over the posterosuperior iliac spine to produce an anterior rotation. This technique will correct a unilateral posterior rotation.

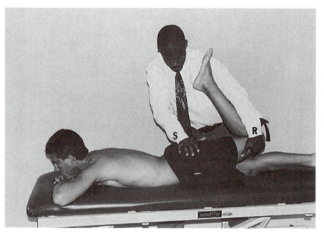

•**Figure 16-43** Anterior innominate rotation. An anterior innominate rotation may also be accomplished by extending the hip, applying upward force on the upper thigh, and stabilizing over the posterosuperior iliac spine. Once again, this technique is used to correct a posterior unilateral innominate rotation.

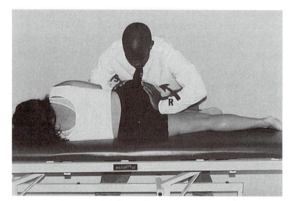

•**Figure 16-44** Posterior innominate rotation. A posterior innominate rotation with the patient in sidelying position is done by flexing the hip, stabilizing the anterosuperior iliac spine, and applying pressure to the ischium in an anterior direction.

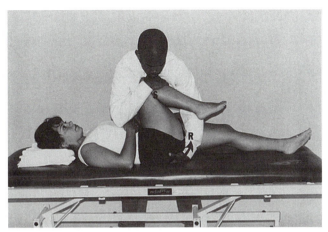

•**Figure 16-45** Posterior innominate rotation. Another posterior innominate rotation with the hip flexed at 90 degrees stabilizes the knee and rotates the innominate anteriorly through upward pressure on the ischium.

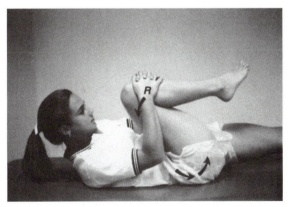

•**Figure 16-46** Posterior innominate rotation self-mobilization (supine). Posterior innominate rotation may be easily accomplished using self-mobilization. In a supine position the patient grasps behind the flexed knee and gently rocks the innominate in a posterior direction.

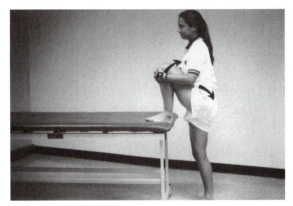

•**Figure 16-47** Posterior rotation self-mobilization (standing). In a standing position the patient can perform a posterior rotation self-mobilization by pulling on the knee and rocking forward.

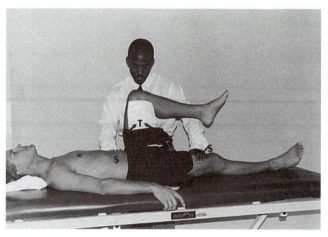

•**Figure 16-48** Lateral hip traction. Since the hip is a very strong, stable joint, it may be necessary to use body weight to produce effective joint mobilization or traction. An example of this would be in lateral hip traction. One strap should be used to secure the patient to the treatment table. A second strap is secured around the patient's thigh and around the therapist's hips. Lateral traction is applied to the femur by leaning back away from the patient. This technique is used to reduce pain and increase hip mobility.

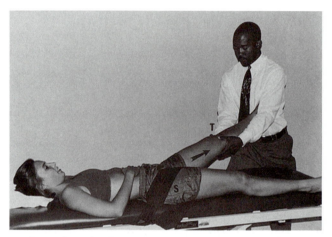

•**Figure 16-49** Femoral traction. Femoral traction with the hip at 0 degrees reduces pain and increases hip mobility. Inferior femoral glides in this position should be used to increase flexion and abduction.

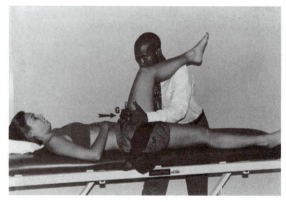

•**Figure 16-50** Inferior femoral glides. Inferior femoral glides at 90 degrees of hip flexion may also be used to increase abduction and flexion.

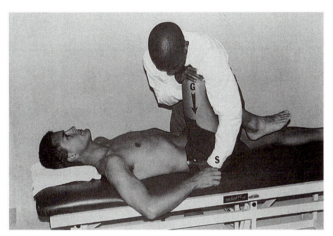

•**Figure 16-51** Posterior femoral glides. With the patient supine, a posterior femoral glide can be done by stabilizing underneath the pelvis and using the body weight applied through the femur to glide posteriorly. Posterior glides are used to increase hip flexion.

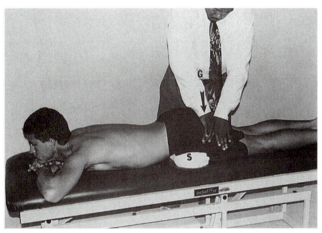

•**Figure 16-52** Anterior femoral glides. Anterior femoral glides increase extension and are accomplished by using some support to stabilize under the pelvis and applying an anterior glide posteriorly on the femur.

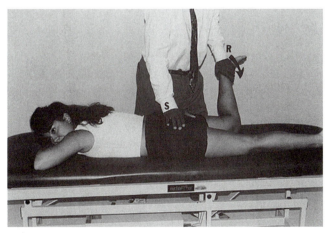

•**Figure 16-53** Medial femoral rotations. Medial femoral rotations may be used for increasing medial rotation and are done by stabilizing the opposite innominate while internally rotating the hip through the flexed knee.

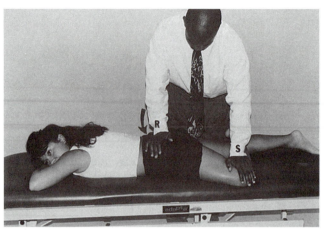

•**Figure 16-54** Lateral femoral rotation. Lateral femoral rotation is done by stabilizing a bent knee in the figure 4 position and applying rotational force to the ischium. This technique increases lateral femoral rotation.

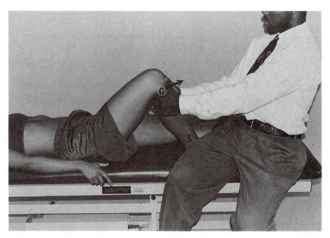

•**Figure 16-55** Anterior tibial glides. Anterior tibial glides are appropriate for the patient lacking full extension. Anterior glides should be done in prone position with the femur stabilized. Pressure is applied to the posterior tibia to glide anteriorly.

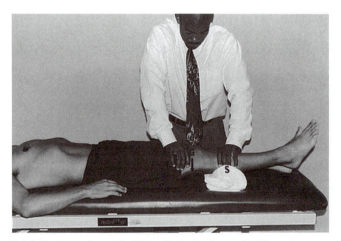

•**Figure 16-56** Posterior femoral glides. Posterior femoral glides are appropriate for the patient lacking full extension. Posterior femoral glides should be done in supine position with the tibia stabilized. Pressure is applied to the anterior femur to glide posteriorly.

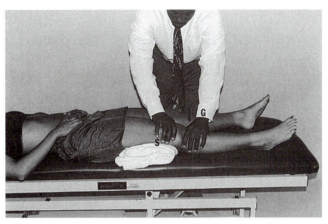

•**Figure 16-57** Posterior tibial glides. Posterior tibial glides increase flexion. With the patient in a supine position, stabilize the femur, and glide the tibia posteriorly.

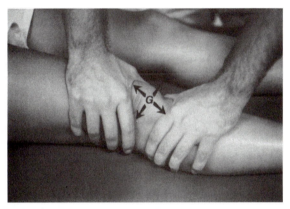

•**Figure 16-58** Patellar glides. Superior patellar glides increase knee extension. Inferior glides increase knee flexion. Medial glides stretch the lateral retinaculum. Lateral glides stretch tight medial structures.

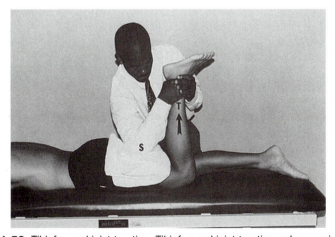

•**Figure 16-59** Tibiofemoral joint traction. Tibiofemoral joint traction reduces pain and hypomobility. It may be done with the patient prone and the knee flexed at 90 degrees. The elbow should stabilize the thigh while traction is applied through the tibia.

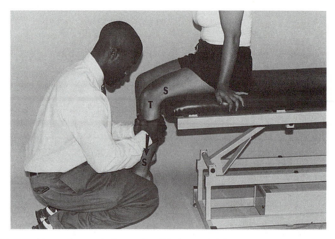

•**Figure 16-60** Alternative techniques for tibiofemoral joint traction. In very large individuals an alternative technique for tibiofemoral joint traction uses body weight of the sports therapist to distract the joint once again for reducing pain and hypomobility.

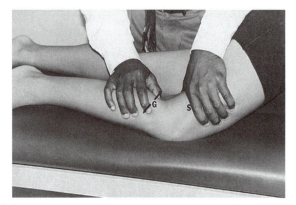

•**Figure 16-61** Proximal anterior and posterior glides of the fibula. Anterior and posterior glides of the fibula may be accomplished proximally. They increase mobility of the fibular head and reduce pain. The femur should be stabilized. With the knee slightly flexed, grasp the head of the femur, and glide it both anteriorly and posteriorly.

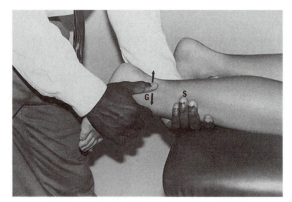

•**Figure 16-62** Distal anterior and posterior fibular glides. Anterior and posterior glides of the fibula may be accomplished distally. The tibia should be stabilized, and the fibular malleolus is mobilized in an anterior or posterior direction.

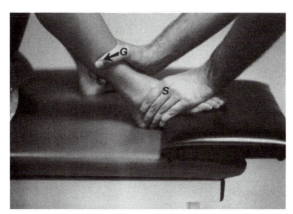

•Figure 16-63 Posterior tibial glides. Posterior tibial glides increase plantarflexion. The foot should be stabilized, and pressure on the anterior tibia produces a posterior glide.

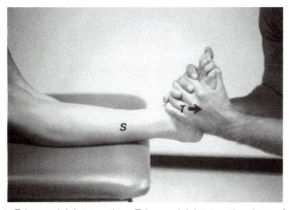

•Figure 16-64 Talocrural joint traction. Talocrural joint traction is performed using the patient's body weight to stabilize the lower leg and applying traction to the midtarsal portion of the foot. Traction reduces pain and increases dorsiflexion and plantarflexion.

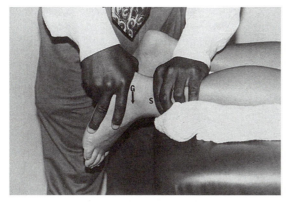

•Figure 16-65 Anterior talor glides. Plantarflexion may also be increased by using an anterior talar glide. With the patient prone the tibia is stabilized on the table, and pressure is applied to the posterior aspect of the talus to glide it anteriorly.

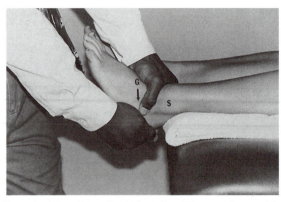

•**Figure 16-66** Posterior talor glides. Posterior talar glides may be used for increasing dorsiflexion. With the patient supine the tibia is stabilized on the table, and pressure is applied to the anterior aspect of the talus to glide it posteriorly.

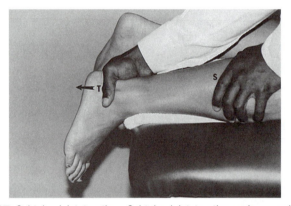

•**Figure 16-67** Subtalor joint traction. Subtalar joint traction reduces pain and increases inversion and eversion. The lower leg is stabilized on the table, and traction is applied by grasping the posterior aspect of the calcaneus.

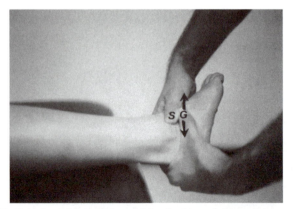

•**Figure 16-68** Subtalor joint medial and lateral glides. Subtalar joint medial and lateral glides increase eversion and inversion. The talus must be stabilized while the calcaneus is mobilized medially to increase inversion and laterally to increase eversion.

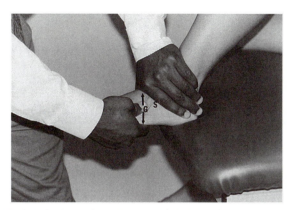

•**Figure 16-69** Anterior/posterior calcaneocuboid glides. Anterior/posterior calcaneocuboid glides may be used for increasing adduction and abduction. The calcaneus should be stabilized while the cuboid is mobilized.

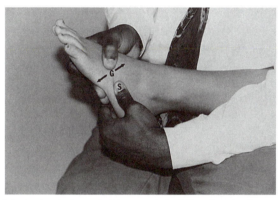

•**Figure 16-70** Anterior/posterior cuboidmetatarsal glides. Anterior/posterior cuboidmetatarsal glides are accomplished with one hand stabilizing the cuboid and the other gliding the base of the fifth metatarsal. They are used for increasing mobility of the fifth metatarsal.

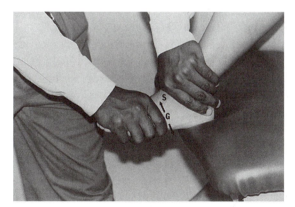

•**Figure 16-71** Anterior/posterior carpometacarpal glides. Anterior/posterior carpometacarpal glides decrease hypomobility of the metacarpals.

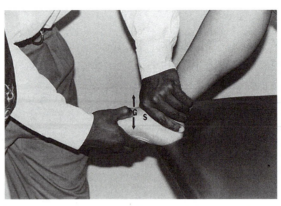

•**Figure 16-72** Anterior/posterior talonavicular glides. Anterior/posterior talonavicular glides also increase adduction and abduction. One hand stabilizes the talus while the other mobilizes the navicular bone.

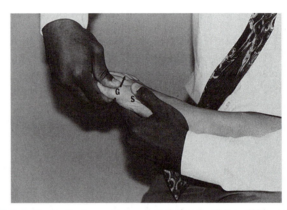

•**Figure 16-73** Anterior/posterior metacarpophalangeal glides. With anterior/posterior metacarpophalangeal glides, the anterior glides increase extension, and posterior glides increase flexion. Mobilizations are accomplished by isolating individual segments.

Treatment Tip
Both joint mobilization and traction should be done with both the patient and the therapist positioned in a comfortable and relaxed manner. The therapist should mobilize one joint at a time. The joint should be stabilized as near one articulating surface as possible, while moving the other segment with a firm, confident grasp. If the therapist is not confident in their technique the patient will quite often sense this, which may make the treatment less effective.

SUMMARY

1. Mobilization and traction techniques increase joint mobility or decrease pain by restoring accessory movements to the joint.
2. Physiological movements result from an active muscle contraction that moves an extremity through traditional cardinal planes.
3. Accessory motions refer to the manner in which one articulating joint surface moves relative to another.
4. Normal accessory component motions must occur for full-range physiological movement to take place.
5. Accessory motions are also referred to as joint arthrokinematics, which include spin, roll, and glide.
6. The Convex-Concave Rule states that if the concave joint surface is moving on the stationary convex surface, gliding will occur in the same direction as the rolling motion. Conversely, if the convex surface is moving on a stationary concave surface, gliding will occur in an opposite direction to rolling.
7. The resting position is one in which the joint capsule and the ligaments are most relaxed, allowing for a maximum amount of joint play.

8. The treatment plane falls perpendicular to a line running from the axis of rotation in the convex surface to the center of the concave articular surface.

9. Maitland has proposed a series of five graded movements or oscillations in the range of motion to treat pain and stiffness.

10. Kaltenborn uses three grades of traction to reduce pain and stiffness.

11. Kaltenborn emphasizes that traction should be used in conjunction with mobilization glides to treat joint hypomobility.

REFERENCES

1. Barak T., Rosen E., Sofer R.: Mobility: passive orthopedic manual therapy. In Gould J., Davies, G., editors: Orthopedic and sports physical therapy, St. Louis, 1990, C.V. Mosby.

2. Basmajian J.: Therapeutic exercise, Baltimore, 1978, Williams & Wilkins.

3. Cookson J.: Orthopedic manual therapy: an overview. II. The spine, J. Am. Phys. Ther. Assoc. 59:259, 1979.

4. Cookson J., Kent, B.: Orthopedic manual therapy: an overview. I. The extremities, J. Am. Phys. Ther. Assoc. 59:136, 1979.

5. Cyriax, J.: Textbook of orthopedic medicine: treatment by manipulation, massage, and injection, vol. 2, Baltimore, 1974, Williams & Wilkins.

6. Donatelli, R., Owens-Burkhart, H.: Effects of immobilization on the extensibility of periarticular connective tissue, J. Orthop. Sports Phys. Ther. 3:67, 1981.

7. Edmond, S.: Manipulation and mobilization: extremity and spinal techniques, St. Louis, 1993, C.V. Mosby.

8. Grimsby, O.: Fundamentals of manual therapy: a course workbook, Vagsbygd, Norway, 1981, Sorlandets Fysikalske Institutt.

9. Hollis, M.: Practical exercise, Oxford, 1981, Blackwell Scientific.

10. Kaltenborn, F.: Mobilization of the extremity joints: examination and basic treatment techniques, Norway, 1980, Olaf Norlis Bokhandel.

11. Kisner, C., Colby, L.: Therapeutic exercise: foundations and techniques, Philadelphia, 1997, F.A. Davis.

12. MacConaill, M., Basmajian, J.: Muscles and movements: a basis for kinesiology, Baltimore, 1969, Williams & Wilkins.

13. Maigne, R.: Orthopedic medicine, Springfield, Illinois, 1976, Charles C Thomas.

14. Maitland, G.: Extremity manipulation, London, 1977, Butterworth.

15. Maitland, G.: Vertebral manipulation, London, 1978, Butterworth.

16. Mennell, J.: Joint pain and diagnosis using manipulative techniques, New York, 1964, Little, Brown.

17. Nygard, R.: Manipulation: definition, types, application, In Basmajian, J., Nyberg, R. editors: Rational manual therapies, Baltimore, 1993, Williams & Wilkins.

18. Paris, S.: The spine: course notebook, Atlanta, 1979, Institute Press.

19. Paris, S.: Mobilization of the spine, Phys. Ther. 59:988, 1979.

20. Saunders, D.: Evaluation, treatment and prevention of musculoskeletal disorders, Bloomington, Minnesota, 1985, Educational Opportunities.

21. Schiotz, E., Cyriax, J.: Manipulation past and present, London, 1978, Heinemann.

22. Stoddard, A.: Manual of osteopathic practice, London, 1969, Hutchinson Ross.

23. Taniqawa, M.: Comparison of the hold-relax procedure and passive mobilization on increasing muscle length, Phys. Ther. 52(7):725–735, 1972.

24. Wadsworth, C.: Manual examination and treatment of the spine and extremities, Baltimore, 1988, William & Wilkins.

25. Zohn, D., Mennell, J.: Musculoskeletal pain: diagnosis and physical treatment, Boston, 1976, Little, Brown.

26. Zusman, M.: Reappraisal of a proposed neurophysiological mechanism for the relief of joint pain with passive joint movements, Physiother. Pract. 1:61–70, 1985.

SUGGESTED READINGS

Bukowski, E.: Assessing joint mobility, Clin. Manage. 11(6):48–56, 1991.

Cibulka, M., Rose, S., and Delitto, A.: Hamstring muscle strain treated by mobilizing the sacroiliac joint, Phys. Ther. 66(8): 1220–1223, 1986.

Cochrane, C.: Joint mobilization principles: considerations for use in the child with central nervous system dysfunction, Phys. Ther. 67(7):1105–1109, 1987.

DonTigny, R.: Measuring PSIS movement, Clin. Manage. 10(3): 43–44, 1990.

Eiff, M., Smith, A., and Smith, G.: Early mobilization versus immobilization in the treatment of lateral ankle sprains, Amer. J. Sports Med. 22(1):83–88, 1994.

Gibson, H., Ross, J., and Allen, J.: The effect of mobilization on forward bending range, J. Manual Manipul. Ther. 1(4):142–147, 1993.

Gratton, P.: Early active mobilization after flexor tendon repairs, J. Hand Ther. 6(4):285–289, 1993.

Harris, S., Lundgren, B.: Joint mobilization for children with central nervous system disorders: indications and precautions, Phys. Ther. 71(12):890–896, 1991.

Lee, M., Latimer, J., and Maher, C.: Manipulation: investigation of a proposed mechanism, Clin. Biomechan. 8(6):302–306, 1993.

Lee, R., Evans, J.: Towards a better understanding of spinal posteronaterior mobilization, Physiotherapy 80(2):68–73, 1994.

Levin, S.: Early mobilization speeds recovery, Phys. Sports Med. 21(8):70–74, 1993.

Maitland, G.: Treatment of the glenohumeral joint by passive movement, Physiotherapy 69(1):3–7, 1983.

May, E.: Controlled mobilization after flexor tendon repair in the hand: techniques, methods and results, Aust. Occupat. Ther. J. 41(3):143, 1994.

McCollam, R., Benson, C.: Effects of postero-anterior mobilization on lumbar extension and flexion, J. Manual Manipul. Ther. 1(4):134–141, 1993.

Mulligan, B.: Extremity joint mobilizations combined with movements, NZ J. Physiother. 20(1):28–29, 1992.

Mulligan, B.: Mobilizations with movement (MWM's), J. Manual Manipul. Ther. 1(4):154–156, 1993.

Nield, S., Davis, K., and Latimer, J.: The effect of manipulation on the range of movement at the ankle joint, Scand. J. Rehabil. Med. 25(4):161–166, 1993.

Ottenbacher, K., Difabio, R.: Efficacy of spinal manipulation/mobilization therapy: a meta-analysis, Spine 10(9):833–837, 1985.

Petersen, P., Sites, S., and Grossman, L.: Clinical evidence for the utilization and efficacy of upper extremity mobilization, Br. J. Occupat. Ther. 55(3):112–116, 1992.

Prentice, W.: Techniques of manual therapy for the knee, J. Sport Rehabil. 1(3):249–257, 1992.

Quillen, W., Halle, J., and Rouillier, L.: Manual therapy: mobilization of the motion-restricted shoulder, J. Sport Rehabil. 1(3):237–248, 1992.

Randall, T., Portney, L., and Harris, B.: Effects of joint mobilization on joint stiffness and active motion of the metacarpalphalangeal joint, JOSPT 16(1):30–36, 1992.

Schoensee, S., Jensen, G., and Nicholson, G.: The effect of mobilization on cervical headaches, JOSPT 21(4):184–196, 1995.

Smith, R., Sebastian, B., and Gajdosik, R.: Effect of sacroiliac joint mobilization on the standing position of the pelvis in healthy men, JOSPT 10(3):77–84, 1988.

Stuberg, W.: Manual therapy in pediatrics: some considerations, PT Mag. Phys. Ther. 1(3):54–56, 1993.

Taylor, N., Bennell, K.: The effectiveness of passive joint mobilization on the return of active wrist extension following Colles' fracture: a clinical trial, NZ J. Physiother. 22(1):24–28, 1994.

Wilson, F.: Manual therapy versus traditional exercises in mobilization of the ankle post-ankle fracture: a pilot study, NZ J. Physiother. 19(3):11–16, 1991.

Wise, P.: Mobilization technique improves neural mobility, Aust. J. Physiother. 40(1):51–54, 1994.

Zito, M.: Joint mobilization: stretch specificity using a distraction, JOSPT 23(1):65, 1996.

GLOSSARY

accessory motions Refer to the manner in which one articulating joint surface moves relative to another.

close-packed position There is maximal contact of the articulating surfaces of bones with the capsule and ligaments tight or tense

Convex-Concave Rule Defines the relationship between the shape of articulating joint surfaces and the direction of gliding.

gliding Occurs when a specific point on one articulating surface comes in contact with a series of points on another surface.

joint play The amount of movement in a joint.

loose-packed position The articulating joint surfaces are maximally separated.

physiological movements Result from an active muscle contraction that moves an extremity through traditional cardinal planes.

resting position Position in which the joint capsule and the ligaments are most relaxed.

rolling Occurs when a series of points on one articulating surface comes in contact with a series of points on another articulating surface.

spin Occurs around some stationary longitudinal mechanical axis and may be in either a clockwise or counterclockwise direction.

treatment plane Falls perpendicular to, or at a right angle to, a line running from the axis of rotation in the convex surface to the center of the concave articular surface.

LAB ACTIVITY

JOINT MOBILIZATION

DESCRIPTION:

After an injury to a joint, there usually is some loss of range of motion. The loss of range of motion can result from physiological movement constraints involving the musculotendinous unit or limitation in accessory motions involving joint capsule and ligamentous structures. Joint mobilization techniques are used to improve joint mobility or decrease joint pain by restoring accessory movements to the joint.

Physiological Effects:

Elongation of connective and contractile tissue
Reflexogenic effect of reducing pain, decreasing muscle guarding, inhibiting stretch reflex, and improving kinesthetic awareness

Therapeutic Effects:

Increase in active and passive joint range of motion
Decrease in joint pain

Indications:

The primary indications for joint mobilization are painful, stiff, or hypomobile joints resulting from injury or following surgery and immobilization.

Contraindications:

- Inflammatory arthritis
- Malignancy
- Bone disease
- Neurological involvement
- Unstable fracture
- Congenital bone deformity
- Vascular disorder

JOINT MOBILIZATION			
PROCEDURE	Evaluation		
	1	2	3
1. Check supplies and equipment.			
2. Question patient.			
a. Verify identity.			
b. Verify absence of contraindications.			
c. Ask about previous joint mobilization treatments.			
3. Position patient.			
a. Place patient in a well-supported, comfortable position: prone, supine or seated with joint in loose packed position.			
b. Expose joint to be treated.			

PROCEDURE	Evaluation		
	1	2	3
c. Drape patient to preserve patient's modesty, protect clothing, but allow access to joint.			
4. Inspect joint to be treated.			
a. Check sensation.			
b. Check circulatory status.			
c. Assess active and passive range of motion (ROM) and point of limitation (PL).			
d. Assess joint irritability (pain).			
5. Select indicated joint mobilization technique based on the following.			
a. Convex–Concave Rule			
b. Treatment plane of joint surface			

c. Oscillation amplitude based on severity of pain and joint stiffness
  i. Grade I
  ii. Grade II
  iii. Grade III
  iv. Grade IV			

6. Apply indicated mobilization/traction technique for 20 to 60 seconds for three to six repeated bouts at a rate of one to three oscillations per second.			
7. Assess treatment efficacy.			
a. Ask the patient how treated joint feels.			
b. Reassess active and passive range of motion (ROM), point of limitation (PL), and joint irritability (pain).			
8. Remove draping material and have patient dress.			
9. Instruct the patient in any indicated exercise.			

CHAPTER 17

SEVENTEEN

PROPRIOCEPTIVE NEUROMUSCULAR FACILITATION TECHNIQUES

WILLIAM E. PRENTICE

OBJECTIVES

After completion of this chapter, the student therapist should be able to:

✓ Explain the neurophysiological basis of proprioceptive neuromuscular facilitation (PNF) techniques.

✓ Discuss the rationale for use of the techniques.

✓ Discuss the basic principles of using PNF in rehabilitation.

✓ Identify the various PNF strengthening and stretching techniques.

✓ Describe PNF patterns for the upper and lower extremity, for the upper and lower trunk, and for the neck.

Proprioceptive neuromuscular facilitation (PNF) is an approach to therapeutic exercise based on the principles of functional human anatomy and neurophysiology. It uses proprioceptive, cutaneous, and auditory input to produce functional improvement in motor output and can be a vital element in the rehabilitation process of many sports-related injuries. These techniques have long been recommended for increasing strength, flexibility, and range of motion.[7,10,13,17,18,26] It is apparent that PNF techniques are also useful for enhancing neuromuscular control.[24] This discussion should guide the therapist using the principles and techniques of PNF as a component of a rehabilitation program.

THE NEUROPHYSIOLOGICAL BASIS OF PROPRIOCEPTIVE NEUROMUSCULAR FACILITATION

The therapeutic techniques of PNF were first used in the treatment of patients with paralysis and neuromuscular disorders. Most of the principles underlying modern therapeutic exercise techniques can be attributed to the work of Sherrington, who first defined the concepts of facilitation and inhibition.[23]

PNF Uses
- Proprioceptive input
- Cutaneous input
- Auditory input

Facilitation techniques for strengthening

Inhibition techniques for stretching

Stretch Reflex
- Muscle spindles
- Golgi tendon organs

An impulse traveling down the corticospinal tract or an afferent impulse traveling up from peripheral receptors in the muscle causes an impulse volley, which results in the discharge of a limited number of specific motor neurons, as well as the discharge of additional surrounding (anatomically close) motor neurons in the subliminal fringe area. An impulse causing the recruitment and discharge of additional motor neurons within the subliminal fringe is said to be facilitory. Conversely, any stimulus that causes motor neurons to drop out of the discharge zone and away from the subliminal fringe is said to be inhibitory.[12] Facilitation results in increased excitability, and inhibition results in decreased excitability of motor neurons.[28] Thus, the function of weak muscles is aided by facilitation, and muscle spasticity is decreased by inhibition.[9]

Sherrington attributed the impulses transmitted from the peripheral stretch receptors via the afferent system as being the strongest influence on the alpha motor neurons.[23] Therefore, the therapist should be able to modify the input from the peripheral receptors and thus influence the excitability of the alpha motor neurons. The discharge of motor neurons can be facilitated by peripheral stimulation, which causes afferent impulses to make contact with excitatory neurons and results in increased muscle tone or strength of voluntary contraction. Motor neurons can also be inhibited by peripheral stimulation, which causes afferent impulses to make contact with inhibitory neurons, thus resulting in muscle relaxation and allowing for stretching of the muscle.[23] To indicate any technique in which input from peripheral receptors is used to facilitate or inhibit, PNF should be used.[9]

The principles and techniques of PNF described here are based primarily on the neurophysiological mechanisms involving the stretch reflex. The stretch reflex involves two types of receptors: muscle spindles that are sensitive to a change in length, as well as the rate of change in length of the muscle fiber; and Golgi tendon organs that detect changes in tension (Fig. 17-1).

Stretching a given muscle causes an increase in the frequency of impulses transmitted to the spinal cord from the muscle spindle, which in turn produces an increase in the frequency of motor nerve impulses returning to that same muscle, thus reflexively resisting the stretch. However, the development of excessive tension

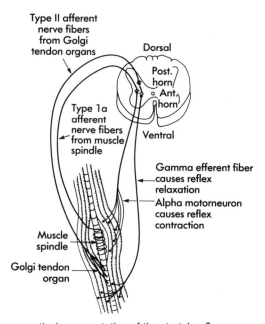

•Figure 17-1 Diagrammatical representation of the stretch reflex.

within the muscle activates the Golgi tendon organs, whose sensory impulses are carried back to the spinal cord. These impulses have an inhibitory effect on the motor impulses returning to the muscles and thus cause that muscle to relax.

Two neurophysiological phenomena help to explain facilitation and inhibition of the neuromuscular systems. The first is known as **autogenic inhibition** and is defined as inhibition mediated by afferent fibers from a stretched muscle acting on the alpha motor neurons supplying that muscle, thus causing it to relax. When a muscle is stretched, motor neurons supplying that muscle receive both excitatory and inhibitory impulses from the receptors. If the stretch is continued for a slightly extended period of time, the inhibitory signals from the Golgi tendon organs eventually override the excitatory impulses and therefore cause relaxation.[14] Because inhibitory motor neurons receive impulses from the Golgi tendon organs while the muscle spindle creates an initial reflex excitation leading to contraction, the Golgi tendon organs apparently send inhibitory impulses that last for the duration of increased tension (resulting from either passive stretch or active contraction) and eventually dominate the weaker impulses from the muscle spindle. This inhibition seems to protect the muscle against injury from reflex contractions resulting from excessive stretch.[1]

A second mechanism, known as **reciprocal inhibition,** deals with the relationships of the agonist and antagonist muscles (Fig. 17-2). The muscles that contract to produce joint motion are referred to as agonists, and the resulting movement is called an agonistic pattern. The muscles that stretch to allow the agonist pattern to occur are referred to as antagonists. Movement that occurs directly opposite to the agonist pattern is called the antagonist pattern.

When motor neurons of the agonist muscle receive excitatory impulses from afferent nerves, the motor neurons that supply the antagonist muscles are inhibited by afferent impulses.[2] Thus, contraction or extended stretch of the agonist muscle must elicit relaxation or inhibit the antagonist. Likewise, a quick stretch of the antagonist muscle facilitates a contraction of the agonist. For facilitating or inhibit-

Muscle spindles = reflex contraction
Golgi tendon organs = reflex relaxation

Autogenic inhibition = Golgi tendon organs

agonist = muscle contracting
antagonist = muscle relaxing

reciprocal inhibition Deals with the relationships of the agonist and antagonist muscles.

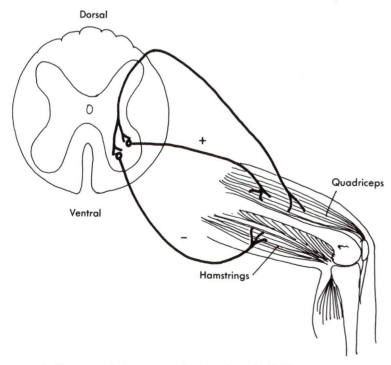

•**Figure 17-2** Diagrammatical representation of reciprocal inhibition.

CASE STUDY 17-1
PROPRIOCEPTIVE NEUROMUSCULAR FACILITATION

Background: A 15-year-old high school volleyball player complained of anterior shoulder pain during the follow through at the completion of her serve. Examination revealed an atraumatic multidirectional right glenohumeral joint instability. Manual muscle test revealed weakness (4-/5) in the rotator cuff and a positive sulcus sign. The patient experienced no sense of apprehension. The remainder of the upper quarter examination was unremarkable.

Impression: Atraumatic multidirectional shoulder instability with secondary rotator cuff muscle weakness.

Treatment Plan: The patient was initiated on a daily regimen of dynamic rotator cuff muscle strengthening exercises utilizing elastic bands. Supplementing this exercise was the provision of manual resistance PNF pattern exercise (D1 flexion/extension, D2 flexion/extension) three times per week for the right upper extremity.

Response: Repeat manual muscle testing at 3 weeks post initiation of exercise demonstrated normalized strength. The patient reported less anterior shoulder pain and a greater "sense" of shoulder stability. She was instructed how to perform the PNF diagonals with elastic bands and continued maintenance exercise throughout the volleyball season without further occurrence of shoulder discomfort.

The rehabilitation professional employs therapeutic agent modalities to create an optimum environment for tissue healing while minimizing the symptoms associated with the trauma or condition.

Discussion Questions

- What tissues were injured or affected?
- What symptoms were present?
- What phase of the injury-healing continuum did the patient present for care in?
- What are the therapeutic agent modality's biophysical effects (direct, indirect, depth, and tissue affinity)?
- What are the therapeutic agent modality's indications and contraindications?
- What are the parameters of the therapeutic agent modality's application, dosage, duration, and frequency in this case study?
- What other therapeutic agent modalities could be utilized to treat this injury or condition? Why? How?

---

ing motion, PNF relies heavily on the actions of these agonist and antagonist muscle groups.

A final point of clarification should be made regarding autogenic and reciprocal inhibition. The motor neurons of the spinal cord always receive a combination of inhibitory and excitatory impulses from the afferent nerves. Whether these motor neurons will be excited or inhibited depends on the ratio of these incoming impulses.

Several different approaches to therapeutic exercise based on the principles of facilitation and inhibition have been proposed. Among these are the Bobath method, Brunnstrom method, Rood method, and the Knott and Voss method, which they called proprioceptive neuromuscular facilitation.[3,4,11,21] Although each of these techniques is important and useful, the PNF approach of Knott and Voss probably makes the most explicit use of proprioceptive stimulation.[11]

RATIONALE FOR USE

As a positive approach to injury rehabilitation, PNF is aimed at what the patient can do physically within the limitations of the injury. It is perhaps best used to decrease deficiencies in strength, flexibility, and coordination in response to demands that are

placed on the neuromuscular system. The emphasis is on selective reeducation of individual motor elements through development of neuromuscular control, joint stability, and coordinated mobility. Each movement is learned and then reinforced through repetition in an appropriately demanding and intense rehabilitative program.[22]

The body tends to respond to the demands placed on it. The principles of PNF attempt to provide a maximal response for increasing strength, flexibility, and coordination. These principles should be applied with consideration of their appropriateness in achieving a particular goal. That continued activity during a rehabilitation program is essential for maintaining or improving strength or flexibility is well accepted. Therefore, an intense program should offer the greatest potential for recovery.

The PNF approach is holistic, integrating sensory, motor, and psychological aspects of a rehabilitation program. It incorporates reflex activities from the spinal levels and upward, either inhibiting or facilitating them as appropriate.

The brain recognizes only gross joint movement and not individual muscle action. Moreover, the strength of a muscle contraction is directly proportional to the activated motor units. Therefore, to increase the strength of a muscle, the maximum number of motor units must be stimulated to strengthen the remaining muscle fibers.[10,11] This "irradiation," or overflow effect, can occur when the stronger muscle groups help the weaker groups in completing a particular movement. This cooperation leads to the rehabilitation goal of return to optimal function.[2,11] The following principles of PNF should be applied to reach that ultimate goal.

Principles of PNF should be applied to techniques of PNF.

BASIC PRINCIPLES OF PROPRIOCEPTIVE NEUROMUSCULAR FACILITATION

Margret Knott, in her text on PNF, emphasized the importance of the principles rather than specific techniques in a rehabilitation program.[11] These principles are the basis of PNF that must be superimposed on any specific technique. The principles of PNF are based on sound neurophysiological and kinesiologic principles and clinical experience.[22] Application of the following principles may assist in promoting a desired response in the patient being treated.

Indications and Contraindications for Using PNF Techniques

Indications
   Increase strength
   Increase flexibility
   Enhance neuromuscular control
   Muscle cocontraction
   Enhance stability
   Muscle reeducation
   Enhance functional movement

Contraindications
   Inflammatory arthritis
   Malignancy
   Bone disease
   Bone fracture
   Congenital bone deformities

1. The patient must be taught the PNF patterns regarding the sequential movements from starting position to terminal position. The therapist has to keep instructions brief and simple. It is sometimes helpful for the therapist to passively move the patient through the desired movement pattern to demonstrate precisely what is to be done. The patterns should be used along with the techniques to increase the effects of the treatment.

2. When learning the patterns, the patient is often helped by looking at the moving limb. This visual stimulus offers the patient feedback for directional and positional control.

3. Verbal cues are used to coordinate voluntary effort with reflex responses. Commands should be firm and simple. Commands most commonly used with PNF techniques are "push" and "pull," which ask for an isotonic contraction; "hold," which asks for an isometric or stabilizing contraction; and "relax."

4. Manual contact with appropriate pressure is essential for influencing direction of motion and facilitating a maximal response because reflex responses are greatly affected by pressure receptors. Manual contact should be firm and confident to give the patient a feeling of security. The manner in which the therapist touches the patient influences patient confidence as well as the appropriateness of the *motor* response or relaxation.[22] A movement response may be facilitated by the hand over the muscle being contracted to facilitate a movement or a stabilizing contraction.

5. Proper mechanics and body positioning of the therapist are essential in applying pressure and resistance. The therapist should stand in a position that is in line with the

direction of movement in the diagonal movement pattern. The knees should be bent and close to the patient such that the direction of resistance can easily be applied or altered appropriately throughout the range.

6. The amount of resistance given should facilitate a maximal response that allows smooth, coordinated motion. The appropriate resistance depends to a large extent on the capabilities of the patient. It may also change at different points throughout the range of motion. Maximal resistance may be used with those techniques that use isometric contractions to restrict motion to a specific point; it may also be used in isotonic contractions throughout a full range of movement.

7. Rotational movement is a critical component in all of the PNF patterns because maximal contraction is impossible without it.

8. Normal timing is the sequence of muscle contraction that occurs in any normal motor activity resulting in coordinated movement.[11] The distal movements of the patterns should occur first. The distal movement components should be completed by no later than halfway through the total PNF pattern. To accomplish this, appropriate verbal commands should be timed with manual commands. Normal timing may be used with maximal resistance or without resistance from the therapist.

9. Timing for emphasis is used primarily with isotonic contractions. This principle superimposes maximal resistance, at specific points in the range, on the patterns of facilitation, allowing overflow or irradiation to the weaker components of a movement pattern. Thus, the stronger components are emphasized to facilitate the weaker components of a movement pattern.

10. Specific joints may be facilitated by using traction or approximation. Traction spreads apart the joint articulations, and approximation presses them together. Both techniques stimulate the joint proprioceptors. Traction increases the muscular response, promotes movement, assists isotonic contractions, and is used with most flexion antigravity movements. Traction must be maintained throughout the pattern. Approximation increases the muscular response, promotes stability, assists isometric contractions, and is used most with extension (gravity-assisted) movements. Approximation may be quick or gradual and may be repeated during a pattern.

11. Giving a quick stretch to the muscle before muscle contraction facilitates a muscle to respond with greater force through the mechanisms of the stretch reflex. It is most effective if all the components of a movement are stretched simultaneously. However, this quick stretch may be contraindicated in many orthopedic conditions because the extensibility limits of a damaged musculotendinous unit or joint structure may be exceeded, thus exacerbating the injury.

TECHNIQUES OF PROPRIOCEPTIVE NEUROMUSCULAR FACILITATION

Each of the principles described in the preceding should be applied to the specific techniques of PNF. These techniques may be used in a rehabilitation program either to strengthen or facilitate a particular agonistic muscle group or to stretch or inhibit the antagonistic group. The choice of a specific technique depends on the deficits of a particular patient. Specific techniques or combinations of techniques should be selected on the basis of the patient's problem.

STRENGTHENING TECHNIQUES

The following techniques are most appropriately used for the development of muscular strength, endurance, and coordination.

The rhythmic initiation technique involves a progression of initial passive, then active-assistive, followed by active movement against resistance through the agonist

PNF Strengthening Techniques
• Repeated contraction
• Slow reversal
• Slow reversal-hold
• Rhythmic stabilization
• Rhythmic initiation

pattern. Movement is slow, goes through the available range of motion, and avoids activation of a quick stretch. It is used for patients who are unable to initiate movement and who have a limited range of motion because of increased tone. It may also be used to teach the patient a movement pattern.

Repeated contraction is useful when a patient has weakness either at a specific point or throughout the entire range. It is used to correct imbalances that occur within the range by repeating the weakest portion of the total range. The patient moves isotonically against maximal resistance repeatedly until fatigue is evidenced in the weaker components of the motion. When fatigue of the weak components becomes apparent, a stretch at that point in the range should facilitate the weaker muscles and result in a smoother, more coordinated motion. Again, quick stretch may be contraindicated with some musculoskeletal injuries. The amount of resistance to motion given by the therapist should be modified to accommodate the strength of the muscle group. The patient is commanded to push by using the agonist concentrically and eccentrically throughout the range.

Slow reversal involves an isotonic contraction of the agonist followed immediately by an isotonic contraction of the antagonist. The initial contraction of the agonist muscle group facilitates the succeeding contraction of the antagonist muscles. The slow reversal technique can be used for developing active range of motion of the agonists and normal reciprocal timing between the antagonists and agonists, which is critical for normal coordinated motion. The patient should be commanded to push against maximal resistance by using the antagonist and then to pull by using the agonist. The initial agonistic push facilitates the succeeding antagonist contraction.

Slow reversal-hold is an isotonic contraction of the agonist followed immediately by an isometric contraction, with a hold command given at the end of each active movement. The direction of the pattern is reversed by using the same sequence of contraction with no relaxation before shifting to the **antagonistic pattern.** This technique can be especially useful in developing strength at a specific point in the range of motion.

Rhythmic stabilization uses an isometric contraction of the agonist, followed by an isometric contraction of the antagonist to produce co-contraction and stability of the two opposing muscle groups. The command given is always "hold," and movement is resisted in each direction. Rhythmic stabilization results in an increase in the holding power to a point where the position cannot be broken. Holding should emphasize co-contraction of agonists and antagonists.

STRETCHING TECHNIQUES

The following techniques should be used to increase range of motion, relaxation, and inhibition.

Contract-relax is a stretching technique that moves the body part passively into the agonist pattern. The patient is instructed to push by contracting the antagonist (muscle that will be stretched) isotonically against the resistance of the therapist. The patient then relaxes the antagonist while the therapist moves the part passively through as much range as possible to the point where limitation is again felt. This contract-relax technique is beneficial when range of motion is limited by muscle tightness.

Hold-relax is very similar to the contract-relax technique. It begins with an isometric contraction of the antagonist (muscle that will be stretched) against resistance, followed by a concentric contraction of the agonist muscle combined with light pressure from the therapist to produce maximal stretch of the antagonist. This technique is appropriate when there is muscle tension on one side of a joint and may be used with either the agonist or antagonist.

agonist pattern The direction of movement caused by agonist contraction.

agonists Muscles that contract to produce joint motion.

PNF Stretching Techniques
- Contract-relax
- Hold-relax
- Slow reversal-hold-relax

antagonist pattern Movement that occurs directly opposite to the agonist pattern.

antagonists Muscles that stretch to allow the agonist pattern to occur are referred to as antagonists.

Slow reversal-hold-relax technique begins with an isotonic contraction of the agonist, which often limits range of motion in the agonist pattern, followed by an isometric contraction of the antagonist (muscle that will be stretched) during the push phase. During the relax phase, the antagonists are relaxed while the agonists are contracting, causing movement in the direction of the agonist pattern and thus stretching the antagonist. The technique, like the contract-relax and hold-relax, is useful for increasing range of motion when the primary limiting factor is the antagonistic muscle group.

Because the goal of rehabilitation in most injuries is restoration of strength through a full, nonrestricted range of motion, several of these techniques are sometimes combined in sequence to accomplish this goal. Figure 17-3 shows a PNF stretching technique in which the therapist is stretching the injured patient.

TREATING SPECIFIC PROBLEMS WITH PROPRIOCEPTIVE NEUROMUSCULAR FACILITATION TECHNIQUES

Proprioceptive neuromuscular facilitation strengthening and stretching techniques may be useful in a variety of different conditions.[20] To some extent the choice of the most effective technique to use in a given situation is dictated by the state of the existing condition and by the capabilities and limitations of the individual patient. There are some advantages to using PNF techniques in general.

Relative to strengthening, the PNF techniques are not encumbered by the design constraints of commercially designed exercise machines. With the PNF patterns movement can occur in three planes simultaneously, thus more closely resembling a functional movement pattern. The amount of resistance applied by the therapist can be easily adjusted and altered at different points through the range of motion to meet patient capabilities. The therapist can choose to concentrate on strengthening through the entire range of motion or through a very specific range. Combinations of several strengthening techniques can be used concurrently within the same PNF pattern.[15] Rhythmic initiation is useful in the early stages of rehabilitation when the patient is having difficulty in moving actively through a pain-free arc. Passive movement can allow the patient to maintain a full range while using an active contraction to move through the available pain-free range. Slow reversal

Treatment Tip
PNF strengthening and stretching techniques may be useful in a variety of different conditions. To some extent the choice of the most effective technique to use in a given situation will be dictated by the state of the existing condition and by the capabilities and limitations of the individual patient.

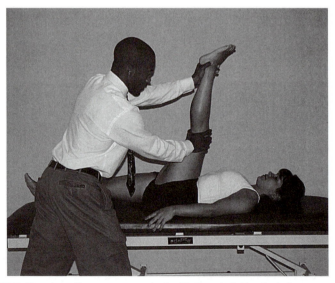

•**Figure 17-3** Proprioceptive neuromuscular facilitation stretching technique.

CASE STUDY 17-2
PROPRIOCEPTIVE NEUROMUSCULAR FACILITATION TECHNIQUES

Background: A 22-year-old woman sustained a traction injury (axonotmesis) of the upper brachial plexus (Erb's palsy) 4 months ago when she fell while rock climbing. She experienced partial paralysis of the affected myotomes, but is now recovering some function, which indicates regeneration of the ruptured axons. All musculature is now innervated, to varying degrees. Her passive range of motion is full, and she has no other deficits. Her major complaints now are weakness and loss of proprioception.

Impression: Axonotmesis of the upper brachial plexus, with partial reinnervation and loss of strength and motor control.

Treatment Plan: To assist in regaining both strength and motor control, a regimen of active and resistive exercise was initiated, along with sensory reorganization training. An element of the treatment is proprioceptive neuromuscular facilitation (PNF). The patient was treated on a 3-day-per-week schedule; each session of PNF lasted approximately 20 minutes. Various patterns were used, with emphasis on those that required external rotation and abduction of the shoulder. The patient was treated for 6 weeks, then discharged to a home program. At the time of discharge, she had at least 4+/5 strength of all muscle groups, full active and passive range of motion, and fair to good proprioceptive ability. Four months later, she had normal function of the neuromuscular system of the affected limb.

The rehabilitation professional employs therapeutic agent modality to create an optimum environment for tissue healing while minimizing the symptoms associated with the trauma or condition.

Discussion Questions

- What tissues were injured or affected?
- What symptoms were present?
- What phase of the injury-healing continuum did the patient present for care in?
- What are the therapeutic agent modality's biophysical effects (direct, indirect, depth, and tissue affinity)?
- What are the therapeutic agent modality's indications and contraindications?
- What are the parameters of the therapeutic agent modality's application, dosage, duration, and frequency in this case study?
- What other therapeutic agent modalities could be used to treat this injury or condition? Why? How?

should be used to help improve muscular endurance. Slow reversal hold is used to correct existing weakness at specific points in the range of motion through isometric strengthening.[19]

Rhythmic stabilization is used to achieve stability and neuromuscular control around a joint.[8] This techniques requires co-contraction of opposing muscle groups and is useful in creating a balance in the existing force couples.

PROPRIOCEPTIVE NEUROMUSCULAR FACILITATION PATTERNS

The PNF patterns are concerned with gross movement as opposed to specific muscle actions. The techniques identified previously may be superimposed on any of the PNF patterns. The techniques of PNF are composed of both rotational and diagonal exercise patterns that are similar to the motions required in most sports and in normal daily activities.

PNF Patterns Include
- Upper extremity
- Lower extremity
- Upper trunk
- Lower trunk
- Neck

The exercise patterns are three component movements: flexion-extension, abduction-adduction, and internal-external rotation. Human movement is patterned and rarely involves straight motion because all muscles are spiral in nature and lie in diagonal directions.

The PNF patterns described by Knott and Voss involve distinct diagonal and rotational movements of the upper extremity, lower extremity, upper trunk, lower trunk, and neck.[11] The exercise pattern is initiated with the muscle groups in the lengthened or stretched position. The muscle group is then contracted, moving the body part through the range of motion to a shortened position.

The upper and lower extremities each have two separate patterns of diagonal movement for each part of the body, which are referred to as the diagonal 1 (D1) and diagonal 2 (D2) patterns. These diagonal patterns are subdivided into D1 moving into flexion, D1 moving into extension, D2 moving into flexion, and D2 moving into extension.[16] Figures 17-4 and 17-5 diagram the PNF patterns for the upper and lower extremities, respectively. The patterns are named according to the proximal pivots at either the shoulder or the hip (e.g., the glenohumeral joint or femoral-acetabular joint).

Tables 17-1 and 17-2 describe specific movements in the D1 and D2 patterns for the upper extremities. Figures 17-6 through 17-13 show starting and terminal positions for each of the diagonal patterns in the upper extremity.

Tables 17-3 and 17-4 describe specific movements in the D1 and D2 patterns for the lower extremities. Figures 17-14 through 17-21 show the starting and terminal positions for each of the diagonal patterns in the lower extremity.

Table 17-5 describes the rotational movement of the upper trunk moving into extension (also called chopping) and moving into flexion (also called lifting). Figures 17-22 and 17-23 show the starting and terminal positions of the upper extremity chopping pattern moving into flexion to the right. Figures 17-24 and 17-25 show the starting and terminal positions for the upper extremity lifting pattern moving into extension to the right.

Table 17-6 describes rotational movement of the lower extremities moving into positions of flexion and extension. Figures 17-26 and 17-27 show the lower extrem-

Upper and Lower Extremity Patterns
- D1 moving into flexion
- D1 moving into extension
- D2 moving into flexion
- D2 moving into extension

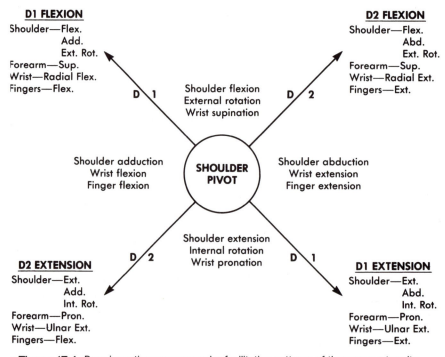

•**Figure 17-4** Proprioceptive neuromuscular facilitation patterns of the upper extremity.

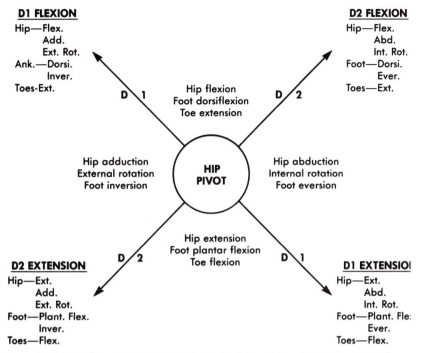

•**Figure 17-5** Proprioceptive neuromuscular facilitation patterns of the lower extremity.

ity pattern moving into flexion to the left. Figures 17-28 and 17-29 show the lower extremity pattern moving into extension to the left.

The neck patterns involve simply flexion and rotation to one side (Figs. 17-30 and 17-31) with extension and rotation to the opposite side (Figs. 17-32 and 17-33). The patient should follow the direction of the movement with the eyes.

The principles and techniques of PNF, when used appropriately with specific patterns, can be an extremely effective tool for rehabilitation of injury.[25] They may be used to strengthen weak muscles or muscle groups and improve the range of motion around an injured joint. Specific techniques selected for use should depend on individual patient needs and may be modified accordingly.[5,6]

TABLE 17-1
D1 Upper Extremity Movement Patterns

Body Part	Moving into Flexion		Moving into Extension	
	Starting Position (Figure 11-6)	Terminal Position (Figure 11-7)	Starting Position (Figure 11-8)	Terminal Position (Figure 11-9)
Shoulder	Extended	Flexed	Flexed	Extended
	Abducted	Adducted	Adducted	Abducted
	Internally rotated	Externally rotated	Externally rotated	Internally rotated
Scapula	Depressed	Flexed	Elevated	Depressed
	Retracted	Protracted	Protracted	Retracted
	Downwardly rotated	Upwardly rotated	Upwardly rotated	Downwardly rotated
Forearm	Pronated	Supinated	Supinated	Pronated
Wrist	Ulnar extended	Radially flexed	Radially flexed	Ulnar extended
Finger and thumb	Extended	Flexed	Flexed	Extended
	Abducted	Adducted	Adducted	Abducted
Hand position for sports therapist*	Left and inside volar surface of hand Right hand underneath arm in cubital fossa of elbow		Left hand on back of elbow on humerus Right hand on dorsum of hand	
Verbal command	Pull		Push	

*For athlete's right arm.

TABLE 17-2
D2 Upper Extremity Movement Patterns

Body Part	Moving into Flexion		Moving into Extension	
	Starting Position (Figure 11-10)	Terminal Position (Figure 11-11)	Starting Position (Figure 11-12)	Terminal Position (Figure 11-13)
Shoulder	Extended	Flexed	Flexed	Extended
	Adducted	Abducted	Abducted	Adducted
	Internally rotated	Externally rotated	Externally rotated	Internally rotated
Scapula	Depressed	Elevated	Elevated	Depressed
	Protracted	Retracted	Retracted	Protracted
	Downwardly rotated	Upwardly rotated	Upwardly rotated	Downwardly rotated
Forearm	Pronated	Supinated	Supinated	Pronated
Wrist	Ulnar flexed	Radially extended	Radially extended	Ulnar flexed
Finger and thumb	Flexed	Extended	Extended	Flexed
	Adducted	Abducted	Abducted	Adducted
Hand position for sports therapist*	Left hand on back of humerus Right hand on dorsum of hand		Left hand on volar surface of humerus Right hand on cubital fossa of elbow	
Verbal command	Push		Pull	

*For athlete's right arm.

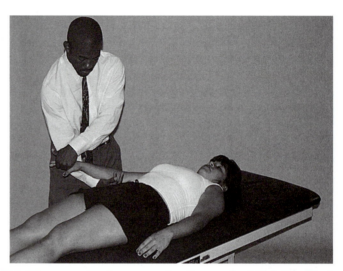

•**Figure 17-6** D1 upper extremity movement pattern moving into flexion. Starting position.

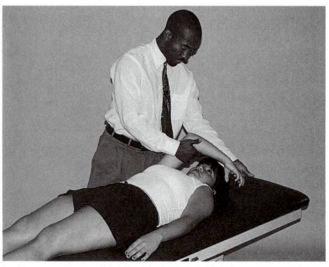

•**Figure 17-7** D1 upper extremity movement pattern moving into flexion. Terminal position.

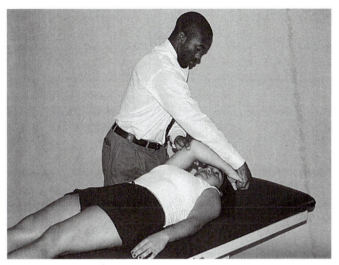

•**Figure 17-8** D1 upper extremity movement pattern moving into extension. Starting position.

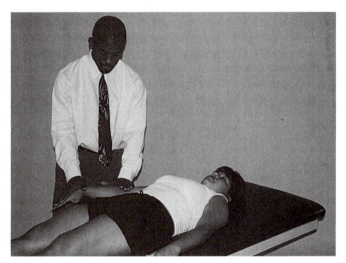

•**Figure 17-9** D1 upper extremity movement pattern moving into extension. Terminal position.

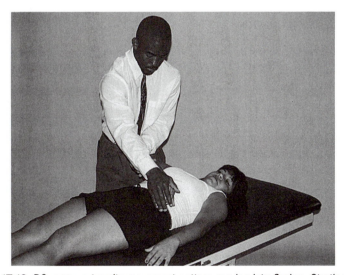

•**Figure 17-10** D2 upper extremity movement pattern moving into flexion. Starting position.

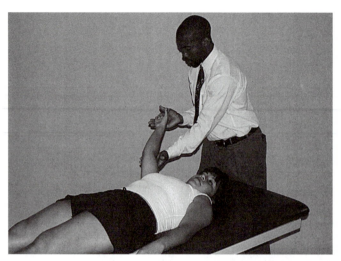

•**Figure 17-11** D2 upper extremity movement pattern moving into flexion. Terminal position.

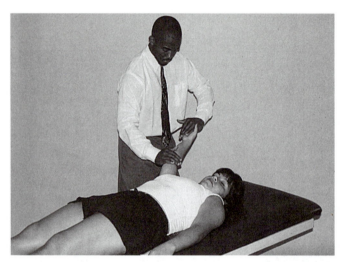

•**Figure 17-12** D2 upper extremity movement pattern moving into extension. Starting position.

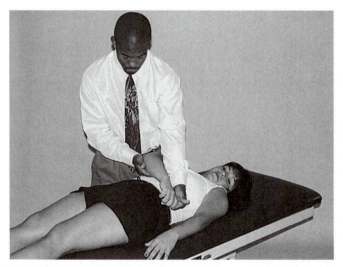

•**Figure 17-13** D2 upper extremity movement pattern moving into extension. Terminal position.

TABLE 17-3
D1 Lower Extremity Movement Patterns

Body Part	Moving into Flexion		Moving into Extension	
	Starting Position (Figure 11-14)	Terminal Position (Figure 11-15)	Starting Position (Figure 11-16)	Terminal Position (Figure 11-17)
Hip	Extended Abducted Internally rotated	Flexed Adducted Externally rotated	Flexed Adducted Externally rotated	Extended Abducted Internally rotated
Knee	Extended	Flexed	Flexed	Extended
Position of tibia	Externally rotated	Internally rotated	Internally rotated	Externally rotated
Ankle and foot	Plantar flexed Everted	Dorsiflexed Inverted	Dorsiflexed Inverted	Plantar flexed Everted
Toes	Flexed	Extended	Extended	Flexed
Hand position for sports therapist*	Right hand on dorsimedial surface of foot Left hand on anteromedial thigh near patella		Right hand on lateralplantar surface of foot Left hand on posteriolateral thigh near popliteal crease	
Verbal command	Pull		Push	

*For athlete's right leg.

TABLE 17-4
D2 Lower Extremity Movement Patterns

Body Part	Moving into Flexion		Moving into Extension	
	Starting Position (Figure 11-18)	Terminal Position (Figure 11-19)	Starting Position (Figure 11-20)	Terminal Position (Figure 11-21)
Hip	Extended Adducted Externally rotated	Flexed Abducted Internally rotated	Flexed Abducted Internally rotated	Extended Adducted Externally rotated
Knee	Extended	Flexed	Flexed	Extended
Position of tibia	Externally rotated	Internally rotated	Internally rotated	Externally rotated
Ankle and foot	Plantar flexed Inverted	Dorsiflexed Everted	Dorsiflexed Everted	Plantar flexed Inverted
Toes	Flexed	Extended	Extended	Flexed
Hand position for sports therapist*	Right hand on dorsilateral surface of foot Left hand on anterolateral thigh near patella		Right hand on medialplantar surface of foot Left hand on posteriomedial thigh near popliteal crease	
Verbal command	Pull		Push	

*For athlete's right leg.

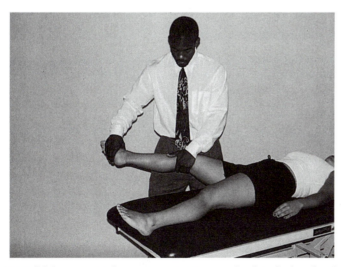

•Figure 17-14 D1 lower extremity movement pattern moving into flexion. Starting position.

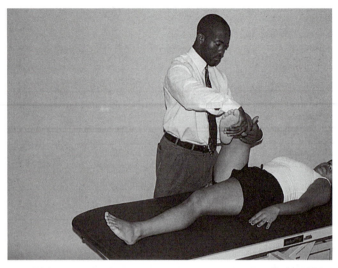

•**Figure 17-15** D1 lower extremity movement pattern moving into flexion. Terminal position.

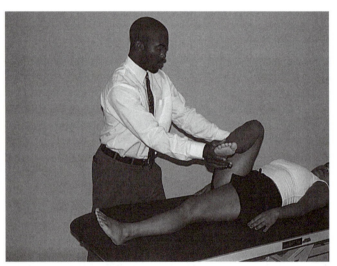

•**Figure 17-16** D1 lower extremity movement pattern moving into extension. Starting position.

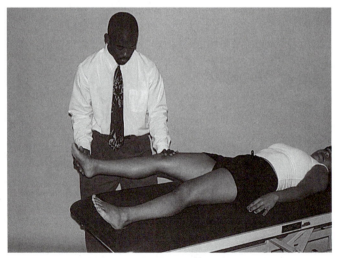

•**Figure 17-17** D1 lower extremity movement pattern moving into extension. Terminal position.

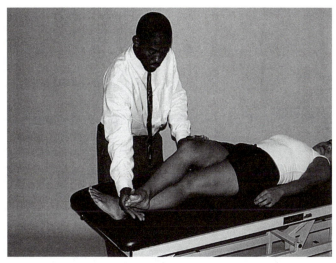

•**Figure 17-18** D2 lower extremity movement pattern moving into flexion. Starting position.

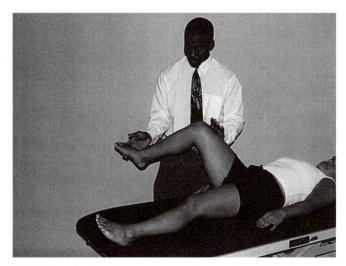

•**Figure 17-19** D2 lower extremity movement pattern moving into flexion. Terminal position.

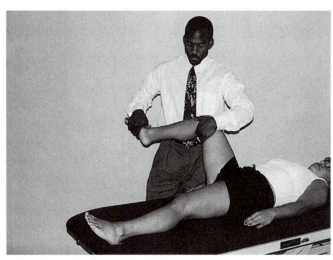

•**Figure 17-20** D2 lower extremity movement pattern moving into extension. Starting position.

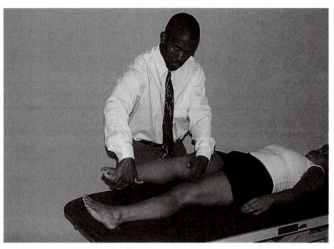

•Figure 17-21 D2 lower extremity movement pattern moving into extension. Terminal position.

TABLE 17-5
Upper Trunk Movement Patterns

Body Part	Moving into Extension (Chopping)*		Moving into Flexion (Lifting)*	
	Starting Position (Figure 11-22)	Terminal Position (Figure 11-23)	Starting Position (Figure 11-24)	Terminal Position (Figure 11-25)
Right upper extremity	Flexed Adducted Internally rotated	Extended Abducted Externally rotated	Extended Adducted Internally rotated	Flexed Abducted Externally rotated
Left upper extremity (left hand grasps right forearm)	Flexed Abducted Externally rotated	Extended Adducted Internally rotated	Extended Abducted Externally rotated	Flexed Adducted Internally rotated
Trunk	Rotated and extended to left	Rotated and flexed to right	Rotated and flexed to left	Rotated and extended to right
Head	Rotated and extended to left	Rotated and flexed to right	Rotated and flexed to left	Rotated and extended to right
Hand position of sports therapist	Left hand on right anterolateral surface of forehead Right hand on dorsum of right hand		Right hand on dorsum of right hand Left hand on posteriolateral surface of head	
Verbal command	Pull down		Push up	

*Athletes rotation is to the right.

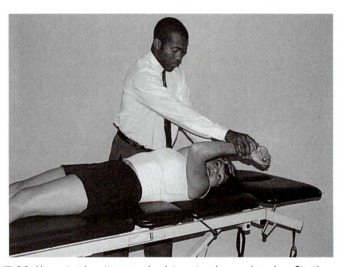

•Figure 17-22 Upper trunk pattern moving into extension or chopping. Starting position.

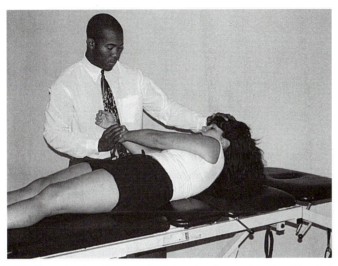

•**Figure 17-23** Upper trunk pattern moving into extension or chopping. Terminal position.

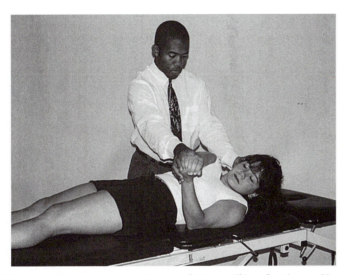

•**Figure 17-24** Upper trunk pattern moving into flexion or lifting. Starting position.

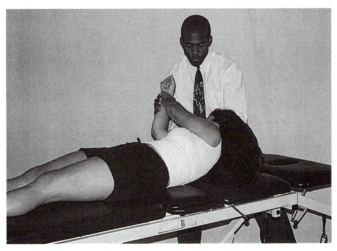

•**Figure 17-25** Upper trunk pattern moving into flexion or lifting. Terminal position.

TABLE 17-6
Lower Trunk Movement Patterns

Body Part	Moving into Flexion*		Moving into Extension†	
	Starting Position (Figure 11-26)	Terminal Position (Figure 11-27)	Starting Position (Figure 11-28)	Terminal Position (Figure 11-29)
Right hip	Extended	Flexed	Flexed	Extended
	Abducted	Adducted	Adducted	Abducted
	Externally rotated	Internally rotated	Internally rotated	Externally rotated
Left hip	Extended	Flexed	Flexed	Extended
	Adducted	Abducted	Abducted	Adducted
	Internally rotated	Externally rotated	Externally rotated	Internally rotated
Ankles	Plantar flexed	Dorsiflexed	Dorsiflexed	Plantar flexed
Toes	Flexed	Extended	Extended	Flexed
Hand position of sports therapist	Right hand on dorsum of feet Left hand on anterolateral surface of left knee		Right hand on plantar surface of foot Left hand on posteriolateral surface of right knee	
Verbal command	Pull up and in		Push down and out	

*Athlete's rotation is to the left in flexion.
†Athlete's rotation is to the right in extension.

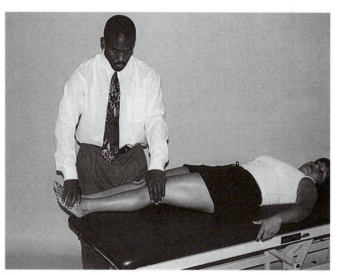

•**Figure 17-26** Lower trunk pattern moving into flexion to the left. Starting position.

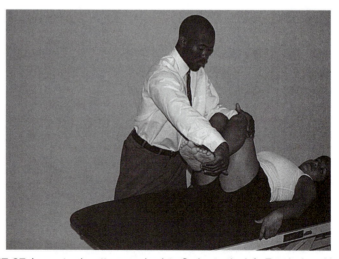

•**Figure 17-27** Lower trunk pattern moving into flexion to the left. Terminal position.

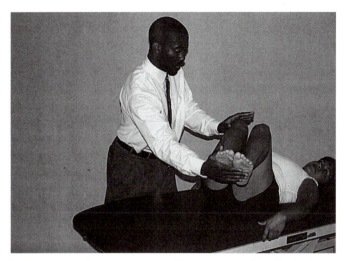

•**Figure 17-28** Lower trunk pattern moving into extension to the left. Starting position.

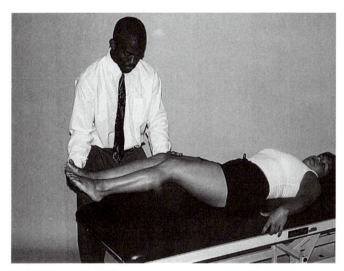

•**Figure 17-29** Lower trunk pattern moving into extension to the left. Terminal position.

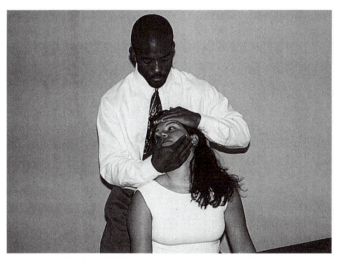

•**Figure 17-30** Neck flexion and rotation to the left. Starting position.

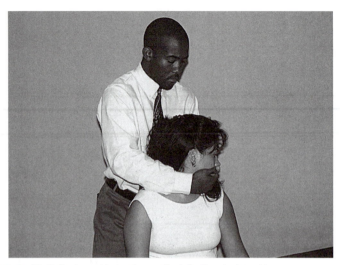

•**Figure 17-31** Neck flexion and rotation to the left. Terminal position.

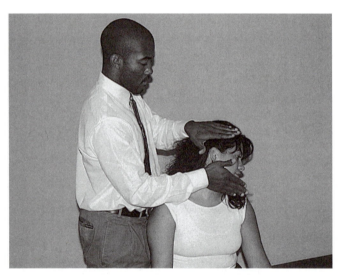

•**Figure 17-32** Neck extension and rotation to the right. Starting position.

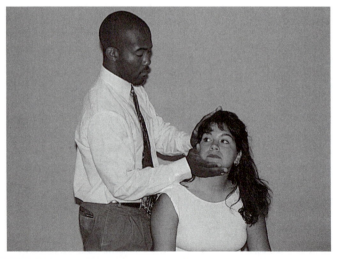

•**Figure 17-33** Neck extension and rotation to the right. Terminal position.

SUMMARY

1. Proprioceptive neuromuscular facilitation techniques may be used to increase both strength and range of motion and are based on the neurophysiology of the stretch reflex.

2. The motor neurons of the spinal cord always receive a combination of inhibitory and excitatory impulses from the afferent nerves. Whether these motor neurons will be excited or inhibited depends on the ratio of the two types of incoming impulses.

3. Proprioceptive neuromuscular facilitation techniques emphasize specific principles that may be superimposed on any of the specific techniques.

4. Proprioceptive neuromuscular facilitation strengthening techniques include repeated contraction, slow-reversal, slow-reversal hold, rhythmic stabilization, and rhythmic initiation.

5. Proprioceptive neuromuscular facilitation stretching techniques include contract-relax, hold-relax, and slow-reversal-hold-relax.

6. The techniques of PNF are rotational and diagonal movements in the upper extremity, lower extremity, upper trunk, and the head and neck.

REFERENCES

1. Barak, T., Rosen, E., and Sofer, R.: Mobility: passive orthopedic manual therapy. In Gould, J., Davies, G., editors: Orthopedic and sports physical therapy, St. Louis, 1985, C.V. Mosby.

2. Basmajian, J.: Therapeutic exercise, Baltimore, 1978, Williams & Wilkins.

3. Bobath, B.: The treatment of motor disorders of pyramidal and extrapyramidal tracts by reflex inhibition and by facilitation of movement, Physiotherapy 41:146, 1955.

4. Brunnstrom, S.: Movement therapy in hemiplegia, New York, 1970, Harper & Row.

5. Cookson, J.: Orthopedic manual therapy: an overview. II. The spine, J. Am. Phys. Ther. Assoc. 59:259, 1979.

6. Cookson, J., Kent, B.: Orthopedic manual therapy: an overview. I. The extremities, J. Am. Phys. Ther. Assoc. 59:176, 1979.

7. Cornelius, W., Jackson, A.: The effects of cryotherapy and PNF on hip extension flexibility, J. Ath. Train. 19(3):184, 1984.

8. Engle, R., Canner, G.: Proprioceptive neuromuscular facilitation (PNF) and modified procedures for anterior cruciate ligament (ACL) instability, J. Orthop. Sports Phys. Ther. 11(6): 230–236, 1989.

9. Harris, F.: Facilitation techniques and therapeutic exercise. In Basmajian, J., editor: Therapeutic exercise, Baltimore, 1978, Williams & Wilkins.

10. Hollis, M.: Practical exercise, Oxford, 1981, Blackwell Scientific.

11. Knott, M., Voss, D.: Proprioceptive neuromuscular facilitation: patterns and techniques, New York, 1968, Harper & Row.

12. Lloyd, D.: Facilitation and inhibition of spinal motorneurons, J. Neurophysiol. 9:421, 1946.

13. Markos, P.: Ipsilateral and contralateral effects of proprioceptive neuromuscular facilitation techniques on hip motion and electromyographic activity, Phys. Ther. 59(11)P:1766–1773, 1979.

14. Osternig, L., Robertson, R., Troxel, R., et al.: Differential responses to proprioceptive neuromuscular facilitation stretch techniques, Med. Sci. Sports Exerc. 22:106–111, 1990.

15. Osternig, L., Robertson, R., Troxel, R., and Hansen, P.: Muscle activation during proprioceptive neuromuscular facilitation (PNF) stretching techniques: stretch-relax (SR), contract-relax (CR) and agonist contract-relax (ACR), Am. J. Phys. Med. 66(5):298–307, 1987.

16. Prentice, W.: Proprioceptive neuromuascular facilitation (videotape), St. Louis, 1993, C.V. Mosby.

17. Prentice, W.: An electromyographic analysis of heat and cold and stretching for inducing muscular relaxation, J. Orthop. Sports Phys. Ther. 3:137–140, 1982.

18. Prentice, W.: A comparison of static stretching and PNF stretching for improving hip joint flexibility, J. Ath. Train. 18(1):56–59, 1983.

19. Prentice, W.: A manual resistance technique for strengthening tibial rotation, J. Ath. Train. 23(3):230–233, 1988.

20. Prentice, W., Kooima, E.: The use of proprioceptive neuromuscular facilitation techniques in the rehabilitation of sport-related injuries, J. Ath. Train. 21:26–31, 1986.

21. Rood, M.: Neurophysiologic reactions as a basis of physical therapy, Phys. Ther. Rev. 34:444, 1954.

22. Saliba, V., Johnson, G., and Wardlaw, C.: Proprioceptive neuromuscualr facilitation. In Basmajian, J. Nyberg, R.: Rational manual therapies, Baltimore, 1993, Williams & Wilkins.

23. Sherrington, C.: The integrative action of the nervous system, New Haven, Connecticut, 1947, Yale University Press.

24. Surburg, P., Schrader, J.: Proprioceptive neuromuscular facilitation techniques in clinical: a reassessment, J. Ath. Train. 32(1):34–39, 1997.

25. Surberg, P.: Neuromuscular facilitation techniques in sports-medicine, Phys. Ther. Rev. 34:444, 1954.
26. Taniqawa, M.: Comparison of the hold-relax procedure and passive mobilization on increasing muscle length, Phys. Ther. 52(7):725–735, 1972.
27. Worrell, T., Smith, T., and Winegardner, J.: Effect of hamstring stretching on hamstring muscle performance, J. Orthop. Sports Phys. Ther. 20(3):154–159, 1994.
28. Zohn, D., Mennell, J.: Musculoskeletal pain: diagnosis and physical treatment, Boston, 1976, Little, Brown.

SUGGESTED READINGS

Blakely, R., Palmer, M.: Analysis of shoulder rotation accompanying a proprioceptive neuromuscular facilitation approach, Phys. Ther. 66(8):1224–1227, 1986.

Cornelius, W., Craft-Hamm, K.: Proprioceptive neuromuscular facilitation flexibility techniques: acute effects on arterial blood pressure,. Phys. Sports Med. 16(4):152–157, 160–161, 1988.

Engle, R., Canner, G.: Proprioceptive neuromuscular facilitation (PNF) and modified procedures for anterior cruciate ligament (ACL) instability. JOSPT 11(6):230–236, 1989.

Osternig, L., Robertson, R., and Troxel, R.: Muscle activation during proprioceptive neuromuscular facilitation (PNF) stretching techniques: stretch-relax (SR), contract-relax (CR), Amer. J. Phys. Med. 66(5):298–307, 1987.

Segal, R.: Depression of Hoffmann reflexes following voluntary contraction and implications for proprioceptive neuromuscular facilitation therapy, Phys. Ther. 71(4):329–331, 1991.

Sundquist, R., Harter, R.: Comparative effects of static and proprioceptive neuromuscular facititation stretching techniques in increasing hip flexion range of motion, J. Ath. Train. 31 (Suppl):S-5, 1996.

Svendsen, D., Matyas, T.: Facilitation of the isometric maximum voluntary contraction with traction: a test of PNF predictions: Proprioceptive Neuromuscular Facilitation, Amer. J. Phys. Med. 62(1):27–37, 1983.

Waddington, P.: Proprioceptive neuromuscular facilitation techniques and plasticity, Physiotherapy 70(8):295–296, 1984.

Wang, R.: Effect of proprioceptive neuromuscular facilitation on the gait of patients with hemiplegia of long and short duration, Phys. Ther. 74(12):1108–1115, 1994.

GLOSSARY

agonist pattern The direction of movement caused by agonist contraction.

agonists Muscles that contract to produce joint motion.

antagonist pattern Movement that occurs directly opposite to the agonist pattern.

antagonists Muscles that stretch to allow the agonist pattern to occur.

approximation Compresses joint articulations together.

autogenic inhibition Inhibition that is mediated by afferent fibers from a stretched muscle acting on the alpha motor neurons supplying that muscle, thus causing it to relax.

reciprocal inhibition Deals with the relationships between the agonist and antagonist muscles.

stretch reflex Causes either a reflex contraction or relaxation of a muscle being stretched.

traction Spreads apart the joint articulations.

LAB ACTIVITY

PROPRIOCEPTIVE NEUROMUSCULAR FACILITATION

DESCRIPTION:

Proprioceptive neuromuscular facilitation (PNF) is a rehabilitation technique that attempts to normalize neuromuscular function (and therefore joint motion) via input to the central nervous system from cutaneous and joint receptors. Proprioceptive neuromuscular facilitation techniques may be adapted to enhance whatever element of normal joint motion is dysfunctional; coordination, range of motion, or strength.

There are many elements to PNF, including facilitation of weak muscle to encourage strength development, stimulation of hypotonic muscles, inhibition of hypertonic muscles, and stretch of tight muscles. Terms such as "hold-relax," "slow reversal-hold," and "contract-relax," are used to describe the techniques. All PNF techniques are therapist-intensive; unlike the classical physical agent modalities, the presence of the therapist is required for the duration of the session.

Because there are so many PNF techniques, the checklist for this treatment is extremely generic. It may be adapted readily to any of the specific techniques.

PHYSIOLOGICAL EFFECTS:

Enhanced force developing capacity of the muscle
Remodeling of articular connective tissue
Normalization of muscle tone

THERAPEUTIC EFFECTS:

Increased muscle strength
Increased range of joint motion
Normalization of joint motion

INDICATIONS:

Proprioceptive neuromuscular facilitation is indicated for use with patients who have either a neurological or orthopaedic (musculoskeletal) disorder that results in abnormal motion. Whether the abnormal motion is owing to insufficient power, abnormal joint motion, or a lack of coordination between sensory and motor elements of the nervous system, PNF may play an effective role in rehabilitation of the patient.

CONTRAINDICATIONS:

There are no specific established contraindications to PNF, but common sense should prevail. A PNF pattern involving vigorous contraction of the muscles would not be appropriate for use with the right upper member of a patient who has an unstable fracture of the right upper member. However, PNF could be useful for this patient's lower members or uninjured upper member.

PROPRIOCEPTIVE NEUROMUSCULAR FACILITATION

PROCEDURE	Evaluation		
	1	2	3
1. Check supplies.			
a. Obtain towels or sheets for draping.			
b. Wash hands, remove jewelry from patient (if warranted) and therapist.			
2. Question patient.			

PROCEDURE	Evaluation		
	1	2	3
a. Verify identity of patient (if not already verified).			
b. Verify the absence of contraindications.			
c. Ask about previous therapeutic exercise regimens, check treatment notes.			
3. Position patient.			
a. Place patient in a well-supported, comfortable position.			
b. Expose body part to be treated.			
c. Drape patient to preserve patient's modesty, protect clothing, but allow access to body part.			
4. Inspect body part to be treated.			
a. Check light touch perception.			
b. Assess function of body part (e.g., ROM, irritability).			
5. Apply PNF technique.			
a. Determine the methods and patterns to be used.			
b. If increasing muscle strength is the goal, establish the principal motions to use.			
c. If increasing range of motion is the goal, establish the direction of the limitation; the direction to stretch will be opposite.			
d. If increasing coordination is the goal, determine the optimum levels of resistance and assistance to achieve the goal.			
e. If the patient reports anything unusual, such as pain or joint locking, discontinue treatment.			
f. Continue to monitor the patient during the duration of the treatment.			
6. Complete treatment.			
a. When the treatment is completed, decrease intensity of resistance or stretch for a few more repetitions to allow the patient to cool down.			
b. Remove material used for draping, assist the patient in dressing as needed.			
c. Clean the treatment area according to normal protocol.			
7. Assess treatment efficacy.			
a. Ask the patient how the treated area feels.			
b. Visually inspect the treated area for any adverse reactions.			
c. Perform functional tests as indicated.			

APPENDICES

Appendix A-1

Locations of the Motor Points

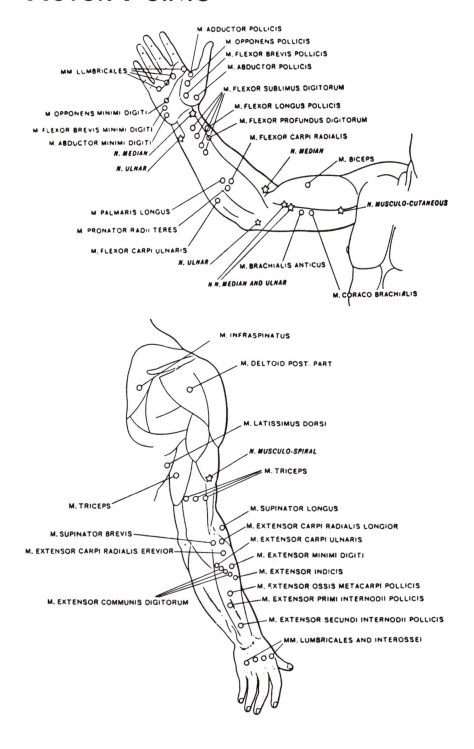

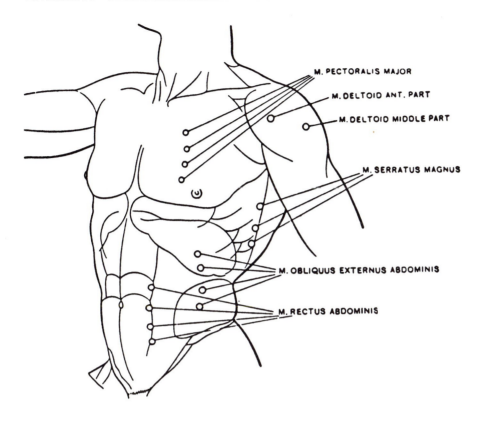

M. PECTORALIS MAJOR
M. DELTOID ANT. PART
M. DELTOID MIDDLE PART
M. SERRATUS MAGNUS
M. OBLIQUUS EXTERNUS ABDOMINIS
M. RECTUS ABDOMINIS

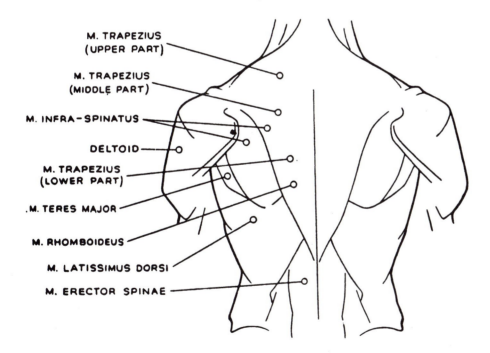

M. TRAPEZIUS (UPPER PART)
M. TRAPEZIUS (MIDDLE PART)
M. INFRA-SPINATUS
DELTOID
M. TRAPEZIUS (LOWER PART)
.M. TERES MAJOR
M. RHOMBOIDEUS
M. LATISSIMUS DORSI
M. ERECTOR SPINAE

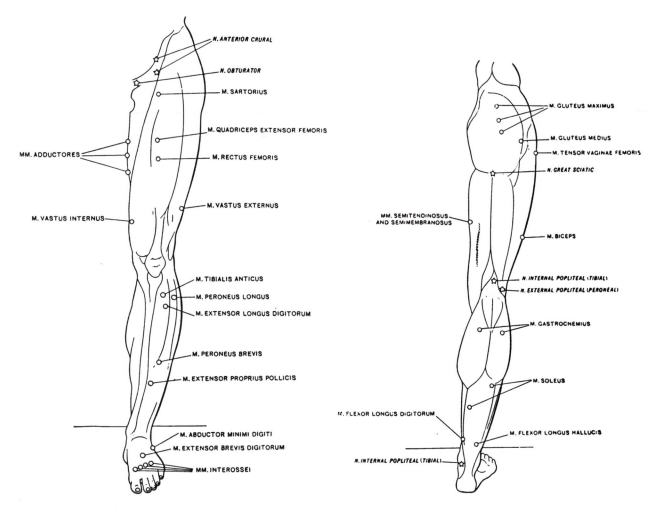

M = Muscle
N = Nerves

Appendix A-2

List of Therapeutic Modality Equipment Manufacturers and Distributors

ELECTROTHERAPY

Electrodes

AdvanTeq Development Corp
12509 Crenshaw Blvd
Hawthorne, CA 90250
800/234-7846

AliMed Inc.
297 High St
Dedham, MA 02026
617/329-2900

American Imex
16520 Aston St
Irvine, CA 92714
800/521-8286
714/553-8885

Amrex-Zetron, Incorporated
641 East Walnut Street
Carson, California 90746
800/221-9069

Anodyne Inc.
7300 France Ave S, Ste 403
Edina, MN 55435
800/736-8367
612/831-6130

Austin Medical Equipment Inc
5947 S Oak Park Ave
Chicago, IL 60638
800/382-0300

BioMedical Life Systems Inc
1120 Sycamore Ave, Ste F
Vista, CA 92085
800/726-8367
619/727-5600

Chattanooga Group Inc
4717 Adams Rd
PO Box 489
Hixson, TN 37343
800/592-7329
615/870-2281

Comfort Technologies Inc
PO Box 7
Pittstown, NJ 08867
800/321-STIM
908/735-0344

CONMED Corp
310 Broad St
Utica, NY 13501
315/797-8375

Davicon Inc
79 Second Ave
Burlington, MA 01803
800/DAVICON
617/229-2800

AR Davis Co Inc
PO Box 219
Irvington, AL 36544
800/872-5804
205/957-3214
FAX: 205/957-2031

Dynatronics
470 W Lawndale Dr
Bldg D
Salt Lake City, UT 84115
801/485-4739

DynaWave Corp
2520 Kaneville Ct
Geneva, IL 60134
708/232-4945
FAX: 708/232-7042

The Electrode Store
PO Box 188
Enumclaw, WA 98022
800/537-1093
206/735-9259
FAX: 206/735-9343

Electro-Med Health Industries
11601 Biscayne Blvd, Ste 200A
Miami, FL 33181
305/892-2866
FAX: 305/892-2980

Electronic Waveform Lab Inc
15683 Chemical Ln
Huntington Beach, CA 92649
800/874-9283

ELMED Inc
60 W Fay Ave
Addison, IL 60101
312/543-2792

Empi Inc
1275 Grey Fox Rd
St Paul, MN 55112
800/328-2536
612/636-6600

Excel Tech Ltd
1200-11 Aerowood Dr
Mississauga, Ontario, Canada
L4W 2S7
800/387-7516

Henley International, A Division of Maxxim Medical
104 Industrial Blvd
Sugar Land, TX 77478
800/477-7342
FAX: 713/240-2577

IOMED Inc
1290 W 2320 S
Salt Lake City, UT 84119
800/621-3347
801/975-1191

Life-Tech Inc
10920 Kinghurst
Houston, TX 77099
713/495-9411

William B McBeth Co
PO Box 267
Telford, PA 18969
800/346-2171
215/723-0824

MECI Electrotherapeutics
810-B NW Main St
PO Box 1149
Lee's Summit, MO 64063
800/527-0748

Medical Devices Inc
833 Third St SW
St Paul, MN 55112
800/328-0875

Medical Science Products Inc
PO Box 381
Canal Fulton, OH 44614
800/456-1971

Mettler Electronics Corp
1333 S Claudina St
Anaheim, CA 92805
800/854-9305
714/533-2221
FAX: 714/635-7539

Monad Corp
908 E Holt Ave
Pomona, CA 91767
800/34MONAD
800/233MENS (in CA)

Nemectron Medical Inc
28069 Diaz Rd, Unit A
Temecula, CA 92590
800/428-4010

Physical Health Devices Inc
417 Corporate Sq
1500 W Cypress Creek Rd
Ft Lauderdale, FL 33309
305/351-0303
FAX: 305/351-0598

JA Preston Corp
PO Box 89
Jackson, MI 49204
800/631-7277
517/787-1600

Promatek Medical Systems Inc
1851 Black Rd
Joliet, IL 60435
800/327-3422
815/725-6766

PTI
PO Box 19005
Topeka, KS 66619-0005
80/255-3554

Rich-Mar Corp
PO Box 879
Inola, OK 74036
800/762-4665
918/543-2222

Self Regulation Systems Inc (SRS)
14770 NE 95th St
Redmond, WA 98052
800/345-5642
206/882-1101
FAX: 206/882-1935

Sentry Medical Products Inc
17171 Murphy Ave
Irvine, CA 92714
800/854-6004 (outside CA)
714/250-0233

Sparta Surgical Corp
26602 Corporate Ave
Hayward, CA 94545
510/887-7717

Staodyn Inc
1225 Florida Ave
PO Box 1379
Longmont, CO 80502-1379
800/525-2114
303/772-3631

TC Medical Inc
6565 City W Pkwy
Minneapolis, MN 55344-3248
800/826-3342
FAX: 612/829-8284

Thera-Kinetics Inc
1300 Rte 73
Mount Laurel, NJ 08054
800/234-0900

3M Health Care/Electrotherapy Products
3M Ctr, Bldg 275-4W-02
St Paul, MN 55144-1000
800/228-3957

TMD, A Division of Staodyn Inc
3625 Queen Palm Dr
PO Box 30244
Tampa, FL 33630-3244
800/343-0488

Uni-Patch Inc
1313 Grant Blvd W
PO Box 271
Wabasha, MN 55981
800/328-9454
612/565-2601

Verimed Inc
1401 E Broward Blvd
Ste 200
Ft Lauderdale, FL 33301
800/999-9797
305/768-9990

Electrotherapy Equipment

AdvanTeq Development Corp
12509 Crenshaw Blvd
Hawthorne, CA 90250
800/234-7846

American Imex
16520 Aston St
Irvine, CA 92714
800/521-8286
714/553-8885

Anodyne Inc
7300 France Ave S, Ste 403
Edina, MN 55435
800/736-8367
612/831-6130

Austin Medical Equipment Inc
5947 S Oak Park Ave
Chicago, IL 60638
800/382-0300

BioMedical Life Systems Inc
1120 Sycamore Ave, Ste F
Vista, CA 92085
800/726-8367
619/727-5600

Chattanooga Group Inc
4717 Adams Rd
PO Box 489
Hixson, TN 37343
800/592-7329
615/870-2281

Comfort Technologies Inc
PO Box 7
Pittstown, NJ 08867
800/321-STIM
908/735-0344

Davicon Inc
79 Second Ave
Burlington, MA 01803
800/DAVICON
617/229-2800

Dynatronics
470 W Lawndale Dr
Bldg D
Salt Lake City, UT 84115
801/485-4739

DynaWave Corp
2520 Kaneville Ct
Geneva, IL 60134
708/232-4945
FAX: 708/232-7042

Electro-Med Health Industries
11601 Biscayne Blvd
Ste 200A
Miami, FL 33181
305/892-2866
FAX: 305/892-2980

Electro Medical Inc
18433 Amistad
Fountain Valley, CA 92708
800/422-8726
714/964-6776
FAX: 714/968-0712

Electronic Waveform Lab Inc
15683 Chemical Ln
Huntington Beach, CA 92649
800/874-9283

ELMED Inc
60 W Fay Ave
Addison, IL 60101
312/543-2792

Empi Inc
1275 Grey Fox Rd
St Paul, MN 55112
800/328-2536
612/636-6600

Ergometrics Inc
3753 Varsity Dr
Ann Arbor, MI 48014
800/447-3009
313/971-7111

Excel Tech Ltd
1200-11 Aerowood Dr
Mississauga, Ontario, Canada
L4W 2S7
800/387-7516

GNR Health Systems Inc
1203 SW 12th St
Bldg H
Ocala, FL 32674
800/523-0912

Ideal Medical Products Inc
County Rd 623
Rte 1, PO Box 56
Broseley, MO 63932
800/321-5490
314/686-0003

IOMED Inc
1290 W 2320 S
Salt Lake City, UT 84119
800/621-3347
801/975-1191

I-REP Inc
29885 Second St, #G
Lake Elsinore, CA 92532
800/828-0852

Med Labs Inc
28 Vereda Cordillera
Goleta, CA 93117
805/968-2486

Mettler Electronics Corp
1333 S Claudina St
Anaheim, CA 92805
800/854-9305
714/533-2221
FAX: 714/635-7539

Microcurrent Research Inc
10443 N Cave Creek Rd
Ste 211
Phoenix, AZ 85020
800/872-6789
FAX: 602/943-6409

Monad Corp
908 E Holt Ave
Pomona, CA 91767
800/34MONAD
800/233MENS (in CA)

David Nelson, PT
1602 35th Ave
Vero Beach, FL 32960
407/562-5316

Nemectron Medical Inc
28069 Diaz Rd, Unit A
Temecula, CA 92590
800/428-4010

JA Preston Corp
PO Box 89
Jackson, MI 49204
800/631-7277
517/787-1600

Promatck Medical Systems Inc
1851 Black Rd
Joliet, IL 60435
800/327-3422
815/725-6766

PTI
PO Box 19005
Topeka, KS 66619-0005
800/255-3554

Rich-Mar Corp
PO Box 879
Inola, OK 74036
800/762-4665
918/543-2222

Rothhammer International
PO Box 5579
Santa Maria, CA 93456
800/235-2156

Thera-Kinetics Inc
1300 Rte 73
Mount Laurel, NJ 08054
800/234-0900

TMD, A Division of Staodyn Inc
3625 Queen Palm Dr
PO Box 30244
Tampa, FL 33630-3244
800/343-0488

Verimed Inc
1401 E Broward Blvd
Ste 200
Ft Lauderdale, FL 33301
800/999-9797
305/768-9990

Galvanic Stimulators

Anodyne Inc
7300 France Ave S, Ste 403
Edina, MN 55435
800/736-8367
612/831-6130

BioMedical Life Systems Inc
1120 Sycamore Ave, Ste F
Vista, CA 92085
800/726-8367
619/727-5600

Comfort Technologies Inc
PO Box 7
Pittstown, NJ 08867
800/321-STIM
908/735-0344

DynaWave Corp
2520 Kaneville Ct
Geneva, IL 60134
708/232-4945
FAX: 708/232-7042

Electro-Med Health Industries
11601 Biscayne Blvd, Ste 200A
Miami, FL 33181
305/892-2866
FAX: 305/892-2980

ELMED Inc
60 W Fay Ave
Addison, IL 60101
312/543-2792

Excel Tech Ltd
1200-11 Aerowood Dr
Mississauga, Ontario, Canada
L4W 2S7
800/387-7516

William B McBeth Co
PO Box 267
Telford, PA 18969
800/346-2171
215/723-0824

MECI Electrotherapeutics
810-B NW Main St
PO Box 1149
Lee's Summit, MO 64063
800/527-0748

Medical Devices Inc
833 Third St SW
St Paul, MN 55112
800/328-0875

Med Labs Inc
28 Vereda Cordillera
Goleta, CA 93117
805/968-2486

Mettler Electronics Corp
1333 S Claudina St
Anaheim, CA 92805
800/854-9305
714/533-2221
FAX: 714/635-7539

Physio Therapeutix Inc
3500 N Causeway Blvd
Ste 160
Metairie, LA 70002
800/274-9746

Rich-Mar Corp
PO Box 879
Inola, OK 74036
800/762-4665
918/543-2222

Staodyn Inc
1225 Florida Ave
PO Box 1379
Longmont, CO 80502-1379
800/525-2114
303/772-3631

Thera-Kinetics Inc
1300 Rte 73
Mount Laurel, NJ 08054

TMD, A Division of Staodyn Inc
3625 Queen Palm Dr
PO Box 30244
Tampa, FL 33630-3244
800/343-0488

Gels/Sprays

AdvanTeq Development Corp
12509 Crenshaw Blvd
Hawthorne, CA 90250
800/234-7846

AliMed Inc
297 High St
Dedham, MA 02026
617/329-2900

AloeTran Products Inc
PO Box 337
Farmerville, LA 71241
800/328-8367
318/368-7266

American Imex
16520 Aston St
Irvine, CA 92714
800/521-8286
714/553-8885

CONMED Corp
310 Broad St
Utica, NY 13501
315/979-8375

AR Davis Co Inc
PO Box 219
Irvington, AL 36544
800/872-5804
205/957-3214
FAX: 205/957-2031

Dynatronics
470 W Lawndale Dr
Bldg D
Salt Lake City, UT 84115
801/485-4739

The Electrode Store
PO Box 188
Enumclaw, WA 98022
800/537-1093
206/735-9259
FAX: 206/735-9343

Electro-Med Health Industries
11601 Biscayne Blvd, Ste 200A
Miami, FL 33181
305/892-2866
FAX: 305/892-2980

Electronic Waveform Lab Inc
15683 Chemical Ln
Huntington Beach, CA 92649
800/874-9283

ELMED Inc
60 W Fay Ave
Addison, IL 60101
312/543-2792

Excel Tech Ltd
1200-11 Aerowood Dr
Mississauga, Ontario, Canada
L4W 257
800/387-7516

Ideal Medical Products Inc
County Rd 623
Rte 1, PO Box 56
Broseley, MO 63932
800/321-5490
314/686-0003

William B McBeth Co
PO Box 267
Telford, PA 18969
800/346-2171
215/723-0824

Medical Devices Inc
833 Third St SW
St Paul, MN 55112
800/328-0875

Mecical Science Products Inc
PO Box 381
Canal Fulton, OH 44614
800/456-1971

Parker Laboratories Inc
307 Washington St
Orange, NJ 07050
201/676-5000
FAX: 201/676-0784

Pharmaceutical Innovations Inc
897 Frelinghuysen Ave
Newark, NJ 07114
201/242-2900
FAX: 201/242-0578

Rich-Mar Corp
PO Box 879
Inola, OK 74036
800/762-4665
918/543-2222

Self Regulation Systems Inc (SRS)
14770 NE 95th St
Redmond, WA 98052
800/345-5642
206/882-1101
FAX: 206/882-1935

TC Medical Inc
6565 City West Pkwy
Minneapolis, MN 55344
800/826-3342
FAX: 612/829-8284

Thera-Kinetics Inc
1300 Rte 73
Mount Laurel, NJ 08054
800/234-0900

Uni-Patch Inc
1313 Grant Blvd W
PO Box 271
Wabasha, MN 55981
800/328-9454
612/565-2601

Interferential Therapy

AdvanTeq Development Corp
12509 Crenshaw Blvd
Hawthorne, CA 90250
800/234-7846

American Imex
16520 Aston St
Irvine, CA 92714
800/521-8286
714/553-8885

Anodyne Inc
7300 France Ave S, Ste 403
Edina, MN 55435
800/736-8367
612/831-6130

Austin Medical Equipment Inc
5947 S Oak Park Ave
Chicago, IL 60638
800/382-0300

BioMedical Life Systems Inc
1120 Sycamore Ave, Ste F
Vista, CA 92085
800/726-8367
619/727-5600

Chattanooga Group Inc
4717 Adams Rd
PO Box 489
Hixson, TN 37343
800/592-7329
615/870-2281

Comfort Technologies Inc
PO Box 7
Pittstown, NJ 08867
800/321-STIM
908/735-0344

Dynatronics
470 W Lawndale Dr
Bldg D
Salt Lake City, UT 84115
801/485-4739

ELMED Inc
60 W Fay Ave
Addison, IL 60101
312/543-2792

Excel Tech Ltd
1200-11 Aerowood Dr
Mississauga, Ontario, Canada
L4W 2S7
800/387-7516

Ideal Medical Products Inc
County Rd 623
Rte 1, PO Box 56
Broseley, MO 63932
800/321-5490
314/686-0003

I-REP Inc
29885 Second St, #G
Lake Elsinore, CA 92532
800/828-0852

William B McBeth Co
PO Box 267
Telford, PA 18969
800/346-2171
215/723-0824

Medical Devices Inc
833 Third St SW
St Paul, MN 55112
800/328-0875

Mettler Electronics Corp
1333 S Claudina St
Anaheim, CA 92805
800/854-9305
714/533-2221
FAX: 714/635-7539

Microcurrent Research Inc
10443 N Cave Creek Rd
Ste 211
Phoenix, AZ 85020
800/872-6789
FAX: 602/943-6509

Monad Corp
908 E Holt Ave
Pomona, CA 91767
800/34MONAD
800/233MENS (in CA)

Nemectron Medical Inc
28069 Diaz Rd, Unit A
Temecula, CA 92590
800/428-4010

Promatek Medical Systems Inc
1851 Black Rd
Joliet, IL 60435
800/327-3422
815/725-6766

PTI
PO Box 19005
Topeka, KS 66619-0005
800/255-3554

Rich-Mar Corp
PO Box 879
Inola, OK 74036
800/762-4665
918/543-2222

Iontophoretic Systems

Anodyne Inc
7300 France Ave S, Ste 403
Edina, MN 55435
800/736-8367
612/831-6130

ELMED Inc
60 W Fay Ave
Addison, IL 60101
312/543-2792

Empi Inc
1275 Grey Fox Rd
St Paul, MN 55112
800/328-2536
612/636-6600

General Medical Co
1935 Armacost Ave
Los Angeles, CA 90025-5296
310/820-5881

General Medical Manufacturing Co
8741 Landmark Rd
Richmond, VA 23228
804/264-7500

Henley International, A Division of Maxxim Medical
104 Industrial Blvd
Sugar Land, TX 77478
800/477-7342
FAX: 713/240-2577

IOMED, Inc
1290 W 2320 S
Salt Lake City, UT 84119
800/621-3347
801/975-1191

Life-Tech Inc
10920 Kinghurst
Houston, TX 77099
713/495-9411

William B McBeth Co
PO Box 267
Telford, PA 18969
800/346-2171
215/723-0824

Medical Science Products Inc
PO Box 381
Canal Fulton, OH 44614
800/456-1971

Monad Corp
908 E Holt Ave
Pomona, CA 91767
800/34MONAD
800/233MENS (in CA)

Muscle Stimulators

AdvanTeq Development Corp
12509 Crenshaw Blvd
Hawthorne, CA 90250
800/234-7846

American Imex
16520 Aston St
Irvine, CA 92714
800/521-8286
714/553-8885

Anodyne Inc
7300 France Ave S, Ste 403
Edina, MN 55435
800/736-8367
612/831-6130

Austin Medical Equipment Inc
5947 S Oak Park Ave
Chicago, IL 60638
800/382-0300

Ballert International Inc
3645 Woodhead Dr
Northbrook, IL 60062-1816
800/345-3456
FAX: 312/480-1088

BioMedical Life Systems Inc
1120 Sycamore Ave, Ste F
Vista, CA 92085
800/726-8367
619/727-5600

Chattanooga Group Inc
4717 Adams Rd
PO Box 489
Hixson, TN 37343
800/592-7329
615/870-2281

Comfort Technologies Inc
PO Box 7
Pittstown, NJ 08867
800/321-STIM
908/735-0344

Complete Medical Products Inc
2052 N Decatur Rd
Decatur, GA 30033
800/525-4119

Dynatronics
470 W Lawndale Dr
Bldg D
Salt Lake City, UT 84115
801/485-4739

DynaWave Corp
2520 Kaneville Ct
Geneva, IL 60134
708/232-4945
FAX: 708/232-7042

Electro-Med Health Industries
11601 Biscayne Blvd, Ste 200A
Miami, FL 33181
305/892-2866
FAX: 305/892-2980

Electro Medical Inc
18433 Amistad
Fountain Valley, CA 92708
800/422-8726
714/964-6776
FAX: 714/968-0712

Electronic Waveform Lab Inc
15683 Chemical Ln
Huntington Beach, CA 92649
800/874-9283

ELMED Inc
60 W Fay Ave
Addison, IL 60101
312/543-2792

Empi Inc
1275 Grey Fox Rd
St Paul, MN 55112
800/328-2536
612/636-6600

Excel Tech Ltd
1200-11 Aerowood Dr
Mississauga, Ontario, Canada
L4W 2S7
800/387-7516

General Physiotherapy Inc
13222 Lakefront Dr
St Louis, MO 63045-1504
800/237-1832
314/291-1442

Ideal Medical Products Inc
County Rd 623
Rte 1, PO Box 56
Broseley, MO 63932
800/321-5490
314/686-0003

MECI Electrotherapeutics
810-B NW Main St
PO Box 1149
Lee's Summit, MO 64063
800/527-0748

Med Labs Inc
28 Vereda Cordillera
Goleta, CA 93117
805/968-2486

Mettler Electronics Corp
1333 S Claudina St
Anaheim, CA 92805
800/854-9305
714/533-2221
FAX: 714/635-7539

Nemectron Medical Inc
28069 Diaz Rd, Unit A
Temecula, CA 92590
800/428-4010

JA Preston Corp
PO Box 89
Jackson, MI 49204
800/631-7277
517/787-1600

Promatek Medical Systems Inc
1851 Black Rd
Joliet, IL 60435
800/327-3422
815/725-6766

PTI
PO Box 19005
Topeka, KS 66619-0005
800/255-3554

Rich-Mar Corp
PO Box 879
Inola, OK 74036
800/762-4665
918/543-2222

Sparta Surgical Corp
26602 Corporate Ave
Hayward, CA 94545
510/887-7717

Sportmaster
PO Box 5000
Pittsburgh, PA 15206
412/441-0200

Staodyn Inc
1225 Florida Ave
PO Box 1379
Longmont, CO 80502-1379
800/525-2114
303/772-3631

Sutter Corp
9425 Chesapeake Dr
San Diego, CA 92123
800/854-2216
619/569-8148

TC Medical Inc
6565 City West Pkwy
Minneapolis, MN 55344-3248
800/826-3342
FAX: 612/829-8284

Thera-Kinetics Inc
1300 Rte 73
Mount Laurel, NJ 08054
800/234-0900

TMD, A Division of Staodyn Inc
3625 Queen Palm Dr
PO Box 30244
Tampa, FL 33630-3244
800/343-0488

Neuromuscular Stimulators

AdvanTeq Development Corp
12509 Crenshaw Blvd
Hawthorne, CA 90250
800/234-7846

American Imex
16520 Aston St
Irvine, CA 92714
800/521-8286
714/553-8885

Anodyne Inc
7300 France Ave S, Ste 403
Edina, MN 55435
800/736-8367
612/831-6130

BioMedical Life Systems Inc
1120 Sycamore Ave, Ste F
Vista, CA 92085
800/726-8367
619/727-5600

Chattanooga Group Inc
4717 Adams Rd
PO Box 489
Hixson, TN 37343
800/592-7329
615/870-2281

Comfort Technologies Inc
PO Box 7
Pittstown, NJ 08867
800/321-STIM
908/735-0344

Electro-Med Health Industries
11601 Biscayne Blvd, Ste 200A
Miami, FL 33181
305/892-2866
FAX: 305/892-2980

Electro Medical Inc
18433 Amistad
Fountain Valley, CA 92708
800/422-8726
714/964-6776
FAX: 714/968-0712

Electronic Waveform Lab Inc
15683 Chemical Ln
Huntington Beach, CA 92649
800/874-9283

ELMED Inc
60 W Fay Ave
Addison, IL 60101
312/543-2792

Empi Inc
1275 Grey Fox Rd
St Paul, MN 55112
800/328-2536
612/636-6600

Excel Tech Ltd
1200-11 Aerowood Dr
Mississauga, Ontario, Canada
L4W 2S7
800/387-7516

Henley International, A Division of Maxxim Medical
104 Industrial Blvd
Sugar Land, TX 77478
800/477-7342
FAX: 713/240-2577

Ideal Medical Products Inc
County Rd 623
Rte 1, PO Box 56
Broseley, MO 63932
800/321-5490
314/686-0003

MECI Electrotherapeutics
810-B NW Main St
PO Box 1149
Lee's Summit, MO 64063
800/527-0748

Medical Devices Inc
833 Third St SW
St Paul, MN 55112
800/328-0875

Med Labs Inc
28 Vereda Cordillera
Goleta, CA 93117
805/968-2486

Mettler Electronics Corp
1333 S Claudina St
Anaheim, CA 92805
800/854-9305
714/533-2221
FAX: 714/635-7539

Monad Corp
908 E Holt Ave
Pomona, CA 91767
800/34MONAD
800/233MENS (in CA)

NAPCOR
9852 Crescent Ctr Dr
Ste 801
Rancho Cucamonga, CA 91730
909/989-1641

Nemectron Medical Inc
28069 Diaz Rd, Unit A
Temecula, CA 92590
800/428-4010

Promatek Medical Systems Inc
1851 Black Rd
Joliet, IL 60435
800/327-3422
815/725-6766

PTI
PO Box 19005
Topeka, KS 66619-0005
800/255-3554

Rich-Mar Corp
PO Box 879
Inola, OK 74036
800/762-4665
918/543-2222

Sparta Surgical Corp
26602 Corporate Ave
Hayward, CA 94545
510/887-7717

Sportmaster
PO Box 5000
Pittsburgh, PA 15206
412/441-0200

Staodyn Inc
1225 Florida Ave
PO Box 1379
Longmont, CO 80502-1379
800/525-2114
303/772-3631

Thera-Kinetics Inc
1300 Rte 73
Mount Laurel, NJ 08054
800/234-0900

TMD, A Division of Staodyn Inc
3625 Queen Palm Dr
PO Box 30244
Tampa, FL 33630-3244
800/343-0488

Verimed Inc
1401 E Broward Blvd
Ste 200
Ft Lauderdale, FL 33301
800/999-9797
305/768-9990

TENS Units

AdvanTeq Development Corp
12509 Crenshaw Blvd
Hawthorne, CA 90250
800/234-7846

AGAR USA Inc
1915 Eye St, #500
Washington, DC 20006
202/296-1111

American Imex
16520 Aston St
Irvine, CA 92714
800/521-8286
714/553-8885

Anodyne Inc
7300 France Ave S, Ste 403
Edina, MN 55435
800/736-8367
612/831-6130

Austin Medical Equipment Inc
5947 S Oak Park Ave
Chicago, IL 60638
800/382-0300

BioMedical Life Systems Inc
1120 Sycamore Ave, Ste F
Vista, CA 92085
800/726-8367
619/727-5600

Comfort Technologies Inc
PO Box 7
Pittstown, NJ 08867
800/321-STIM
908/735-0344

AR Davis Co Inc
PO Box 219
Irvington, AL 36544
800/872-5804
205/957-3214
FAX: 205/957-2031

Electro-Med Health Industries
11601 Biscayne Blvd, Ste 200A
Miami, FL 33181
305/892-2866
FAX: 305/892-2980

Electro Medical Inc
18433 Amistad
Fountain Valley, CA 92708
800/422-8726
714/964-6776
FAX: 714/968-0712

Electronic Research Devices Corp
9320 SW Barbur Blvd
Ste 150
Portland, OR 97219
800/547-0366
503/245-7241
FAX: 503/245-4863

ELMED Inc
60 W Fay Ave
Addison, IL 60101
312/543-2792

Empi Inc
1275 Grey Fox Rd
St Paul, MN 55112
800/328-2536
612/636-6600

Excel Tech Ltd
1200-11 Aerowood Dr
Mississauga, Ontario, Canada
L4W 2S7
800/387-7516

Henley International, A Division of Maxxim Medical
104 Industrial Blvd
Sugar Land, TX 77478
800/477-7342
FAX: 713/240-2577

MECI Electrotherapeutics
810-B NW Main St
PO Box 1149
Lee's Summit, MO 64063
800/527-0748

Medical Devices Inc
833 Third St SW
St Paul, MN 55112
800/328-0875

Medical Science Products Inc
PO Box 381
Canal Fulton, OH 44614
800/456-1971

Monad Corp
908 E Holt Ave
Pomona, CA 91767
800/34MONAD
800/233MENS (in CA)

JA Preston Corp
PO Box 89
Jackson, MI 49204
800/631-7277
517/787-1600

Sparta Surgical Corp
26602 Corporate Ave
Hayward, CA 94545
510/887-7717

Sportmaster
PO Box 5000
Pittsburgh, PA 15206
412/441-0200

Staodyn Inc
1225 Florida Ave
PO Box 1379
Longmont, CO 80502
800/525-2114
303/772-3631

TC Medical Inc
6565 City West Pkwy
Minneapolis, MN 55344-3248
800/826-3342
FAX: 612/829-8284

Thera-Kinetics Inc
1300 Rte 73
Mount Laurel, NJ 08054
800/234-0900

3M Health Care/Electrotherapy Products
3M Ctr, Bldg 275-4W-02
St Paul, MN 55144-1000
800/228-3957

TMD, A Division of Staodyn Inc
3625 Queen Palm Dr
PO Box 30244
Tampa, FL 33630-3244
800/343-0488

Uni-Patch Inc
1313 Grant Blvd W
PO Box 271
Wabasha, MN 55981
800/328-9454
612/565-2601

Biofeedback Instrumentation

Anodyne Inc
7300 France Ave S, Ste 403
Edina, MN 55435
800/736-8367
612/831-6130

BioMedical Life Systems Inc
1120 Sycamore Ave, Ste F
Vista, CA 92085
800/726-8367
619/727-5600

Davicon Inc
79 Second Ave
Burlington, MA 01803
800/DAVICON
617/229-2800

Ergometrics Inc
3753 Varsity Dr
Ann Arbor, MI 48014
800/447-3009
313/971-7111

Innovative Systems for Rehabilitation (ISR)
1711 W County Rd B
Ste 208 N
St Paul, MN 55113
612/636-8212

Lafayette Instrument Co
3700 Sagamore Pkwy N
PO Box 5729
Lafayette, IN 47903
800/428-7545
317/423-1505

William B McBeth Co
PO Box 267
Telford, PA 18969
800/346-2171
215/723-0824

NeuroCom International Inc
9570 SE Lawnfield Rd
Clackamas, OR 97015
800/767-6744
503/653-2144
FAX: 503/653-1992

Physical Health Devices Inc
417 Corporate Sq
1500 W Cypress Creek Rd
Ft Lauderdale, FL 33309
305/351-0303
FAX: 305/351-0598

Self Regulation Systems Inc (SRS)
14770 NE 95th St
Redmond, WA 98052
800/345-5642
206/882-1101
FAX: 206/882-1935

Tekdyne Corp
550-3 California Rd
Quakertown, PA 18951
800/747-1824
215/538-1826
FAX: 215/338-3059

Thera-Kinetics Inc
1300 Rte 73
Mount Laurel, NJ 08054
800/234-0900

Universal Gym Equipment Inc
PO Box 1270
Cedar Rapids, IA 52406
800/843-3906
319/365-7561

Verimed Inc
1401 E Broward Blvd
Ste 200
Ft Lauderdale, FL 33301
800/999-9797
305/768-9990

CRYOTHERAPY

Ice Packs, Disposable

Austin Medical Equipment Inc
5947 S Oak Park Ave
Chicago, IL 60638
800/382-0300

Biomark Inc
PO Box 340
Edmonds, WA 98040
800/633-3034
206/745-9200

DeRoyal Orthopedic Group
200 DeBusk Ln
Powell, TN 37849
800/251-9864

Medical Science Products Inc
PO Box 381
Canal Fulton, OH 44614
800/456-1971

Mueller Sports Medicine Inc
One Quench Dr
Prairie du Sac, WI 53578
800/356-9522
608/643-8530

Pelton Shepherd Industries
PO Box 30218
Stockton, CA 95213
800/BLUEICE
209/983-0893

Rolliture Systems
4231 Pacific St, #31
Rocklin, CA 95677
916/652-7887
FAX: 916/652-8188

Rothhammer International
PO Box 5579
Santa Maria, CA 93456
800/235-2156

Slim Ez/Mr America Mfg Inc
Ooltewah Industrial Park
Ooltewah, TN 37363
800/251-6040

Southwest Technologies Inc
2018 Baltimore
Kansas City, MO 64108
800/247-9951

Ice Packs, Reusable

Anodyne Inc
7300 France Ave S, Ste 403
Edina, MN 55435
800/736-8367
612/831-6130

Aqua-Cel Corp
PO Box 26827
Santa Ana, CA 92799
714/962-2776

Biomark Inc
PO Box 340
Edmonds, WA 98040
800/633-3034
206/745-9200

Bird & Cronin Inc
2601 E 80th St
Minneapolis, MN 55425
800/328-1095
612/854-5626

Bodyline Comfort Systems
3730 Kori Rd
Jacksonville, FL 32257
800/874-7715
904/262-4068

Chattanooga Group Inc
4717 Adams Rd
PO Box 489
Hixson, TN 37343
800/592-7329
615/870-2281

DePuy Inc
700 Orthopaedic Dr
PO Box 988
Warsaw, IN 46581-0988
800/366-8143

Dura-Kold Corp
1117 Cornell Pkwy
Oklahoma City, OK 73108
405/943-8811

Elgin Exercise Equipment Corp
270 N Eisenhower Ln
Unit 4-A
Lombard, IL 60148
800/279-3762
708/268-1000

Medical Science Products Inc
PO Box 381
Canal Fulton, OH 44614
800/456-1971

Mueller Sports Medicine Inc
One Quench Dr
Prairie du Sac, WI 53578
800/356-9522
608/643-8530

Northwest Orthopaedic Products Corp
12300 SW Sidney Rd
Port Orchard, WA 98366
800/331-8188

Orthopedic Physical Therapy Products
PO Box 47009
Minneapolis, MN 55447-0009
800/367-7393
612/553-0452
FAX: 612/553-9355

Pelton Shepherd Industries
PO Box 30218
Stockton, CA 95213
800/BLUEICE
209/983-0893

JA Preston Corp
PO Box 89
Jackson, MI 49204
800/631-7277
517/787-1600

Rich-Mar Corp
PO Box 879
Inola, OK 74036
800/762-4665
918/543-2222

Rothhammer International
PO Box 5579
Santa Maria, CA 93456
800/235-2156

Slim Ez/Mr America Mft Inc
Ooltewah Industrial Park
Ooltewah, TN 37363
800/251-6040

Southwest Technologies Inc
2018 Baltimore
Kansas City, MO 64108
800/247-9951

Sports Supports Inc
400 Union Bower Ct, #410
Irving, TX 75061
800/527-5273
214/554-1174

Sportsware West
415 E Figueroa St, Ste A
Santa Barbara, CA 93101
805/962-7454
FAX: 805/966-3631

SUB IP Inc
1545 N Verdugo Rd
Glendale, CA 91208
818/242-7546

Sutter Corp
9425 Chesapeake Dr
San Diego, CA 92123
800/854-2216
619/569-8148

Therabite Corp
6 S Bryn Mawr Ave
Ste 100
Bryn Mawr, PA 19010
800/322-2650

TMD, A Division of Staodyn Inc
3625 Queen Palm Dr
PO Box 30244
Tampa, FL 33630-3244
800/343-0488

Uni-Patch Inc
1313 Grant Blvd W
PO Box 271
Wabasha, MN 55981
800/328-9454
612/565-2601

Sprays, Vapocoolants

Austin Medical Equipment Inc
5947 S Oak Park Ave
Chicago, IL 60638
800/382-0300

Gebauer Co
9410 St Catherine Ave
Cleveland, OH 44104
216/271-5252

Mueller Sports Medicine Inc
One Quench Dr
Prairie du Sac, WI 53578
800/356-9522
608/643-8530

THERMOTHERAPY

Fluidotherapy

AquaSoothe International Inc
2016 Concord Lake Rd
Kannapolis, NC 28083
704/784-4620

Henley International, A Division of Maxxim Medical
104 Industrial Blvd
Sugar Land, TX 77478
800/477-7342
FAX: 713/240-2577

Thera-Kinetics Inc
1300 Rte 73
Mount Laurel, NJ 08054
800/234-0900

Heating Pads

American Imex
16520 Aston St
Irvine, CA 92714
800/521-8286
714/553-8885

Battle Creek Equipment Co
307 W Jackson St
Battle Creek, MI 49017-2385
800/253-0854

Southwest Technologies Inc
2018 Baltimore
Kansas City, MO 64108
800/247-9951

Hot Packs

American Imex
16520 Aston St
Irvine, CA 92714
800/521-8286
714/553-8885

Aqua-Cel Corp
PO Box 26827
Santa Ana, CA 92799
714/962-2776

Austin Medical Equipment Inc
5947 S Oak Park Ave
Chicago, IL 60638
800/382-0300

Battle Creek Equipment Co
307 W Jackson St
Battle Creek, MI 49017-2385
800/253-0854

Biomark Inc
PO Box 340
Edmonds, WA 98040
800/633-3034
206/745-9200

Bird & Cronin Inc
2601 E 80th St
Minneapolis, MN 55425
800/328-1095
612/854-5626

Bodyline Comfort Systems
3730 Kori Rd
Jacksonville, FL 32257
800/874-7715
904/262-4068

Contour Form Products
12 N Diamond St
PO Box 328
Greenville, PA 16125
800/223-8808
412/588-4452

Ferno Ille, A Division of
Ferno-Washington Inc
70 Weil Way
Wilmington, OH 45177
513/382-1451

Ideal Medical Products Inc
County Rd 623
Rte 1, PO Box 56
Broseley, MO 63932
800/321-5490
314/686-0003

Logan Inc
3041 S Shannon St
Santa Ana, CA 92704
714/556-6441

Medical Science Products Inc
PO Box 381
Canal Fulton, OH 44614
800/456-1971

Orthopedic Physical Therapy Products
PO Box 47009
Minneapolis, MN 55447-0009
800/367-7393
612/553-0452
FAX: 612/553-9355

Pelton Shepherd Industries
PO Box 30218
Stockton, CA 95213
800/BLUEICE
209/983-0893

JA Preston Corp
PO Box 89
Jackson, MI 49204
800/631-7277
517/787-1600

Re-Heater Inc
15828 S Broadway
Garden, CA 90248
310/719-9582

Paraffin Baths

American Imex
16520 Aston St
Irvine, CA 92714
800/521-8286
714/553-8885

Austin Medical Equipment Inc
5947 S Oak Park Ave
Chicago, IL 60638
800/382-0300

Bird & Cronin Inc
2601 E 80th St
Minneapolis, MN 55425
800/328-1095
612/854-5626

Complete Medical Products Inc
2052 N Decatur Rd
Decatur, GA 30033
800/525-4119

Ferno Ille, A Division of
Ferno-Washington Inc
70 Weil Way
Wilmington, OH 45177
513/382-1451

Grimm Scientific Industries Inc
Newport Pike
PO Box 2143
Marietta, OH 45750
800/223-5395
614/374-3412

The Hygenic Corp
1245 Home Ave
Akron, OH 44310-2575
800/321-2135
216/633-8460

I-REP Inc
29885 Second St, #G
Lake Elsinore, CA 92532
800/828-0852

William B McBeth Co
PO Box 267
Telford, PA 18969
800/346-2171
215/723-0824

JA Preston Corp
PO Box 89
Jackson, MI 49204
800/631-7277
517/787-1600

Thermo-Electric Co
455 Rte 30
Imperial, PA 15126
800/633-8088
412/695-1890

WR Medical Electronics Co
123 N Second St
Stillwater, MN 55082
800/321-6387
612/430-1200

HYDROTHERAPY

Hydrotherapy Equipment

AquaSoothe International Inc
2016 Concord Lake Rd
Kannapolis, NC 28083
704/784-4620

AquaTherapeutics™
PO Box 5775
Asheville, NC 28813
800/237-0469

Bailey Manufacturing Co
118 Lee St
PO Box 130
Lodi, OH 44254
800/321-8372
216/948-1080
FAX: 216/948-4439

Ferno Ille, A Division of
Ferno-Washington Inc
70 Weil Way
Wilmington, OH 45177
513/382-1451

GNR Health Systems Inc
1203 SW 12th St
Bldg H
Ocala, FL 32674
800/523-0912

Good Sports
6031 Broad St Mall
Pittsburgh, PA 15206
412/661-9500

Hospital Therapy Products Inc
757 N Central Ave
Wood Dale, IL 60191
708/766-7101

I-REP Inc
29885 Second St, #G
Lake Elsinore, CA 92532
800/828-0852

Jetta Products Inc
217 Altamonte Commerce Blvd, #1218
Altamonte Springs, FL 32714
800/775-3882
FAX: 407/774-7260

Rothhammer International
PO Box 5579
Santa Maria, CA 93456
800/235-2156

Sportmaster
PO Box 5000
Pittsburgh, PA 15206
412/441-0200

Stewart Medical
70 NE Loop 410
Ste 675
San Antonio, TX 78216
800/437-8216

Stranco
PO Box 389
Bradley, IL 60915
800/882-6466
815/932-8154

Whitehall Manufacturing Inc
15058 Proctor Ave
City of Industry, CA 91746
818/968-6681

ULTRASOUND

Gels

AloeTran Products Inc
PO Box 337
Farmerville, LA 71241
800/328-8367
318/368-7266

Anodyne Inc.
7300 France Ave S, Ste 403
Edina, MN 55435
800/736-8367
612/831-6130

Ari-Med Pharmaceuticals
1615 W University Dr
Ste 125
Tempe, AZ 85281
800/527-4923
602/966-9802
FAX: 602/966-9806

AR Davis Co Inc
PO Box 219
Irvington, AL 36544
800/872-5804
205/957-3214
FAX: 205/957-2031

Echo Ultrasound
RR 2, PO Box 118
Reedsville, PA 17084-9772
800/233-0261

ELMED Inc
60 W Fay Ave
Addison, IL 60101
312/543-2792

Excel Tech Ltd
1200-11 Aerowood Dr
Mississauga, Ontario, Canada
L4W 2S7
800/387-7516

Fairway King Co
3 E Main St
Oklahoma City, OK 73104
405/528-8571

Ideal Medical Products Inc
County Rd 623
Rte 1, PO Box 56
Broseley, MO 63932
800/321-5490
314/686-0003

William B McBeth Co
PO Box 267
Telford, PA 18969
800/346-2171
215/723-0824

Mettler Electronics Corp
1333 S Claudina St
Anaheim, CA 92805
800/854-9305
714/533-2221
FAX: 714/635-7539

North Coast Medical Inc
187 Stauffer Blvd
San Jose, CA 95125-1042
800/821-9319
408/283-1900
FAX: 408/283-1950

Parker Laboratories Inc
307 Washington St
Orange, NJ 07050
201/676-5000
FAX: 201/676-0784

Pelton Shepherd Industries
PO Box 30218
Stockton, CA 95213
800/BLUEICE
209/983-0893

Pharmaceutical Innovations Inc
897 Frelinghuysen Ave
Newark, NJ 07114
201/242-2900
FAX: 201/242-0578

Rich-Mar Corp
PO Box 879
Inola, OK 74036
800/762-4665
918/543-2222

Third Millennium Science
2195 Faraday Ave, Ste F
Carlsbad, CA 92008
619/431-7181

Uni-Patch Inc
1313 Grant Blvd W
PO Box 271
Wabasha, MN 55981
800/328-9454
612/565-2601

Ultrasound Equipment

Anodyne Inc
7300 France Ave S, Ste 403
Edina, MN 55435
800/736-8367
612/831-6130

Arjo-Century Inc
8130 Lehigh Ave
Morton Grove, IL 60053
800/323-1245
708/967-0360

Austin Medical Equipment Inc
5947 S Oak Park Ave
Chicago, IL 60638
800/382-0300

Chattanooga Group Inc
4717 Adams Rd
PO Box 489
Hixson, TN 37343
800/592-7329
615/870-2281

Complete Medical Products Inc
2052 N Decatur Rd
Decatur, GA 30033
800/525-4119

Dynatronics
470 W Lawndale Dr
Bldg D
Salt Lake City, UT 84115
801/485-4739

ELMED Inc
60 W Fay Ave
Addison, IL 60101
312/543-2792

Excel Tech Ltd
1200-11 Aerowood Dr
Mississauga, Ontario, Canada
L4W 2S7
800/387-7516

GNR Health Systems Inc
1203 SW 12th St
Bldg H
Ocala, FL 32674
800/523-0912

Good Sports
6031 Broad St Mall
Pittsburgh, PA 15206
412/661-9500

Huntleigh Healthcare
227 Rte 33 E
Manalapan, NJ 07726
800/223-1218

Ideal Medical Products Inc
County Rd 623
Rte 1, PO Box 56
Broseley, MO 63932
800/321-5490
314/686-0003

I-REP Inc
29885 Second St, #G
Lake Elsinore, CA 92532
800/828-0852

William B McBeth Co
PO Box 267
Telford, PA 18969
800/346-2171
215/723-0824

Mettler Electronics Corp
1333 S Claudina St
Anaheim, CA 92805
800/854-9305
714/533-2221
FAX: 714/635-7539

Nemectron Medical Inc
28069 Diaz Rd, Unit A
Temecula, CA 92590
800/428-4010

Promatek Medical Systems Inc
1851 Black Rd
Joliet, IL 60435
800/327-3422
815/725-6766

PTI
PO Box 19005
Topeka, KS 66619-0005
800/255-3554

Rich-Mar Corp
PO Box 879
Inola, OK 74036
800/762-4665
918/543-2222

Rothhammer International
PO Box 5579
Santa Maria, CA 93456
800/235-2156

LIGHT THERAPY

Infrared Lamps

I-REP Inc
29885 Second St, #G
Lake Elsinore, CA 92532
800/828-0852

Lasers, Helium-Neon

Dynatronics
470 W Lawndale Dr
Bldg D
Salt Lake City, UT 84115
801/485-4739

I-REP Inc
29885 Second St, #G
Lake Elsinore, CA 92532
800/828-0852

North Coast Medical Inc
187 Stauffer Blvd
San Jose, CA 95125-1042
800/821-9319
408/283-1900
FAX: 408/283-1950

Smith & Nephew Rolyan Inc
N93W14475 Whittaker Way
PO Box 555
Menomonee Falls, WI 53051
800/558-8633

Ultraviolet Lamps

I-REP Inc
29885 Second St, #G
Lake Elsinore, CA 92532
800/828-0852

DIATHERMY

Microwave Diathermy

Nemectron Medical Inc
28069 Diaz Rd, Unit A
Temecula, CA 92590
800/428-4010

Shortwave Diathermy

ELMED Inc
60 W Fay Ave
Addison, IL 60101
312/543-2792

International Medical Electronics Ltd
3939 Broadway
Ste 100
Kansas City, MO 64111-2516
800/432-8003

I-REP Inc
29885 Second St, #G
Lake Elsinore, CA 92532
800/828-0852

Mettler Electronics Corp
1333 S Claudina St
Anaheim, CA 92805
800/854-9305
714/533-2221
FAX: 714/635-7539

TRACTION EQUIPMENT

Akron Therapy Products/Electro-Medical Equipment Inc
PO Box 7671
Marietta, GA 30065
800/235-2952

AliMed Inc
297 High St
Dedham, MA 02026
617/329-2900

AquaSoothe International Inc
2016 Concord Lake Rd
Kannapolis, NC 28083
704/784-4620

Austin Medical Equipment Inc
5947 S Oak Park Ave
Chicago, IL 60638
800/382-0300

Ballert International Inc
3645 Woodhead Dr
Northbrook, IL 60062-1816
800/345-3456
FAX: 312/480-1088

Care • a • peutics
10850 White Oak Ave
Granada Hills, CA 91344
818/831-1361

INTERMITTENT COMPRESSION UNITS

Chattanooga Group Inc
4717 Adams Rd
PO Box 489
Hixson, TN 37343
800/592-7329
615/870-2281

Complete Medical Products Inc
2052 N Decatur Rd
Decatur, GA 30033
800/525-4119

Huntleigh Healthcare
227 Rte 33 E
Manalapan, NJ 07726
800/223-1218

The Jobst Institute Inc
653 Miami St
PO Box 653
Toledo, OH 43697
419/698-1611

Ideal Medical Products Inc
County Rd 623
Rte 1, PO Box 56
Broseley, MO 63932
800/321-5490
314/686-0003

Sammons
145 Tower Dr, Dept 966
Burr Ridge, IL 60521
708/325-1700

Schaefer Products
PO Box 450208
Garland, TX 75045
214/238-9368

Sportsware West
415 E Figueroa St, Ste A
Santa Barbara, CA 93101
805/962-7454
FAX: 805/966-3631

SUB IP Inc
1545 N Verdugo Rd
Glendale, CA 91208
818/242-7546

MASSAGERS

AquaSoothe International Inc
2016 Concord Lake Rd
Kannapolis, NC 28083
704/784-4620

Battle Creek Equipment Co
307 W Jackson St
Battle Creek, MI 49017-2385
800/253-0854

Foot Management Inc
Rte 1, 30-A Friendship Rd
PO Box 100
Pittsville, MD 21850-0100
800/468-3668
301/835-3668

General Physiotherapy Inc
13222 Lakefront Dr
St Louis, MO 63045-1504
800/237-1832
314/291-1442

GMG Enterprises Inc
3536 Ctr Circle Dr
Fort Mill, SC 29715
800/848-3985
803/548-1131

APPENDIX A-3

UNITS OF MEASURE

Milliseconds (msec)   = $\frac{1}{1000}$ of a second
Microseconds (μsec) = $\frac{1}{1,000,000}$ of a second
Nanosecond (nsec)   = $\frac{1}{1,000,000,000}$ of a second
Milliamp (mamp)   = $\frac{1}{1,000}$ of an amp
Microamp (μamp)   = $\frac{1}{1,000,000}$ of an amp
Angstrom (Å)   = $\frac{1}{10,000,000,000}$ of a meter
Nanometer (nm)   = $\frac{1}{1,000,000,000}$ of a meter
Hertz (Hz)   = 1 cycle per second
Kilohertz (KHz)   = 1,000 cycles per second
Megahertz (MHz)   = 1,000,000 cycles per second

INDEX

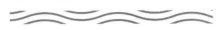

Note: Page numbers followed by *f* indicate figures. Page numbers followed by *t* indicate tables.

ISBN 0-07-050771-6
90000